MASTER TECHNIQUES IN OTOLARYNGOLOGY

Head and Neck Surgery

RECONSTRUCTIVE SURGERY

MASTER TECHNIQUES IN OTOLARYNGOLOGY

Head and Neck Surgery

RECONSTRUCTIVE SURGERY

Series Editor

Eugene N. Myers, MD, FACS, FRCS Edin (Hon)

Distinguished Professor and Emeritus Chair
Department of Otolaryngology
University of Pittsburgh School of Medicine
Professor
Department of Oral Maxillofacial Surgery
University of Pittsburgh School of Dental Medicine
Pittsburgh, Pennsylvania

Editor

Eric M. Genden, MD, FACS

The Isadore Friesner Professor of Otolaryngology–Head and Neck Surgery
Department of Otolaryngology
Professor of Neurosurgery and Immunology
The Mount Sinai School of Medicine
Director, The Head, Neck, and Thyroid Center
The Icahn School of Medicine at Mount Sinai
New York, New York

Wolters Kluwer
Health

Philadelphia • Baltimore • New York • London
Buenos Aires • Hong Kong • Sydney • Tokyo

Acquisitions Editor: Ryan Shaw
Product Developmental Editor: Brendan Huffman
Production Project Manager: Alicia Jackson
Director of Creative Services: Doug Smock
Senior Manufacturing Manager: Beth Welsh
Marketing Manager: Daniel Dressler
Production Service: SPi Global

Two Commerce Square
2001 Market Street
Philadelphia, PA 19103 USA
LWW.com

Printed in China

Library of Congress Cataloging-in-Publication Data
Head and neck surgery (Genden)
Head and neck surgery : reconstructive surgery / editor, Eric M. Genden. — 1st edition.
p. ; cm. — (Master techniques in otolaryngology)
Includes index.
ISBN 978-1-4511-7586-8
I. Genden, Eric M., editor of compilation. II. Title. III. Series: Master techniques in otolaryngology.
[DNLM: 1. Head—surgery. 2. Neck—surgery. 3. Oral Surgical Procedures—methods. 4. Otorhinolaryngologic Surgical Procedures—methods. 5. Reconstructive Surgical Procedures—methods. 6. Surgical Flaps. WE 705]
RD521
617.5'1059—dc23

2014001714

Care has been taken to confirm the accuracy of the information presented and to describe generally accepted practices. However, the authors, editors, and publisher are not responsible for errors or omissions or for any consequences from application of the information in this book and make no warranty, expressed or implied, with respect to the currency, completeness, or accuracy of the contents of the publication. Application of the information in a particular situation remains the professional responsibility of the practitioner.

The authors, editors, and publisher have exerted every effort to ensure that drug selection and dosage set forth in this text are in accordance with current recommendations and practice at the time of publication. However, in view of ongoing research, changes in government regulations, and the constant flow of information relating to drug therapy and drug reactions, the reader is urged to check the package insert for each drug for any change in indications and dosage and for added warnings and precautions. This is particularly important when the recommended agent is a new or infrequently employed drug.

Some drugs and medical devices presented in the publication have Food and Drug Administration (FDA) clearance for limited use in restricted research settings. It is the responsibility of the health care provider to ascertain the FDA status of each drug or device planned for use in their clinical practice.

To purchase additional copies of this book, call our customer service department at (800) 638–3030 or fax orders to (301) 223–2320. International customers should call (301) 223–2300.

Visit Lippincott Williams & Wilkins on the Internet: at LWW.com. Lippincott Williams & Wilkins customer service representatives are available from 8:30 am to 6 pm, EST.

10 9 8 7 6 5 4 3 2 1

RRS1404

This series of books is dedicated to Barbara, my wife and best pal.

Our daughter, Marjorie Fulbright, her husband, Cary, and their sons, Alexander F. Fulbright and Charles J. Fulbright.

Our son, Jeffrey N. Myers, MD, PhD, his wife, Lisa, and their sons, Keith N. Myers, Brett A. Myers, and Blake D. Myers.

All of whom we love and cherish.

Eugene N. Myers

The masters *who have contributed to this project have dedicated their life's work to helping those in need. I applaud their dedication and commitment and I owe them my gratitude for inspiring me. I dedicate this work to my loving family, my wife, Audrey, my son, Eric Jr, and my daughters, Sophia and Isabelle. I could not have accomplished this work without your love and support.*

Eric M. Genden

Contributors

Keith E. Blackwell, MD
Professor
Department of Head and Neck Surgery
David Geffen School of Medicine at University of California
Los Angeles, California

James S. Brown, MD, FRCS, FDSRCS, LRCP, MRCS, BDS
Professor
Department of Head and Neck Surgery
Liverpool University
Consultant
Department of Head and Neck Surgery
Aintree University Hospital
Liverpool, United Kingdom

Brian B. Burkey, MD, MEHP
Vice-Chairman and Section Head, Head and Neck Surgery/Oncology Position
Head and Neck Institute
Cleveland Clinic Foundation
Cleveland, Ohio

Douglas B. Chepeha, MD, MSPH, FRCS
Professor
Department of Otolaryngology–Head and Neck Surgery
University of Michigan
Ann Arbor, Michigan

Francisco J. Civantos, MD, FACS
Associate Professor
Department of Otolaryngology–Head and Neck Surgery
The University of Miami
Miami, Florida

Peter D. Costantino, MD, FACS
Professor
Department of Otolaryngology
Hofstra North Shore-LIJ School of Medicine
Chairman, Department of Otolaryngology–Head and Neck Surgery
Lenox Hill Hospital
Manhattan Eye, Ear and Throat Hospital
Executive Director and Senior Vice President
The New York Head and Neck Institute
The Otolaryngology–Head and Neck Surgery Service Line
North Shore-LIJ Health System
New York, New York

Terry A. Day, MD, FACS
Professor
Vice Chair
Department of Otolaryngology–Head and Neck Surgery
Wendy and Keith Wellin Chair in Head and Neck Surgery
Director, Head and Neck Tumor Center
Medical University of South Carolina
Charleston, South Carolina

Frederic W.-B. Deleyiannis, MD, FACS, MPhil, MPH
Professor
Department of Surgery, Plastic and Reconstructive Surgery and Pediatric Surgery
University of Colorado School of Medicine
Aurora, Colorado

Daniel G. Deschler, MD, FACS
Professor
Department of Otology and Laryngology
Harvard Medical School
Director, Division of Head and Neck Surgery
Department of Otolaryngology
Massachusetts Eye and Ear Infirmary
Boston, Massachusetts

Paul Donald, MD, FRCS (C)
Professor Emeritus
Center for Skull Base Surgery
UC Davis Health System
Sacramento, California

Neal D. Futran, MD, DMD
Allison T. Wanamaker Professor and Chair
Department of Otolaryngology–Head and Neck Surgery
Director, Head and Neck Surgery
University of Washington
Seattle, Washington

Eric M. Genden, MD, FACS
The Isadore Friesner Professor of Otolaryngology–Head and Neck Surgery
Department of Otolaryngology
Professor of Neurosurgery and Immunology
The Mount Sinai School of Medicine
Director, The Head, Neck, and Thyroid Center
The Icahn School of Medicine at Mount Sinai
New York, New York

Ralph W. Gilbert, MD, FRCSC
Professor
Department of Otolaryngology–Head and Neck Surgery
University of Toronto
Toronto, Ontario, Canada

D. Gregory Farwell, MD, FACS
Professor
Director of Head and Neck Oncology, Microvascular Surgery
Department of Otolaryngology–Head and Neck Surgery
University of California, Davis
Sacramento, California

Patrick J. Gullane, CM, MB, FRCSC, FACS, FRACS(Hon), FRCS(Hon), FRCSI(Hon)
Professor
Department of Otolaryngology–Head and Neck Surgery
University of Toronto
University Health Network
Toronto, Ontario, Canada

Bruce H. Haughey, MBChB, FACS, FRACS
Kimbrough Professor
Department of Otolaryngology–Head and Neck Surgery
Director, Head and Neck Surgical Oncology
Washington University School of Medicine
Barnes-Jewish Hospital
St. Louis, Missouri

Richard E. Hayden, MD
Professor
Department of Otolaryngology–Head and Neck Surgery
The Mayo Clinic
Scottsdale, Arizona

Kevin M. Higgins, MD, MSc, FRCSC
Assistant Professor
Department of Otolaryngology–Head and Neck Surgery
Faculty of Medicine
University of Toronto
Staff Surgeon
Department of Otolaryngology–Head and Neck Surgery
Sunnybrook Health Sciences Center
Toronto, Ontario, Canada

William Lawson, MD, DDS
Professor
Department of Otolaryngology–Head and Neck Surgery
The Icahn School of Medicine at Mount Sinai
New York, New York

Derrick T. Lin, MD
Associate Professor
Department of Otology and Laryngology
Harvard Medical School
Co-Director, Cranial Base Center
Co-Director, Head and Neck Oncology Fellowship
Department of Otology and Laryngology
Massachusetts Eye and Ear Infirmary
Massachusetts General Hospital
Boston, Massachusetts

Brett A. Miles, DDS MD FACS
Assistant Professor
Department of Otolaryngology–Head and Neck Surgery
Assistant Professor of Oral and Maxillofacial Surgery
The Icahn School of Medicine at Mount Sinai
New York, New York

Eric J. Moore, MD
Professor
Department of Otolaryngology–Head and Neck Surgery
Mayo Clinic–Rochester
Rochester, Minnesota

Peter C. Neligan, MD
Professor
Department of Surgery
University of Washington School of Medicine
Director, Center for Reconstructive Surgery
Seattle, Washington

Joseph A. Paydarfar, MD
Associate Professor
Division of Otolaryngology–Head and Neck Surgery
Geisel School of Medicine at Dartmouth
Attending Physician
Division of Otolaryngology–Head and Neck Surgery
Dartmouth-Hitchcock Medical Center
Lebanon, New Hampshire

Rod Rezaee, MD, FACS
Assistant Professor
Head and Neck Surgery
Ear, Nose, and Throat Institute
Case Western Reserve University School of Medicine
Director, Microvascular Head and Neck Reconstructive Surgery
Ear, Nose, and Throat Institute
University Hospitals Case Medical Center/Seidman Cancer Center
Cleveland, Ohio

Elliott H. Rose, MD
Associate Clinical Professor
Plastic and Reconstructive Surgery
The Icahn School of Medicine at Mount Sinai
New York, New York

Eben L. Rosenthal, MD
John S. Odess Professor
Director, Division of Otolaryngology
Department of Surgery
University of Alabama at Birmingham
Birmingham, Alabama

Jesse C. Selber, MD, MPH, FACS
Associate Professor
Department of Plastic Surgery
MD Anderson Cancer Center
Houston, Texas

Marita S. Teng, MD, FACS
Associate Professor
Department of Otolaryngology–Head and Neck Surgery
Director, Residency Training Program
The Icahn School of Medicine at Mount Sinai
New York, New York

Terance T. Tsue, MD, FACS
Endowed Professor of Head and Neck Surgical Oncology
Vice Chairman
Department of Otolaryngology–Head and Neck Surgery
University of Kansas School of Medicine
Physician in Chief
University of Kansas Cancer Center
University of Kansas Hospital
Kansas City, Kansas

Mark A. Varvares, MD, FACS
Professor
Department of Otolaryngology–Head and Neck Surgery
The Donald and Marlene Jerome Endowed Chair in Otolaryngology–Head and Neck Surgery
The Saint Louis University
Director, Cancer Center
The Saint Louis University
Co-Director, Center for Cancer Prevent, Research and Outreach
Saint Louis University
St. Louis, Missouri

Mark K. Wax, MD FACS FRCS(C)
Professor
Otolaryngology and Oral Maxillofacial Surgery
Program Director
Director Microvascular Reconstruction
Past President American Head and Neck Society
Oregon Health Sciences University
Portland, Oregon

Donald T. Weed, MD, FACS
Associate Professor
Department of Otolaryngology
Vice Chairman for Academic Affairs
University of Miami Miller School of Medicine
Miami, Florida

Peak Woo, MD
Clinical Professor
Department of Otolaryngology–Head and Neck Surgery
Ichan School of Medicine at Mount Sinai
New York, New York

Series Preface

Since its inception in 1994, the *Master Techniques in Orthopedic Surgery* series has become the go-to text for surgeons in training and in practice. The user-friendly style of providing and illustrating authoritative information on a broad spectrum of techniques of orthopedic surgery obviously filled a need in orthopedic educational materials. The format has become a standard against which others are compared, and there are now 13 volumes in the series with other volumes in the planning phase.

When I was approached to be the series editor, I already knew what a daunting task it would be from my previous experience with editing surgical texts, but I felt that this unique approach could become a valuable fixture in the catalogue of literature on surgery in all the subspecialty fields of Otolaryngology. This first edition includes volumes on Head and Neck Oncology which was published earlier this year. Reconstructive Surgery of the Head and Neck, Cranial Base Surgery, Rhinology, Aesthetic Surgery, and Otology and Lateral Skull Base Surgery.

I have recruited real masters to be volume editors including Robert L. Ferris, Eric M. Genden, Carl H. Snyderman and Paul Gardner, David Kennedy, Wayne Larrabee and James Ridgeway, and Thomas J. Roland, respectively. Having a separate volume on Reconstructive Surgery of the Head and Neck as a separate companion piece for the volume on Head and Neck Oncology is somewhat nontraditional but enabled us to include more topics.

I do hope that you will find the Master Techniques to be a useful addition to your surgical armamentarium for the benefit of your patients.

Eugene N. Myers, MD
Series Editor

Preface

Arguably, head and neck cancer is the most merciless of maladies. Deficits in form and function that commonly follow ablative surgery can be functionally and socially devastating. Hence, there is no other field where reconstruction is such an integral aspect of care. Prior to World War II, reconstructive techniques were limited to skin grafts and local flaps. While these techniques were satisfactory for modest defects, larger more complex defects remained a dilemma. In 1959, Seidenberg knocked on the door of the "modern era" of reconstruction, but in spite of his early success with microvascular free tissue transfer, it was not until two decades later that this technique became commonplace. During the interim period, Bekamjian's deltopectoral flap (1965) and Biller and Lawson's pectoralis flap (1979) became the "workhorse" flaps for reconstruction of the head and neck. However, in spite of these staple techniques, regional flaps were inadequate for defects of the mandible, central skull base, and pharyngoesophagus. Buncke and Panje recognized these limitations, and their work in microsurgery was pivotal in eventually ushering in the age of microvascular reconstruction.

Since this initial work, a select few have been instrumental in refining the techniques of head and neck reconstruction. The work herein is authored by many of the masters who were instrumental in driving forward the discipline of head and neck reconstruction. Each has had a profound impact on the field and each shares his techniques, pearls, and pitfalls.

Head and neck reconstruction is as much an art as a science. The techniques discussed within this volume range from local flaps to free tissue transfer. The contributing authors have done an extraordinary job articulating the art of head and neck reconstruction for the purpose of benefiting our patients and inspiring their colleagues. I am profoundly grateful to the authors for their contribution. I hope this work will inspire the readership as it has inspired me.

Eric M. Genden, MD, FACS

Acknowledgments

I would like to acknowledge Jonas T. Johnson, MD, for providing me the stimulus to take on the task of editing a new project—*Master Techniques in Otolaryngology—Head and Neck Surgery*. It has proved to be a daunting task, but the positive impact that this book will have on those doing head and neck surgery and their patients will make the effort well worthwhile.

I also acknowledge the dedicated assistance of Agnes C. Zachoszcz in the preparation of the book.

I also gratefully acknowledge Robert Hurley who recruited me into the project and Ryan Shaw, his successor, for his strong support. Brendan Huffman has done a fine job with the technical backup and organizing the book.

Eugene N. Myers, MD

Contents

PART IV: RECONSTRUCTION OF THE PALATOMAXILLARY COMPLEX 151

PART V: RECONSTRUCTION OF THE LARYNX/ TRACHEA 215

PART VI: RECONSTRUCTION OF THE HYPOPHARYNX/CERVICAL ESOPHAGUS 233

PART VII: RECONSTRUCTION OF THE SKIN AND SCALP 295

PART I: RECONSTRUCTION OF THE ORAL CAVITY

1 MANAGEMENT OF THE MAJOR LIP DEFECT

William Lawson

INTRODUCTION

Defects of the lips present the reconstructive surgeon with the complex problem of tissue restoration requiring both cosmetic and functional optimization. The etiology of lip defects is most commonly the result of trauma or the resection of malignant tumors. Aesthetically the lips are a focal point of facial balance and beauty. In this regard, the upper lip offers additional reconstructive difficulty because of the presence of a central dimple and its surrounding philtral columns. Functionally, the lips are of particular importance in facial expression, oral competence, and communication. The challenge of reconstituting aesthetic symmetry while maintaining functionality with large lip defects presents the reconstructive surgeons with a major challenge.

Historically, efforts at lip reconstruction were directed toward the repair of small defects. In particular, the cross-lip procedure in which a lower lip flap was transferred to the upper lip was described separately by Sabattini, Estlander, and Stein in Europe in the early 19th century. However, the technique was popularized by the American surgeon, Robert Abbe, and the flap continues to bear his name. This flap continues to be used to provide bulk and a functional component as they have been shown to have reinnervation in 6 to 12 months. Newer techniques were directed to the repair of subtotal lip defects by advancing or rotating full-thickness local flaps of adjacent cheek tissue by Gillies, Bernard, and von Burow in the period from 1850 to 1950 and by Karapandzic in 1974.

Regional flaps are not suitable for reconstruction of larger defects involving 80% or more of the lip horizontally and which extend past the labiomental sulcus in the vertical plane into the cheek and extend into the oral cavity and involve the maxilla because an adequate lip sulcus and oral aperture cannot be maintained. Thus, in recent times, nonregional tissue transfer has become the mainstay for total lip reconstruction. Some examples include the deltopectoral flap, sternocleidomastoid musculocutaneous flap, and the radial forearm free flap. Unfortunately, it is difficult to preserve sphincter competence with distant flaps, which has led to modifications in free tissue transfer to include the addition of vascularized palmaris longus tendon or tensor fascial lata grafts to contribute a static component to reconstruction. Furthermore, enhanced dynamic reconstruction options combining an innervated depressor anguli oris, temporalis, or masseter muscle flap transfer to a radial forearm free flap have been reported, demonstrating muscle activity on electromyography at 6-month postoperative follow-up.

Reconstruction of large defects of the upper lip including maintenance of oral competence and avoiding microstomia remains a technical challenge for the head and neck surgeon. The numerous techniques described for reconstruction of near-total full-thickness lip defects underscores the fact that while soft tissue replacement can be achieved, functional restoration is elusive. Flaps that recruit the remaining orbicularis oris provide the potential for motor and sensory function but are limited by the development of postoperative microstomia, which often requires secondary commissuroplasty to facilitate oral feeding, hygiene, and placement of dentures.

Alternatively, techniques that do not involve local musculocutaneous tissue transfer, such as local and regional cutaneous flaps or free microvascular tissue transfer reconstruction, allow for replacement of greater amounts of tissue for repair of defects but increase the likelihood of oral incompetence. Consequently, they find their greatest application in reconstruction of large composite lip perioral defects where a large volume of tissue is necessary.

The use of the nasolabial or melolabial transposition flap has been extensively described in lip reconstruction for both cutaneous and full-thickness defects. Its blood supply is from a random subdermal plexus of vessels, with contributions from the facial, infraorbital, and transverse facial arteries and can be superiorly or inferiorly based. Superiorly based flaps have been used for reconstruction of nose, cheek, lower eyelid, and central upper lip defects, while the inferiorly based flap is most commonly used for repair of the lateral upper and lower lip, oral commissure, and anterior oral cavity.

The fan flap reported by Gillies in 1957 is the prototypical rotation–advancement nasolabial flap for reconstruction of upper and lower lip defects. In its original form, it entailed full-thickness incision of the lip and cheek, with the flap based on a narrow vascular pedicle at the oral commissure. Gillies cautioned that the limit of correction was one-half of the upper lip because of the development of microstomia, lip eversion, and intraoral scarring. Having the pivot point at the oral commissure caused the distortion. Additionally, the through and through division of skin, muscle, and mucosa resulted in transection of the nerve supply and the creation of an adynamic lip segment. A later modification by McGregor created a rectangular flap also pedicled on the labial artery compared to Nakajima's flap that had the facial artery as its vascular pedicle. Both employed full-thickness incisions to transfer cheek tissue to the lip.

While this flap design creates a potentially denervated and adynamic flap, there are reports of patients who regained sensory and motor function.

HISTORY

The patient's history is an important aspect of the reconstructive planning. A history of prior surgery or radiotherapy may limit the options. In such cases, radiation and/or surgery can impair the use of local flaps because the blood supply may be compromised. In such cases, free tissue transfer may be indicated. Another aspect of the patient history that should be sought is a history of collagen vascular disease that may impair healing. When a careful preoperative history is obtained, the chances of an optimal outcome are maximized and the risks of complications are minimized.

PHYSICAL EXAMINATION

Anatomically, the lips are a central feature of the lower third of the face. When approaching defects of either the upper or lower lip, a thorough evaluation of its location and extent visually and by palpation is critical in selecting the most appropriate reconstructive option. Defects can involve the upper or lower lip individually or may include a portion of each. They may also be either medially or more laterally based and can involve the oral commissure, which may significantly alter the reconstructive approach. Cancer involving the commissure has a propensity for cervical lymph node metastasis making careful evaluation of the neck mandatory. In addition to location, accurately evaluating the extent and depth of the defect on physical examination is of utmost importance. The lips are composed of skin, muscle, mucosa, and underlying skeletal bone of the maxilla, mandible, and alveolus that may be deficient to varying degrees. The tissue components involved will dictate the most suitable reconstructive technique or whether additional tissue will be indicated. A key aesthetic boundary is the vermilion border delineating the mucocutaneous junction of the lip, and if this landmark is violated, careful approximation can be planned. Defects may also extend across the nasolabial and labiomandibular creases to involve surrounding structures such as the base of the nose, cheek, and chin necessitating more complex reconstructive planning and techniques.

INDICATIONS

Defects of the lip most commonly result from trauma, congenital malformation, or malignancy. Traumatic injury to the upper and lower lip can often be repaired primarily after the freshening of wound edges and careful realignment of aesthetic boundaries, but more extensive soft tissue damage may call for the use of various locoregional flaps or even microvascular free tissue transfer. Congenital defects from unilateral and bilateral cleft lip with or without palatal involvement certainly may pose distinct challenges to the reconstructive surgeon but are not specifically addressed in this chapter.

The most frequent indication for reconstruction of major defects of the lip is following resection of skin cancer. Cutaneous malignancies including basal cell carcinoma, squamous cell carcinoma, and malignant melanoma are among the most prevalent cancers today. Due to their exposure to direct sunlight, the lips are particularly vulnerable to solar insults. This is especially true of the lower lip, which harbors the majority of sun-induced cancers due to its more exposed position. Smoking and the use of tobacco-containing products can also increase the risk of developing lip cancer. Fortunately, its prominent location lends itself to manifesting visible signs and symptoms and therefore typically leads to earlier clinical detection and treatment. Still, some lesions may present in later stages due to patient neglect or misdiagnosis necessitating more aggressive surgical resection and therefore larger defects. Even with the advent of Mohs surgery, resulting defects are often larger than at first expected, and reconstruction of these complex postablative subtotal and total lip defects will be required.

CONTRAINDICATIONS

There are no contraindications to the reconstruction of major lip defects other than the availability of suitable donor tissue and patient-related factors. Particularly, patients who are not candidates for microvascular free tissue transfer due to the presence of extensive peripheral vascular disease, active smoking, or other significant comorbidities may be better served with a less aggressive type of reconstruction despite the possibility of inferior aesthetic and functional outcomes. Recent advances in microvascular techniques and the use of two-team approaches have reduced surgical time so that performing a radial forearm free flap may actually be faster than the more complex locoregional reconstructive flaps in some settings. Additionally, a radical resection may not be reasonable in the presence of distant metastatic disease, although there may be a role for palliative debulking at the primary tumor site in some cases. Certainly, all local and patient-related factors must be carefully considered in open discourse between the patient and surgeon in order to select the most reasonable and appropriate treatment option.

PREOPERATIVE PLANNING

Imaging Studies

Imaging studies, in general, are not necessary when evaluating more superficial lesions of the lip; however, there are instances in which a contrast-enhanced CT scan may be very useful. Examples include extensive tumors that involve neighboring structures, recurrent neoplasms, or those that are highly aggressive in nature (e.g., malignant melanoma). In addition to the primary site, it is prudent in such cases to evaluate for metastatic lymphadenopathy by cervical CT scan. Any lymph nodes detected can undergo fine needle aspiration (FNA) to determine whether they represent metastatic cancer or an inflammatory response to large lesions, which also tend to be superficially ulcerated and infected. CT scan may also help to determine the presence or extent of underlying bone involvement from deeply invasive lip lesions to allow for appropriate preoperative planning. For instance, if microvascular free tissue transfer is indicated, the most common flap used is the radial forearm flap, which typically requires only a reliable Allen test.

Although not as commonly used in major lip reconstruction, magnetic resonance angiography of the lower extremities would be indicated prior to harvesting of a fibular free flap. PET/CT is now routinely used for accurate staging of more extensive or aggressive malignancies to evaluate for distant metastases prior to any definitive surgical intervention.

Biopsy

Due to the readily accessible nature of the lips, biopsy of lesions is typically performed in an outpatient setting under topical or local anesthetic. When dealing with a possible cutaneous malignancy, it is important to perform either a small wedge excisional biopsy or an adequate punch biopsy in order to accurately determine the depth of the lesion, which has prognostic significance and may alter the subsequent surgical approach. A biopsy in the center of the lesion is preferable. Bleeding following biopsy is generally negligible and can be controlled with direct pressure, chemical cautery using silver nitrate sticks, dissolvable hemostatic agents, handheld electrocautery, or an absorbable suture used to approximate the edges of the defect. Histopathologic analysis will confirm the diagnosis and dictate whether further diagnostic studies or intervention is indicated.

Due to their aesthetic and functional importance, the lips are also amenable to Mohs excision to ensure clear margins while conserving the maximum amount of native tissue. If metastatic lymphadenopathy is suspected either clinically or radiographically, an FNA may also be performed in clinic by the surgeon or cytopathologist. Image-guided FNA may help in cases where cervical lymph nodes are not palpable.

SURGICAL TECHNIQUE

Nasolabial (Melolabial) Transposition Flap

The advantages of the nasolabial flap for repair of the upper lip include its close proximity to the defect and adequate color match. Donor site morbidity is generally minimal due to the redundancy of tissue in the nasolabial fold, allowing for reasonable camouflage of the scar. However, drawbacks to the use of the nasolabial flap include the absence of function of the oral sphincter following reconstruction. Reconstitution of the oral

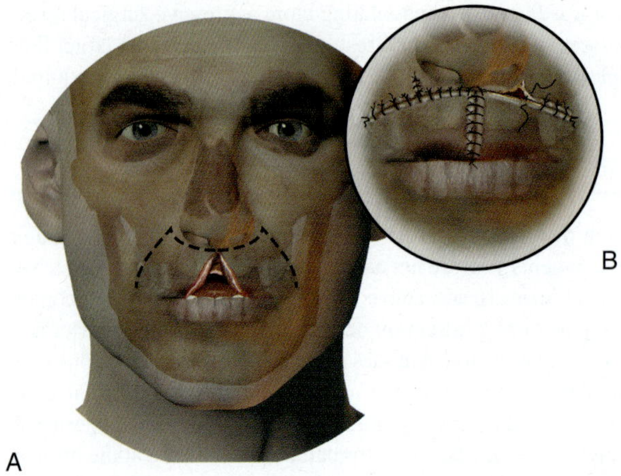

FIGURE 1.1 Diagram of bilateral nasolabial transposition flaps. The flaps are designed with incisions lying in the melolabial folds and flaps transposed over the adjacent alar bases to meet in the midline of the upper lip. **A.** Bilateral nasolabial flaps outlined. **B.** Flaps advanced and sutured together to create a new vermilion border and fill the defect.

mucosa is an important consideration when employing cutaneous flaps for lip reconstruction. Buccal mucosal advancement flaps have the advantage of providing like-appearing mucosa to recreate the vermilion border and of being sensate. The potential downside with the advancement of large amounts of buccal mucosa is the potential loss of lip fullness, lip inversion, and loss of the gingivobuccal sulcus.

Description of Technique: Nasolabial (Melolabial) Transposition Flap

The patient is placed under general anesthesia and may be intubated transorally; however, a nasotracheal tube secured superiorly away from the surgical field is preferable in order to avoid distortion of the tissues. The patient is then prepped and draped in standard sterile fashion with the lower two-thirds of the face and upper neck exposed. The flap is designed to incorporate the nasolabial fold and subalar crease to improve aesthetic results (Fig. 1.1). Surgical technique involves incisions based along the nasolabial folds. The flap is then raised in a plane deep to the skin and subcutaneous tissue and superficial to the facial musculature. The rotation point of the inferiorly based flap should be just superior and lateral to the oral commissure to minimize dog-ear formation. This case depicts the use of bilateral nasolabial flaps to reconstruct a large central defect of the upper lip extending to the base of the nose (Fig. 1.2A–C).

Reconstruction of a subtotal and total defect of the upper lip requires two local regional flaps. Bilateral nasolabial flaps provide ample tissue but, unfortunately, are adynamic. On the side of less involvement, the reverse Karapandzic flap is used to transfer innervated elements of the remaining orbicularis oris to restore some sphincteric function. The original fan flap has been modified by eliminating the through and through incision and instead creating two advancement-rotation flaps. The cutaneous–subcutaneous flap provides external coverage of the new lip, while the mucosal muscular flap replaces the internal lining of the lip and creates a new vermilion border. The skin component is preplanned while the internal component is created by making sequential mucosal incisions as necessary to achieve flap advancement and coverage. Moreover, this flap transfers with it the modiolus (which is 1.5 cm beyond the anterior commissure), which carries elevator and depressor muscles and the buccinator muscle providing some dynamic activity.

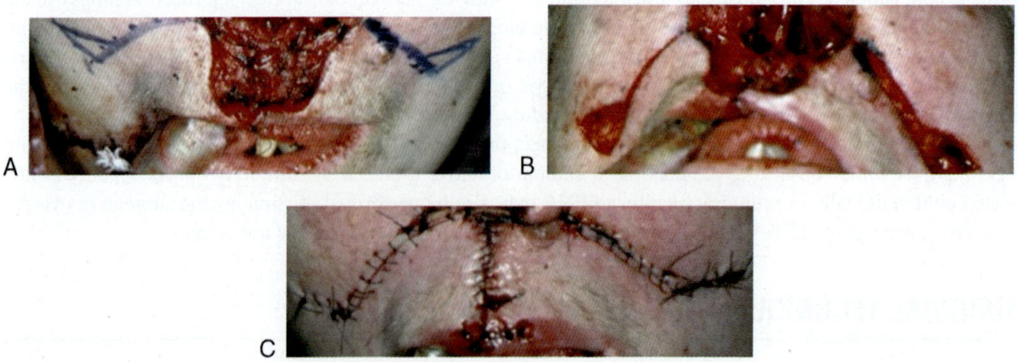

FIGURE 1.2 **A.** Central defect of the upper lip involving entire philtrum and extending superiorly to the nasal base. Incisions are marked for bilateral nasolabial transposition flap reconstruction. **B.** Bilateral nasolabial transposition flaps are raised after incisions through the melolabial creases and excision of partial-thickness triangles inferiorly. Flaps are raised in a subcutaneous plane taking care not to violate the underlying mucosa. **C.** Flaps are advanced toward the midline and closed in layers with careful realignment of the vermilion border and subnasale. Note that bilateral incisions lie within the melolabial creases to help with eventual camouflage of the scar.

When nasolabial flaps are used, a new oral commissure is created unilaterally or bilaterally. The two flaps are advanced and sutured together, and the cheek flap is sutured to the opposite lip at the point where the new commissure is to be created. This entails a deep suture of 3-0 Vicryl. The skin is attached with a 5-0 nylon suture and 4-0 chromic sutures after the mucosal flap has been advanced to create a new vermilion border. Care must be taken to ensure that the new vermilion border is correctly realigned. Closure should be performed in three layers consisting of mucosa, subcutaneous tissue, and skin using 4-0 chromic, 3-0 Vicryl, and 5-0 nylon sutures, respectively. Steri-Strips can be used to reinforce the incision if under moderate tension; otherwise, bacitracin ointment may be applied following closure.

Circumoral Rotation–Advancement Flap: Karapandzic Flap

The Karapandzic flap is an advancement–rotation flap based on the superior and inferior labial arteries and nasoseptal artery branches. A distinguishing feature of this flap is the preservation of the neurovascular innervation of the orbicularis oris muscle during transfer to reconstitute a functional oral sphincter. This flap also transfers with it the modiolus of the lip, with its attached muscles and adjacent decussating fibers, which while producing misdirection of muscular fibers and proprioceptive elements, nevertheless recreates a functional oral unit. Its greatest application is with unilateral flaps to reconstruct small to moderate defects of the lower lip although a modification can be used for upper lip reconstruction (reverse Karapandzic). The Karapandzic flap is generally not used to reconstruct defects of the lateral lip and oral commissure.

Good functional outcomes have been reported in case series of patients undergoing Karapandzic reconstruction of lip defects with up to 75% of patients regaining normal postoperative speech and oral competence. When rotational flaps are used as the exclusive method of reconstruction in the repair of large defects, commissuroplasty and commissurotomy are necessary to correct the resultant severe microstomia. Other disadvantages relate to aesthetic concerns, including the potential for an unsightly perioral scar as well as rounding of the commissure.

Description of Technique: Karapandzic Flap

The patient is placed under general anesthesia and may be intubated transorally; however, a nasotracheal tube secured superiorly away from the surgical field is preferable. The patient is then prepped and draped in standard sterile fashion with the lower two-thirds of the face and upper neck exposed. Surgical technique involves bilateral circumoral incisions around the defect along the nasolabial folds from the lower to upper lip (Fig. 1.3). Blunt dissection is then carried out within the orbicularis oris to mobilize muscle fibers while preserving the major neurovasculature bundles typically located near the oral commissures. The mucosa should not be violated during the course of dissection until the flaps are completely raised and advanced together under appropriate tension. Care must be taken to ensure that the new vermilion border is correctly realigned. Closure should be performed in three layers consisting of mucosa, subcutaneous tissue, and skin using 4-0 chromic, 3-0 Vicryl, and 5-0 nylon sutures, respectively. Steri-Strips can be used to reinforce the incision if under moderate tension; otherwise, Bacitracin ointment may be applied following closure.

Transoral Cross-Lip Flaps: Abbe and Estlander Flaps

The transoral cross-lip or lip-switch flaps were devised in the mid 1800s and are still used today for reconstruction of the lip (Figs. 1.4 and 1.5). They provide a reliable method of restoring medium-sized lip defects with or without oral commissure involvement and can also be used in combination with other locoregional flaps for subtotal and total lip reconstruction. Advantages include good color match and skin texture from the opposing lip as well as the ability to position the incision in a natural skin crease, which leads to more favorable scar formation. Drawbacks are the need for a two-stage procedure when using the Abbe flap for central lip defects, possible distortion of upper lip subunits when using this as a donor site for lower lip repair, and the potential need for a revision commissuroplasty with the Estlander flap. Overall, even 200 years after its initial development, the transoral cross-lip flap has endured the test of time and is still commonly employed in major lip repair by today's reconstructive surgeons.

Description of Technique: Abbe and Estlander Flaps

The patient is placed under general anesthesia with a nasotracheal tube secured superiorly away from the surgical field; nasal intubation is preferred due to the need of the flap pedicle to cross over the lips. This procedure can also be done under local with IV sedation. The patient is then rotated 180 degrees and prepped and draped in standard sterile fashion with the lower two-thirds of the face and upper neck exposed. The flap should be designed to incorporate the nasolabial crease for improved cosmesis with its length approximating that of the defect. Incisions are made sharply through the skin and subcutaneous tissues taking care not to disrupt the vascular pedicle based either medially or laterally off the labial artery. After complete elevation, the flap may be rotated into the corresponding defect and closed in layers. Abbe flaps used to close more centrally based

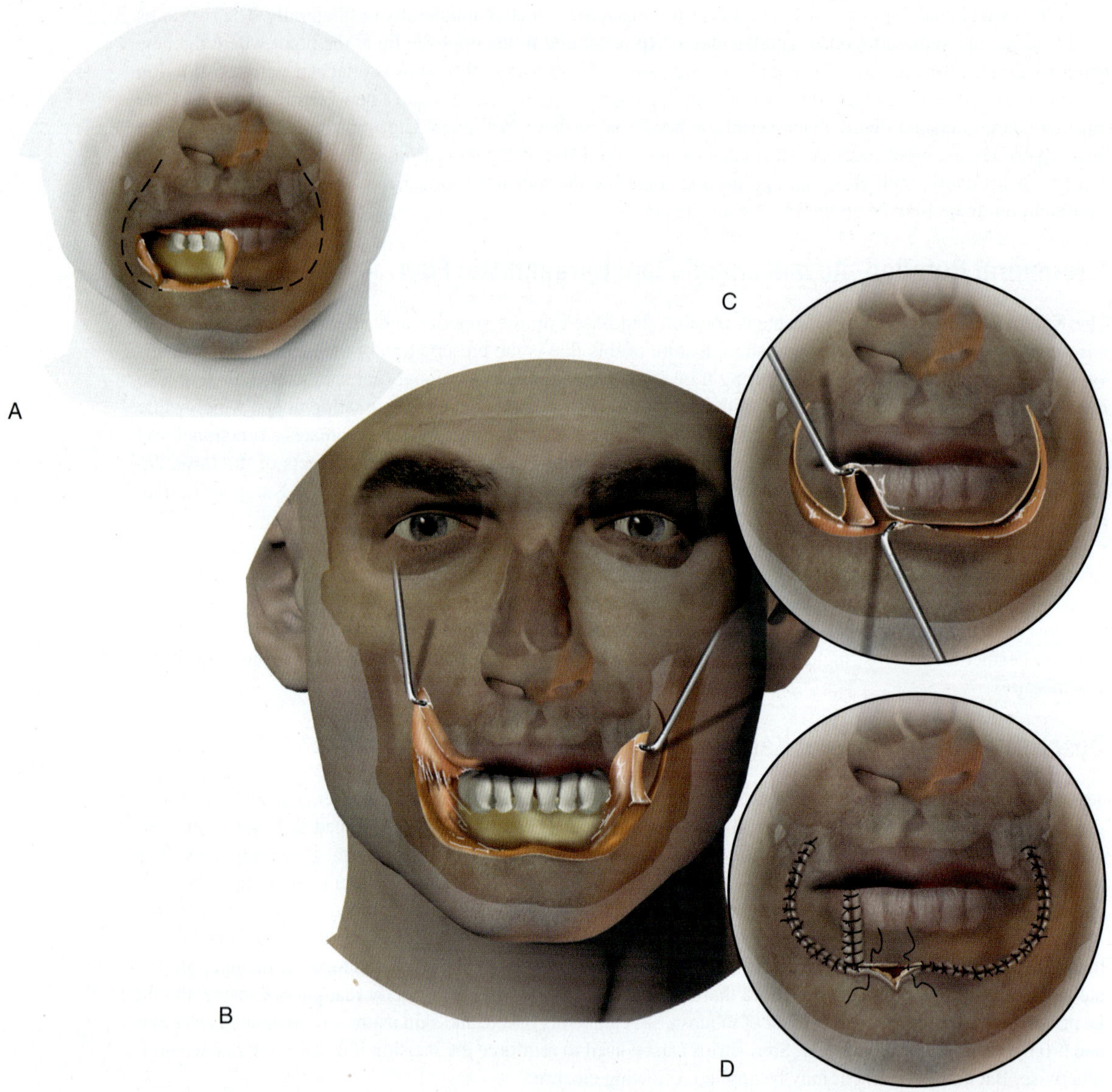

FIGURE 1.3 Diagram of proposed Karapandzic flap for repair of right subtotal defect of the lower lip. **A.** Bilateral circumoral incisions outlined. **B.** Orbicularis oris muscle bluntly dissected to expose nerve. **C.** Flaps advanced and vermilion border aligned. **D.** Completed layered closure.

defects will require a second-stage procedure for pedicle division in 2 to 3 weeks, while the Estlander flap used to reconstruct the oral commissure laterally typically will not require a second surgery unless revision commissuroplasty is indicated. The incisions should be kept clean and moist with antibiotic ointment postoperatively, and patients should adhere to a modified diet until healing is complete.

Bilateral Cheek Advancement Flap: Bernard-Webster Flap

Lower lip subtotal defects can be reconstituted with a combined Karapandzic and Bernard-Webster–type flap to maximize dynamic function. With total defects of the lower lip, bilateral Bernard-Webster flaps are necessary for adequate tissue mass. The Bernard-Webster flap is a modification of the original Bernard-von Burow flap described in the 1850s used for reconstruction of total full-thickness defects of the upper or lower lip. The technique involves the excision of partial-thickness triangles from the nasolabial creases to facilitate advancement superiorly and inferiorly of the adjacent local tissue. Similar to the modified fan flap used for upper lip reconstruction, the Bernard-Webster flap is not created by full-thickness incisions through the adjacent cheek tissue but divided into an outer cutaneous and inner mucosal portion. While the outer component is preset, the intraoral component is incised incrementally to achieve adequate advancement and to resurface the mucosal aspect of the neolip and vermilion border.

Transferring the modiolus forward with its attached depressor and elevator muscles as well as the buccinator muscle adds a dynamic component and provides some sphincteric function. I modify this method further by making bilateral labiomandibular incisions rather than excising triangles in this region (Fig. 1.6).

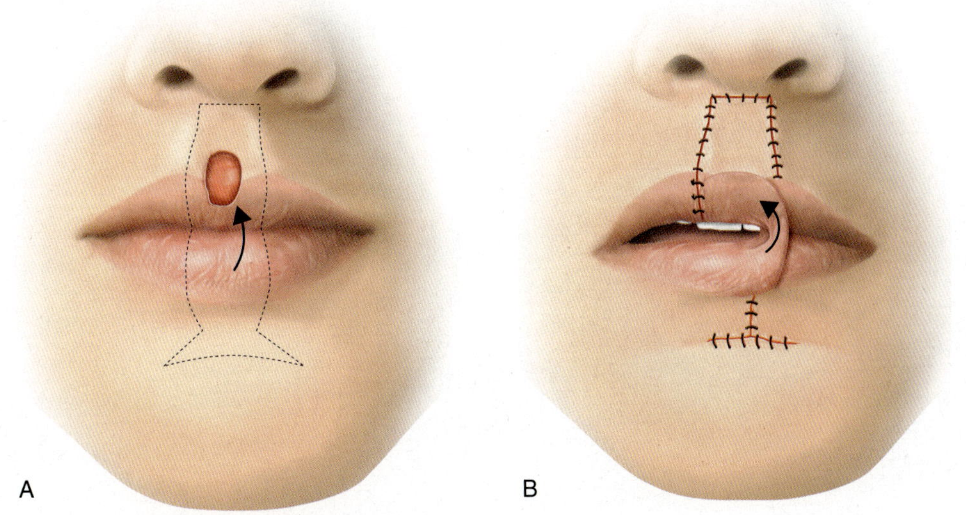

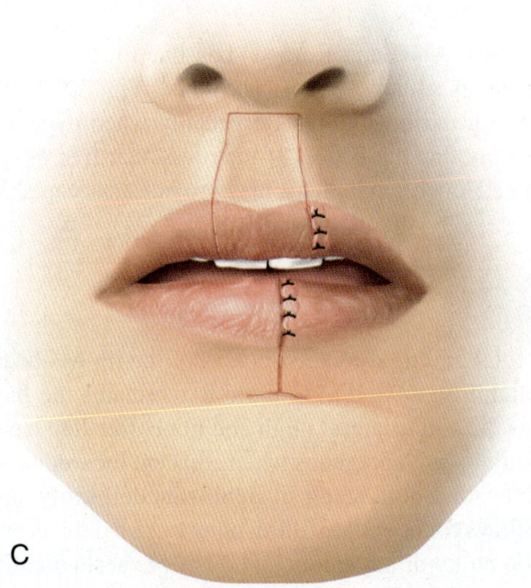

FIGURE 1.4
Abbe flap. **A.** Central area of resection of upper lip outlined. Area of lower lip to be transposed outlined. **B.** Lower lip donor flap sutured into upper lip defect. **C.** Pedicle divided after 2–3 weeks. (From Thorne CH (ed). *Grabb and Smith's Plastic Surgery, 7th ed.* Philadelphia, PA: Lippincott Williams & Wilkins, 2014.)

Typically, the flap innervation is not preserved with this technique with possible functional postoperative deficits. For this reason, I prefer microvascular free flaps as a more reliable reconstruction option for larger defects; however, bilateral cheek advancement technique may still play a role in patients who cannot undergo free tissue transfer or when used in combination with related locoregional flaps.

Locoregional Flap Combinations

When one type of locoregional flap is insufficient to repair a larger lip defect, a combination of various reconstructive techniques may be employed. These may include the use of a modified Bernard-Webster flap with either a transoral cross-lip flap or a circumoral rotation–advancement flap such as the Karapandzic (Fig. 1.7A

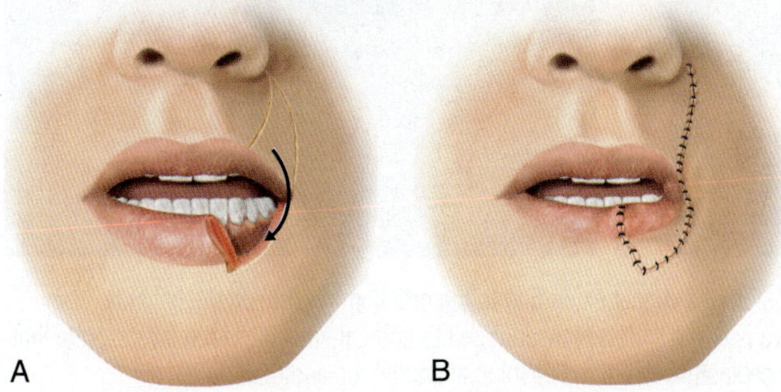

FIGURE 1.5
Estlander flap. **A.** Donor flap from upper lip including the commissure is outlined for lateral defect. **B.** Flap transfered into long lip defect. Note rounding of commissure. (From Thorne CH (ed). *Grabb and Smith's Plastic Surgery, 7th ed.* Philadelphia, PA: Lippincott Williams & Wilkins, 2014.)

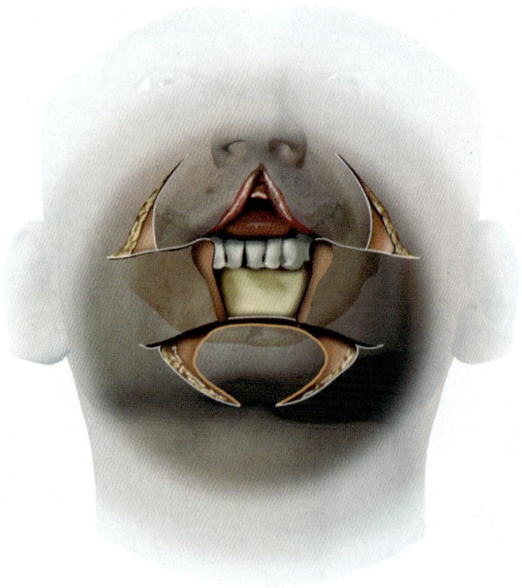

FIGURE 1.6 Diagram of modified Bernard-Webster flap for reconstruction of total lower lip defect. Bilateral partial-thickness nasolabial triangles are excised along with labiomandibular incisions inferiorly.

and B). This case illustrates the utility in performing a combined Abbe and Karapandzic flap to reconstruct a subtotal upper lip defect after excision of a recurrent cutaneous squamous cell carcinoma (Fig. 1.8A–D). Excellent postoperative outcomes have been demonstrated using these techniques especially when dynamic function is maintained through neurovascular preservation during flap dissection. If microvascular free tissue transfer is not available or is contraindicated, the use of combined locoregional flaps may provide an acceptable alternative to the repair of major lip defects.

Microvascular Free Tissue Transfer

The application of microvascular free tissue transfer to subtotal and total reconstruction of the lip has been reported since the 1980s. Due to its thin skin paddle and pliability, the radial forearm flap remains the flap most commonly used to repair the lip although others such as the anterolateral thigh and fibula free flap have also been used. Free tissue transfer from distant sites is particularly advantageous when adjacent locoregional tissue flaps are not available, may be invaded with malignancy, or would result in significant deformity and microstomia. The ability to harvest large amounts of tissue allows for adequate filling of extensive defects but has also led to concerns that such reconstructions may be too bulky or adynamic and therefore aesthetically and functionally deficient. Further developments such as the incorporation of the palmaris longus tendon and fascia lata sling for static suspension as well as simultaneous free muscle transfer including the depressor anguli oris, temporalis, and masseter have improved overall outcomes for these patients. In the presence of composite bone defects, osteofasciocutaneous flaps such as the scapula, iliac crest, and fibula free flap may also be used. As the techniques of microvascular free tissue transfer and facial reanimation evolve, they will no doubt continue to play a large role in the reconstruction of major defects of the lip.

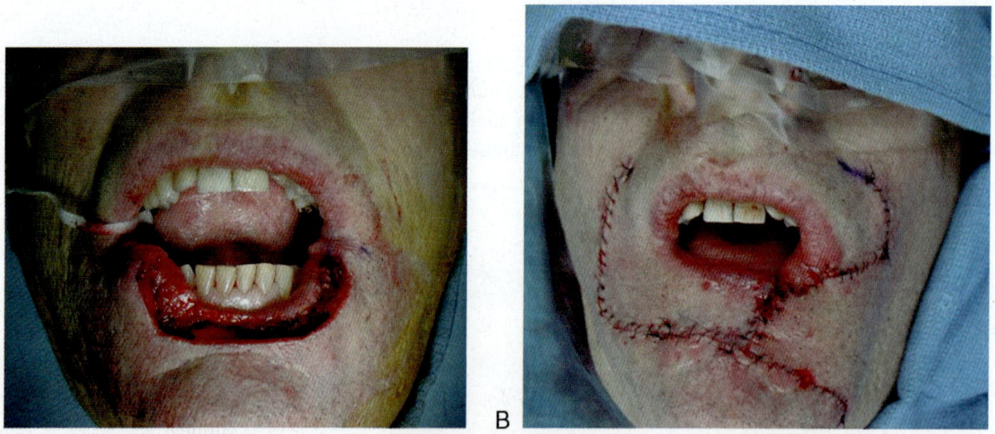

A B

FIGURE 1.7 A. Subtotal lower lip defect after excision of a cancer extending to the oral commissure on the left side. **B.** Combined Karapandzic and modified Bernard-Webster flaps are advanced together and carefully closed in layers. Note that resulting circumoral incisions lie in cosmetically acceptable areas of the nasolabial and labiomandibular folds.

Description of Technique: Radial Forearm Free Flap with Palmaris Longus Tendon

The patient is placed under general anesthesia preferably with a nasotracheal tube secured superiorly away from the surgical field and appropriate lines and monitors are placed. The patient is then rotated 180 degrees and prepped and draped in standard sterile fashion with the lower two-thirds of the face and entire neck exposed along with the upper and lower extremity donor sites. A tourniquet is placed around the upper arm, which is laid outstretched on an arm board. Resection is then carried out with confirmation of clear margins by frozen section (Fig. 1.9A). When neck dissection is also performed, it is important to identify and preserve vasculature such as the facial artery and vein that can potentially be used for the microvascular anastomosis.

In preparation for free flap harvesting, the forearm must be exsanguinated and the tourniquet inflated. The skin paddle should be appropriately measured based on the size of the corresponding lip defect keeping in mind that some flap reabsorption and wound contraction will be expected to occur over time. The forearm flap may be harvested in typical fashion with ligating of the radial artery, cephalic veins, and distal vena comitans. Vessels can be traced further proximally if additional length of the vascular pedicle is needed. In this case, a palmaris longus tendon was harvested along with the radial forearm free flap to create a static sling for the lower lip; fascial connections may remain attached or it can be separated for use as a free graft (Fig. 1.9B). Prior to detachment of the flap, the ulnar collateral circulation should be checked to ensure that the hand remains well perfused.

A subcutaneous tunnel is then made from the lip defect into the neck and widened sufficiently to permit easy passage of the vascular pedicle. The radial forearm flap is then inset into the defect using 3-0 Vicryl circumdental sutures placed intraorally. Microvascular anastomosis is next performed with the operating microscope using 8-0 nylon microsuture; in this case, the facial artery was used. The venous anastomosis was then carried out using a 3.5-mm coupling device to establish continuity between the confluence of the cephalic and radial veins with the common facial vein. At this point, the patency of both arterial and venous anastomoses should be confirmed as well as perfusion of the microvascular flap assessed. Clinically, the flap should be bleeding well upon gentle needle prick and have good color, warmth, and tone (Fig. 1.9C and D).

Closure of the neck is performed in a standard manner with particular care when overlying the vascular pedicle. The platysma is typically closed with interrupted 3-0 or 4-0 Vicryl sutures and skin reapproximated with 4-0 or 5-0 nylon. A number 10 Jackson-Pratt drain is placed in the neck to self-suction and brought out through a small stab incision just lateral to the closure; it should not directly overlie the anastomotic site. Bacitracin ointment and thin xeroform strips may be placed over the neck incision as well as sterile gauze and drain sponge.

Closure of the radial forearm donor site can be performed either during the microvascular anastomosis or simultaneous with closure of the neck wound. Careful attention should be paid to ensure adequate hemostasis prior to closure of the proximal forearm with 3-0 Vicryl sutures and a running 4-0 nylon suture along the skin; insertion of a drain is typically not required. A split-thickness (0.17 mm) skin graft can be harvested from the anterolateral thigh using a dermatome after measuring the appropriate size of the donor site defect. An epinephrine-soaked lap pad may be placed over the skin graft donor site for temporary hemostasis. The skin graft can then be laid onto the radial forearm defect, trimmed accordingly, and secured using 4-0 chromic sutures. A standard dorsal splint should then be placed for postoperative immobilization along with successive layers of web-roll, Kerlix, and ace bandage.

After closure, the patient may either be extubated or remain sedated overnight on the ventilator in an ICU setting depending on patient factors, surgeon preference, and institutional protocol.

POSTOPERATIVE MANAGEMENT

Depending upon the extent of the lip defect and subsequent reconstruction, the patient is either maintained on a modified diet or kept NPO for approximately 5 to 7 days following surgery. In the latter case, a nasogastric tube may be placed and secured at the time of surgery to facilitate postoperative feeding. Following microvascular free tissue transfer, patients are generally kept in an inpatient setting for flap monitoring for a minimum of 3 to 5 days. Aspirin 81 mg is typically administered daily throughout the first postoperative month. All suture lines are meticulously cleaned and kept moist with bacitracin or petroleum ointment; sutures are removed within 5 to 7 days or longer if the patient has previously received radiation therapy or if wound tension is a concern.

COMPLICATIONS

Complications of major lip reconstruction may be classified as either anatomic or surgical. Certainly, aesthetic compromise is of great concern to the patient, and it is important to set reasonable expectations preoperatively through careful and honest patient counseling. Poor color match and contour of the flap, asymmetric healing, excess tissue bulk, scarring, and contracture all may occur with some degree of unpredictability. Incomplete

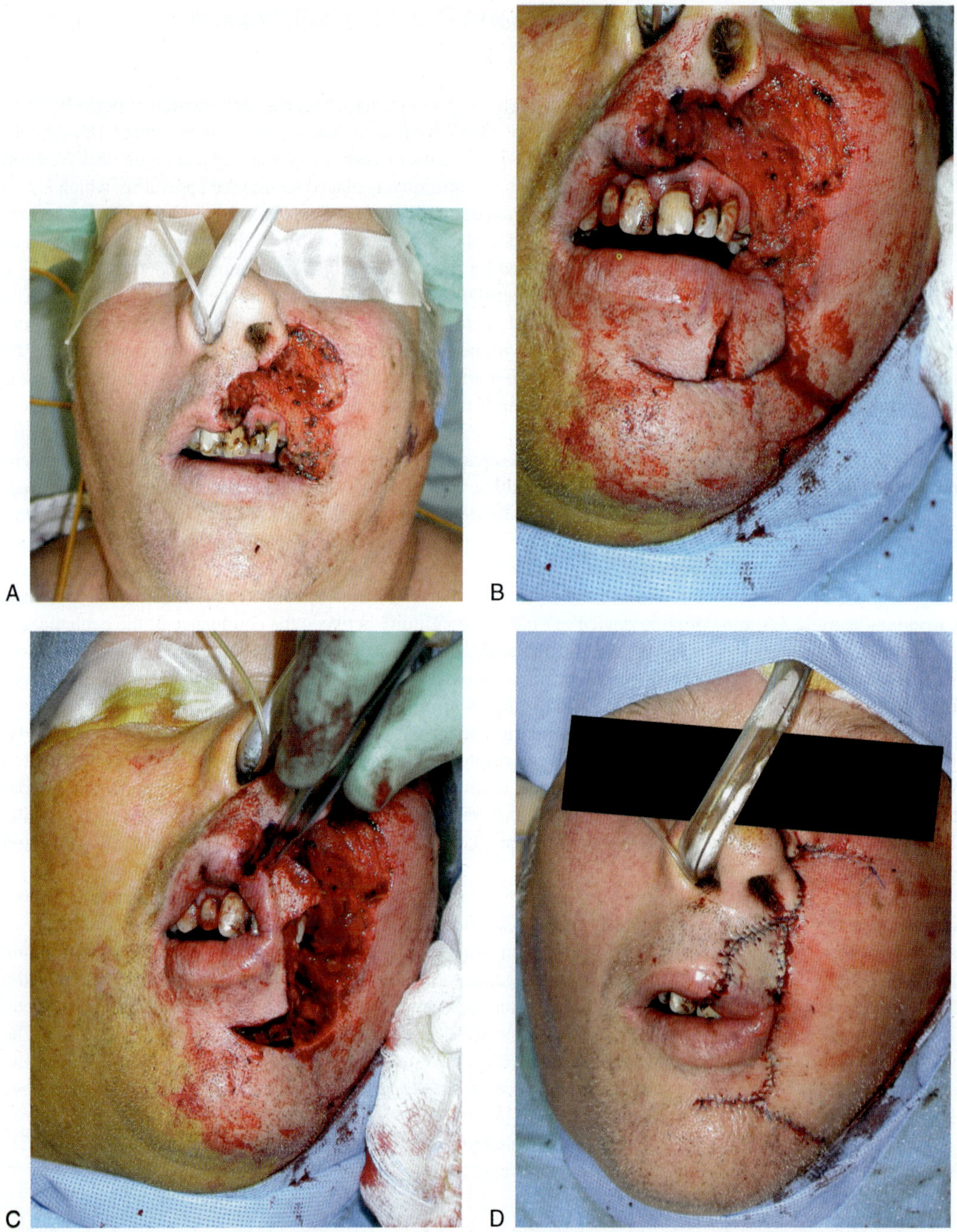

FIGURE 1.8 **A.** Extensive upper lip defect after excision of recurrent squamous cell carcinoma. Defect involves entire left hemilip and extends across the philtrum and left nasolabial fold superiorly onto the cheek and alar base as well as within the left oral commissure. **B.** Incisions made for an inferiorly based Estlander flap along with a modified Karapandzic flap to repair defect of the left upper lip. **C.** Estlander flap rotated transorally into position to meet remainder of the upper lip. The Karapandzic flap will slide circumorally to close the Estlander donor site and oral commissure. Broad undermining is necessary to avoid excess tension on the wound and postoperative microstomia. **D.** Result after closure with combined Estlander and Karapandzic flaps for reconstruction of subtotal defect of the upper lip.

deep volume may result in retraction and notching of the new lip at the point of junction of the flaps. These aesthetic issues can typically be managed more successfully in the postoperative setting when understood beforehand by the patient.

In addition to cosmesis, functional problems can include oral incompetence, dysarthria, and dysphagia that may result from microstomia and adynamic reconstruction. Oral competence may be compromised, and spoon-feeding may be required for several weeks. With the Karapandzic flap, some degree of microstomia and the need for commissuroplasty are to be anticipated. With nasolabial flaps, a new commissure is created. The upper lip has greater volume and distensibility than does the lower lip, and the correction of microstomia is necessary infrequently. The flap is elevated in a plane superficial to the mimetic muscle, and no significant

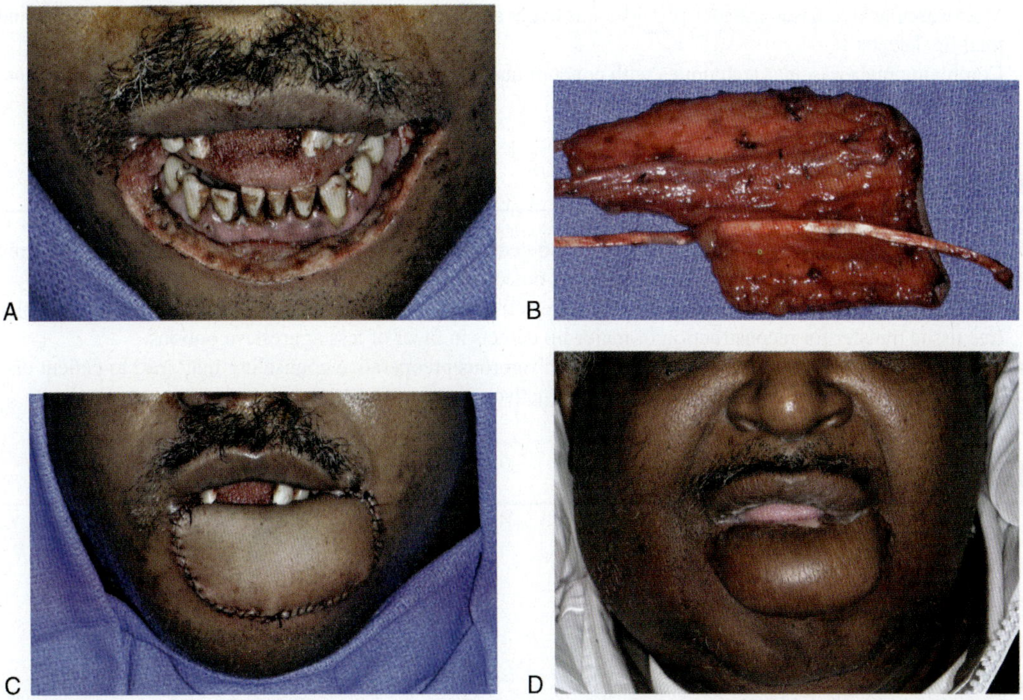

FIGURE 1.9 **A.** Total lower lip defect following excision of malignant melanoma. **B.** Radial forearm free flap harvested with palmaris longus tendon for total lower lip reconstruction with static reanimation sling. **C.** Immediate postoperative view after radial forearm flap anastomosis and insetting. Nylon sutures were used for the skin while Vicryl circumdental sutures were placed to secure the flap internally. **D.** 6-month postoperative result. Note the good color match and bulk to prevent oral incompetence and achieve excellent functional outcome.

facial nerve injury is incurred. Selecting the proper reconstructive method based on the size of the defect and using dynamic tissue when possible is critical to avoiding these postoperative problems.

Surgical complications at the primary site include infection, bleeding, hematoma, seroma, and wound breakdown. Additional risks inherent to microvascular free tissue transfer will become relevant when this reconstructive technique is employed. These include flap failure, donor site morbidity, and increased overall hospital stay and costs. Complications can be avoided or minimized by thorough preoperative planning, meticulous operative technique, and diligent postoperative care. Integral to this is explicit preoperative patient counseling with realistic expectations regarding the ultimate aesthetic and functional outcomes.

RESULTS

Despite over 200 years of advances in reconstructive techniques, the repair of major lip defects remains a formidable challenge to even the most experienced reconstructive surgeon. As defects progressively increase in size and complexity, the task of restoring a functional and aesthetically pleasing lip becomes ever more elusive. Certainly the advent of microvascular transfer along with free tissue grafting for static suspension has greatly enhanced our ability to provide coverage after extensive ablative surgery or trauma. Surprisingly, in spite of these technologic advances, age-old methods of lip reconstruction including variations of the circumoral rotation–advancement, transoral cross-lip, and bilateral cheek advancement flaps continue to be employed today. This not only speaks to the ingenuity of their original creators but also the truly dynamic challenge that subtotal and total lip reconstruction poses. Only by continued reconstructive creativity and progressive thinking will the primary goal of patient satisfaction with cosmetic and functional outcomes following major lip restoration ultimately be achieved.

PEARLS

- Proper evaluation of the upper and lower lip defect includes a careful analysis of its extent and location with a focus on aesthetic subunits, functional musculature, and tissue composition.
- Preoperative biopsy and imaging are important to confirm the diagnosis and accurately assess the extent of particularly large, aggressive, or recurrent cancer of the lip.
- Meticulous dissection of neurovascular structures and surrounding musculature is critical to maintaining a dynamic reconstructive result when utilizing complex locoregional flaps.

- Microvascular free tissue transfer provides a reliable and versatile option for reconstruction of subtotal and total lip defects.
- Combining microvascular techniques with concomitant tendon or fascial grafts as well as free muscle transfer may improve overall functional outcomes.

PITFALLS

- Attempting to reconstruct subtotal and total lip defects with locoregional flaps may result in microstomia along with unacceptable aesthetic and functional outcomes for the patient.
- Patient comorbidities or malignancies that require active surveillance may preclude the use of microvascular free tissue transfer for reconstruction of major lip defects in favor of less aggressive options.
- Failing to establish realistic expectations through rigorous preoperative counseling may lead to patient dissatisfaction despite technically adequate reconstructive efforts.

INSTRUMENTS TO HAVE AVAILABLE

- Standard head and neck surgical instruments
- Microsurgical instrumentation
- Operating microscope

ACKNOWLEDGMENT

I gratefully acknowledge the contributions of Andrew Klienberger and Vijay Mukija.

SUGGESTED READING

Renner GJ. Reconstruction of the lip. In: Baker SR, ed. *Local flaps in facial reconstruction*, 2nd ed. St. Louis, MO: Mosby/Elsevier, 2007;19:475–524.

Ferris RL, Gillman GS. Cancer of the lip. In: Myers EN, ed. *Operative otolaryngology—head and neck surgery*, 2nd ed. Philadelphia, PA: Saunders/Elsevier, 2008;24:183–193.

DeFatta RJ, Williams EF. Lip reconstruction. In: Papel ID, ed. *Facial plastic and reconstructive surgery*, 3rd ed. Stuttgart, NY: Thieme, 2009;61:841–854.

2 MANAGEMENT OF THE DEFECT OF THE FLOOR OF THE MOUTH: SPLIT THICKNESS SKIN GRAFT

Derrick T. Lin

INTRODUCTION

The floor of the mouth (FOM) is an anatomic subsite of the oral cavity defined anteriorly by the inferior alveolar ridge, extending posteriorly to the ventral surface of the tongue medially and the anterior tonsil pillar laterally. This area overlies the paired sublingual glands, which are situated on the mylohyoid and hyoglossus muscles.

A split-thickness skin graft (STSG) by definition is a graft that incorporates only a portion of the dermis, in contrast to a full-thickness skin graft (FTSG) that includes the entire dermis. STSG may range anywhere from 0.012 to 0.030 inch in depth. STSG is usually preferred over FTSG for FOM defects since they require less ideal conditions for survival.

Defects of the FOM requiring reconstruction are usually the result of resection of a cancer. Cancer of the oral cavity accounts for 2% to 6% of all cancers in the United States and 30% of all cancers of the head and neck. The goals of reconstruction of this area include preservation of the mobility of the tongue and establishment of a sulcus between the mandible and tongue. The use of an STSG is one of several reconstructive options for small, superficial defects in the FOM.

HISTORY

A general history should be performed prior to considering reconstructive surgery. Patients with medical comorbidities such as high-risk heart disease, chronic obstructive lung disease, or other significant systemic illness should be carefully evaluated before surgery to determine if they can tolerate general anesthesia. Additionally, a history of infection, poor healing, or keloid scarring should be considered. A history of radiation therapy of the oral cavity should be sought.

PHYSICAL EXAMINATION

The physical examination should be focused on the size and depth of the cancer and resultant extent of the defect of the oral cavity. Larger defects involving the FOM and the tongue may be managed with a radial forearm free flap to prevent contractures and tethering of the tongue. Donor site must be inspected to rule out infection, previous trauma or surgical scars.

INDICATIONS

STSGs for the defect in the FOM are generally reserved for defects resulting from the resection of small, superficial cancers (T1, T2). Either the periosteum of the mandible must be intact or healthy cancellous bone present in the setting of a marginal mandibulectomy. The integrity of the musculature of the FOM cannot have been violated, and the overall size of the defect should be no more than 4 cm in diameter.

CONTRAINDICATIONS

Free tissue reconstruction or a rotational pedicled flap should be considered in defects larger than 4 cm to prevent significant contracture and tethering of the tongue. STSG should not be considered for defects in which the musculature of the FOM is no longer intact or when a segmental mandibulectomy is necessary.

Previous irradiation or recurrence after prior surgical resection would be considered relative contraindications to the use of an STSG for the defect in the FOM, especially if a marginal mandibulectomy is to be included in the ablative plan.

PREOPERATIVE PLANNING

STSGs donor sites are usually chosen based on areas that are easily concealed such as the upper anterior or lateral thigh. These sites should be free of infections, other skin lesions or previous surgery, radiation or trauma. Preparation of the recipient wound bed is critical for the survival of the STSG. In general, STSG will survive on muscle, fascia, cancellous bone, periosteum, perichondrium, or granulation tissue. The wound needs to be free of necrotic tissue and infection, and hemostasis must be complete.

Postoperative endoscopy and examination of the cancer under general anesthesia is important in determining the extent and resectability of the cancer. Second primary cancers must be ruled out.

SURGICAL TECHNIQUE

The STSG is usually taken from the upper thigh. The donor site is inspected to ensure that there is no infection, lesions, eschar, or granulation tissue. The area is prepped and draped in the usual sterile fashion.

Gauze soaked with 1:100,000 epinephrine is placed on the proposed donor site. Mineral oil is then placed over the site in preparation for the dermatome. The dermatome is set at a depth of 0.0185 inch (range of 0.012 to 0.030 inch). A no. 15 blade may be used to simulate the thickness by placing the beveled edge in the dermatome. Using a tongue blade on the thigh to maintain constant pressure, the dermatome is then applied at a 30- to 45-degree angle and activated (Fig. 2.1). When the appropriate size is achieved, the dermatome is tilted away from the skin and the base of the graft is separated from the donor site using either a scalpel or scissors (Fig. 2.2).

Before suturing the graft into the FOM defect, the graft is "pie-crusted" to allow for egress of any possible fluid accumulation. This is achieved by making small longitudinal incisions with a no. 15 blade. A nasogastric tube is inserted prior to suturing the graft into the defect.

The graft is sutured into the defect using 3-0 Vicryl sutures. A Xeroform gauze bolster is placed over the graft and sutured into place. 2-0 silk sutures are tied over the bolster to immobilize the graft. If there is significant edema of the FOM or retropulsion of the tongue, a tracheostomy should be considered.

Donor-site hemostasis is achieved by placing 1:100,000 epinephrine–soaked gauze. Once hemostasis is achieved, a Tegaderm is placed.

POSTOPERATIVE MANAGEMENT

Postoperatively, the patient receives his or her nutrition through a nasogastric tube. The bolster is left in place for 7 days. Revascularization of the graft usually begins after 2 to 3 days with full circulation achieved by 6 to 7 days.

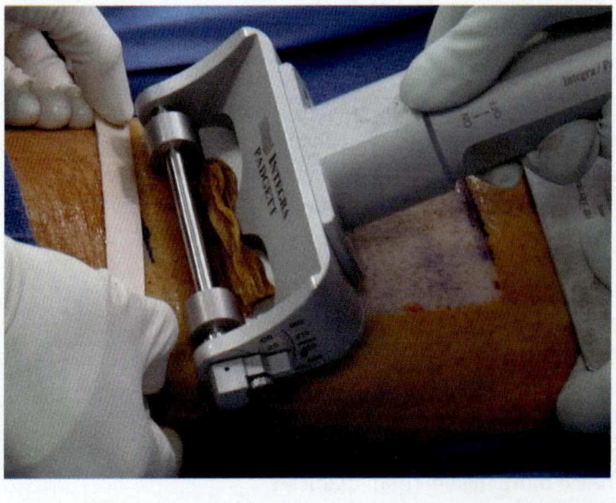

FIGURE 2.1
Using a tongue blade on the thigh to maintain constant pressure, the dermatome is then applied at a 30- to 45-degree angle and activated.

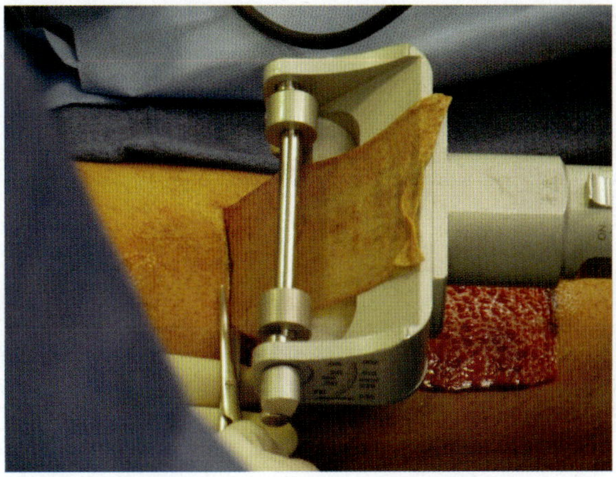

FIGURE 2.2
When the appropriate size of the skin graft is achieved, the dermatome is tilted away from the skin and the base of the graft is separated from the donor site using either a scalpel or scissors.

After the bolster is removed, the patient may begin an oral diet. Oral hygiene with Peridex rinse is begun at this time. If there is any wound breakdown, continual NPO with nasogastric tube feeding is recommended. Primary contracture of 10% to 20% is expected in the use of an STSG.

COMPLICATIONS

In patients who are carefully selected, postoperative complications are rare. Hematoma under the skin graft needs to be watched for since an unrecognized hematoma would compromise the integrity of the graft. The development of excessive edema of the area should also be carefully monitored. This could lead to airway compromise necessitating a temporary tracheostomy. A keloid may develop in the donor site in those patients predisposed with a history of keloid formation.

RESULTS

The use of an STSG for the reconstruction of the oral cavity is safe, simple, and reliable. However, careful patient selection is essential. Patients with a large defect, resection of the musculature of the FOM, segmental mandibulectomy, and previous radiation therapy should be excluded.

In my experience, the risk of hematoma is small and a tracheostomy is rarely needed. The expected take rate is about 80% to 100% initially with complete healing in about 4 weeks. Contraction of approximately 10% to 20% of the wound is expected and should be taken into account when assessing the use of STSG. The majority of patients begin an oral diet 7 days after surgery when the bolster is removed. In well-selected patients, long-term cosmesis and function should be excellent (Figs. 2.3 and 2.4).

PEARLS

- Rigorous evaluation of the defect and donor site preoperatively is essential for successful reconstruction.
- Use a dermatome depth of 0.012 to 0.030 inch.

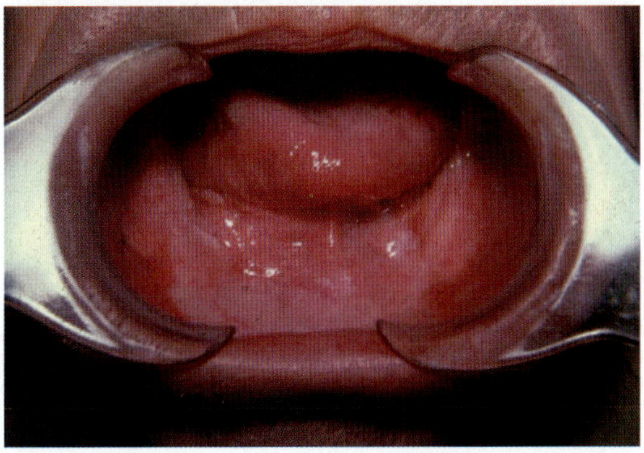

FIGURE 2.3
Long-term results demonstrate a well-healed skin graft and a natural contour to the FOM.

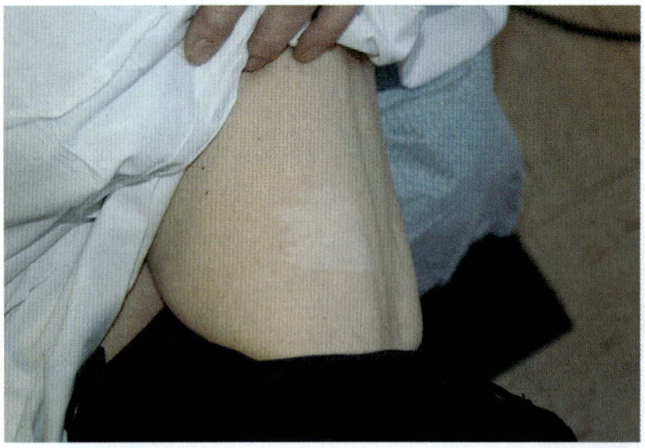

FIGURE 2.4
The donor site defect is acceptable.

- Expect 10% to 20% contraction of the skin graft.
- Keep the bolster in place for 1 week to allow for vascularization of the STSG.
- Inspect for donor site lesions.

PITFALLS

- Contraindicated in large defects or defects with resection of FOM musculature
- Contraindicated in previously radiated patients who will have a marginal mandibulectomy
- Contraindicated in exposed mandibular bone without periosteum or cancellous bed

INSTRUMENTS TO HAVE AVAILABLE

- Dermatome
- Standard head and neck surgical instruments

SUGGESTED READING

Branham GH, Thomas JR. Skin grafts. *Otolaryngol Clin North Am* 1990;23(5):889–897.

Feldman DL. Which dressing for split-thickness skin graft donor sites? *Ann Plast Surg* 1991;27(3):288–291.

Petruzelli GJ, Johnson JT. Skin grafts. *Otolaryngol Clin North Am* 1994;27(1):25–37.

Tran LE, Berry GJ, Fee WE Jr. Split-thickness skin graft attachment to bone lacking periosteum. *Arch Otolaryngol Head Neck Surg* 2005;131(2):124–128.

Hartig GK. Free flaps in oral cavity reconstruction: when you need them and when you don't. *Int J Radiat Oncol Biol Phys* 2007;69:S19–S21.

de Bree R, Rinaldo A, Genden E, et al. Modern reconstruction for oral and pharyngeal defects after tumor resection. *Eur Arch Otorhinolayngol* 2008;265:1–9.

3 THE FLOOR OF THE MOUTH DEFECT: RADIAL FOREARM FREE FLAP

Eben L. Rosenthal

INTRODUCTION

Reconstruction of the oral cavity, particularly the floor of the mouth, can be a challenging task for numerous reasons. The complex anatomy of this area as well as its spatial relationship to surrounding structures, in particular the mandible and tongue, are definite obstacles for the reconstructive surgeon. The goals of reconstruction of the floor of the mouth are to separate the oral cavity from the neck, to restore unrestricted mobility of the tongue, and to construct a platform for bolus preparation to assist with oral intake.

An adequate reconstruction can be accomplished in numerous ways depending on the size of the defect. Smaller defects with residual, viable soft tissue can be closed primarily or with a split-thickness skin graft, which can provide a water-tight closure. Various regional flaps have been described for larger defects, the most common of which is the submental island pedicled flap, the facial artery musculomucosal flap, or the platysma flap. The radial forearm fasciocutaneous flap is the free flap most frequently used for the reconstruction of the oral cavity. The focus of this chapter is to describe the use of the radial forearm free flap for reconstruction of the floor of the mouth.

HISTORY

A positive history of tobacco and alcohol exposure is typically present in patients with cancer of the oral cavity. The smoking is thought to interfere with healing due to small vessel obliteration. Patients often present with pain, dysphagia, and weight loss resulting from limited oral intake.

PHYSICAL EXAMINATION

The physical findings in patients with cancer of the floor of the mouth may include ulcerative, exophytic lesions or simply irregular mucosa with subtle surface changes. In more extensive lesions, limited mobility of the tongue or disruption of dentition may be present. The physical examination should always evaluate two important factors: involvement of the tongue and invasion of the mandible. The degree of bone invasion is important to determine preoperatively in order to plan for possible mandibulectomy requiring bone reconstruction. The findings on physical examination are also helpful for the reconstructive surgeon in predicting the size of the defect. The forearm donor site should be examined, taking into account the handedness of the patient and any previous surgery or trauma. An Allen test should be performed on the donor arm to assess for patency of the collateral circulation to the hand via the ulnar artery. Venipuncture should not be performed on the planned donor arm, and any evidence of intravenous drug abuse, recent radial artery puncture, or failure of the Allen test is a contraindication to harvesting a radial forearm flap from that arm. The neck must be evaluated for possible cervical lymph node metastasis. A neck dissection is usually necessary and may impact the reconstruction options.

INDICATIONS

The main goals of reconstruction of the floor of the mouth are to separate the oral cavity from the neck, restore unrestricted mobility to the tongue, and provide a solid platform upon which bolus preparation can occur. Adequate postoperative function of speech and swallowing remains a major challenge for the reconstructive surgeon. Ideally, reconstruction should be performed with an adequate amount of soft, mobile tissue with the anticipation of some degree of contracture upon healing. Radial forearm fasciocutaneous free flaps are particularly useful due to their thin, pliable nature.

CONTRAINDICATIONS

The only contraindications to reconstruction of the floor of the mouth using the radial forearm free flap are related to those patients with an inadequate Allen test (incomplete vascular palmar arch).

PREOPERATIVE PLANNING

Routine anatomic imaging, in the form of CT or MRI, is usually performed preoperatively to assess the size of the primary tumor or depth of invasion into the tongue or mandible. An MRI is typically superior to CT in evaluation of soft tissue and nerve involvement; however, CT scans can more accurately predict invasion of the mandible. A CT scan can also be useful in preoperative modeling of the contour of the mandible to define the architecture of the titanium plate that will be used in the reconstruction.

Regardless of the preoperative evaluation, one should always be prepared to deviate from the plan as new information is presented from intraoperative findings. This may be due to numerous factors including growth of the cancer prior to surgery or false-negative/-positive physical or radiographical findings. For intermediate-size defects of the floor of the mouth, it is often best to consider several options for reconstruction.

Patient selection is important in determining whether they are a candidate for free tissue transfer. Advanced age alone is not a contraindication to this procedure, but age-related comorbidities, particularly significant atherosclerosis with poor cardiac function, should be considered prior to surgery. Patients with coagulopathies, collagen vascular diseases, and other vascular disorders are not good candidates for free tissue transfer. Malnutrition should also be addressed because of its detrimental effects on wound healing.

Prior radiation therapy to the head and neck often results in decreased patency of vessels secondary to vessel fibrosis and endothelial cell disruption. Hypothyroidism may also occur following radiation to the neck.

The availability of the appropriate surgical and nursing personnel should also be addressed during preoperative planning. These individuals play critical roles in both the initial procedure as well as the postoperative period. This varies based on the institution, but the patient should have a monitored bed available for at least the first 24 to 48 hours for hourly flap assessments. Either a conventional intensive care unit or "step-down" intensive care bed should be arranged prior to the day of the procedure.

SURGICAL TECHNIQUE

The blood supply to the radial forearm flap is based on the radial artery and is a well-vascularized and pliable flap that has a low incidence of failure when used for reconstruction of the floor of the mouth. Outflow from the flap is via the paired venae comitantes, which accompany the artery as well as various subcutaneous veins of the forearm. Generally, the vascular pedicle may be up to 18 cm in length, and the vessel diameters are usually large (2 to 4 mm). A common radial vein can usually be identified to allow a single venous outflow microvascular anastomosis. The medial and lateral antebrachial cutaneous nerves can be harvested to create a sensate flap, although the added benefit of this technique remains controversial. A bilobed design in the flap design creating a flap in the shape of a mitten has been described to improve mobility of the tongue. The vascular pedicle can be easily identified and marked at the beginning of the procedure prior to the elevation of the flap.

The skin paddle should be fashioned to overlie the distal radial artery and usually encompasses numerous muscular perforators of the radial artery. The flap design should be with the distal and proximal end tapered to allow the flap to inset into the V-shaped defect of the lateral gingivolingual sulcus on either side of the defect. It is best to fashion the skin paddle wider (add 1.5 to 3 cm) and slightly longer than the measured defect because contracture of the graft results in significant tongue immobility (Fig. 3.1). Loss of a segment of the mandible can be managed by harvesting a portion of the distal aspect of the radius.

Although the distal aspect of the flap should be set proximal enough to be covered by the shirt sleeve, thinner tissue is often present in the distal aspect of the arm and may be required in obese patients. The arm is

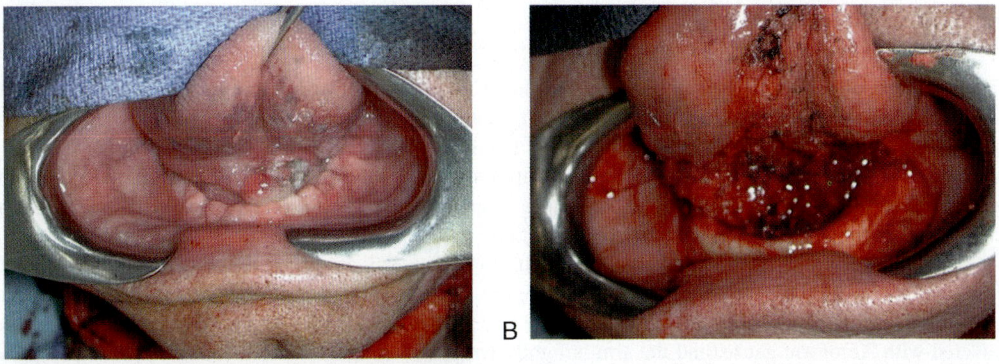

A B

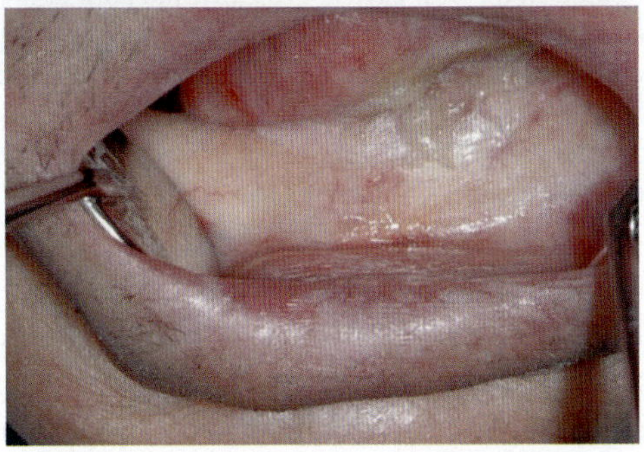

C

FIGURE 3.1
Floor of the mouth repair using the radial forearm free flap. The cancer is demonstrated **(A)** prior to resection. The defect included the floor of the mouth with invasion of the gingival surface with exposed bone and a connection into the neck **(B)**. The 6-month postoperative appearance of the flap with blunting of the alveolus and appropriate healing **(C)**.

then exsanguinated, and a tourniquet is inflated to approximately 250 mm Hg. The first skin incision is made at the distal end of the skin paddle along the ulnar border down to fascia, and a subfascial dissection is performed toward the flexor carpi radialis tendon. Care should be taken to preserve paratenon over the tendon to prevent loss of the skin graft. The use of suprafacial dissection has been described that results in improved take of the split-thickness skin graft without vascular compromise to the skin paddle. The distal ends of the radial artery and venae comitantes are isolated and ligated with suture, and the radial margin of the flap is incised down to brachioradialis preserving the distal branches of the radial nerve. The lateral intermuscular septum is identified, and the flap is raised from distal to proximal following the course of the vascular pedicle to the antecubital fossa. Small branches from the pedicle are isolated and taken along the way with bipolar cautery and/or small vascular clips. The ulnar artery is identified and preserved and a common radial vein isolated where possible and the tourniquet lowered and hemostasis obtained using bipolar cautery and clips on the pedicle. The vascularity of the thumb and forefingers should be assessed prior to dividing the pedicle. The flap is transferred to the recipient site for inset. Total ischemia time should be less than 6 hours for optimum flap survival.

The distal forearm defect can be closed in a number of ways. A split-thickness skin graft harvested from the forearm prior to raising the graft or from the lateral thigh is pie crusted and inset into the donor site defect. This is typically held in position with absorbable suture. The skin graft site is bolstered into place with a nonadherent dressing and the forearm splinted with the wrist slightly extended for 5 days. This improves survival of the split-thickness skin graft by limiting movement between the skin graft and the underlying muscles and tendons. Other options for repair of the distal forearm defect have been described. These include cadaveric skin grafting or placement of a skin graft with a negative pressure dressing to improve take rate. The advantage of a negative pressure dressing is elimination of a splint, which allows better postoperative monitoring of the distal extremity; however, it is associated with significantly higher costs. The negative pressure dressing is typically left in place for 3 to 5 days. Take rates are relatively equivalent, although significant contracture of the wound can occur with the negative pressure dressing resulting in overall improved appearance.

The recipient site is prepared, and the flap is transferred to the floor of the mouth. The harvested forearm tissue is arranged in a manner so as to fully fill the defect and inset is begun. The flap is sutured to the mucosa of the oral cavity with interrupted Vicryl suture using great effort to provide a watertight seal. If no mucosa remains on the surface of the mandible, suture can be placed around the base of the remaining teeth or small holes can be drilled directly into the mandible to hold the flap securely in place.

Once the flap is inset or nearly so, attention is turned to the neck for the microvascular anastomosis. The facial, lingual, or superior thyroid arteries are preferred based on vessel size for the arterial anastomosis. Venous anastomosis is usually performed end to end with any of the branches from the internal jugular vein. My preference is the use of the continuous suture technique using 8-0 nylon suture, which involves placement of two interrupted sutures placed opposite each other and then a simple running suture applied around the vessel. A drain can be placed through the mylohyoid muscle to lie underneath the closure to monitor for a salivary leak postoperatively. A microvascular coupler is most commonly used to anastomose the veins in an end-to-end fashion.

POSTOPERATIVE MANAGEMENT

Patients are monitored in a specialty nursing "step-down" type of intensive care unit for 24 hours where the flap can be checked hourly. The pedicle vasculature can be monitored via external or implantable Doppler. The skin paddle is typically easily visible in the floor of the mouth for visual and tactile assessment of flap viability as well. The average hospital stay is 5 to 7 days. Patients are given 3 doses of perioperative antibiotics (clindamycin or piperacillin–tazobactam) and daily low-dose aspirin therapy for 3 weeks. The wounds and drains are carefully monitored for signs of salivary contamination.

The splint is removed from the donor site on postoperative day 4 or 5, and a lightweight plastic splint is fashioned and worn for 10 to 14 days after which aggressive passive and active range of motion exercises are performed to prevent limitation of movement even if tendon exposure does occur. The skin graft site is kept covered with Xeroform gauze, and the arm is lightly wrapped with gauze underneath the splint. The patient should resume oral intake only once a complete seal is assured in the oral cavity. Typically, the patient is fed via nasogastric or gastrostomy tube for the first 5 days while swallowing therapy is initiated. Management of patients in the hospital and anticipated complications can be predicted depending on the postoperative day (Fig. 3.2). Aggressive postoperative speech therapy is critical in ensuring a safe return to an oral diet. A modified barium swallow may be required, especially in elderly patients, who are more likely to have silent aspiration and significant pulmonary sequelae as a complication. The majority of patients are discharged home on pureed or soft oral diets.

COMPLICATIONS

The most significant complications associated with radial forearm free flap reconstruction of the floor of the mouth are dependent on flap viability. Early flap failures should be noted immediately and taken to the operating room for management. Microvascular complications are typically reported to be between 4% and 6% with approximately half of those being salvageable. Occasionally, leech therapy is used to assist with venous congestion if the anastomosis has been explored and no thrombus was seen and/or the patient's medical comorbidities do not allow for another general anesthetic.

Salivary leak into the neck is another complication and can be managed based on severity. Treatment options range from conservative observation with oral antibiotics to aggressive debridement and irrigation. A fistula can be managed with a Penrose drain in place or negative pressure dressings (Fig. 3.3). I have found that application of the negative pressure dressings to rapidly promote granulation tissue in severely compromised wounds and placement of the dressing directly over the pedicle or carotid to be safe. Drains should be left in the neck until a salivary leak is of minimal threat to wound healing.

Donor site tendon exposure is reported in approximately 10% to 30% of forearm defects, but these wounds usually heal over a period of 2 to 6 weeks. To prevent long-term complications, movement of the wrist should be encouraged with passive and active range of motion. Limited functional deficits of the donor site are reported even in the presence of significantly delayed healing secondary to tendon exposure (Fig. 3.4). Typically, patients will have measurably decreased strength in the donor arm in comparison to the contralateral side; however, this does not tend to interfere with daily activities of life.

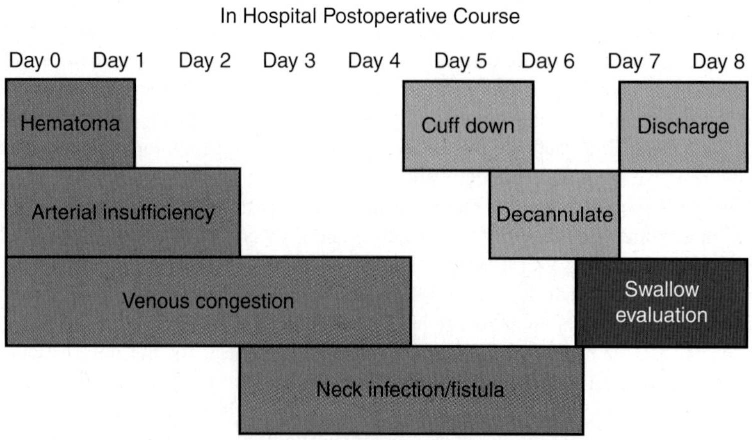

FIGURE 3.2 In-hospital management of patient and anticipated complications of patients undergoing radial forearm free flap reconstruction. Typically, the first 24 hours are at highest risk for hematoma, and anytime in the first 3 days, there is a risk of vascular complications. After postoperative management follows a relatively routine course in the absence of a surgical or medical event.

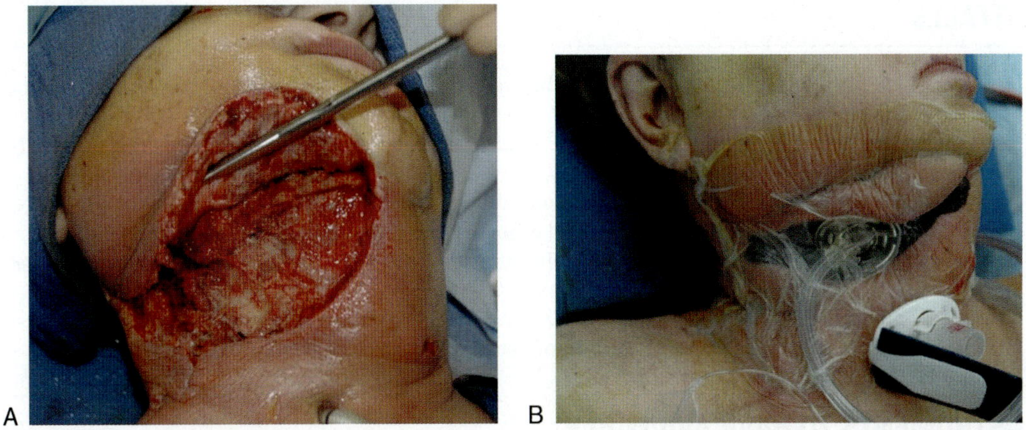

FIGURE 3.3 Use of negative pressure dressings to manage fistulas after floor of the mouth reconstructions. The patient had viable tissue in the neck but developed a salivary leak in the floor of the mouth **(A)**. Application of a negative pressure dressing within the defect for a limited period of time (3 to 7 days) allows for contraction of the wound site and promotes healing **(B)**.

RESULTS

The results with this technique are excellent. The pliable nature of the radial forearm skin makes it an ideal choice for reconstruction of the floor of the mouth.

PEARLS

- Limited mobility of the tongue is difficult to treat secondarily, and management is often delayed for 4 to 12 months after completion of radiation therapy.
- Tethering of the tongue can be improved by releasing the tongue with placement of a split-thickness skin graft in the floor of the mouth as a secondary procedure.
- In large cancers of the floor of the mouth, it may be best to wait until pathology reports indicate that the cancer has been completely resected because there may be unrecognized involvement of deep tongue and/or bone, which can significantly change the choice of the flap.
- Harvesting a flap slightly larger than the size of the defect is helpful in preventing tethering of the tongue.
- Thinning of the flap may be required postoperatively to improve control of oral secretions.
- The remaining mucosa of the gingiva, if available, can provide sufficient strength to hold sutures. If dentition is present, sutures placed circumferentially around the teeth can be used intermittently to relieve tension on the relatively thin mucosa of the floor of the mouth.
- If the deep tongue muscle attachments to the mandible are resected, their reattachment can be helpful in preventing retraction of the posterior tongue, which can limit the diameter of the oropharyngeal airway.
- A tracheostomy is not always required in limited resections of the floor of the mouth.
- If the patient has undergone previous radiation therapy, however, he or she may experience unpredictable postoperative edema making a tracheostomy necessary.

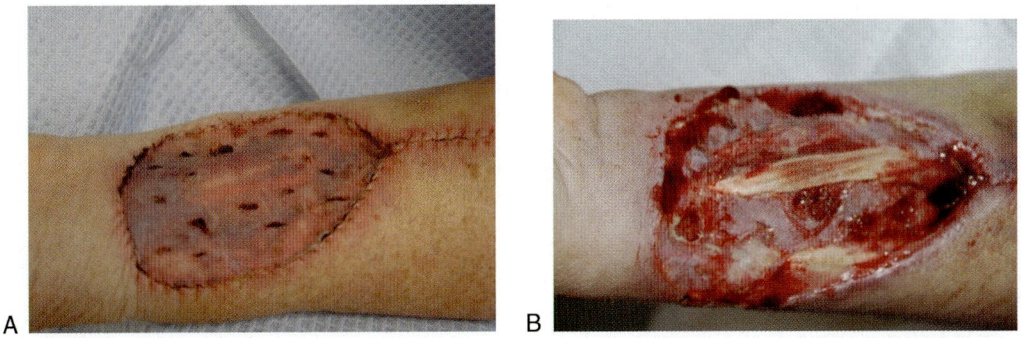

FIGURE 3.4 Tendon exposure after radial forearm free flap. Immediate postoperative view at 1 week demonstrates some discoloration of the graft, but otherwise appropriate healing **(A)**. However, at 3 weeks, significant loss of the graft has occurred particularly over the flexor carpi radialis **(B)**, which is the most common site for loss due to the mobility of this surface tendon and low vascularity.

PITFALLS

- Excessive bulk in the reconstructed tissue should be avoided anteriorly to avoid glossoptosis and/or obliteration of the lower lip sulcus.
- Scar contracture may tether the tongue; therefore, ample tissue should be transferred to the defect primarily, which can be debulked at a later time if necessary.
- Injury to the lingual nerve during the ablative operation may limit tongue sensation or mobility that is perceived as decreased mobility by the patient but cannot be surgically corrected.
- Premature return to oral intake may compromise the integrity of the wound in the floor of the mouth and lead to salivary fistula.
- Dental rehabilitation in the floor of the mouth defects remains controversial and costly to the patients. It may be best to defer in-depth preoperative discussion of options until several months after surgery.

INSTRUMENTS TO HAVE AVAILABLE

- Standard head and neck surgical set
- Dermatome

ACKNOWLEDGMENT

I gratefully acknowledge the contributions of Hillary White, MD.

SUGGESTED READING

Ko AB, Lavertu P, Rezaee RP. Double bilobed radial forearm free flap for anterior tongue and floor-of-mouth reconstruction. *Ear Nose Throat J* 2010;89(4):177–179.

Huang JJ, Wu CW, Lam WL, et al. Anatomical basis and clinical application of the ulnar forearm free flap for head and neck reconstruction. *Laryngoscope* 2012;122(12):2670–2676.

4 MANAGEMENT OF THE DEFECT IN THE BUCCAL MUCOSA

Mark K. Wax

INTRODUCTION

The buccal mucosa is an integral part of the cheek. Pathologic processes that involves it may require consideration of reconstruction of the cheek complex. Consequently, this chapter focuses on the reconstruction of defects in the buccal mucosa but takes into consideration the entire cheek complex. The cheek is one of the major contributors to normal upper aerodigestive tract physiologic function, cosmesis, and the perception of oneself as well as what others think of you as an individual. Normal cheek function is important in the ability of individuals to eat, drink, and talk. Defects of this important anatomic area will result in a decrease in these functions. The face is the first structure that we see in the mirror, and others see when we interact with the outside world. Any abnormality in appearance is immediately fixed upon and can lead to severe social repercussions.

The most common cancer arising in the buccal mucosa is squamous cell carcinoma. In North America, lesions arising from the buccal mucosa are uncommon and may present as a visible mass in the cheek or as a mass distorting the buccal mucosa. In Southeast Asia where chronic exposures to carcinogens is part of the culture, squamous cell carcinoma is the most common cancer of the oral cavity. Even though the majority of cancers are squamous cell, a precise diagnosis by biopsy is needed. A detailed history, clinical examination, and imaging studies are essential in defining the location and extent of these cancers.

There are several options for reconstruction of the buccal mucosa including skin graft, local flaps, and free flap reconstruction. The size and depth of the defect will determine the optimal reconstructive option. A split-thickness skin graft (STSG) can be used for many of the defects in the buccal mucosa; however, this approach may be associated with scar contracture and trismus. The radial forearm skin tends to resist scar contracture and can be used for all defects, including those that penetrate through and through.

HISTORY

Reconstruction of the buccal mucosal defect can be achieved through a variety of techniques. Obtaining a history from the patient is essential to understand if the patient is medically frail, in which case, a simple technique such as an STSG is the most appropriate choice. In medically stable patients, a radial forearm free flap may provide a more appropriate reconstruction option. Although both techniques are effective, the history may impact my decision. I have found that patients with a history of betel nut use tend to suffer from scar contracture when a skin graft is used. In contrast, the radial forearm reconstruction provides a source of tissue that is less inclined to contract. A history is often helpful in identifying such factors that may influence your decisions on reconstructive approach.

PHYSICAL EXAMINATION

A thorough physical examination should then be undertaken focusing on depth of the tumor involvement as well as the local tissues affected by the cancer, such as bone, orbit, ear, and other subsets of the oral cavity and oropharynx.

After a history and physical is obtained, a diagnosis is necessary, and this can be accomplished with a punch biopsy or an incisional biopsy. Once the diagnosis is established, staging, as is done for any cancer of the oral cavity, must be performed. This will allow determination of the best oncologic treatment and planning for possible reconstructive options. Laryngoscopy may be needed to determine the anatomic extent of the tumor. Since the buccal mucosa is so thin and the area is often secondarily involved, some form of imaging is helpful in determining the anatomic extent of the tumor. Both CT and MRI have been used, and whichever modality is used depends on the preference of the surgeon and the institutional bias.

The cheek is considered to extend from the inferior border of the mandible superiorly to the inferior orbital rim, although some surgeons will consider the superior extent to be a line drawn from the level of the brow to the superior attachment of the helix. Medially, it arises at the lateral aspect of the nasolabial line and extends to the preauricular area. Considered as an anatomic subunit, the cheek is composed of skin, subcutaneous tissue, muscle, and the buccal mucosal lining on the inside of the oral cavity.

The areas of interest are the buccal adipose tissue, which is the deepest layer and is separated from the oral cavity by a thin layer of buccal mucosa. The only nonneurovascular structure that passes through this area is the parotid duct. This structure courses through the cheek, penetrating the buccinator muscle. The papilla of Stensen duct can be seen opposite the second maxillary molar. The anatomical structures involved in the defect will help to dictate what type of reconstructive procedure is performed. Composite tissue loss will mandate reconstruction using a composite tissue flap.

Sensory supply to the cheek is provided primarily by the second and third divisions of the trigeminal nerve; the mental nerve and the infraorbital nerve are the terminal branches. There is a marked degree of overlap and should one of these sensory nerves be severed or interfered with, ingrowth from the adjacent dermatome will allow for recovery of sensation to a great degree. The superficial facial muscles are supplied by the seventh cranial nerve as it exits the parotid gland.

Finally, the arterial supply comes mainly through the external carotid artery via the facial artery. Venous drainage is by way of the anterior facial vein into the internal jugular venous system. The vascular supply is richly anastomotic with connections from deeper structures and from the contralateral vasculature. Ligation of major vessels, such as the facial artery bilaterally, will not have a detrimental effect on healing.

The function of the cheek and its musculature is to assist in deglutition and vocalization. Its role in deglutition is multifold. The ability to open one's mouth fully without any degree of trismus depends on the integrity of the internal lining of the buccal mucosa. We usually think of trismus as involving the muscles of mastication. However, in patients who are missing a large portion of the internal lining of the buccal mucosa, the maxilla–mandible complex will not be able to separate and function normally. Anything that affects this relationship will cause trismus because of scar formation. Evaluation of the neck is critical since frequently metastases to the cervical lymph nodes are present. A neck dissection is usually required, which may impact the reconstructive options or techniques.

INDICATIONS

Reconstruction of the buccal mucosa can be classified into three categories: (1) Lesions involving the buccal mucosa only; (2) lesions involving the buccal mucosa, the buccal adipose tissue, and contiguous structures; and (3) full-thickness cheek lesions or large lesions or lesions that infiltrate the skin.

CONTRAINDICATIONS

The contraindications to using this technique for reconstruction of the buccal defect are limited to defects that involve extensive mandibular defects. These defects often require a vascularized osteocutaneous free flap.

PREOPERATIVE PLANNING

Occasional small cancers of the buccal mucosa are encountered, and because of the looseness of the buccal mucosa and the redundancy of the tissue, primary reconstruction or reconstruction using a local advancement flap to the buccal mucosa can be used. Areas of up to 3 × 3 cm usually will heal quite well without any trismus developing.

STSG can be used in many patients. Meshed or not, these grafts are sewn in and held in place with a bolster for 5 days, and in my practice, the take rate of an intraoral skin graft has been found to be acceptable without an intraoral bolster. In recent years, more and more of these patients are presenting with deeper lesions that will need to be or have been radiated. In this circumstance, I have found that an STSG is not adequate. It will often still scar over. Other forms of reconstruction must be considered. This also holds true for patients who are going to undergo postoperative radiation. The skin graft will often shrink a great deal after being radiated, and trismus may result.

Lesions of the buccal mucosa are usually squamous cell carcinoma. In the majority of cases, the buccal mucosa is involved secondary to a cancer arising in another anatomic subsite in the oral cavity. Consequently, the reconstruction of the buccal lining must take into consideration the retromolar trigone, the mandible, or the anterior floor of the mouth lesion. In the majority of these cases, free tissue transfer is used whether it is with bone reconstruction or simply a soft tissue reconstruction, and the reconstruction of the buccal mucosa is addressed at that time.

For the patient who has been previously radiated or had an extensive resection of the buccal mucosa, reconstruction with surfacing of the area with a thin fasciocutaneous free flap is often warranted. The radial forearm flap has been my preferred method of reconstruction due to the supple three-dimensionally pliable thin tissue. The size is usually adequate for reconstruction in both a superior–inferior as well as an anterior–posterior dimension. If the tissue turns out to be too thick or the volume is too heavy with subsequent "chewing" on the flap, it can always be debulked and revised at a later date. The anterior lateral thigh flap as well as the latissimus muscle flap with STSG have been used in reconstructing these defects. These flaps offer a larger surface area than the forearm flap but can be too bulky and limit the function of the reconstruction, but are good alternatives in settings where increased bulk is needed, that is, reconstruction of the tongue. Careful attention must be paid to the condition of the donor site in order to rule out prior injury, radiation, cutaneous lesion, or infection. An Allen test must be done to evaluate the collateral circulation.

SURGICAL TECHNIQUE

When reconstructing the defect in the buccal mucosa with a free tissue transfer, it is important to consider the size of the defect (Fig. 4.1) and the pliability of the transferred tissue and to ensure that adequate tissue is harvested and inset in order to prevent posttreatment trismus (Fig. 4.2). When harvesting the flap, an additional 20% is added to the size of the defect in order to ensure that adequate amount of tissue is harvested. The flap is secured to the surrounding mucosal defect with a running 3-0 Vicryl (polyglactin 910, Ethicon) suture (Fig. 4.3).

The vascular pedicle is typically positioned in the ipsilateral neck, and a microvascular anastomosis with a running 9-0 Nurolon (Nylon, Ethicon) suture is performed on the arterial system. The facial artery is preferred given its location, size, and geometry. The venous anastomosis is accomplished with a venous coupling device (Synovis), although there are occasions given the final flap/pedicle geometry or size mismatch of the veins that a sutured venous anastomosis is required. One or two implantable Dopplers are then placed on the arterial system, venous system, or both for continuous monitoring of the vascularity of the free tissue transfer.

POSTOPERATIVE MANAGEMENT

Postoperatively, the patient should be NPO for 1 week unless the patient has received radiation in which case, I recommend 2 weeks.

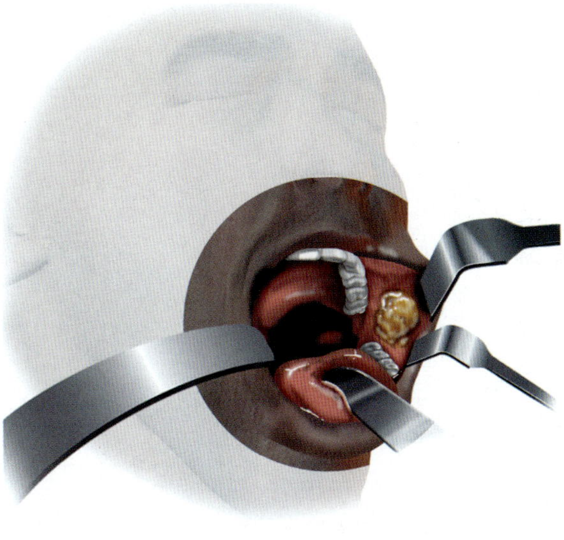

FIGURE 4.1
Cancer may arise from the buccal mucosa but more frequently arise from the alveolus or tongue and extend onto the buccal mucosa. The defect should be carefully measured to design the flap appropriately.

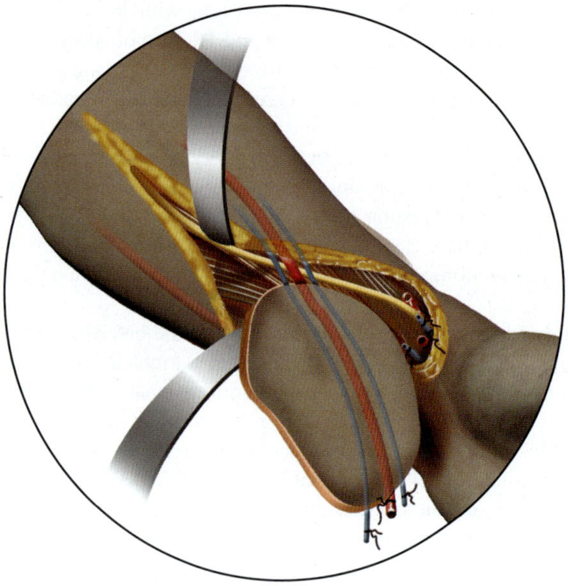

FIGURE 4.2
The radial forearm free flap is designed to accommodate the defect.

COMPLICATIONS

Complications include flap failure or fistula. Both are rare, but both may pose a significant problem when they occur. Other complications include donor site morbidity or scar contracture leading to trismus.

RESULTS

Lesions of the buccal mucosa involve a multitude of differing pathologies and surgical technique. The cheek plays an essential role in one's perception of oneself as well as the physiologic process of chewing and speaking. Reconstruction of the majority of defects is adequately performed with local regional tissue transfer that allows for excellent cosmetic and matching with functional results. Occasionally, one will encounter a patient who has extensive surface area defect in a previously radiated field that is not amenable to local tissue movement so that free tissue transfer is required. Through-and-through tissue defects of the cheek and those involving composite tissues of the mandible or maxilla require free tissue transfer for reconstruction, and patients can oftentimes be rehabilitated with adequate cosmesis and function.

PEARLS

- The ultimate reconstruction of a buccal mucosal defect should offer enough tissue to reconstruct the defect, vascularized as well as innervated tissue, and rapid return of function, at the same time maintaining normal oral competence and minimal donor site morbidity.

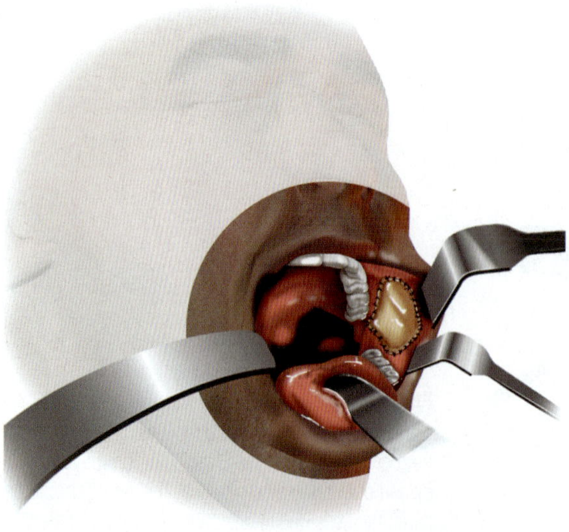

FIGURE 4.3
The flap is sutured into the defect with mild redundancy to prevent trismus as the tissue contracts during healing.

- Each reconstructive decision is based on the patient's preoperative goals and function as well as his or her projected posttreatment function.
- Appropriate evaluation and planning of the reconstructive procedure must be performed prior to surgery.
- If only internal lining is required, primary closure, local rotational flaps, or thin pliable free flaps should be considered depending on the size of the defect.
- Larger composite resections and through-and-through defects will require free tissue transfer.
- Remember to reconstruct the inside dimensions as close to the original defect size whenever possible. But also consider that it is easier to debulk a large soft tissue flap than it is to take care of the complications (wound breakdown, fistulas, or stenosis) resulting in too little tissue to repair the defect.
- Postoperative radiation therapy is one of the most effective means of debulking a flap, so it is important to take into consideration the overall oncologic treatment of each patient.
- Patients with cancer of the head and neck require a multidisciplinary team to ensure not only proper treatment of their cancer but also their posttreatment function. Speech therapy, physical therapy, and dental care are all essential components of the overall care of these patients.

PITFALLS

- If the free flap is not of adequate size, trismus as a result of contracture may ensue.
- If the defect and reconstruction involve the parotid duct, it is important to marsupialize the duct to prevent parotitis.

INSTRUMENTS TO BE AVAILABLE

- Standard head and neck surgery set

SUGGESTED READING

Alvi A, Myers EN. Skin graft reconstruction of the composite resection defect. *Head Neck* 1996;18(6):538–543; discussion 543–544.

Chhetri DK, Rawnsley JD, Calcaterra TC. Carcinoma of the buccal mucosa. *Otolaryngol Head Neck Surg* 2000;123(5):566–571.

Ducci Y, Herford A. The use of a palatal Island flaps as an adjunct to microvascular free tissue transfer for reconstruction of complex oromandibular defects. *Laryngoscope* 2001;111:1666.

Deleyiannis FW, Dunklebarger J, Lee E, et al. Reconstruction of the marginal mandibulectomy defect: an update. *Am J Otolaryngol* 2007;28(6):363–366.

Girod D, Sykes K, Jorgensen J, et al. Acellular dermis compared to skin grafts in oral cavity reconstruction. *Laryngoscope* 2009;119:2141.

5 MANAGEMENT OF THE PARTIAL GLOSSECTOMY DEFECT: SPLIT THICKNESS SKIN GRAFT

D. Gregory Farwell

INTRODUCTION

Cancer of the oral tongue is typically treated by surgical resection. Optimal reconstruction of the partial glossectomy defect recreates a functional tongue that allows for oral diet and normal articulation. Several techniques are available to reconstruct the tongue including healing by secondary intention, skin grafting, allografting, pedicled local and regional flaps, and free tissue transfer.

Split-thickness skin grafting is a time-honored technique that allows for the rapid reconstruction of select defects. This technique is straightforward and does not require additional specialized surgical techniques but is not appropriate for every defect. Smaller defects in a healthy, well-vascularized wound bed are best for this technique. Larger defects and hostile wounds are less appropriate for this technique and are typically better reconstructed with vascularized free flaps.

HISTORY

The typical patient in need of split-thickness skin graft (STSG) reconstruction of the oral tongue has been diagnosed with cancer of the tongue (Fig. 5.1). With improvements in dental education, many patients may be referred from a dentist for an asymptomatic lesion noted on routine dental evaluation.

Other patients may present with a lesion on the tongue that is often painful locally or has referred pain to the ear or is bleeding. The patient may complain of being "tongue-tied" (dysarthria). If the cancer has impeded their diet, they may complain of either dysphagia or frank weight loss. Because of the robust lymphatics of the ventral tongue and floor of the mouth, even small cancers may have already metastasized. In these cases, the patient may notice a mass in the neck.

A careful history should be elicited, documenting known risk factors such as the use of tobacco and alcohol, recurring trauma from a dental or prosthetic source, and preexisting lesions such as erosive lichen planus. Questions should be asked about other symptoms such as dysgeusia or paresthesias of the tongue, lips, or cheek. Other symptoms to look for include dental issues with pain in the teeth or loose teeth. Additionally, a history that evaluated the patient's comorbidities is important.

A careful diagnostic evaluation including a staging examination is critical before embarking on aggressive surgical therapy. Any suggestion of cervical lymphadenopathy should be carefully noted and evaluated. As many of these patients have been smokers, a systematic evaluation should include a careful history of pulmonary disease or other coexisting medical conditions that might complicate treatment.

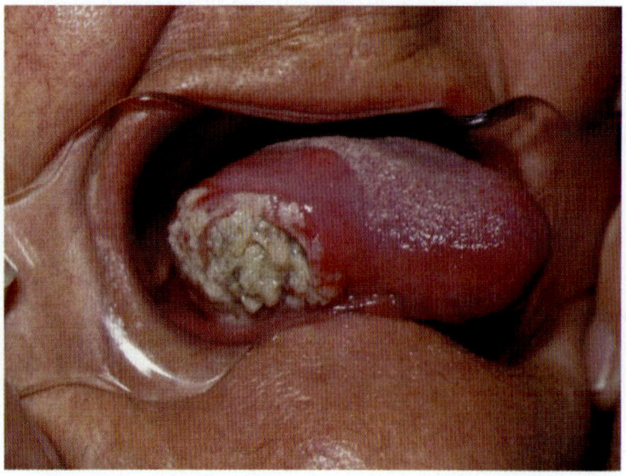

FIGURE 5.1
Squamous cell cancer of the tongue appropriate for STSG reconstruction.

PHYSICAL EXAMINATION

A comprehensive examination of the head and neck is performed with special attention to the tongue including the size of the lesion, the thickness of the lesion, deviation of the tongue on protrusion, tethering of the tongue or reduced mobility, and the cranial nerve examination. Fixation of the cancer to the mandible may imply bone invasion that may influence the reconstructive choices other than the skin graft. Any suggestion of hypoglossal nerve weakness or lingual nerve involvement suggests a larger and more extensive tumor and may imply a more extensive resection, less appropriate for an STSG. A careful assessment of the rest of the aerodigestive tract is indicated to rule out a second primary cancer in patients with a smoking history. The submental, submandibular, and jugulodigastric chains are most commonly involved with cervical metastasis; therefore, a complete examination of the neck is also critical to document lymphatic metastasis. The donor site must be inspected to rule out infection, cutaneous lesions, or indications of previous surgery or radiation.

INDICATIONS

Indications for the STSG include small- or moderate-sized defects with limited involvement of the floor of the mouth. Large defects managed with a skin graft will scar and tether the tongue, which leads to an impairment of speech and swallowing.

CONTRAINDICATIONS

Contraindications to split-thickness skin grafting include tumor-specific and patient-specific factors. Larger tumors are best treated with other techniques such as free tissue transfer with an anterolateral thigh or radial forearm free flap. The complication rate is higher with STSG reconstruction of large oral defects. Specifically, large skin graft reconstructions are prone to wound breakdown, fistula, wound contracture, and poorer functional outcomes such as dysarthria and dysphagia. STSG reconstruction is contraindicated in previously radiated patients. Patient-specific factors such as diffuse skin disease, significant sun exposure, and lack of an appropriate donor site may be rare contraindications to the use of a skin graft.

PREOPERATIVE PLANNING

Imaging Studies

Computed tomography (CT) and/or magnetic resonance imaging (MRI) scans may be used to evaluate the extent of the primary cancer and the regional lymphatics. Historically, the contrast-enhanced CT is the most frequently used form of imaging for evaluating the oral cavity due to its resolution and ability to evaluate for bone invasion. However, dental artifact from metal fillings or prosthesis may compromise its quality in the area of interest. MRI scanning may provide excellent soft tissue resolution of the tongue when there is unacceptable artifact found on the CT scan.

For cancers with advanced T and N stages, examination of the chest and abdomen is important. Historically, CT of the chest and abdomen were frequently used. Currently, PET–CT is increasingly used to stage cancers of the head and neck. This modality is especially useful in lesions with multiple metastatic lymph nodes or inferior level IV lymph nodes where the likelihood of distant metastasis is increased.

Staging Endoscopy

Preoperative endoscopy and examination under anesthesia is important in determining the extent of the lesion and the resectability of the cancer. The extent of the cancer is mapped, and the extension into the mandible or adjacent structures is analyzed. The expected size of the defect is determined to guide the choice of the optimal reconstruction technique. Unexpected second primary cancers may be discovered, which will probably influence the timing of additional procedures.

Preoperative Testing

No additional testing is required for split-thickness skin grafting beyond the tumor assessment as listed above.

SURGICAL TECHNIQUE

An STSG is typically harvested from the thigh or abdomen depending upon the quality of the skin and the patient preference. Selecting a donor site that can be easily hidden with clothing is ideal. Using a dermatome with settings of approximately 0.015 inch, the skin is stretched flat with a tongue blade, malleable, or other flat instrument to minimize the redundancy of the skin and maximize the chance of an optimal graft. Often a skin lubricant such as mineral oil is applied to allow the dermatome to advance smoothly. The dermatome is then advanced against the skin and the appropriate-sized graft is harvested. My preferred technique is to have the dermatome at full speed and then engage the skin at an acute angle. The graft is harvested with the dermatome flat against the skin with the tongue blade advancing just ahead of the dermatome to flatten the skin and then lifting the dermatome off of the skin at the angle. This approach has been likened to an airplane doing a "touch and go" where it lands, rolls along the runway, and then takes off again.

The graft is then placed in a moist sponge until ready to be inset. Once the glossectomy defect is created and the margins are confirmed as free of cancer, the graft may be inset. Typically, an absorbable suture such as a 4-0 chromic is used to inset the graft circumferentially. Care should be taken to stretch out the defect (Fig. 5.2) and use a graft that is at least as large as the defect. The graft will often contract with healing, and in order to maximize the mobility of the tissues, the graft is often slightly oversized before inset. Another technique is to perform small fenestrations through the graft. These holes allow the serum and exudate to escape from under the graft and not lift up the graft like a bulla (Fig. 5.3). If these bulla form, the graft is less likely to achieve a blood supply and adhere to the wound bed leading to failure of the graft. The graft is then bolstered to the wound with a dressing made from petroleum-based gauze, cotton balls, or other dressing material (Fig. 5.4). Sutures from the periphery of the tongue are then tied over the graft to apply gentle downward pressure on the graft, increasing the chances of adherence to the underlying muscle and good healing. Approximately a week later, the bolster is removed and the graft is inspected. Minimization of tissue trauma is ideal on the new graft. Therefore, a soft diet is typically recommended for a short period of time to allow for healing. Careful oral hygiene with saline rinses or chlorhexidine gluconate rinses are often used.

Care of the split-thickness graft site centers on an occlusive dressing and monitoring for signs of infection. There are several commercial dressings that have been used from petroleum-based products to newer products that are gel based. Surgeon preference will determine the optimal choice of dressing material. The wound is often painful, and appropriate analgesics are required.

POSTOPERATIVE MANAGEMENT

Postoperatively, the patient is followed for wound healing and signs of infection. In defects where there is continuity with the neck, such as after a neck dissection, the wound is watched closely for signs of a fistula. Once

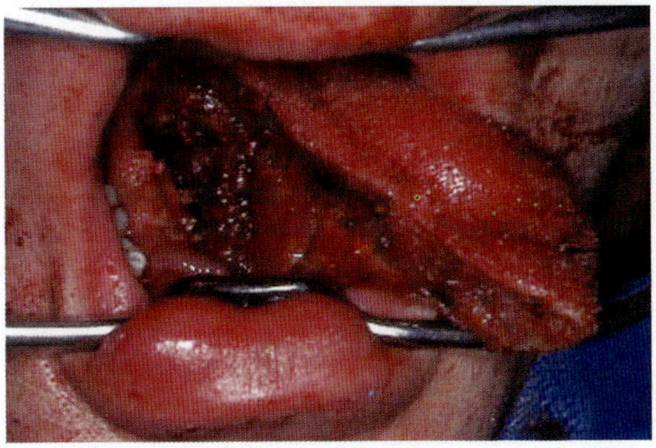

FIGURE 5.2
Defect after tumor resection with healthy, well-vascularized surgical bed.

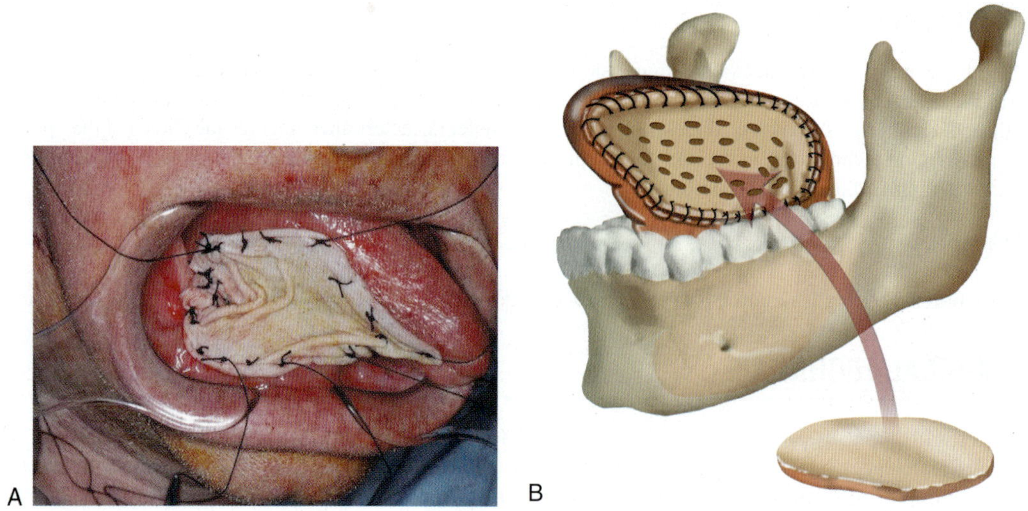

FIGURE 5.3 **A.** STSG of appropriate size is sutured into place. **B.** Illustration of graft placement. Small fenestrations are made to avoid bulla formation.

the bolster is removed on approximately the 7th postoperative day, the skin graft is inspected for its viability. Any blebs are opened to allow the graft to adhere to the wound and prevent additional accumulation that might lift off adjacent portions of the graft. Oral hygiene is continued as the patient's diet is advanced. The skin graft donor site is also monitored during the healing period. Typically, an occlusive dressing is applied while the donor site reepithelializes.

COMPLICATIONS

Fortunately, complications from skin graft reconstruction of partial glossectomy defects happen infrequently. While complete necrosis of the graft is rare, partial necrosis of a portion of the graft may happen if the graft does not adhere to the underlying vascularized tissue. Nonadherence of the graft can be minimized by fenestration of the graft and bolster placement, but due to the convexities and concavities of the three-dimensional tongue, it can be difficult to get complete adaptation of the graft to the graft bed. The necrotic portion of the skin graft should be debrided, and the tissue beneath the graft will typically heal by second intention. Rarely, patients cannot tolerate the bolster due to discomfort, globus sensation, or airway concerns. In these patients, the graft can usually be successfully adapted to the bed with quilting sutures throughout the graft to the underlying soft tissue. Infections of the donor site are rare and can be managed with local wound care and antibiotics as necessary.

More commonly, complications are related to contracture. Depending upon the location of the graft, the wound may contract and restrict the mobility of the oral tissues. Attempting to control for this by stretching the wound bed and sizing the graft to the maximum size of the defect can help minimize this problem. Similarly, trying to use the skin graft technique for larger and more complex defects will be associated with more failures including fistulas. Utilizing alternative techniques such as microvascular tissue transfer will minimize these complications.

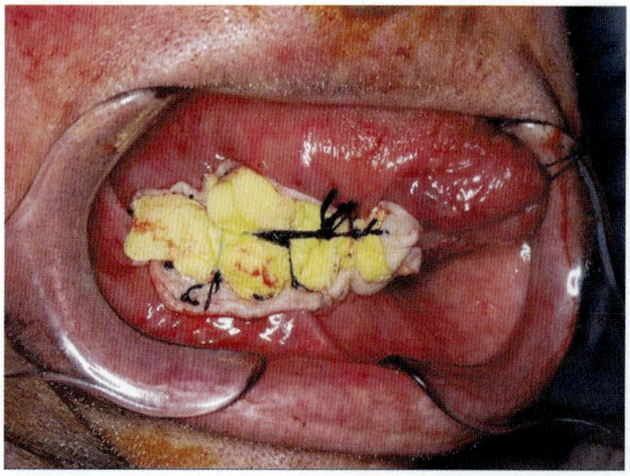

FIGURE 5.4 Bolster in place.

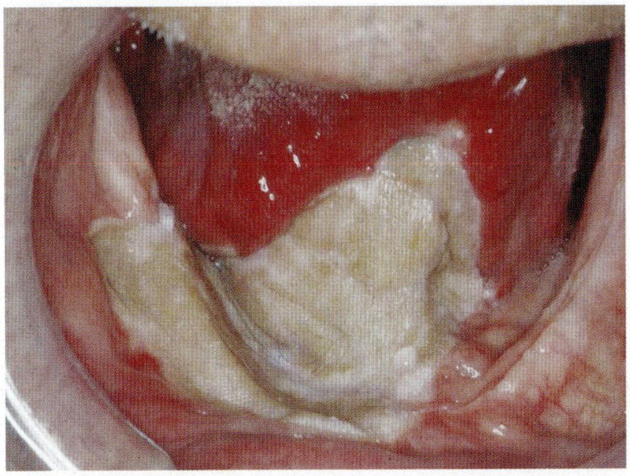

FIGURE 5.5
Healed split-thickness skin graft.

RESULTS

Surgical reconstruction of partial glossectomy defects with STSGs is a time-tested technique that when applied to appropriate defects can successfully achieve the goals of wound closure and return to function (Fig. 5.5). McConnel et al. in 1982 evaluated the functional results of STSG compared to tongue flaps and regional myocutaneous flaps and found that STSG reconstructions had superior results compared to the alternatives studied. Since that time, microvascular reconstruction has revolutionized oral cavity reconstruction and improved our ability to reliably close larger defects with superior functional results.

Steiner and others have demonstrated excellent functional results with limited complications using transoral laser resection with healing by secondary intention with the potential advantage of not "burying" residual tumor thereby allowing for earlier detection of recurrences. However, for small defects, an STSG offers a straightforward technique for rapid closure of partial glossectomy defects and is an appropriate and reasonable choice in these defects.

PEARLS

- Appropriate tumor sizing and staging of the cancer is critical to choosing the appropriate reconstructive technique. Small cancers and smaller defects are most appropriately treated with an STSG.
- Stretching the defect to its maximum dimension will allow the appropriate sizing of the skin graft. The skin graft should be the maximum size of the defect to avoid contracture and maximize mobility of the residual tongue.
- Fenestration and bolstering of the graft to its underlying vascularized bed will maximize skin graft take and successful reconstruction.

PITFALLS

- Choosing the skin graft technique for larger defects will give a suboptimal result compared to other techniques such as microvascular reconstruction.
- Undersizing STSGs can result in wound contracture and limited mobility.

INSTRUMENTS TO HAVE AVAILABLE

- Standard head and neck surgery set
- Dermatome

SUGGESTED READING

Schramm VL, Myers EN. Skin grafts in oral cavity reconstruction. *Arch Otolaryngol* 1980;106:528–532.

McConnel FMS, Teichgraeber JF, Adler RK. A comparison of three methods of oral reconstruction. *Arch Otolaryngol Head Neck Surg* 1987;113:496–500.

Zuydam AC, Lowe D, Brown JS, et al. Predictors of speech and swallowing function following primary surgery for oral and oropharyngeal cancer. *Clin Otolaryngol* 2005;30(5):428–437.

Ellies M, Steiner W. Peri- and postoperative complications after laser surgery of tumors of the upper aerodigestive tract. *Am J Otolaryngol* 2007;28(3):168–172.

6 MANAGEMENT OF THE PARTIAL GLOSSECTOMY DEFECT: RADIAL FOREARM FREE FLAP

Kevin M. Higgins

INTRODUCTION

The radial forearm flap, remains a popular flap in the management and reconstruction of the partial glossectomy defect, especially where the base of tongue and suprahyoid musculature has been preserved, and reconstructive bulk is unnecessary (Fig. 6.1). Numerous studies have shown the utility afforded by the thin pliable nature of the fasciocutaneous radial forearm free flap (RFFF). It facilitates and maintains the mobility of the remaining oral tongue, which is of major importance for deglutition and articulation. Furthermore, the antebrachial cutaneous nerve of the forearm has sensory reinnervation capability using a microneural anastomosis with the lingual nerve that affords a high degree of sensory recovery and enhanced function.

HISTORY

The second most common site of oral cancer is in the mobile portion of the oral tongue, anterior to the circumvallate line. Patients with cancer of the oral tongue may present with odynophagia, often with referred otalgia, with or without dysarthria, and with dysgeusia. The cancer typically manifests as a noduloulcerative lesion affecting the lateral border of the tongue as the most common subsite with associated metastasis to levels 1, 2, 3, and occasionally 4. There is often an associated history of the long-term habits of smoking cigarettes, using smokeless tobacco, and drinking alcohol. Additional pertinent risk factors include human papillomavirus infection, chronic inflammatory conditions affecting the mucosal surfaces such as lichen planus, long-standing erythroleukoplakia, and poor oral hygiene.

PHYSICAL EXAMINATION

A complete examination of the head and neck should be carried out with a combination of inspection, palpation, indirect mirror examination, and direct endoscopy. Careful visualization for any irregularities of the mucosal lining of the upper aerodigestive tract is critical in order to effectively map out the extent of disease and to examine for any suspicious coincidental synchronous primary cancers. An examination of cranial nerve function is important and should include ipsilateral tongue deviation with protrusion, loss of power, tone and bulk as well as any fasciculation seen with lower motor neuron lesions is vitally important. Examination of the status of the dentition for obvious caries, loose teeth, root exposures, and gross gingival involvement or periodontal disease should be undertaken. An assessment of sensation of the teeth of the lower arch and the lower lip is important for assessment of trigeminal nerve function. In addition, palpation of the lesion is critical in order to assess the depth of invasion, relationship to the floor of the mouth, midline tongue raphe, and base of the tongue. Finally, one should carefully palpate the cervical nodal basins especially levels 1, 2, and 3 that are the primary echelon lymph nodes for metastasis from a primary cancer of the oral tongue. A neck dissection is usually carried out that may impact the reconstruction options or technique.

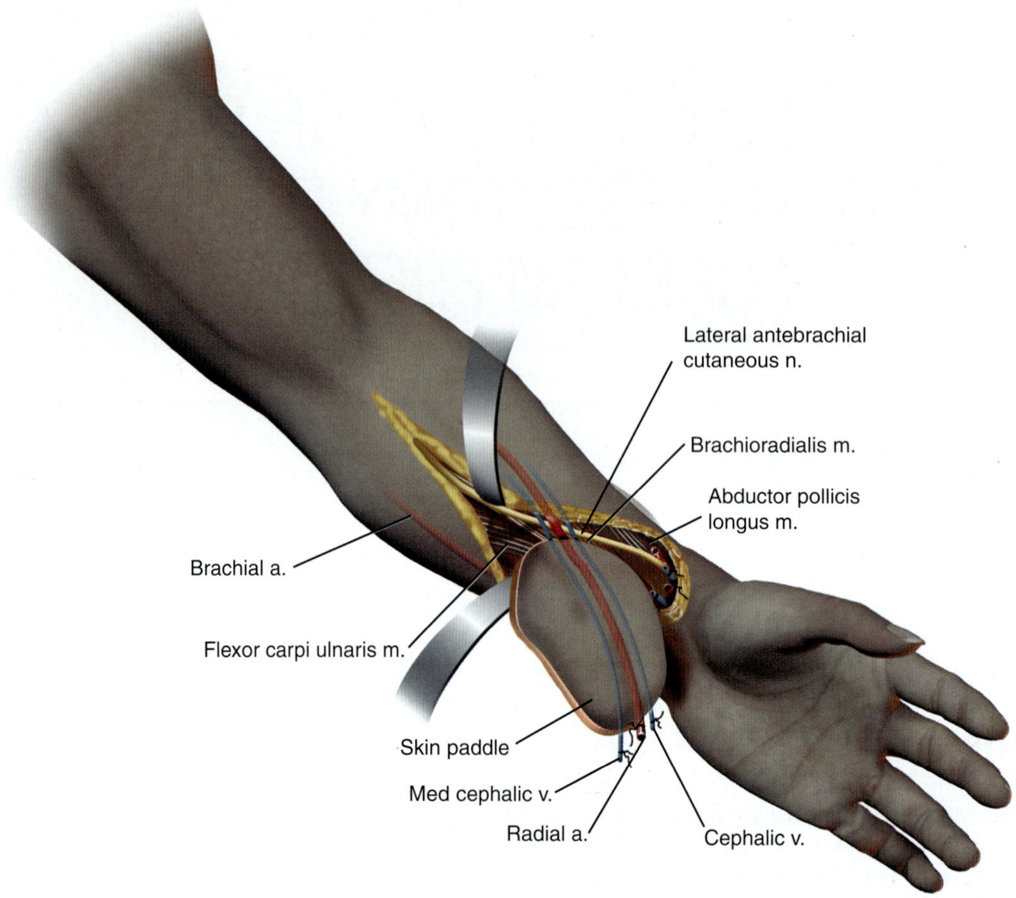

FIGURE 6.1 An elevated radial forearm free flap.

INDICATIONS

As with other head and neck malignancies, cancer of the oral cavity must be staged according to the American Joint Committee on Cancer TNM staging system. In general, surgery is the recommended first-line treatment for cancer of the oral tongue. Patients in whom surgery is contraindicated may have the options of brachytherapy or external beam radiation therapy.

CONTRAINDICATIONS

Contraindications for surgical management with the RFFF include inability to tolerate anesthesia due to medical illness, a negative Allen test, or patient refusal.

PREOPERATIVE PLANNING

A detailed metastatic survey with computed tomography (CT) with contrast of the head/neck and chest is routine. The CT is widely used to assess for bone invasion and cervical lymph node metastasis, while magnetic resonance imaging can complement CT scanning by providing better visualization of soft tissue structures, invasion of the tongue musculature, and extension to the base of the tongue as well as perineural invasion.

During the preoperative planning phase, testing the vasculature of the nondominant hand can provide information on the viability of the donor hand following RFFF transfer. This is assessed with the Allen test to ensure patency of the ulnar and radial forearm vessels but more importantly to ensure adequate anastomotic channels and completeness of the superficial and deep palmer arches (Fig. 6.2). Anatomic variants such as the superficial ulnar artery and incomplete palmar arches are extremely uncommon. If the Allen test is equivocal, a pulse oximeter can be placed on the thumb or index finger (the digits at greatest risk for potential ischemia with anatomic variants) and an arterial pressure trace observed. Significant flattening and loss of the anacrotic notch (normal triphasic pattern) should prompt formal digital plethysmography or a search for another reconstructive flap option such as the anterolateral thigh or lateral arm flap.

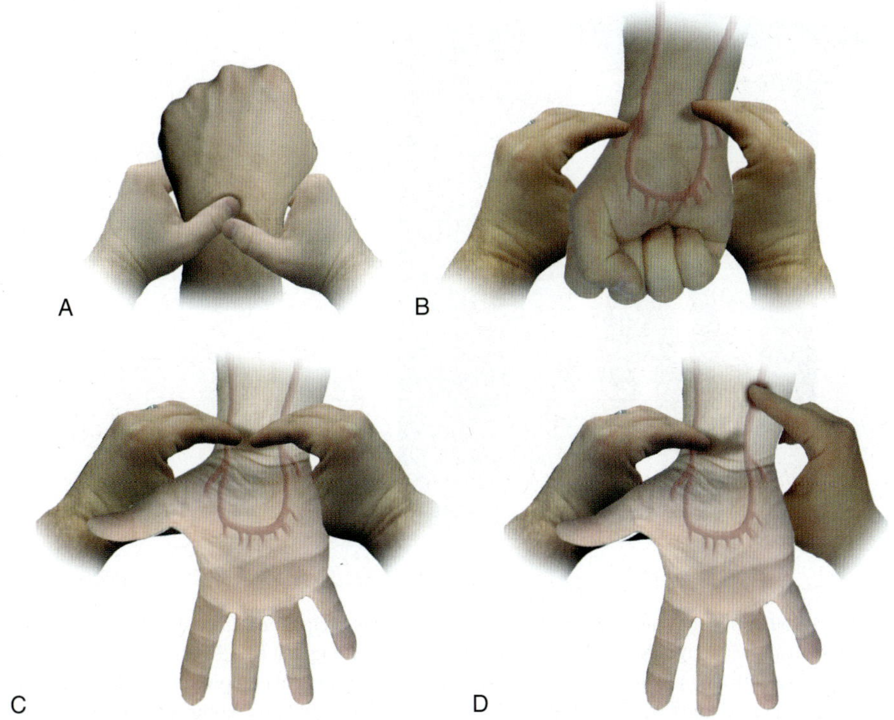

FIGURE 6.2
The modified Allen test. A positive test is demonstrated by reperfusion of the palm within 7 to 10 seconds of release of pressure on the ulnar artery. A negative test is demonstrated by lack of reperfusion within 7 to 10 seconds and indicates poor collateral ulnar circulation to the hand.

Office-based duplex ultrasonography is becoming increasingly performed by head and neck surgeons. This technology allows a detailed assessment of cervical node status and availability and location of suitable recipient vessels in the neck, and with a fingertip probe, an assessment of the depth of invasion. In addition, it can facilitate the ability to perform US-guided fine needle aspirations.

SURGICAL TECHNIQUE

Oral cavity defects can often be approached transorally with the exposure maximized by the judicious use of multiarmed retractors such as the Dingman Gag (Fig. 6.3). Retraction sutures inserted into the remaining tip of the tongue and dorsum help to facilitate triangulation for excision and insetting of the flap. Novel techniques such as transoral robotic surgery also have a role in primary ablative surgery, with robotic assistance in the insetting of more posteriorly located defects that can potentially minimize the need for mandibular swing or lingual release approaches that tend to add to overall patient morbidity and length of stay. An additional key consideration is hemostasis after completing the ablation. Lingual vessels should be controlled with vascular clips and bipolar

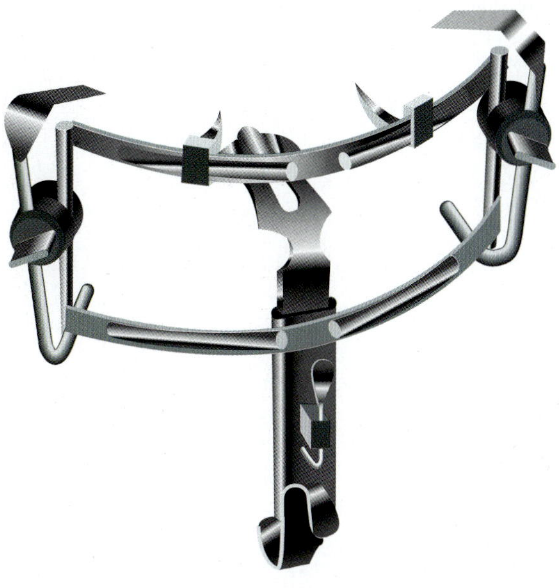

FIGURE 6.3
The Dingman retractor provides exposure for transoral reconstruction.

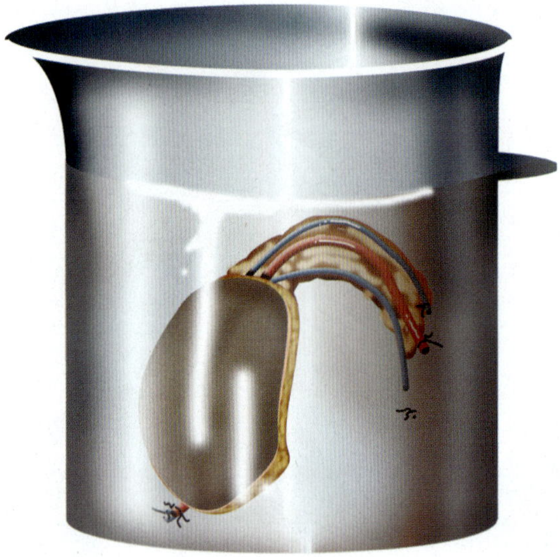

FIGURE 6.4
The Archimedes volume displacement technique is used to determine the approximate volume of the radial forearm free flap.

cautery or other novel closure systems such as the harmonic scalpel or Ligasure™ device. A Valsalva maneuver to 30 cm H_2O allows for the identification of occult venous bleeding that could open up with buried inset, causing flap compromise with a hematoma of the floor of the mouth and potential compromise of the oral airway. Oozing from the defect can be controlled with Surgicel that can be combined with recombinant thrombin to enhance the hemostatic effect. A moistened laparotomy sponge is left in the oral cavity while the flap is harvested. One potential pitfall is the access to the neck recipient vessels. It often helps to divide a portion of the mylohyoid muscle to avoid potential strangulation of the microsurgical pedicle. The tunnel should be enlarged with serial dilatation to allow easy accommodation of at least two gloved fingers and maintained with a moistened 1-inch Penrose drain.

The RFFF is designed based on the dimensions of the defect in the tongue. It is extremely important to avoid overfilling the defect as it negatively impacts mobility and requires secondary debulking procedures. One should not measure the defect based on the ablative dead space volume as it typically overestimates the overall requirement. This is especially true when the jaw has been split and swung open with a mandibulotomy approach. A foil template can be fashioned based on the resection specimen and unfolded on the forearm to allow for two-dimensional mapping. I routinely use an overflow cylinder with a modified Archimedes technique to obtain a volume measurement as well that helps to ensure overall like-for-like volume matching (Fig. 6.4). The nondominant forearm is selected. The palpable radial arterial pulse line is marked, as is the course of the superficial cephalic vein. The arm should be free draped and the flap harvested ideally under tourniquet control. An Esmark bandage can be wrapped from distal to proximal around the forearm prior to cuff inflation to exsanguinate the forearm, while other authors prefer to leave some blood in the vascular channels to aid in their identification and control. The tourniquet is then inflated with the hand elevated to 250 mm Hg. The flap design should ideally allow the pedicle to exit either posteriorly or inferiorly. Smaller defects (typically <3 cm × 3 cm) can be incorporated into an ulnar "hatchet"-style flap to avoid skin graft coverage (Fig. 6.5). The long axis of the flap needs to be oriented in a transverse direction to facilitate a hatchet flap closure of the distal wrist

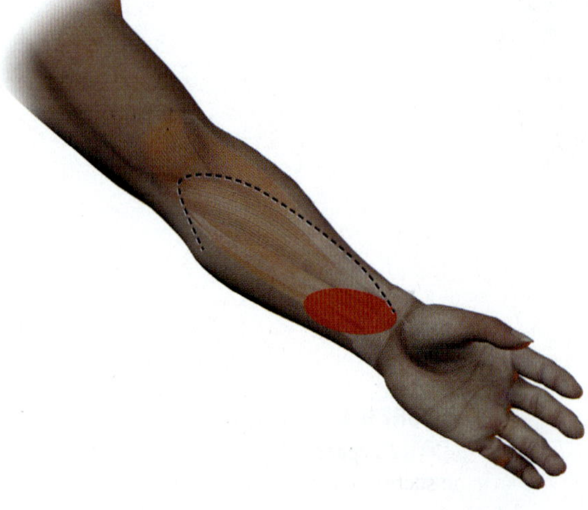

FIGURE 6.5
RFFF donor defect can be corrected with an ulnar hatchet flap.

crease margin. Additional local bilobed flaps based on ulnar septocutaneous perforators can also be designed. These local flaps have been shown to prevent donor site morbidity especially as it relates to overall wrist mobility; however, they may complicate exposure of the pedicle.

The flap can be raised in either the suprafascial or subfascial plane. Suprafascial technique and elevation protects the paratenon and helps enhance skin graft take; however, for novice surgeons, it can endanger the septal perforators that are extremely small yet numerous, as the intermuscular septum is approached from the radial and ulnar direction between the flexor carpi radialis and the brachioradialis. It is ideal to incorporate the cephalic vein in the flap design and elevation. Even if it seems divergent based on the superficial anatomical course, one is typically able to capture a side branch draining the flap distally toward the wrist crease. This facilitates microvascular anastomosis in that the cephalic vein usually affords a 3- to 4-mm vessel caliber, whereas the major vena comitans that accompanies the radial artery is seldom larger than 2.5 mm unless a communicating branch between the deep and superficial venous system is traced proximally toward the antecubital fossa. The radial sensory nerve has to be preserved throughout its forearm course as damage to it can result in problematic dermatomal deficits and potentially traumatic neuromata. It is carefully protected as it emerges beneath the brachioradialis muscle belly and courses over its tendon. It typically ramifies in close proximity to the cephalic vein, and its most medial branch is often intimate to the microsurgical pedicle and the delicate septocutaneous perforators to the skin paddle. However, despite these anatomical challenges, it seldom if ever requires sacrifice with jeweled microsurgical instruments and a nerve clinging technique, to safely separate the most medial branch from the microsurgical pedicle.

Different authors advocate elevation of subcutaneous adipose tissue along with the antebrachial fascia to protect the pedicle from salivary contamination or neck cutaneous breakdown in postchemoradiation salvage operations. This bulk is not a problem with large volume defects with mandible swing approaches. For smaller transoral approaches, this added bulk can cause strangulation of the flap in the floor of the mouth tunnel. It is safer to restrict the pedicle to the cephalic vein, antebrachial cutaneous nerve of the forearm, and the radial artery and its minor and major *venae comitantes* in this situation. Harvesting the flap can be accelerated with automatic clip appliers or clamp, seal, and cut devices such as the Ligasure™ and Harmonic Focus™. The pedicle is most safely approached from ulnar and radial as opposed to a distal-to-proximal dissection technique. This allows release of the flexor retinaculum, protection of the median nerve, and avoidance of delicate septocutaneous perforator destabilization by inadvertent suprafascial dissection planes that can be inadvertently developed by novice surgeons. In addition, the deep periosteal branches in the area of the radial styloid can be ligated more easily as they are seen earlier or can be more readily incorporated into an osteocutaneous flap design. As the pedicle is dissected toward the antecubital fossa, it is often helpful to follow the venae comitantes toward a confluent common vena comitans, which is typically seen at the emergence of the communicating branch. This dissection can be tedious as there are multiple deep perforator branches into the deep flexor muscles such as the pronator teres. This additional dissection is obviated with a reliable and robust cephalic vein that is draining the marked skin paddle. The tourniquet is deflated and the pedicle copiously irrigated with warmed heparinized saline solution and carefully inspected along its length and along the undersurface of the skin paddle for any obvious bleeding points. An exhaustive search for bleeders from the forearm donor site is also undertaken at the same time. Color and capillary refill are then observed in the hand and especially in the area of the thenar eminence. The flap should be allowed to drink for 10 to 15 minutes after primary ischemia time to minimize reperfusion injury after secondary ischemia and microsurgical anastomosis. This gives the surgeon time to comfortably prepare the recipient vessels for anastomosis. The facial artery and common facial vein are typically the best size match for the radial artery and cephalic vein or major vena comitans. The vessels should be prepared under loupe magnification with vessel dilatation and excess adventitial trimming. Approximating microvascular clamps are very helpful in maintaining vessel orientation during anastomosis. The harvested flap is then detached by interrupting arterial inflow first and allowing the venous blood to run out prior to venous clamp and tie. A surgical marker should be used to draw a straight vertical line along the pedicle axis. This allows any helical spiraling to be identified as the pedicle is drawn through the premoistened 1-inch Penrose drain into the neck. Careful insetting is then performed. It is often helpful to leave the ends of each previously placed suture long in order to facilitate traction and to avoid any fistula created by buried suture material. The anterior sutures often need to be left long and parachuted after any locking low-profile titanium plate is replaced. Circumdental sutures should be considered laterally, as the floor of the mouth mucosa is extremely thin and prone to tearing. Microvascular anastomosis is then undertaken with an operating microscope with 9-0 or 10-0 microsurgical nylon material (Fig. 6.6). An anastomotic coupler device, such as the 3 M Unilink, can be used to reduce anastomotic time (Fig. 6.7).

Care should be taken with arterial coupling as it requires generous arterial vessel caliber, greater than 2.5 mm, and stiff atherosclerotic vessel walls often tear or pop off the ring pin collars. Once the microsurgical clamps are removed, visible thrill and palpable pulse should be confirmed. Venous strip test should be performed with microsurgical dilator instruments to demonstrate complete microsurgical loop with anterograde venous runoff, and then finally, the flap should be scratched to examine for bright red bleeding with delay of 1 to 3 seconds commensurate with capillary refill. Excess pedicle length can become dependent and kink, and this should be avoided with stay sutures or microsurgical clips to keep the pedicle in an appropriate resting position. Once the vessels are reapproximated, the neck and arm are reapproximated with layered closure. I routinely employ a suction drain system with care to place the suction away from the microsurgical pedicle.

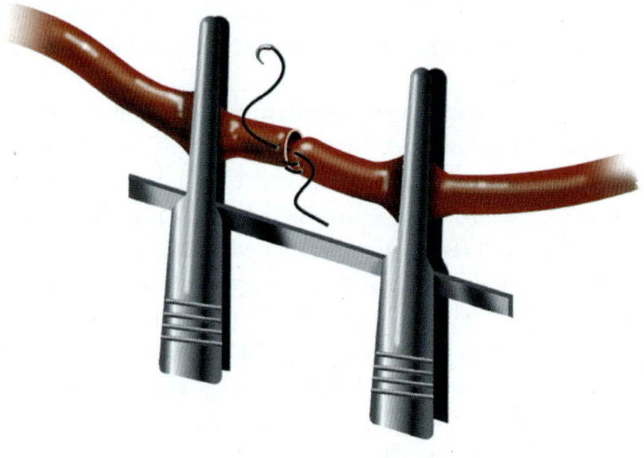

FIGURE 6.6
Microvascular vessel clamps allow for suturing the vessels together.

Fast-dissolving sutures such as Vicryl Rapide can be used to secure the suction drain away from the microsurgical pedicle, with Gelfoam slabs also being used to protect the microsurgical anastomoses.

POSTOPERATIVE MANAGEMENT

As with management of other free flaps, clinical bedside check is essential in the immediate postoperative period for detecting flap failure. For the intraoral tongue flap, this includes assessing flap color, capillary refill, and any dehiscence of the incision line.

After the initial postoperative period, frequent close surveillance of patients for the first 3 to 5 years posttreatment is currently being advised. Postoperative imaging can be obtained if clinically indicated, and patients should be educated of any signs and symptoms of tumor recurrence, such as hoarseness, pain, dysphagia, referred otalgia, oral bleeding, and enlarged lymph nodes.

COMPLICATIONS

As with other operations, the risk of bleeding and infection is present. Hematoma in the neck needs to be carefully managed and a low index of suspicion for vascular pedicle compromise as being the cause with venous outflow obstruction. There are also risks of loss of tongue function, including airway obstruction, dysarthria, dysphagia with impaired oral preparatory, and oropharyngeal initiation of a functional swallow (temporary G-tube dependence), as well as free flap failures. With the radial forearm flap, the issue with flap compromise tends to relate to geometry issues with a long redundant pedicle causing kinking or helical twisting of the venae comitantes or a tight floor of the mouth tunnel causing strangulation of the venous outflow rather than arterial compromise as the intimal diameter with the radial artery and the facial artery or superior thyroid is usually 2.5 to 3 mm.

RESULTS

The tongue remains a difficult structure to reconstruct in the oral cavity, given its central role in articulation, deglutition, and airway protection. In this chapter, I have highlighted the microvascular techniques for RFFF

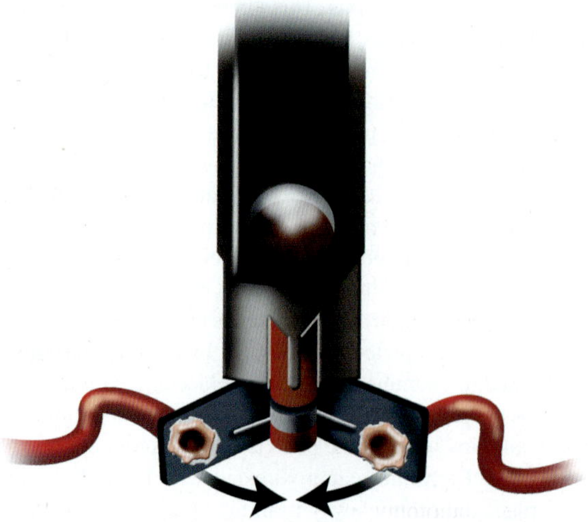

FIGURE 6.7
An anastomotic device (3 M Unilink) can be used to expedite connection of microvascular vessels.

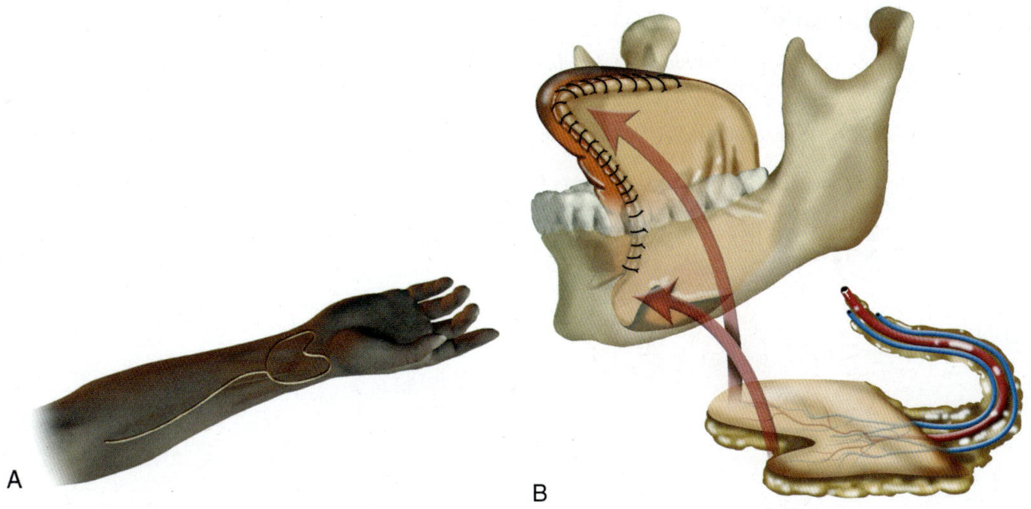

FIGURE 6.8
A, B. Bilobed flaps allow for reconnection of the tongue and floor of the mouth.

reconstruction of a partial glossectomy. The RFFF is robust and versatile. In one comparison between the RFFF and the anterolateral thigh flap, there were no reported differences in speech intelligibility, tongue mobility, or deglutition scores.

PEARLS

- Depending on the location and size of the defect, there is typically a floor of the mouth component that needs to be managed to effectively seal off the oral cavity from the neck compartment. Separation of the floor of the mouth subunit from the lateral and ventral tongue surface is also important in maintaining overall tongue mobility and, in particular, to facilitate tongue protrusion.
- These goals of separation and seal are facilitated with a bilobed design with a longer curvilinear lobe for the dorsum and tip and the shorter lobe for the floor of the mouth (Fig. 6.8A and B).
- Additional bulk to fill in the tongue and restore some bulk to the base of the tongue if necessary or to recreate the tongue mound can be achieved with an additional "beaver-tail" modification with the additional forearm adipose tissue and fascia placed in a jelly-roll configuration under the skin paddle.
- Issues involving skin graft take can be mitigated with careful preservation of the paratenon investing the forearm tendon sheathes.

PITFALLS

- Placement of the skin paddle more proximally over the forearm muscle bellies results in less tendon exposure. This does have the drawback of shortening effective pedicle length.
- Bolster dressing application and effective volar forearm splinting in the position of function also assist in minimizing shearing forces. Adjunctive measures such as application of platelet-rich plasma and VAC dressing application are currently being investigated by several groups, especially with problematic donor sites.
- If there are issues with reperfusion of the flap or forearm donor site, the following sequence should be followed; one needs to ensure that the patient is normothermic and has sufficient perfusion pressure. Hemoglobin and hematocrit should be optimized. Pulsed irrigation with papaverine should be used to combat and counteract vasospasm. Trial evidence and experimental model would suggest limited effect on sympathectomized free flaps with inotropic support in order to optimize overall perfusion pressure once volume has been expanded. I use ephedrine and dopamine and avoid selective alpha agonists such as phenylephrine. On very rare occasions, an interposition vein graft may be required to replace the transplanted radial artery.

INSTRUMENTS TO HAVE AVAILABLE

- Basic neck tray
- Armoured/flexible endotracheal tubes that are low profile and keep the anesthetic circuit out of the operative field (adult number 7 or 8)
- Mouth gags (Davis, Dingman, props)
- Spandex self-retaining double-lip retractor
- Dental set (periosteal elevators, gouges, extractors)
- 2.0 low-profile mandibular locking plating system (if mandibulotomy is required)

SUGGESTED READING

Guofan Y, Baoque C, Yuzhi G, et al. Forearm free skin flap transplantation. *Natl Med J China* 1981;61:139–141.

Soutar DS, McGregor IA. The radial forearm flap in intraoral reconstruction: a versatile method for intra-oral reconstruction. *Br J Plast Surg* 1983;36:1–8.

Dubner S, Heller KS. Reinnervated radial forearm free flaps in head and neck reconstruction. *J Reconstr Microsurg* 1992;8:467–468.

Genden EM, Desai S, Sung CK. Transoral robotic surgery for the management of head and neck cancer: a preliminary experience. *Head Neck* 2009;31:283–289.

Mukhija VK, Sung CK, Desai SC, et al. Transoral robotic assisted free flap reconstruction. *Otolaryngol Head Neck Surg* 2009;140:124–125.

7 MANAGEMENT OF THE TOTAL GLOSSECTOMY DEFECT: PECTORALIS MAJOR MYOCUTANEOUS FLAP

Patrick J. Gullane

INTRODUCTION

The pectoralis major myocutaneous flap was first described by Ariyan in 1979. It is a reliable, robust, and easily harvested pedicled flap that was the most popular technique for head and neck reconstruction prior to the introduction of free tissue transfer. Though widely used in the past for reconstruction following total glossectomy, it has now been replaced almost entirely by free tissue microvascular flaps, such as radial forearm fasciocutaneous flap, anterolateral thigh fasciocutaneous flap, latissimus dorsi myocutaneous flap, rectus abdominis myocutaneous flap, and gracilis myocutaneous flap. However, for select patients in whom free tissue transfer is not an option, the pectoralis major myocutaneous flap offers a reliable reconstructive procedure following both primary and salvage surgery.

The tongue serves three main functions: deglutition, articulation, and airway protection. Reconstruction of a total glossectomy defect must take these functions into consideration. The ideally reconstructed neotongue must have adequate dorsal height, bulk, anterior length, and support in order to enable the patient to swallow. Dorsal height is necessary to allow contact of the neotongue to the palate, so as to propel the food bolus posteriorly. Bulk is required for better quality of speech. The neotongue must also have sufficient anterior length to contact teeth to allow for articulation. Since the floor of the mouth and extrinsic tongue musculature is often resected, the neotongue must be adequately supported across the mandibular arch to prevent ptosis. Lastly, the suprahyoid and extrinsic tongue musculature act to elevate the larynx. Because these muscles are usually detached or excised during the ablation, laryngeal suspension to the mandible or a reconstruction plate in the anterosuperior vector is required to minimize postoperative aspiration.

HISTORY

A careful history is essential to understand the prior exposure to external beam radiotherapy, systemic chemotherapy, and prior surgery. When the patient has a history of prior radiotherapy, healing is often compromised. The pectoralis flap provides a vascularized muscle flap that is helpful in aiding healing. All prior exposures can impact on wound healing and the availability of donor vessels for microvascular reconstruction. In those patients with a history of prior neck dissection, the neck may be depleted of vessels for microvascular free tissue transfer. In such cases, regional flap reconstruction may be indicated. In addition, a careful review of the patient's comorbidities can help determine if there are limitations to free tissue transfer or regional flap reconstruction.

PHYSICAL EXAMINATION

Physical examination should entail a review of the defect and the chest wall to make sure that the anatomy of the chest wall is appropriate for reconstruction of the defect within the oral cavity. In the repair of the anterior aspect of the floor of the mouth, the pectoralis major myocutaneous may be inadequate in length to reconstruct a total glossectomy defect so that a tension free closure is achieved. In such a case, an alternative donor site will need to be used. Evidence of previous surgery in this area may eliminate the pectoralis flap as an option.

Examination of the defect is important to determine if laryngeal preservation can be accomplished with the glossectomy reconstruction. Glossectomy resections that involve the supraglottic larynx are poorly tolerated because aspiration is common. Pure total glossectomy defects can be reconstructed with the pectoralis flap; however, bulk is essential to protect the airway.

INDICATIONS

The indications for this technique are when a microvascular option is not available. Free tissue transfer offers an excellent option for the total glossectomy defect, but there are times when this cannot be achieved and a pectoralis flap is necessary.

CONTRAINDICATIONS

The contraindications for this flap are when there is a concomitant mandible defect or if the skin paddle will not reach the anterior aspect of the oral tongue defect because of anatomic restrictions. Previous surgery, trauma, and radiation to the chest wall are also contraindications.

PREOPERATIVE PLANNING

Total glossectomy is a life-altering procedure, and therefore, the patient's capacity and motivation for rehabilitation must first be taken into consideration. The indication for concurrent total glossectomy and laryngectomy is dependent on the extent of disease or a patient's pulmonary and functional status. Their pulmonary function may predict whether they will be able to tolerate some possible post operative mild aspiration if the larynx is preserved. The addition of a total laryngectomy is associated with greater morbidity and should only be considered in appropriately selected patients (Fig. 7.1). Nonoperative management, such as chemoradiation or, in some cases, palliative care, should also be discussed with these patients as alternate options.

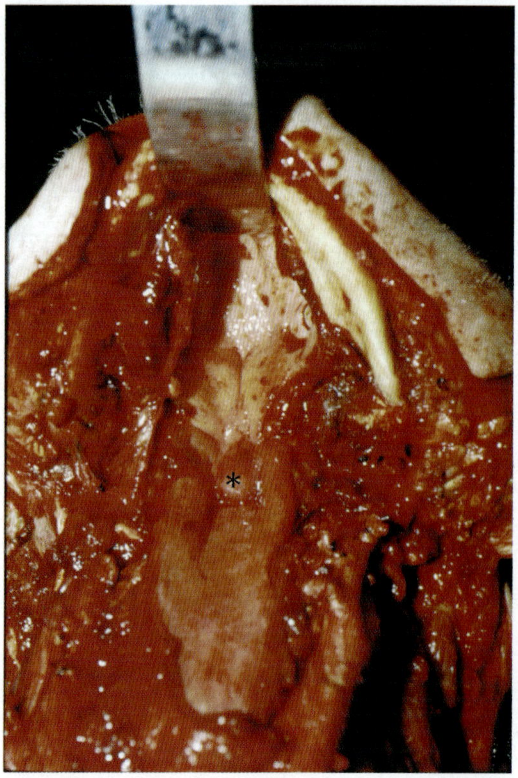

FIGURE 7.1
Total glossectomy and total laryngectomy defect. Note uvula (*asterisk*). (Figure © Patrick J. Gullane.)

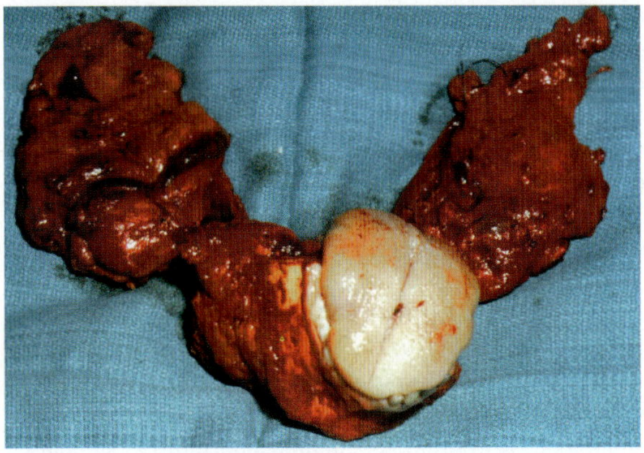

FIGURE 7.2
Total glossectomy, segmental mandibulectomy, bilateral neck dissection specimen. (Figure © Patrick J. Gullane.)

SURGICAL TECHNIQUE

A tracheostomy is performed first to control the airway. Intraoral access can be achieved through a lip split and midline mandibulotomy/mandibulectomy or a lingual release into the neck. To avoid the confusion in the literature regarding the extent of a total glossectomy, we define a "total glossectomy" as resection of the entire oral tongue and base of tongue as far posteriorly as the epiglottis (Fig. 7.2). However, in situations where a subtotal glossectomy can be performed, attempts are made to preserve the hypoglossal and superior laryngeal nerves, and as much floor of the mouth mucosa and native tongue as is oncologically sound.

Using a flexible ruler, the longitudinal dimension is measured from the mandibular symphysis to the posterior extent of the resection (base of tongue, vallecula, or supraglottic larynx), allowing for dorsal curvature of the flap. The transverse dimension is measured from mandibular arch to mandibular arch, again allowing for dorsal curvature so that the flap contacts the hard palate.

Based on the thoracoacromial artery, the pectoralis major flap can be raised as a myocutaneous or fasciocutaneous flap. The skin paddle is designed over the inferomedial aspect of the flap vasculature. In women, the skin paddle is designed medial to the breast (to minimize the incorporation of mammary tissue into the flap), and a laterally based incision is still used, which then extends inferior to the breast along the inframammary fold to connect with the skin paddle.

The skin is incised with a scalpel to minimize thermal necrosis to the skin paddle. Using the monopolar cautery, the dissection is then carried down through subcutaneous tissue to expose the lateral and inferior borders of the pectoralis major muscle. Once the pectoralis major muscle is identified, the superior and inferior skin paddle incisions can be made so that the same paddle is positioned completely over the muscle to maximize the number of musculocutaneous perforators (Fig. 7.3A and B). The flap is then elevated off the chest wall

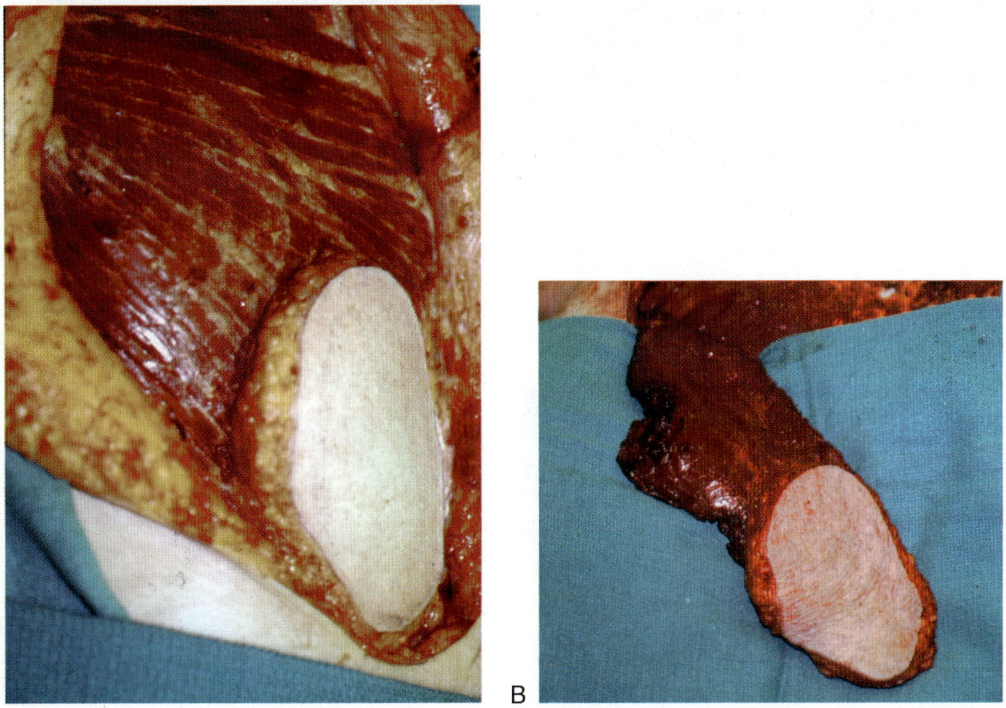

A B

FIGURE 7.3
A. Pectoralis major myocutaneous flap in situ.
B. Harvested pectoralis major myocutaneous flap. (Figures © Patrick J. Gullane.)

fascia and the pectoralis minor muscle. Care is taken to avoid injury to the vascular pedicle, which lies on the deep surface of the pectoralis major muscle. Some have advocated suturing the skin paddle to the underlying muscle to prevent shearing injury during the harvesting process; however, in my experience, this is not necessary. Medially, perforators of the internal mammary artery must be preserved in case a deltopectoral flap is ever required for a subsequent soft tissue reconstruction. Laterally, the humeral attachment of the pectoralis major muscle must be released to permit rotation of the flap. Often, the lateral thoracic artery and lateral pectoral nerve must be divided to increase rotation and length and to decrease tethering of the flap. A broad subcutaneous tunnel is then created over the clavicle, and the flap is carefully delivered into the neck. The chest incision is closed over suction drains.

The pectoralis major myocutaneous flap is brought through the floor of the mouth with the proximal portion of the skin paddle forming the anterior aspect of the neotongue/floor of the mouth. The neotongue is then suspended across the mandibular arch by either suturing to the pterygoid musculature or securing to the mandible using drill holes. The flap is then sutured to the remaining mucosa from posterior to anterior (Fig. 7.4A). If there is not sufficient floor of the mouth mucosa to suture to, circumdental sutures can be used to support and secure the flap. Bunching up of excess tissue in the transverse and longitudinal dimension is favorable, so as to create a "mound" shape to the neotongue/floor of the mouth (Fig. 7.4B). If an anterior reconstruction plate is used, the pectoralis major muscle can then be wrapped around and secured to the plate to minimize plate exposure (Fig. 7.4C and D). Laryngeal suspension is then achieved by drilling holes in the thyroid cartilage and mandibular symphysis and suspending the larynx in an anterosuperior vector with heavy, permanent sutures.

POSTOPERATIVE MANAGEMENT

Postoperative wound care is essential. I recommend placement of a gastrostomy tube during or prior to the procedure to help maintain nutrition during the healing process. All patients undergoing total glossectomy require aggressive speech and swallowing therapy after surgery. Studies reporting outcomes of total glossectomy reconstructed with pectoralis major myocutaneous flap are limited. However, the following can be concluded from my own experience: (1) Most patients regain oral intake; however, they are limited to liquid diet, (2) articulation is adequate, and (3) a small number of patients will ultimately require total laryngectomy due to aspiration.

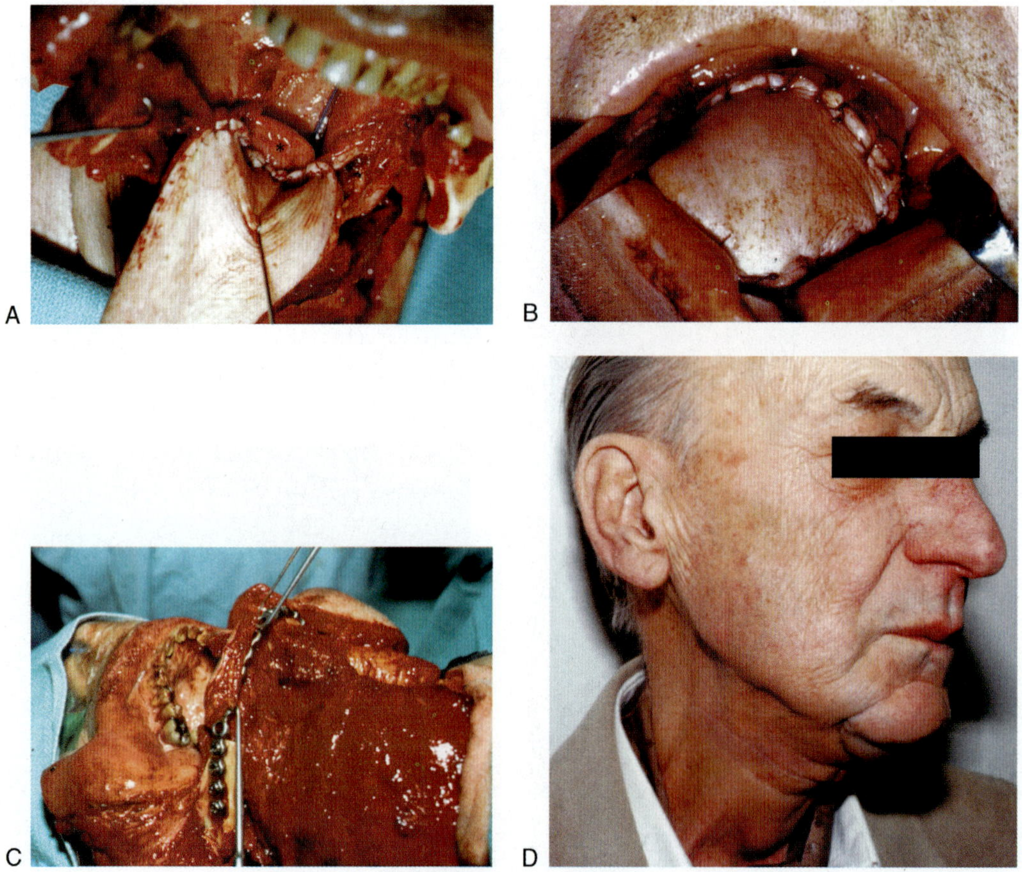

FIGURE 7.4
A. Inset of pectoralis major myocutaneous flap. Note epiglottis posteriorly (*asterisk*). **B.** Intraoral view of inset pectoralis major myocutaneous flap. **C.** Flap inset with mandibular plate reconstruction. Note pectoralis major muscle secured to plate. **D.** Postoperative photograph at 1 year. (Figures © Patrick J. Gullane.)

COMPLICATIONS

There are few donor site complications; however, wound breakdown at the primary site is not uncommon. The weight of the pedicled flap and the very nature of a muscular pedicle can lead to breakdown of the oral wound. I use heavy absorbable sutures (2-0) to decrease the risk of wound dehiscence.

RESULTS

The potential advantages to the pectoralis major myocutaneous flap are the reliability of vessels and vascular pattern, ease of harvesting, robustness of the flap with good vascularity, and the fact that it is a regional flap not requiring vascular anastomosis in vessel-depleted necks. The disadvantages to the pectoralis major myocutaneous flap are the donor site defect, the loss of muscle bulk in the flap over time, excessive subcutaneous adipose tissue, and distal necrosis of the skin paddle. Additionally, in some patients, there may not be adequate length to position the pectoralis major myocutaneous flap in the oral cavity and remain tension free. The complication rate with the pectoralis major myocutaneous flap (flap or donor site) is reported to be approximately 35%. The prevalence of partial thickness skin sloughing ranges between 8% and 26%.

Though total glossectomy reconstruction has largely been replaced by microvascular free tissue transfer, the pectoralis major myocutaneous flap remains a reliable option for patients in whom free tissue transfer is not feasible. All head and neck oncologic surgeons should be able to use the pectoralis major myocutaneous flap for total glossectomy and other head and neck defects.

In my experience, the range of successful deglutition is 67% to 100%, with the average time to swallowing being 4.5 weeks (range 1 to 14). Since tongue movement is absent, the food bolus cannot be propelled posteriorly, so the diet is usually limited to full liquids. There was no difference in swallowing performance between pectoralis major myocutaneous flap and radial forearm free flap reconstruction. The range of adequate articulation is 92% to 100%; however, when compared to radial forearm free flap reconstruction, patients reconstructed with the pectoralis flap had better speech. The use of palatal augmentation prosthesis to facilitate contact of the palate and neotongue was shown to improve articulation. Subsequent total laryngectomy was required in 0% to 7.4% of patients for persistent aspiration.

PEARLS

- Make sure that the skin paddle is large enough to accommodate the defect.
- Lengthen the pedicle as much as possible to limit the drag on the skin paddle.
- Use heavy absorbable suture to secure the skin paddle in the oral cavity defect.

PITFALLS

- The oral wound breakdown should be recognized early and treated.
- The pectoralis is a reliable flap, but the distal random aspect of the skin paddle may undergo necrosis. This should be carefully monitored.

INSTRUMENTS TO HAVE AVAILABLE

- Standard head and neck surgical set

ACKNOWLEDGMENT

I gratefully acknowledge the contributions of Jason Rich and David Goldstein.

SUGGESTED READING

Ariyan S. The pectoralis major myocutaneous flap: a versatile flap for reconstruction in the head and neck. *Plast Reconstr Surg* 1979;63:73–81.

Gullane PJ. Primary mandibular reconstruction: analysis of 64 cases and evaluation of interface radiation dosimetry on bridging plates. *Laryngoscope* 1991;101(54S):1–24.

Davidson J, Brown D, Gullane P. A re-evaluation of radical total glossectomy. *J Otolaryngol* 1993;22(3):160–164.
Haughey B. Tongue reconstruction: concepts and practice. *Laryngoscope* 1993;103:1132–1141.
Liu R, Gullane P, Brown D, et al. Major myocutaneous pedicled flap in head and neck reconstruction: retrospective review of indications and results in 244 consecutive cases at the Toronto General Hospital. *J Otolaryngol* 2001;30(1):34–40.
Su W, Hsia Y, Chang Y, et al. Functional comparison after reconstruction with a radial forearm free flap or a pectoralis major flap for cancer of the tongue. *Otolaryngol Head Neck Surg* 2003;128:412–418.

8 MANAGEMENT OF THE TOTAL GLOSSECTOMY DEFECT: LATISSIMUS DORSI FREE FLAP/ANTEROLATERAL THIGH FLAP

Bruce H. Haughey

INTRODUCTION

Complete oncologic clearance of advanced cancer of the tongue may require a total glossectomy: the end result of this procedure in itself may cause life-threatening loss of function and marked reduction in quality of life. Reconstructive techniques aim to create a neotongue that potentially restores the fundamental functions of airway protection, swallowing, and articulation. In this context, free tissue transfer has evolved as a standard technique for reconstruction of the tongue. A variety of musculocutaneous and fasciocutaneous donor tissues have been described including gracilis, rectus abdominis, latissimus dorsi, radial forearm, and anterolateral thigh (ALT) flaps. Reconstruction with sensate fasciocutaneous flaps has also been proposed, seeking better functional results.

In my practice, the flap of choice for reconstruction of total glossectomy defects is the motor-innervated musculocutaneous latissimus dorsi flap. Acceptable outcomes for swallowing and speech intelligibility have been achieved with the use of this flap. Techniques of latissimus dorsi and ALT free flap reconstruction are described below. The descriptions herein assume and facilitate preservation of the larynx.

Anatomy and Physiology of the Tongue

The tongue is a unique anatomic structure with a complex array of extrinsic and intrinsic muscles and a rich neurovascular supply. The extrinsic muscles include the genioglossus, hyoglossus, styloglossus, and the palatoglossus. The genioglossus and hyoglossus insert into the tongue from their bony origins inferiorly, while the styloglossus and palatoglossus insert from superior and lateral. These muscles are responsible for positioning the tongue in protrusion, retraction, elevation, and depression movements. By contraction of the digastric muscles (via the hyoid bone) and the muscular diaphragmatic floor, created by mylohyoid, along with the suprahyoid muscles, these extrinsic muscles elevate the tongue toward the base of the skull, lifting it high into the oral cavity.

The intrinsic musculature of the tongue is arranged in two bundles of interwoven fibers. One bundle runs across the entire length of the tongue and consists of the superior longitudinal and inferior longitudinal muscle fibers, while the other contributes to the main bulk of the tongue and consists of vertical and transverse fibers. The intrinsic muscles, partly assisted by extrinsic muscles, contract to produce changes in the shape of the tongue, critically important for articulation and swallowing.

The groove behind the row of circumvallate papillae or *sulcus terminalis* divides the tongue into an anterior two-thirds, mobile or oral tongue, and a posterior one-third or the base of the tongue, with bilateral lingual tonsils. The oral tongue is instrumental in the production of intelligible speech. Fine coordination of its contractions and movements helps to manipulate and propel the food bolus toward the pharynx during the oral phase of deglutition. The posterior part of the base of the tongue provides the driving force for initiation of the pharyngeal phase of deglutition. The tongue contributes to the critical function of airway protection by its strategic location in the oral cavity and the oropharynx, above the epiglottis, and also by providing dynamic laryngeal support via the geniohyoid to the mandible and via the styloglossus to the base of the skull.

The hypoglossal nerve provides motor innervation to both the intrinsic and extrinsic muscles except the palatoglossus muscle, which is innervated by the pharyngeal branch of the vagus nerve. General sensory supply from the oral tongue is mediated by the lingual nerve and from the posterior third of the tongue by the glossopharyngeal nerve. Special taste afferents from the oral tongue and the base of the tongue also travel to the central nervous system via the lingual nerve and the glossopharyngeal nerve, respectively.

The extraordinarily unique, multifunctional properties of the human tongue create a predicament following total glossectomy that is difficult to overcome.

Goals of Reconstruction

After total glossectomy, the defect extends from the nadir of the vallecula forward and superiorly to include the entire tongue and partial or entire floor of the mouth. The lingual and hypoglossal nerves are sacrificed bilaterally. This results in loss of articulation, oral preparatory and propulsive phases of deglutition, the piston-like action of the base of the tongue for initiation of the pharyngeal phase of deglutition, and the sense of taste. To date, no reconstructive technique has been able to restore the functions incorporated in the complex musculature of a normal tongue. The aim, however, is to create a neotongue that is capable of simulating such actions to an extent that confers, after appropriate rehabilitation, acceptable though modified function and quality of life. The specific objectives of reconstruction are to

- Provide laryngeal protection to minimize the risk of aspiration
- Achieve flap contact with the palate via appropriate tissue bulk and shape
- Facilitate articulation and mastication via suitable shape of the tip and dorsum
- Assist swallowing via passive mobility of the flap, driven by surrounding muscles
- Provide motor innervation for potential active flap contraction
- Provide sensory innervation, if possible

Latissimus Dorsi Free Flap

Described by Tansini in 1896, the latissimus dorsi flap enjoys the distinction of being the first musculocutaneous flap described in the medical literature. As a versatile perforator flap, Quillen first reported its use in head and neck reconstruction in 1978, followed by Watson who described its application as a microvascular free flap in 1979. Conventionally, longitudinally oriented latissimus dorsi flaps have been described for use in head and neck reconstruction. A modification of this conventional technique has been designed and adopted at our institution for total glossectomy reconstruction (Fig. 8.1).

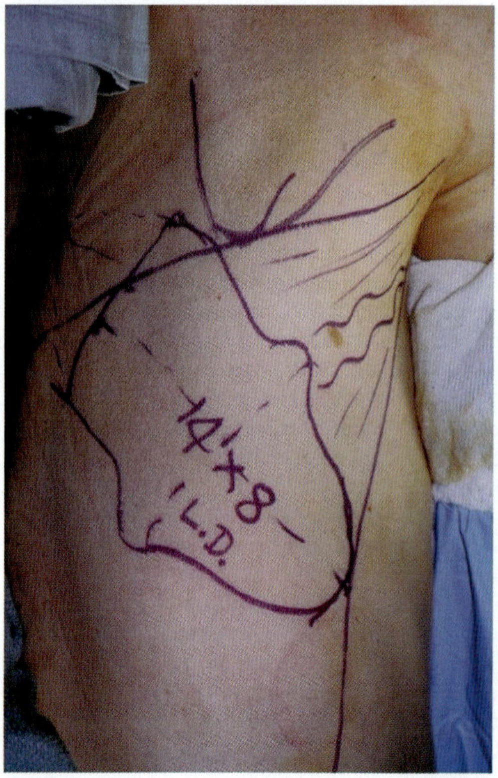

FIGURE 8.1
Design of a right latissimus dorsi musculocutaneous flap for total glossectomy reconstruction. The skin paddle is oriented perpendicular to the axis of the muscle fibers.

Anterolateral Thigh Free Flap

The perforator-based ALT free flap emerged as an option for skin and soft tissue reconstruction after Song et al. described it in 1984. The use of the ALT flap for reconstruction of defects in the head and neck was first reported by Koshima et al. in a cohort of 22 patients. It gained widespread popularity for application in the Asian population, and Wei et al. have described outcomes for 475 patients, the largest series for head and neck reconstruction with the ALT available to date. The reduced application of the ALT flap in the Western population is attributed to a higher incidence of obesity, which causes excess thickness of adipose tissue in the thigh. Furthermore, variability in the vascular anatomy predisposes to difficult dissection. However, experience and expertise acquired by the microvascular surgeons to harvest and thin the flap have rekindled the interest in the application of the ALT flap for reconstruction in the head and neck in many centers.

HISTORY

Evaluation of medical comorbidities is an important component of preoperative history for free tissue transfers since these procedures subject the patient to prolonged anesthesia and fluid imbalance. Hematologic or hepatorenal abnormalities merit a thorough preoperative investigation and correction since these may affect the intraoperative blood loss, postoperative hematoma formation, and thus, the viability of flap. Conditions such as diabetes and active smoking cause small vessel obliteration and are known risk factors for microvascular complications, and necessary measures should be taken to avoid any compromise of the microvascular anastomosis. Preoperative correction of nutritional deficits helps optimize the healing process. Cigarette smoking, administration of more than 7 L crystalloids (approximately 6 mL/kg/h), and weight loss of over 10% prior to surgery have been found to be significant for the overall flap complication rate in our analysis of cases with free tissue transfer.

PHYSICAL EXAMINATION

Assessment of the general body habitus and performance status of the patient is important for any free flap reconstruction to design a plan for harvest, donor site closure, and functional preservation. Furthermore, a complete examination of the head and neck by the microvascular surgeon with prediction of the probable surgical defect following total glossectomy, and careful examination of the donor site are critical in decision-making. Previous traumatic or surgical scars in the head and neck, skin cancer and radiation damage are important considerations in planning the placement of incisions for resection and protection of suitable recipient vessels. Examination of skin and soft tissue bulk, presence of scar, and presence or absence of arterial pulses (axillary, femoral) also influence selection of the donor site. For example, a large, previous thoracotomy incision may have traversed the latissimus dorsi muscle.

INDICATIONS

The latissimus dorsi flap provides suitable bulk and volume for true total glossectomy defects that include the entire base of tongue and oral tongue in the resection. It is also an ideal mode of reconstruction where there is an anticipated need for motor innervation. The ALT flap is more suitable for reconstruction of total oral glossectomy defects and is the flap of choice when a sensate reconstruction is planned. It is also a more conveniently accessed donor site.

CONTRAINDICATIONS

Latissimus Dorsi Flap

Congenital absence of latissimus muscle associated with Poland anomaly or other familial defects of the shoulder girdle is an absolute contraindication. Patients with a scar on their back or with a preexisting disability of the back or shoulder girdle do not make ideal candidates for reconstruction with the latissimus dorsi flap. It is also relatively contraindicated in patients with a history of previous surgery in the axilla due to the risk of possible disruption of the proximal vascular supply to the muscle.

Anterolateral Thigh Flap

Absence of musculofasciocutaneous perforators from the descending branch to the skin paddle is an absolute contraindication to this flap (see below, Pitfalls). Previous injury or surgery of the upper thigh such as vascular bypass procedures are relative contraindications for reconstruction with the ALT flap. Also, atherosclerotic superficial femoral arterial occlusion may result in substantial collateral flow through the profunda femoris and its branches to the distal lower limb. If such a situation pertains, the patient should be evaluated by a vascular surgeon before proceeding to harvest an ALT flap. The presence of a thick saddle bag of adipose tissue in the thigh makes such patients less than ideal candidates for ALT reconstruction because of the excess tissue bulk transferred to the recipient site.

PREOPERATIVE PLANNING

Fundamental to preoperative planning is a thorough knowledge of the anatomy of the donor site, which is critical to the flap harvest and reconstructive technique. Pertinent anatomic details of the latissimus dorsi and ALT flaps are discussed below.

Anatomy of the Latissimus Dorsi Free Flap

The latissimus dorsi muscle originates from the spinous processes of the lower six thoracic vertebrae, posterior iliac crest, the thoracolumbar fascia, last four ribs, and inferior angle of scapula. It inserts at the medial aspect of the intertubercular groove of the humerus. The dominant blood supply of the flap arises from the thoracodorsal artery, which is one of the two branches of the subscapular artery. The latter is the largest branch of the axillary artery and originates from its third part, gives rise to the circumflex scapular artery before continuing as thoracodorsal artery. The thoracodorsal artery enters the upper border of the latissimus dorsi and divides within the muscle into superior and lateral branches. It also gives a branch to the serratus anterior muscle that needs to be ligated during flap harvest. In its inferior half, the muscle receives perforators from the thoracic intercostal and lumbar arteries. The overlying skin is nourished by multiple musculocutaneous perforators that are more abundant over the upper two-thirds of the muscle, making it the preferred site for harvest of the skin paddle.

Venous drainage of the muscle is via the venae comitantes that accompany the thoracodorsal artery during their course along the undersurface of the latissimus dorsi muscle, draining to the axillary vein. The artery may vary in diameter from 1 to 4 mm, and the diameter of the vein may range from 2.5 to 4.5 mm. The motor innervation to the latissimus dorsi is provided by the thoracodorsal nerve (middle subscapular nerve), derived from the posterior cord of the brachial plexus (C6, C7, and C8). The nerve travels distally with the vascular pedicle, but closer to the vein.

Anatomy of the Anterolateral Thigh Flap

For reconstruction following a total glossectomy, the ALT flap is usually harvested as either a perforator-based myocutaneous flap including portions of vastus lateralis muscle or a fasciocutaneous flap (Fig. 8.2).

Fascial and Muscular Anatomy

The superficial fascia of the thigh forms a continuous layer over the thigh and consists of areolar tissue. It may be separated into two or more layers, between which are found the superficial vessels and nerves. The deep fascia of the thigh, the *fascia lata*, varies in thickness in different parts, being thicker in the superior and lateral aspect of the thigh. The muscles encountered during ALT flap harvest include the rectus femoris, vastus lateralis, and the tensor fascia lata. The rectus femoris arises from two tendons: one from the anterior inferior iliac spine and the other from the acetabulum. It occupies the middle of the front of the thigh and ends into a flattened tendon that inserts into the superior patella. The vastus lateralis is the largest part of the quadriceps femoris. It arises by a broad aponeurosis attached mainly to the superior part of the intertrochanteric line and to the anterior and inferior borders of the greater trochanter. The fibers run inferiorly over the lateral side of the thigh and thicken into a flat tendon for insertion into the lateral border of the patella. The tensor fascia lata occupies the lateral border of the thigh. It arises from the posterior part of the iliac crest, anterior superior iliac spine, and the deep surface of the *fascia lata* and gets inserted between the two layers of the *fascia lata* close to the junction of the middle and upper thirds of the thigh.

Vascular Anatomy

The ALT flap is based on the perforating vessels arising from the descending branch of the lateral circumflex femoral artery (LCFA). The LCFA is a branch of the profunda femoris artery and divides into ascending, descending, and transverse branches. The descending branch of LCFA is usually associated with two venae comitantes. It travels obliquely and inferiorly in the intermuscular groove between the rectus femoris and vastus lateralis along with the nerve to the vastus lateralis and terminates in the vastus lateralis just above the knee. The descending branch provides several perforators to the skin of the lateral thigh. These vessels pass in either a septocutaneous or myocutaneous pattern. The septocutaneous perforators run between the rectus femoris and vastus lateralis muscles and traverse the fascia lata to supply the skin of the lateral thigh as *septocutaneous* perforators. Alternatively, the perforators can traverse the vastus lateralis muscle tissue and the deep fascia and supply the skin as *musculocutaneous* perforators.

Septocutaneous perforators are highly inconsistent in their number and origin. The proportion of septocutaneous (vs. musculocutaneous perforators) varies from 10% to 60% across different clinical and cadaveric

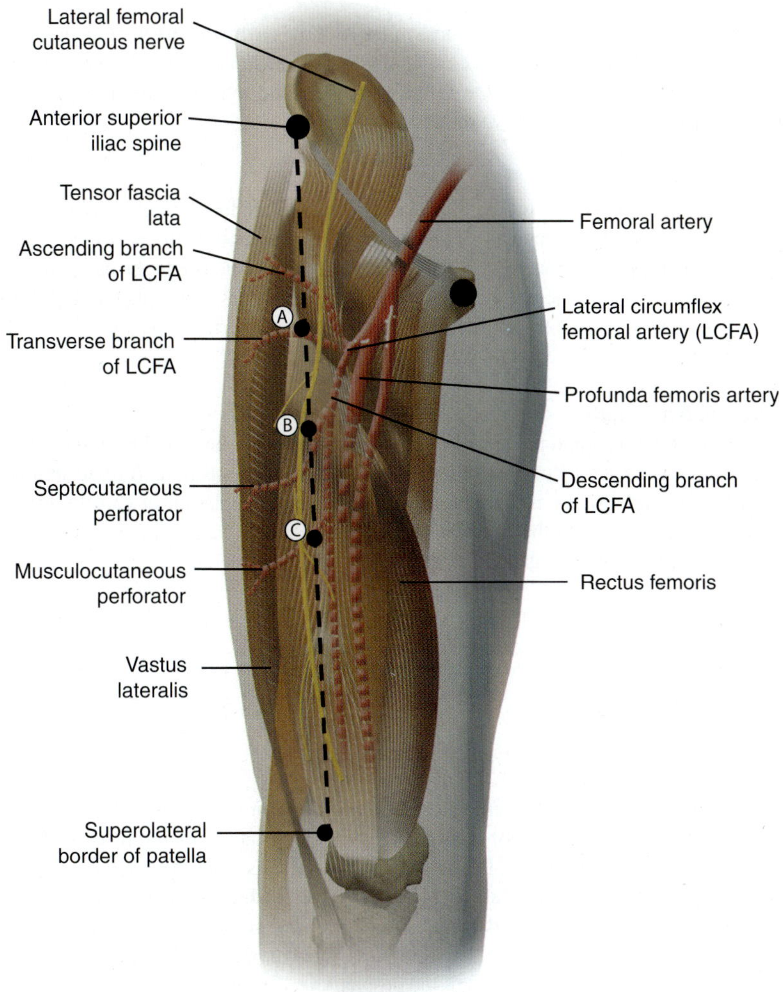

FIGURE 8.2
Anatomy of a right ALT flap. *Black line* represents the intermuscular septum between rectus femoris and vastus lateralis. A, B, and C represent the likely location for proximal, middle (most common), and distal perforators, typically separated by 5 cm. LCFA, lateral circumflex femoral artery.

studies. By contrast, musculocutaneous perforators are more constant, present in 50% to 90% of cases. This variation in vascular anatomy is important to know since elevation of the ALT flap requires meticulous intramuscular dissection for preservation of musculocutaneous perforators.

The average diameters of the vascular pedicle are reported to be 2.1 mm for the artery and 2.6 mm for the vein. These measurements may, however, range from 1.5 to 4 mm and from 1.5 to 5.0 mm, respectively, for the artery and the vein.

Classification of the Perforators

The perforators have been classified by Yu et al. for better identification during flap harvest.

1. *Classification Based on the Pattern of Location:* The cutaneous perforators are usually concentrated within a radius of about 3 cm around the midpoint of the line between the anterior superior iliac spine and superolateral patella. However, more perforators have been discovered that are spread over a larger part of the ALT flap. These are usually present in predictable locations about 5 cm apart and have been named as perforators A (most proximal), B (middle), and C (most distal); Perforators B are present most consistently.
2. *Classification Based on the Origin:* The cutaneous perforators have been classified as types I, II, and III based on their origin from the parent artery.

   Type I: This is the most common type in which perforators originate from the descending branch of the lateral circumflex femoris artery and travel as septocutaneous or musculocutaneous perforators.

   Type II: A single cutaneous perforator derives from the transverse branch of the lateral circumflex femoris artery and travels longitudinally within the vastus lateralis muscle for its entire length before it enters the fasciocutaneous flap.

   Type III: A single perforator derives directly from the profunda femoris artery and pierces through the rectus femoris muscle to reach the fasciocutaneous flap.

Sensory Innervation

The lateral femoral cutaneous nerve is the dominant sensory nerve of the ALT. It is a direct branch of the lumbar plexus (L2, L3) and enters the thigh deep to the lateral aspect of the inguinal ligament near the anterior superior iliac spine. It consistently runs along the line connecting the anterior superior iliac spine and the superolateral patella in the deep subcutaneous tissue immediately above the fascia.

Nerve to the Vastus Lateralis Muscle

The nerve innervating the vastus lateralis muscle is intimately related to the descending branch of the lateral circumflex artery. Two particular variations of the anatomy of the nerve make it susceptible to interruption during harvesting of the ALT flap, thus increasing the risk of denervation of the muscle: One where the motor nerve courses through the vascular pedicle or another where it travels between the perforators supplying the flap. The frequency of the presence of at least one of these unfavorable variations had been reported to be 28% in one of the anatomical studies. However, denervation of the vastus lateralis appears to cause little or no functional loss.

Assessment of Recipient Vessel Availability

Evaluation of the history of previous treatment and physical examination of the entire head and neck will alert the reconstructive surgeon, especially in the setting of previous radiotherapy or neck dissection, to vessel abnormalities. Doppler ultrasonography or angiography in patients with known vessel depletion or carotid artery disease may be required to assess the adequacy of the external carotid artery and its branches for selection of an appropriate recipient vessel for microvascular anastomosis.

SURGICAL TECHNIQUE

Latissimus Dorsi Free Flap

Flap Design

The unique features of my latissimus dorsi flap design include transverse orientation of the skin paddle, demarcation of the skin paddle into two portions—one anterior and another posterior—incorporation of two lateral skin and muscle "wings" (Fig. 8.3), and incorporation of the motor nerve to the latissimus dorsi muscle.

The flap is fashioned in a way so that the musculature forms a transverse sling or "hammock" across the floor of the mouth, and the skin is sufficiently redundant so as to be sculpted vertically at the front of the mouth for articulation. The longitudinal dimensions of the flap allow adequate curvature and suspension of the midportion of the skin and muscle component at the isthmus of the oropharynx. This design facilitates creation

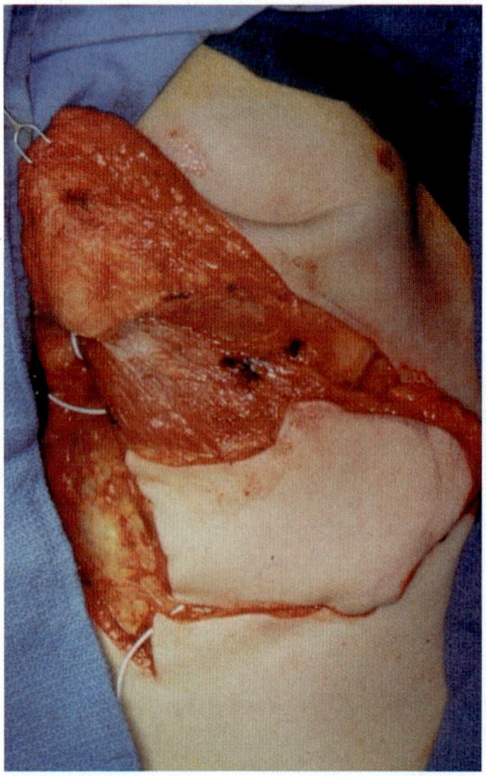

FIGURE 8.3
Right latissimus dorsi free flap harvest. Two silk marker sutures placed on the sides of the muscle component to reference the in situ length–tension relationship.

of oral and pharyngeal portions of the skin paddle that partially simulate oral tongue and the base of tongue, respectively, in structure and function.

Flap Harvest

Harvesting of the latissimus dorsi flap requires a lateral decubitus and a 45-degree shoulder and trunk up position. By rotating the table toward the donor site, resection is facilitated and by rotating the table away from the donor site, harvest is facilitated. This avoids repositioning the patient during the procedure.

Prior to harvesting the flap, using the Doppler flowmeter, the course of the thoracodorsal artery may be marked from its origin from the subscapular artery to the point where it enters the muscle. The skin paddle is carefully marked on the back at the site of flap harvest. The axis of the skin paddle is oriented at a right angle to the underlying muscle fiber axis. The length of the skin paddle equals the distance measured from the anterior floor of the mouth or the mandibular arch, curving superiorly to the palate, and proceeding to the posterior aspect of the defect. The posterior end of the defect is usually the nadir of the vallecula. In cases requiring supraglottic laryngectomy, it may be either the base of the epiglottis or the anterior commissure. The curvilinear transverse dimensions of the flap may be approximated by measuring the width of the mandibular arch and multiplying by $(\pi \times d)/2$, π assuming that the flap will be shaped as a semicircle in the mouth, to resemble the contour of dorsum of oral tongue. Alternatively, for measuring the transverse dimensions, a flexible ruler curved to the desired shape and position of the flap in contact with the hard palate may also be used.

For flap harvest, once scribed on the back, an incision is first made across the anterolateral aspect of the skin paddle, extended superiorly and follows the lateral free border of the muscle into the axilla. Here, the neurovascular pedicle is identified by blunt dissection through the axillary fascia and adipose tissue. Incisions are made on the inferior, medial, and superior aspects of the paddle down to the fascia of the latissimus dorsi muscle. Tacking sutures are then placed between the skin and underlying muscle. The musculature is sharply transected at the distal end of the flap and around the margins of the flap medially and laterally. The neurovascular pedicle is identified entering the muscle on its deep surface underneath, at the lateral border of the muscle, approximately 8 to 10 cm from the midpoint of the axilla. At this stage, two silk marker sutures may be placed across the muscle at a measured distance apart (8 to 10 cm) to allow accurate recreation of the resting length of muscle at inset (Fig. 8.3). The pedicle is dissected and traced into the axilla up to the origin point of the circumflex scapular artery. This requires ligation and division of the artery to the serratus anterior. Finally, the muscle is transected superiorly while carefully preserving the vascular pedicle that is later divided distal to the takeoff of the circumflex scapular artery from the subscapular artery (Fig. 8.4). The free flap is harvested with an intact motor nerve to latissimus dorsi (middle subscapular nerve or long scapular nerve) that is released sharply from its origin at the brachial plexus. The flap can be made sensate by harvesting an intercostal nerve from the chest.

In total glossectomy defects with mandibular resection, the flap may be harvested with the lateral scapular border or the tenth or eleventh rib. These provide a source of vascularized bone for reconstruction of the mandibular ramus in the same surgical sitting.

Closure of the Donor Site. Hemostasis is secured, and suction drains are inserted. The reapposition of the skin edges of the wound defect at the donor site on the back is usually accomplished as a three-limbed closure, resembling a Y shape (Fig. 8.5). Interrupted deep 2-0 sutures are followed by skin closure. Tension is avoided at the skin level of the donor site defect, to prevent wound dehiscence.

Flap Inset

After the recipient vessels are skeletonized and prepared in the neck, the pedicle is detached, and the flap is brought to the neck for performing the microvascular anastomosis. Once the arterial and venous anastomosis is completed and excellent flow is ensured, the nerve graft to the latissimus dorsi is brought into the field. It is anastomosed to the hypoglossal nerve on the side ipsilateral to the microvascular anastomosis. The nerve anastomosis is performed by end-to-end epineural neurorrhaphy using three to four 9-0 nylon sutures. This

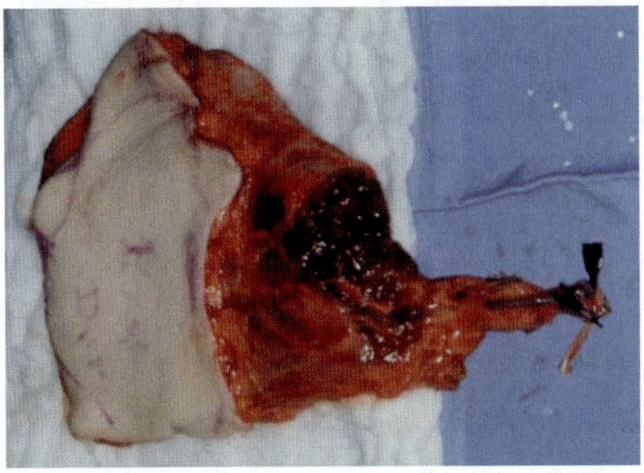

FIGURE 8.4
Latissimus dorsi flap harvested with the musculocutaneous component, vascular pedicle, and thoracodorsal nerve exiting to the right.

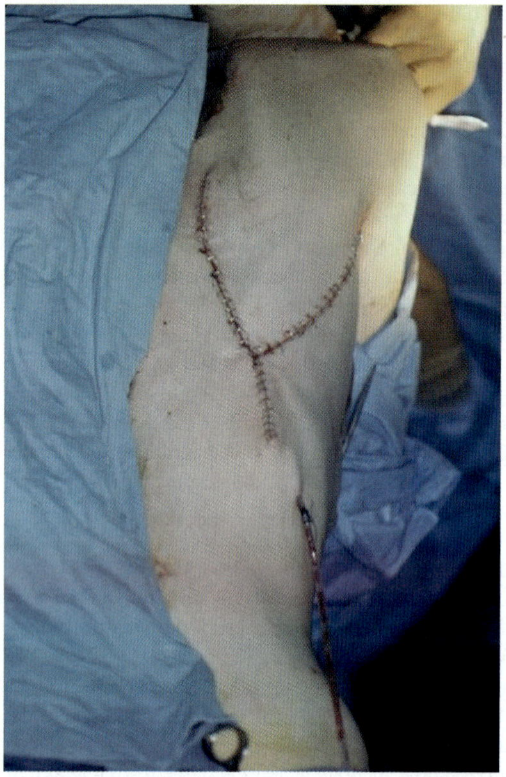

FIGURE 8.5
Three-limbed Y-shaped closure of the donor site after latissimus dorsi flap harvest on the right.

procedure potentially confers to the neotongue, the ability to elevate superiorly toward the palate thus facilitating better swallowing rehabilitation. Occasionally, an interposition nerve graft harvested from the greater auricular or sural nerve may be needed to bridge the distance between the donor nerve and the recipient hypoglossal nerve.

For flap reconstruction, access to the oral cavity and the oropharynx is available from a stepped mandibular osteotomy or a pull-through approach via the neck created by the oncologic resection. During the flap inset, the paddle is rotated such that the skin is oriented with its long axis parallel to the midline. The contouring of the flap tissue is accomplished with a series of suturing and multidimensional folding maneuvers in order to reconstruct the tip and body of the neotongue.

The distal margins of the flap are sutured across the anterior edge of the remnant of the base of the tongue, the mucosa of the vallecula, or the base of the epiglottis. Suturing of the flap to the region of the base of the epiglottis is recommended since it allows for normal downward folding movements during deglutition. Posterolaterally, the flap is sutured to the left and right pharyngeal walls. The two wings of skin and muscle, incorporated at the midpoint of the flap, are set into the tonsil fossae. The direct suturing of the muscle flap to the recipient site muscle may require a tonsillectomy. The muscle is inset as a transverse sling across the isthmus of the oropharynx by suturing it to the remnant of the medial pterygoid, masseter, or superior constrictor muscle depending on the availability (Fig. 8.6A). This maneuver creates an antigravity suspension of the flap from the left to the right skull base, and also a potentially dynamic reinnervated muscle sling to aid in uplifting the flap with swallowing efforts.

In the mouth, the flap is sutured laterally to the alveolar ridges and the cut edges of the mucosa of the floor of the mouth, from posterior to anterior, using an advancement technique. Redundant flap tissue in the anterior midline is elevated superiorly with a skin hook, and the unattached margins of the flap are sutured vertically in the midline. This maneuver helps create a glossomandibular sulcus and a *cupula* of tissue in the anterior aspect of the flap in order to raise the tissue superiorly, for neotongue-to-hard palate contact. Two suspension sutures are placed between the flap tissue and the hard palate to enable correct positioning of the tissue. The anterior flap epithelium is thereafter, de-epithelialized, imbricated, and the margins of the de-epithelialized segment are approximated together with 3-0 Vicryl to create the neotongue tip (Fig. 8.6B). This maneuver traps a core of dermis, which helps in providing bulk and stiffening of the tip (Fig. 8.7).

Finally, the anterior aspect of the floor of the mouth mucosa is closed with 3-0 Vicryl sutures. The muscle flap is further anchored transversely across the floor of the mouth to the anterior digastric bellies if preserved (Fig. 8.8). This gives an excellent tightening of the anterior floor of the mouth component. The mandibular osteotomy is repaired by approximation of the mandibular segments with placement of a precontoured and predrilled reconstruction plate. The anterior belly of the digastric is also reattached to the mandible beneath the flap for reinforcing antigravity support.

Additional support for muscle flap bulk with a transverse Gore-Tex sling below the mandible from one angle to another is recommended to prevent gravitational prolapse of the flap from the oral cavity into the neck. Placement of a heavy monofilament suture between the hyoid bone or thyroid cartilage and anteriorly to the mandible can assist in swallowing and protection of the glottis.

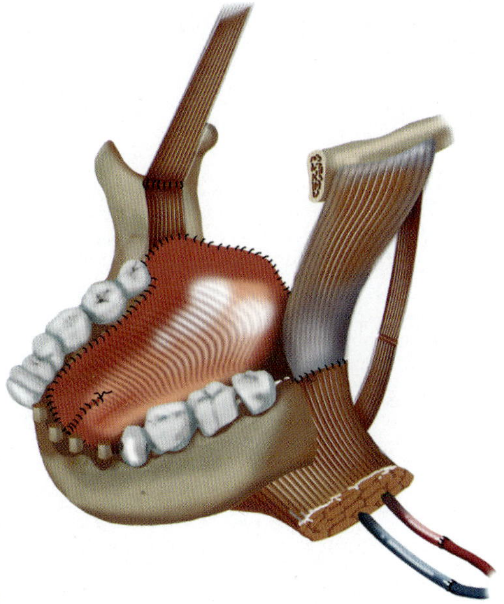

A

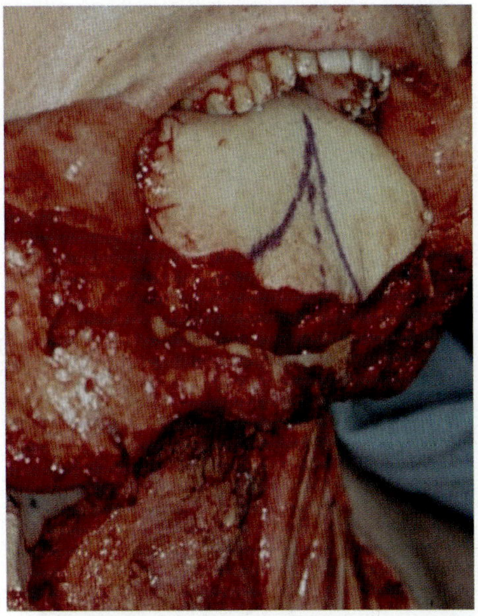

B

FIGURE 8.6 A. Latissimus dorsi free flap inset. Transverse sling created at oral–oropharyngeal isthmus by suturing of muscle flap to medial pterygoid and masseter muscle. **B.** Triangular wedge-shaped area marked anteriorly for de-epithelialization and imbrication for creation of neotongue tip.

Flap Inset After Total Glossectomy and Supraglottic Laryngectomy. In cases where a supraglottic laryngectomy has been performed with total glossectomy, the distal margins of the flap are sutured to the thyroid perichondrium and/or cartilage. Anterior suspension of the laryngeal remnant from the mandible with left and right 2-0 monofilament nylon suture is desirable since this maneuver tilts and transposes the glottis forward beneath the posterior flap and provides static support for minimization of aspiration during swallowing.

Anterolateral Thigh Flap

Flap Design

The intermuscular septum between the rectus femoris and the vastus lateralis muscle is marked by drawing a line between the anterior superior iliac spine and the superolateral border of the patella. The cutaneous perforators are mapped by use of a handheld Doppler probe. They are usually present around the midpoint of the line representing the intermuscular septum within a circle of 3 to 5 cm radius (Perforator B). Perforators A and C can be present at locations further from the midpoint as described earlier (Fig. 8.9).

After completion of the total glossectomy, the exact dimensions of the defect are measured to finalize the design of the flap. The flap is deliberately marked with its center located in the area with maximum number of cutaneous perforators. The long axis is kept parallel to the axis of the thigh. The skin paddle may be fashioned

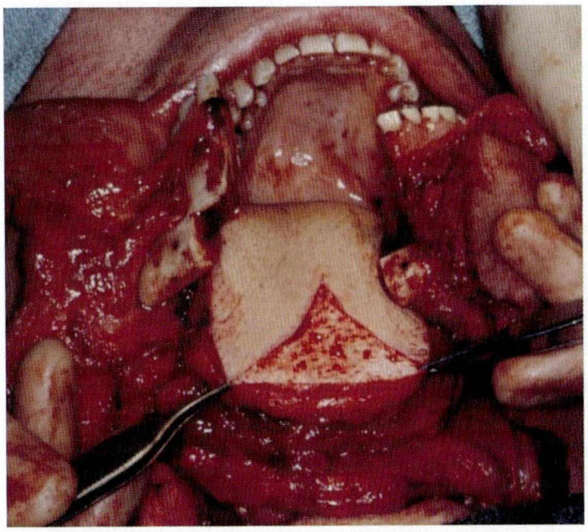

FIGURE 8.7
De-epithelialization of the anterior wedge.

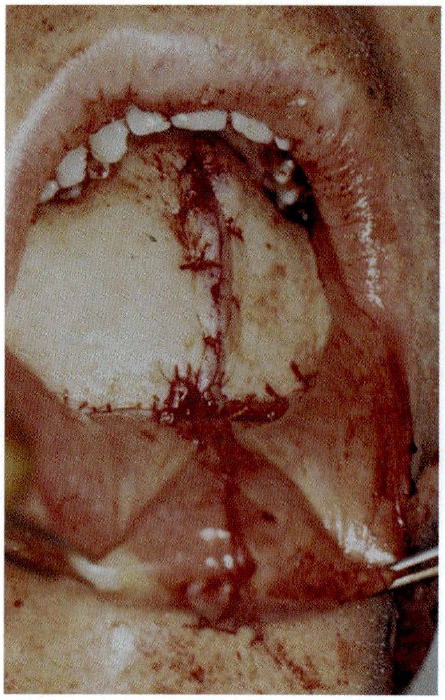

FIGURE 8.8
Margins of de-epithelialized segment sutured together to trap a core of dermis and create a "*cupula*" anteriorly for neo-tongue to hard palate contact.

to incorporate laterally, two wings of skin for suspension, similar to the technique described for the latissimus dorsi myocutaneous flap.

Flap Harvest

The remote location of the donor site from the head and neck defect allows adoption of the simultaneous two-team approach for flap harvest. Proper positioning of the leg facilitates dissection during harvest of the ALT free flap. The ideal position is with slight knee flexion and internal rotation at the hip. The skin incision is initially made on the anteromedial side of the marked skin paddle and is deepened until the fascia lata is reached. The incision is carried through the fascia lata, including it in the flap. Identification of the perforators to the skin requires blunt lateral mobilization of the flap. Once the vessels are located, the skin incisions are completed circumferentially. Subfascially, the dissection is continued toward the septum between the rectus femoris and the vastus lateralis muscles to explore whether the perforator is septocutaneous or myocutaneous. These are traced further proximally until the main pedicle is reached. The pedicle is located by continuing the dissection

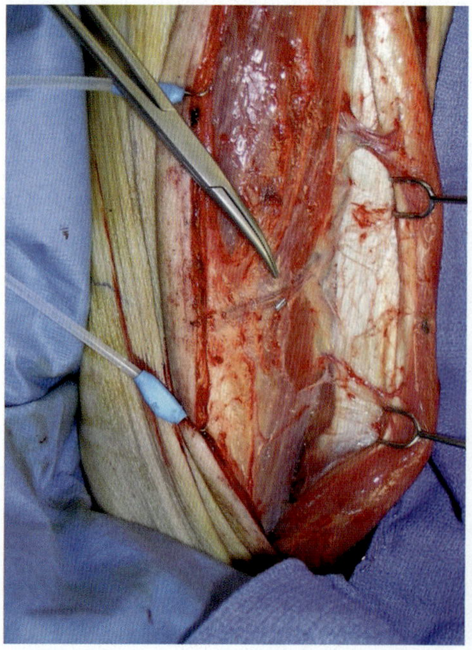

FIGURE 8.9
An intraoperative photograph showing identification of perforators during harvest of a left ALT flap.

between the rectus femoris and vastus lateralis muscles in patients with septocutaneous perforators and through the vastus lateralis muscle in patients with myocutaneous perforators.

The musculocutaneous perforator gives off small branches to the vastus lateralis muscle from the lateral and posterior sides of the vessel and rarely from the anterior aspect. Thus, the course of the perforator is traced by incising the muscle over the perforator followed by ligation of the branches to the muscle from lateral and posterior sides. The perforator is then traced to the descending branch of the LCFA and is further dissected proximally along the descending branch according to the pedicle requirement. A small cuff of muscle may be left around the perforators to facilitate the speed of the harvest.

Ligation of the transverse branch of the LCFA and the branch to the rectus femoris muscle can allow harvesting of a longer pedicle. This may be required for reaching the contralateral neck vessels, if due to previous surgery or irradiation, the ipsilateral neck lacks suitable vessels for anastomosis.

It is important to trace the perforator to the vessel of origin because occasionally, types II and III perforators may be encountered. Type II perforator requires a careful and tedious intramuscular dissection to free the perforator from the vastus lateralis for its entire length. The perforator originates from the transverse branch of the LCFA, and upon entering the muscle superiorly runs in an inferior direction necessitating dissection out of the muscle or extensive muscle harvest. The type III perforator runs to the skin through the rectus femoris and is thus anterior in location. It has both a small caliber and a short pedicle length. When faced with type III perforator, the plan to proceed further with flap harvest should be aborted in favor of other reconstructive options.

In the presence of myocutaneous perforators (the majority), portions of vastus lateralis muscle are included in the flap. It is preferable to elevate the flap such that the muscle is thicker proximally and thinner distally. The thicker portion at the base of the flap can be used to bulk the posterior part and dorsum of the neotongue, while the thinner end can be used to augment the tip. In order to make the flap sensate, the lateral femoral cutaneous nerve of the thigh may be harvested. The nerve is identified below the anterior superior iliac spine when the superior incision of the flap is made. It is possible to harvest an additional 5 cm of nerve by continuing the subcutaneous dissection proximal to the inguinal ligament.

Closure of the Donor Site. Hemostasis is secured, and the wound defect is closed after insertion of suction drain. The drain is carefully placed in the intermuscular space to avoid accumulation of fluid between muscle groups and in the subcutaneous space. In cases where intramuscular dissection has been done to identify the perforators, repair of the muscle segment by loose approximating stitches results in better preservation of function. The donor site can usually be closed primarily without requiring a skin graft. Primary closure of the donor site for a skin paddle as wide as 9 to 12 cm has been reported to be accomplished, but the use of a skin graft is generally recommended for defects exceeding 8 cm.

Flap Inset

Before insetting the flap, the subcutaneous component may require thinning, particularly in the obese patient. Reduction of bulk to the desired thickness requires meticulous dissection under magnification to identify the pattern of the perforators and avoid injuring them. The main perforator usually gives off a few branches that traverse suprafascially, deep in the adipose layer and then to the subdermal plexus. Identification of these branches precedes thinning of the flap. It is advised to preserve 2 mm of adipose tissue on the dermis to ensure that the subdermal plexus is not damaged. Thicker flaps are usually preferred for reconstruction following total glossectomy.

The microvascular anastomosis is carried out in the routine fashion followed by nerve anastomosis in patients undergoing a sensate flap reconstruction. Care should be taken to avoid twisting the pedicle while insetting the flap. The edges of the flap are sutured posteriorly and inferiorly to the base of the tongue or base of the epiglottis, depending on availability. Posterolaterally, the flap is sutured to the pharyngeal mucosa. The lateral skin and fascial processes, if incorporated in the flap design, are elevated and anchored into the tonsil fossae to provide antigravity support. Anteriorly, the edges of the flap are sutured to the gingival mucosa. Additional tissue on the flap may be de-epithelialized and folded beneath the skin paddle to reinforce the floor of the mouth reconstruction. However, in total glossectomy, optimum bulk of tissue is preserved during harvest to restore the height and volume of the neotongue.

Similar to my technique for latissimus dorsi flap inset, advancement sutures can be placed laterally between the edges of the flap and the gingival mucosa. This enables cupula formation anteriorly thus assisting with creation of the neotongue tip. Suture placement with 3-0 Vicryl preferably taking large bites and spacing at every 5 mm is recommended for watertight closure and better wound healing (Fig. 8.10).

A transverse Gore-Tex or preserved acellular cadaver dermis sling underneath the oral portion of flap and anchored to the mandible is useful to prevent tissue sagging. Gore-Tex is biologically well tolerated, although there is concern for possible infection or soft tissue reaction, alternatively acellular cadaveric skin graft may be used. When acellular cadaveric dermis is chosen, it is less rigid and more elastic compared to Gore-Tex. Laryngeal suspension from the mandible with sutures between the hyoid and holes drilled on both sides of the mentum is performed after completion of the flap inset.

Flap Inset After Total Glossectomy of the Oral (Anterior Two-Third) Tongue. In patients who undergo total oral glossectomy that includes no more than 1 cm of tongue base, the final steps of multidimensional folding

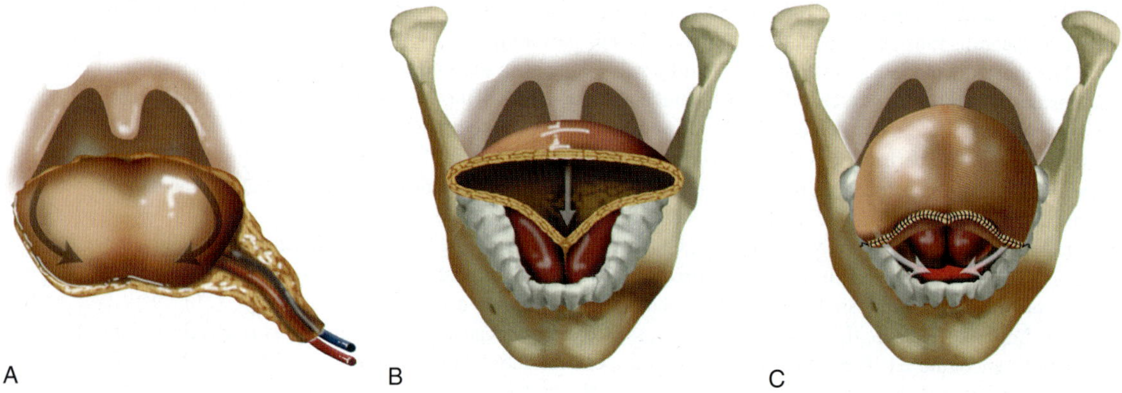

FIGURE 8.10 Multidimensional technique for ALT flap inset used for reconstruction of total *oral* glossectomy defect. **A.** The flap is laid in transversely and sutured bilaterally from posterior to anterior using advancement technique. **B.** Suturing the redundant anterior flap edges to each other vertically in the midline creates anterior neotongue height. The midline of the remaining superior free margin is anchored to the vertical suture line to form a three-point junction. *Arrows* indicate the direction of tissue displacement.
C. Fashioning of right- and left-sided, anterolaterally directed cones that are de-epithelialized (stippled area) and sutured together in the midline thus creating a neotongue. *Curved arrows* indicate arc of rotation of flap corners, to be sutured together in the midline following de-epithelialization.

technique are modified for recreation of the tip of the new oral tongue. After posterior inset across the tongue base and after ensuring adequate height for flap to palate contact, the midline anterior free edge of the skin paddle is depressed inferiorly to create a three-point junction. The right and left corners are sutured onto themselves to form anterolaterally directed cones. These cones are de-epithelialized, swung anteriorly, and sutured together in midline, thus entrapping dermis to stiffen and confer some bulk to the neotongue tip (Fig. 8.8).

POSTOPERATIVE MANAGEMENT

The patient is cared for in an observational unit and preferably kept sedated for 2 to 3 days to avoid neck movement–related shearing stresses on the microvascular anastomoses. Vigilant monitoring of the vital signs, flap viability, nutritional status, and the donor site is essential along with care of the tracheostomy tube and donor site wounds. Donor sites are managed with negative pressure drains and the neck with passive drains.

In patients with latissimus dorsi flap reconstruction, the arm is abducted and flexed often with pillows, to avoid any undue stretch or tension on the donor site wound repair. For tracheostomy management and dietary resumption see "Results."

COMPLICATIONS

The early complications at the recipient site may include anastomotic occlusion, more commonly venous, leading to flap loss. Secondary hemorrhage, infection and, occasionally, wound breakdown and fistula formation may also occur.

Latissimus Dorsi Free Flap

At the donor site, hematoma and wound dehiscence may occur as early complications. The large area of tissue dissection may precipitate late seroma formation. This can be prevented by placing deep tacking sutures between the back skin flaps and the rib cage, pressure dressings, and maintenance of functional suction drains. Inadvertent injury on the lateral chest wall to the long thoracic nerve of Bell may result in "winged scapula."

Anterolateral Thigh Flap

The ALT flap is considered by some to be more prone to venous occlusion or compression of the pedicle, but this is probably due to dissection of small intramuscular perforators versus leaving a more generous muscle cuff. Under these circumstances, loss of the flap due to compression of the muscular perforator may be avoided by reexploration and release of wound pressure. For small caliber perforators, inclusion of the muscle cuff around the vessel is recommended. As with other fasciocutaneous flaps, marginal necrosis may occur in cases where there has been excessive thinning.

Complications at the donor site are reported to be infrequent but include pain and functional morbidity. Extensive fascial elevation of the flap is believed to contribute to prolonged muscular weakness and fatigue.

A higher incidence of complications has been demonstrated to correlate with extent of injury to the vastus lateralis and the need for a skin graft when larger flaps are used. In order to avoid the use of a skin graft, a V–Y perforator–based advancement flap has also been described. The quadriceps femoris muscle is largely composed of the vastus lateralis muscle fibers, and injury of the nerve to the vastus lateralis may compromise the quadriceps function. Quadriceps muscle testing has demonstrated significant deficits in motor function and motion of the range of the knee after flap harvest with an abnormality in gait analyses. A careful knowledge of nerve anatomy and possible variations along with complete skeletonization of the pedicle is believed to preserve the muscle. However, in some cases, the ALT flap cannot be harvested without sacrifice of the nerve.

Seroma formation may occur as in the postoperative period and can be prevented by placement of large bore suction drains. Delayed healing is possible, and contour deformity is customary but mild and easily concealed.

RESULTS

Latissimus Dorsi Flap

The latissimus dorsi myocutaneous free flap provides a large bulk of tissue for neotongue formation with limited donor site functional or cosmetic morbidity. The decrease in the muscle's functions in adduction of the arm, extension, or medial rotation is not a source of significant compromise in the arm movement in the presence of active shoulder girdle muscles. The donor site can usually be closed primarily and does not usually require a skin graft.

The muscle flap provides a reliable and good caliber vascular pedicle with constant anatomical relationships. It can be harvested with portions of rib or scapula for bony reconstruction. The flap can be made sensate and when harvested with its motor nerve can potentially be made to contract for better functional results. Patients are usually decannulated 2 to 3 weeks following surgery, and muscle tissue bulk minimizes the risk of fistula formation. Swallowing rehabilitation can begin soon after decannulation.

In our institutional review of eleven tongue reconstructions with microvascular latissimus dorsi myocutaneous free tissue transfers, one flap failure occurred. Acceptable rates of restoration to oral alimentation, speech intelligibility, and decannulation were observed. Vertical movement of the flap, possibly attributed to successful reinnervation of the latissimus muscle, and initiated voluntarily by the patient, has been documented by video-oropharyngography.

Anterolateral Thigh Flap

The ALT flap is pliable and conforms appropriately to the three-dimensional defect in the oral cavity and oropharynx subsequent to total glossectomy. When endowed with sufficient adipose tissue, it fills the oral cavity and pharynx well enough to provide surface-to-surface contact for swallowing (Fig. 8.11). It offers the

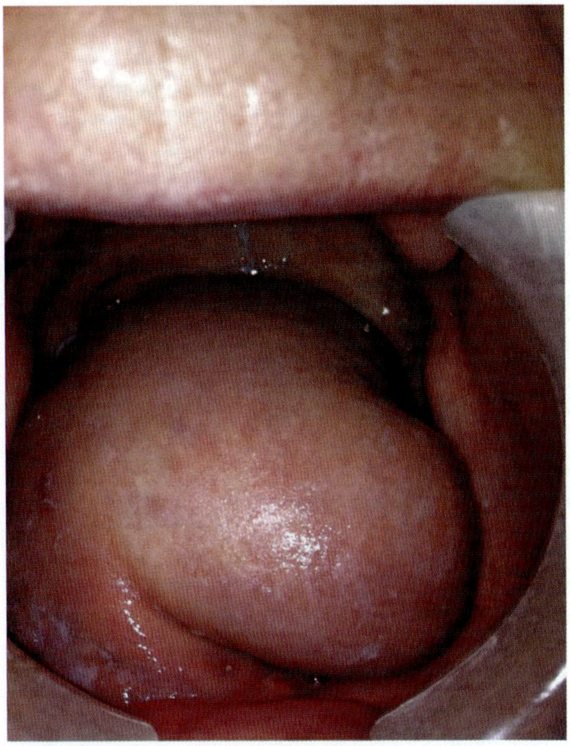

FIGURE 8.11
Neotongue following ALT reconstruction 2 months postoperatively.

advantage of having good caliber vessels and a medium length pedicle. It also has the potential of being used as a sensate flap that has been associated with a higher degree of patient satisfaction; however, the sensory recovery of the neotongue has not been demonstrated to directly translate into better speech and swallowing function.

PEARLS

- Latissimus dorsi free flap: The key to a successful latissimus dorsi free flap reconstruction for total glossectomy includes the following:
  - Preoperative surface marking of the lateral border of the latissimus dorsi is recommended (Fig. 8.2). The muscle contour is palpated and marked after arm elevation. This is important for correct positioning of the skin paddle.
  - Proximal positioning of the donor area avoids a long pedicle (Fig. 8.2). This obviates harvest of excessive muscle and prevents a cumbersome flap inset at the recipient site.
  - The length–tension relationship of muscle can be optimized by careful reinstatement of the resting length of the latissimus dorsi fibers in the recipient site. Failure of muscle contraction will occur if this principle is ignored, that is, shortening the fibers to less than the resting length inhibits adequate contraction. Measured suture placement on the back (Fig. 8.3) at the level of the intended oropharyngeal sling before harvest accomplishes this goal.
- ALT free flap: Dissection and preservation of at least one intact perforator from the lateral circumflex artery to the skin is required to maintain the viability of the flap. To achieve this, along with an adequate knowledge of the perforator anatomy and possible variations, the following keys are helpful.
  - Make the first aspect of the incision on the anterior skin paddle border and proceed in the subfascial plane posteriorly with careful blunt dissection to search for the perforators. Infrequently, anomalous anatomy may be encountered, and search for perforators may need to be directed anteriorly from the groove between the rectus femoris muscle and the vastus lateralis. The skin paddle is accordingly redesigned medial to the incision.
  - Confirm the course of the musculocutaneous perforators in the vastus lateralis muscle by incising the muscle just superficial to the perforators to ensure safe dissection. Maintain 5 mm of muscle on either side of the perforator.
  - In septocutaneous perforators, preservation of a small cuff of fascia around the perforator and intermittent topical use of Xylocaine assist safe dissection.

PITFALLS

- Latissimus dorsi free flap
  - Adequate exposure of the harvest site near the midline of the back requires careful lateral positioning and prepping of the patient.
  - Additional assistance is required for controlling the position of the arm to facilitate appropriate access. In the obese patient, presence of excessive axillary adipose can make identification of the vascular pedicle tedious, requiring a greater depth of dissection and substantial retraction of soft tissue. Prolapsed tissue may be hazardous, obscuring the pedicle, leading to inadvertent damage before identification.
  - The overall flap thickness may limit maneuverability and sculpting of the tissue in situ.
- ALT free flap
  - Dissection of the vascular pedicle poses a major challenge during ALT flap harvest because of the anatomical variability both in origin and course of the perforators supplying the flap. Presence of type II perforator is rare (about 4%) but, when present, may complicate the dissection.
  - Absence of cutaneous perforators on which the flap needs to be based has been reported in up to 5% of cases. In addition to the perforators, the course of the descending branch of the lateral circumflex artery may also vary. Occasionally, it is buried inside the vastus lateralis or is absent. When faced with a situation of unsuitable vascular anatomy, the surgeon should be prepared to abandon the flap and either explore the contralateral thigh or employ an alternative donor site.
  - In the Western population, another source of problem in dissection of vascular pedicle arises from the usually ill-defined septum between the vastus lateralis and rectus femoris muscles. Its presence is indicated by only a line of adipose tissue. Absence of its identification obscures an important landmark because mostly, all reliable perforators are located lateral to the septum.
  - Presence of excessive subcutaneous adipose tissue makes the dissection cumbersome and also creates difficulty in handling the bulky flap during inset.

INSTRUMENTS TO HAVE AVAILABLE

- Standard head and neck surgical set
- Microvascular surgery instruments

ACKNOWLEDGMENT

I gratefully acknowledge the contributions of Parul Sinha.

SUGGESTED READING

Song YG, Chen GZ, Song YL. The free thigh flap: a new free flap concept based on the septocutaneous artery. *Br J Plast Surg* 1984;37:149–159.

Haughey BH, Fredrickson JM. The latissimus dorsi donor site. Current use in head and neck reconstruction. *Arch Otolaryngol Head Neck Surg* 1991;117:1129–1134.

Haughey BH. Tongue reconstruction: concepts and practice. *Laryngoscope* 1993;103:1132–1141.

Koshima I, Fukuda H, Yamamoto H, et al. Free anterolateral thigh flaps for reconstruction of head and neck defects. *Plast Reconstr Surg* 1993;92:421–428, discussion 429–430.

Wei FC, Jain V, Ortho MC, et al. Have we found an ideal soft-tissue flap? An experience with 672 anterolateral thigh flaps. *Plast Reconstr Surg* 2002;109:2219–2226.

9 MANAGEMENT OF THE SOFT PALATE DEFECT

Eric J. Moore

INTRODUCTION

Defects involving the soft palate are usually the by-products of ablative surgery for squamous cell carcinoma of the tonsil fossa or the mucosal lining of the soft palate, during ablative surgery for minor salivary gland neoplasms, or less commonly from posttraumatic, iatrogenic, or congenital defects. The soft palate plays a critical role in velopharyngeal closure during speech and swallowing, and the success of reconstruction of the soft palate defect is judged primarily on the ability to adequately obliterate the velopharyngeal opening on the side of the defect while maintaining free mobility of the remaining functional soft palate.

Small defects of the soft palate and tonsil fossa can be left to heal by second intention or be closed primarily. The distensibility of the soft palate tissues and the excellent vascularity usually result in a successful outcome with either of these options. However, larger defects, particularly those involving more than 50% of the soft palate or those that communicate with the neck will require reconstruction. While regional pedicled flaps and microvascular free flaps have been employed frequently for large defects of the oropharynx, an intermediate level of defect that is too large to close primarily but does not cross the midline extensively can be reconstructed with the use of local pedicle flaps. There are many random and local pedicle flaps that have been described to close defects of the palate. Many of these have applications in primary or secondary closure of cleft palate defects, and they have been adapted for use in reconstruction of oncologic defects of the soft palate. The following section describes the use of the three local pedicle flaps that can be used to close defects of the soft palate: The buccal adipose tissue pad flap, the inferiorly based facial artery musculomucosal (FAMM) flap, and the reverse facial–submental artery island flap. Familiarity with these flaps will allow the surgeon to close intermediate-size defects in the oropharynx without the complexity of creating a separate donor site in a more distant area of the body.

HISTORY

I take a routine history from the patient and focus on determining if the patient has a history of infection, bleeding, an oral mucosal disease, or surgery or radiation of the oral mucosa that may represent a contraindication to reconstruction using a local flap. I am also careful to note that a history of active smoking can impact flap survival. This is particularly true of random flaps.

PHYSICAL EXAMINATION

The physical examination should include a careful surveillance of the oral cavity and the defect in order to ensure that a local flap is an appropriate reconstructive option. Additionally, I like to inspect the donor site and determine if prior surgery or scar in the area may preclude or complicate the surgical reconstruction.

INDICATIONS

Buccal Adipose Tissue Pad

The use of the buccal adipose tissue pad as a pedicle flap was first described by Egyedi in 1977. He advocated its use for closure of oroantral and oronasal fistulae. In that description, a split-thickness skin graft was placed on the oral side, but later descriptions recognized the skin graft as unnecessary since the flap rapidly mucosalizes when placed into the oral cavity. The buccal adipose tissue pad is described as a central body at the posterior maxilla and upper buccinator with four extensions: buccal, pterygoid, superficial, and deep temporal. The adipose tissue pad is prodigious in infants and supports the cheeks during sucking. In adults, it serves to aid in sliding of the masticatory muscles from themselves and the zygomatic arch and mandibular ramus. It is relatively conserved in adults, even in the setting of cachexia. The buccal adipose tissue pad is amply supplied with blood from the maxillary artery, the superficial temporal artery, and the facial artery. It is thinly encapsulated, and the capsule should be preserved with flap harvest to aid in epithelialization and to prevent devascularization. Although the pterygoid extension between the pterygoid musculature and mandibular ramus can be mobilized with flap elevation, mainly the buccal portion is used in reconstruction of the palate.

Facial Artery Musculomucosal Flap

Random buccal flaps have been used for decades to close soft palate defects. Pribaz in 1991 combined the knowledge of random buccal flaps, musculomucosal buccal flaps, and pedicled melolabial flaps to describe an axial buccal flap based on the facial artery that he called the FAMM flap. The added vascularity and the thicker tissue that is transferred with this flap compared to random buccal mucosal flaps make it a versatile local tissue flap to augment oral cavity and oropharyngeal defects.

The buccinator muscle lies just under the mucosa and submucosa of the buccal area. Lateral to the buccinator muscle lie the buccal adipose tissue pad, masseter muscle, ramus of the mandible, buccopharyngeal fascia, terminal buccal branch of the facial nerve, and facial artery and vein. The buccinator is supplied with blood from the buccal artery and branches of the facial artery. Abundant venous drainage flows to the internal maxillary veins and pterygoid plexus posteriorly and to the facial vein anteriorly. After the facial artery crosses the mandible, it runs a tortuous course around the oral commissure under the risorius, zygomaticus major, and lateral orbicularis oris muscles. The artery lies lateral to the buccinator and levator anguli oris muscle. It gives rise to an inferior and superior labial artery that lie medial to the lateral orbicularis oris muscle. The artery continues superiorly as the angular artery. Because of the rich anastomoses between the left and right facial artery and internal maxillary branches, the FAMM flap can be based inferiorly (anterograde) off the more proximal facial artery or superiorly (retrograde) off the distal facial artery. The inferiorly based FAMM flap is favorable for defects of the soft palate, as the pedicle can lie posterior to the maxillary tuberosity and molar teeth (see Fig. 9.1).

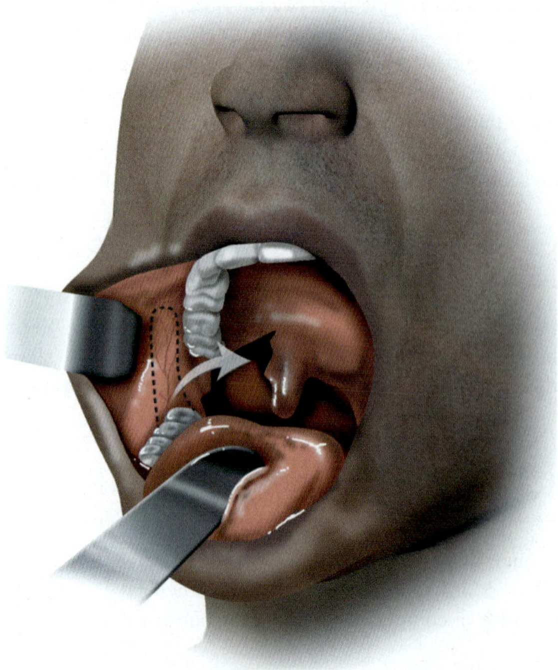

FIGURE 9.1
Design of the inferiorly based FAMM flap.

Reverse Facial–Submental Artery Island Flap

The traditional submental artery flap was first described by Martin in 1993, and the reverse flow facial–submental artery flap was studied anatomically and presented as a new flap by Rojananin et al. in 1996. Possibly because of reports of venous congestion, it did not gain popularity immediately, but multiple reports of large series using this flap to reconstruct oral and oropharyngeal defects have been published in this decade.

After the facial artery leaves the posterior submandibular gland, it gives off the submental branch before it courses over the mandibular notch to continue superiorly into the face. The submental branch runs on the superficial surface of the mylohyoid muscle either deep to the anterior belly of the digastric muscle (70%) or superficial to it (30%). Perforators from the artery come off proximal to the anterior belly of the digastric muscle, through it, and distal to it before piercing the platysma and supplying the overlying submental skin. The facial vein, which has no valves, runs posterior to the facial artery over the mandible, superficial to the submandibular gland, to join the retromandibular vein. The artery and vein have multiple anastomosing branches to arterial and venous vessels in the face. Because of this rich communicating system, there is no significant change in mean intra-arterial pressure in the submental artery after proximal occlusion of the facial artery. Basing the submental artery island flap on this retrograde flow allows a more beneficial axis of rotation and pedicle length to allow the flap to reach the soft palate.

Previous or concurrent neck dissection can interrupt the facial arterial blood supply to the submental island flap both proximally and distally and to the FAMM flap proximally. The anterograde FAMM flap may have adequate blood supply through collateral flow through the inferior labial artery even if the proximal facial artery is ligated. A Doppler should be used intraoperatively to ensure adequate blood supply during the elevation of the flap in this setting.

If the submental island flap is to be used, care must be taken during the neck dissection to preserve the blood supply of the submental artery and the venous outflow. Although this flap has been used in conjunction with a level I neck dissection, the dissection is more tedious. In the situation where there is a high expectation of metastatic cancer in the submental and submandibular triangle, the use of an alternative flap might be prudent. Previous neck dissection does not typically affect the ability to harvest the buccal adipose tissue and FAMM flaps successfully.

CONTRAINDICATIONS

The contraindications for the buccal adipose tissue pad flap, FAMM, and reverse submental island flap are limited to prior surgery that may have impacted the blood supply or tissue flap. In general, these are reliable flaps that have few contraindications.

PREOPERATIVE PLANNING

Careful preoperative history of previous treatment in the head and neck and careful preoperative examination of the oral cavity, oropharynx, and neck will prevent the surgeon from underestimating the extent of the defect or choosing an unfavorable reconstructive option. Even with this planning, the ultimate extent of the defect and the reconstructive challenge cannot always be anticipated preoperatively, and the reconstructive surgeon should discuss several options with the patient and have several reconstructive flaps in mind. As with any ablative and reconstructive surgery, careful communication should be maintained between the ablative and reconstructive team if they are not the same.

SURGICAL TECHNIQUE

Buccal Adipose Tissue Flap

With an oral retractor in place to provide exposure, a horizontal incision is made in the buccal mucosa adjacent to the maxillary molars and below the orifice of the parotid duct. The buccal adipose tissue may prolapse into the incision, or the surgeon may need to bluntly dissect through the buccinator muscle to expose the capsule of the adipose tissue pad. This is mobilized with blunt dissection. Care is taken not to interrupt the capsule as this keeps the buccal adipose tissue pad intact and preserves vascularity, a surface to mucosalized, and the integrity of the flap. After adequate length is obtained, the flap is rotated into or transposed to the defect keeping the lateral soft tissue pedicle intact. The flap can be expanded to a width of approximately 3 cm by gentle manipulation, and then, the capsule of the flap is sutured to the edges of the defect with resorbable sutures. No attempt is made to skin graft the defect, as the surface will mucosalize. If the flap is transposed, it is not tunneled into the defect—the pedicle can be divided in a second stage or left to atrophy. The buccal incision is irrigated and closed loosely around the pedicle.

FAMM Flap

The submucosal course of the facial artery in the buccal area is mapped with a handheld Doppler. For lateral defects in the oropharynx, an inferiorly based flap is designed with a pedicle width of approximately 1 cm and a maximal flap width of 2.5 cm. The maximal length of the flap is approximately 9 cm. The distal portion of the flap is incised through the mucosa and buccinator muscle, taking care to keep the superior edge of the incision inferior and lateral to Stenson orifice. The facial artery is ligated and divided. Dissection proceeds from distal to proximal with care to include the facial artery in the flap. The flap can be converted to an island flap by carefully removing the proximal mucosa, or it can be harvested as a mucosa pedicled flap. Branches of the facial artery are clipped and divided as necessary until adequate mobilization allows rotation or transposition of the flap into the defect. The flap is inset with resorbable horizontal mattress sutures to the edges of the defect (see Fig. 9.2). After irrigation and hemostasis of the donor site, it is closed in layers including the buccinator muscle followed by the mucosa.

Reverse Facial–Submental Artery Flap

The flap is designed with the superior skin incision approximately 1 cm below the inferior edge of the mandible. The inferior, medial, and lateral edges of the incision are then designed based on the extent of the defect. The flap can reliably include the entire submental skin, with the area of the flap primarily determined by the laxity of this skin and the ability to close the neck primarily. The superior edge of the flap is incised, and dissection proceeds down through the platysma to identify and preserve the marginal branch of the facial nerve overlying the facial artery and vein. The medial incisions are then performed, and the flap is raised below the subcutaneous adipose tissue and platysma and over the mylohyoid muscle from medial to lateral until the ipsilateral midline is reached. Although not advocated by all authors, the ipsilateral anterior belly of the digastric muscle should be included in the flap to prevent venous congestion. The facial artery is traced proximally, and downward retraction on the submandibular gland exposes the submental artery behind the gland and the submental vein on its lateral surface.

The proximal facial artery and vein are ligated with care to ensure that the division point is proximal and lateral to the origin of the submental vessels. The flap is then mobilized with division and clipping of the small vascular branches that penetrate the submandibular gland. The reverse flow vascularity of the flap is confirmed, and then the flap is fully mobilized on the distal facial vessel pedicle and gently passed beneath the marginal mandibular nerve to advance the reach of the pedicle. The flap can then be passed intraorally through a mucosal incision in the buccal sulcus. Care is taken to ensure that the pedicle is not kinked or stretched, and then the skin edges of the flap are contoured and sutured to the mucosal edges of the defect with resorbable mattress sutures in a water tight fashion. The donor site is irrigated and closed primarily over a drain.

POSTOPERATIVE MANAGEMENT

The patient is instructed on oral care with saline rinses and antibiotic mouthwash twice daily. Enteral nutrition is provided until the mucosal defect is healed to prevent fistula formation and to discourage dehiscence of the

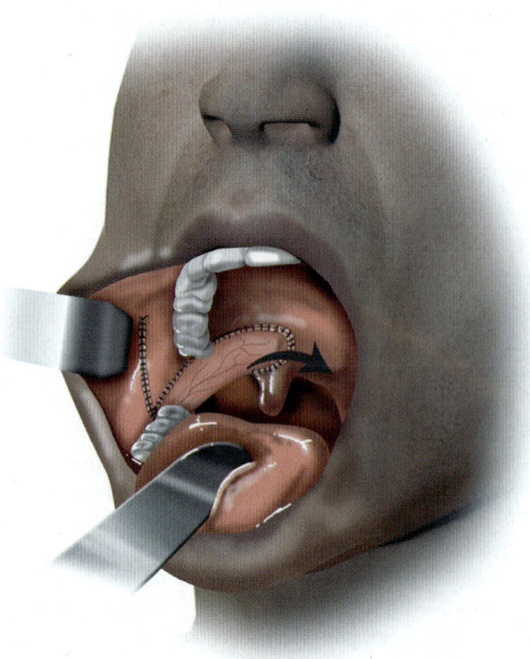

FIGURE 9.2
Inset of the FAMM flap.

flap. The patient is allowed to begin an oral diet once the risk of healing complications has subsided. This period is variable depending on the extent of the defect, the type of reconstruction used, previous treatment effects, and the age of the patient and the preoperative swallowing function.

COMPLICATIONS

Careful design and meticulous technique prevent most complication associated with these flaps. The arterial supply to these flaps is robust, so arterial insufficiency is rare. Venous insufficiency can occur, particularly with the submental island flap. Venous insufficiency is reduced by including the anterior belly of the digastric muscle in the flap design. Venous insufficiency is manifest by bluish discoloration, the flap becoming tense, and eventual skin necrosis and flap dehiscence. In the event of venous congestion, the wound can be explored for hematoma, kinking of the pedicle, or tension on the pedicle. Therapy for venous congestion can include using leeches on the flap, but a new reconstructive treatment may be necessary if the venous congestion cannot be promptly remedied.

RESULTS

The results for these three local flaps are excellent. The blood supply and the tissue are hearty, so the healing is reliable.

PEARLS

- Defects in the oropharynx that involve up to 50% of the palate and are too large to close primarily or to heal by second intention can be managed by using local pedicle flaps.
- Lateral defects of the oropharynx are amenable to buccal adipose tissue pad flaps and FAMM flaps.
- The inferior (anterograde flow) FAMM flap is better suited to a defect in the oropharynx than the superior (retrograde flow) pedicle.
- Larger defects in the oropharynx can be closed with the reverse flow facial–submental artery flap.
- If neck dissection of the submandibular area is performed in conjunction with the submental flap, careful planning and execution are necessary to preserve vascular flow to the flap and venous return.

PITFALLS

- Previous surgery in the distribution of the facial artery may jeopardize the blood supply to the FAMM flap and submental flap.
- Failure to perform careful blunt dissection of the capsule of the buccal adipose tissue pad flap will jeopardize the blood supply and make the flap more difficult to inset.

INSTRUMENTS TO HAVE AVAILABLE

- Standard head and neck surgical set
- Oral maxillofacial surgical tray with Dingman retractor

SUGGESTED READING

Tideman H, Bosanquet A, Scott J. Use of the buccal fat pad as a pedicled graft. *J Oral Maxillofac Surg* 1986;44:435–440.

Pribaz J, Stephens W, Crespo L, et al. A new intraoral flap: facial artery musculomucosal (FAMM) flap. *Plast Reconstr Surg* 1992;90(3):421–429.

Baumann A, Ewers R. Application of the buccal fat pad in oral reconstruction. *J Oral Maxillofac Surg* 2000;58:389–392.

Vural E, Suen J. The submental island flap in head and neck reconstruction. *Head Neck* 2000;22:572–578.

Zhang B, Wang JG, Chen WL, et al. Reverse facial-submental artery island flap for reconstruction of oropharyngeal defects following middle and advanced- stage carcinoma ablation, *Br J Oral Maxillofac Surg* 2011;49:194–197.

10 MANAGEMENT OF THE LATERAL PHARYNGEAL DEFECT: PECTORALIS MAJOR MYOCUTANEOUS FLAP

Terance T. Tsue

INTRODUCTION

Defects in the lateral pharyngeal wall present challenges and difficulties for both the surgeon and the patient. The size of the defect and its location along the vertical and horizontal axis of the pharynx are obvious factors in reconstruction and rehabilitation. Unlike small and/or superficial defects that may be closed primarily or heal by second intention, larger and deeper defects and/or those associated with communication with the neck or exposure of bone and/or major vascular structures require more extensive planning and design. Defects in the superior aspect of the lateral pharynx, such as the nasopharynx, may present the surgeon with difficulties in both approach and exposure for the reconstruction, as opposed to a more inferiorly located lateral pharyngeal defect. Functional outcomes, such as the ability to swallow, speak, and/or breathe, are also a challenge for the patient, depending on the size and location of these lateral defects.

Nearly all defects in the lateral pharyngeal wall are the result of resection of cancer with the remaining few being the result of trauma, and benign tumors. In each case, careful evaluation and preoperative assessment of the defect are necessary in planning the appropriate reconstruction.

In 1979, Ariyan introduced the pedicled pectoralis major myocutaneous flap (PMMF) to head and neck reconstruction. The PMMF was a proven reliable myocutaneous flap for chest wall reconstructions, and it soon became the most popular flap for reconstruction of the head and neck. At the time, compared to microvascular free flaps, the PMMF was more reliable and easier to harvest and did not require expertise in microsurgical techniques. Compared with other contemporary pedicled flaps (e.g., temporal, forehead, deltopectoral (DP), trapezius, sternocleidomastoid, and tongue), the PMMF could be raised in one stage, had a longer arc of rotation, and had less donor site morbidity. With technical advances, better instrumentation, and improved postoperative monitoring, microvascular free flaps have played a more dominant role in head and neck reconstruction. While larger defects are best addressed with a free flap/microvascular reconstruction, there are still many defects in the lateral pharyngeal wall that may be successfully reconstructed with the pedicled PMMF. This is especially true in patients with (1) minimal ipsilateral recipient vasculature as is encountered in patients who have had a radical neck dissection, (2) significant medical comorbidities requiring minimized operative exposure and complexity, (3) severe peripheral vascular disease (PVD) obviating certain free tissue transfer donor sites, and (4) if carotid sheath coverage is concurrently desirable.

HISTORY

When considering the pectoralis donor site for pharyngeal reconstruction, I inquire about a history of shoulder dysfunction or chronic shoulder pain. Patients who relate a history of accessory nerve injury, scapular harvest/trauma, or rotator cuff injury are not ideal candidates for this donor site. A history of previous surgery or trauma in the area of the donor site must be sought.

PHYSICAL EXAMINATION

The physical examination should be focused on the nature of the defect. Patch defects are ideal for this donor site. Circumferential defects and/or defects that involve the nasopharynx are difficult to manage with the pedicled pectoralis flap. The donor site should be inspected for signs of previous surgery or trauma.

INDICATIONS

I consider that the indications for reconstruction of the lateral pharynx defect with the PMMF are dependent on the site. The pectoralis flap is indicated for anterior lateral and/or posterior oropharynx. I find that defects of the nasopharynx are typically difficult to reconstruct with this donor site because it is difficult to reach this remote area from the donor site with a pedicled flap.

CONTRAINDICATIONS

Relative contraindications for using the pectoralis flap include circumferential defects since the rate of fistula is exceptionally high in this situation. Surgical defects in the nasopharynx are also a contraindication. Previous trauma and surgery to the chest wall are also contraindications to the use of this flap.

PREOPERATIVE PLANNING

As in any major reconstructive surgery, careful preparation sets the stage for success. Attention to operative risk assessment, pertinent preoperative imaging, and appropriate swallowing and airway precautions is paramount prior to planned reconstruction with a PMMF. A thorough examination of the head, neck, and chest is required before any decision or treatment plan is begun. Necessary in the assessment is the anticipated location of the defect in the lateral pharyngeal area and its relationship to vital vessels in the neck and the anatomy of the aerodigestive tract. Preoperative or planned CN XI sacrifice with trapezius dysfunction (i.e., concurrent radical neck dissection) and an ipsilateral PMMF harvest can yield some further low neck and shoulder girdle deformity and dysfunction, with subsequent displacement/dysfunction of the medial sternoclavicular joint. It is important to also document baseline speech, swallowing, breathing, and sensory function. The chest should be evaluated for evidence of previous surgery/trauma or congenital bone/muscle deformity that may obviate adequate maintenance of the PMMF vascular pedicle, limit flap adequate bulk, or compromise defect closure/healing. The length of the chest can also influence the arc of the rotation of the PMFF flap and limit its superior reach, although some of this is unpredictable and can only be determined intraoperatively.

Imaging is useful to adequately assess the involvement of the surrounding anatomic structures and the anticipated volume of tissue likely to be needed for reconstruction. Imaging is necessary to evaluate the potential spread of a lateral pharyngeal cancer to the skull base at the level of the nasopharynx, the base of the tongue at the oropharyngeal level, the larynx at the hypopharyngeal level, or the esophagus inferiorly. CT imaging with contrast is especially useful, to map the proximity and course of the vessels of the neck, as well as surrounding anatomy. It is also an excellent predictor of bone involvement should the lesion approach the mandible. MRI can be useful as an adjunct to assess the extent of involvement of the skull base, the base of the tongue, and major vessels. PET/CT is more helpful in defining metastatic cancer.

The role of endoscopy in the operating room setting cannot be underestimated in assisting the surgeon in evaluating the lateral pharyngeal defect, its location, and the feasibility of the planned approach. Direct laryngoscopy, esophagoscopy, and bimanual palpation under general anesthesia assist and confirm the choices made in the decision tree for resection and reconstruction. This is especially important in order to fully evaluate the nasopharynx and the apex of the pyriform sinus, since tumor involvement may not permit a moderate-size resection or laryngeal conservation.

Using this information and one's clinical judgment, a reconstruction ladder or decision tree is used to determine the most ideal reconstruction technique for a given pharyngeal defect based on the information obtained in the preoperative and intraoperative assessment. The patient should be acquainted with the potential multiple reconstruction choices, since the intraoperative findings may require changing of best-laid plans.

Small and/or superficial defects may be closed primarily, heal by second intention, or possibly be reconstructed with a skin graft. Even some moderate-sized "concave" defects in the base of the tongue and/or tonsil fossa may be amenable to healing by second intention and wound contraction with only a small impact on form and function.

Other moderate-sized defects may include a portion of medial oropharyngeal structures with a portion of the lateral pharynx included. Flap reconstruction is often necessary to minimize tethering of the tongue laterally, which can impact speech and swallowing. Inferior moderate-size pharyngeal defects are assessed for potential impact on the larynx. Most inferiorly, defects with extension into the narrower tubed cervical esophagus may require a flap reconstruction that is more pliable than a pedicled pectoralis major flap.

Large defects in the oropharynx usually require flap reconstruction. The decision to use pedicled versus free tissue transfer is dependent on many factors. Some of those factors include (1) patient preference and medical condition, (2) expertise/experience of the surgeon, (3) availability of both donor flap sites and recipient bed vasculature, and (4) other concurrent reconstructive needs, such as the form and character of the reconstruction defect. Frequently, the pedicled PMMF and free tissue transfer are the main choices. I feel that there are several factors that influence the use of a pectoralis flap for reconstruction. These include the following:

1. Reconstruction defects where a bulkier and less pliable PMMF reconstruction does not impact pharyngeal function (i.e., concurrent laryngectomy).
2. Patients' medical conditions that contraindicate microvascular anastomosis (i.e., prothrombotic conditions)
3. Defects that require concurrent coverage of the carotid vasculature.
4. Lack of adequate free flap donor site due to medical disease (i.e., PVD, previous surgery/trauma)
5. Unavailability of microvascular surgeon experience and expertise
6. Patient preference

State-of-the art microvascular free flaps are often required for large defects (larger than acceptable PMMF paddle), with reconstructions requiring different anatomic components (i.e., bone and soft tissue) and/or surgical defects that require complex three-dimensional reconstructions using thin pliable tissue (i.e., multiple plane and/or narrow diameter reconstructions). Successful reconstruction in some of these cases can be achieved with a PMMF, if there remains sufficient pharyngeal mucosa after the ablative resection or a circumferential reconstruction is not required.

SURGICAL TECHNIQUE

Surgical Planning

The pectoralis major muscle is a fan-shaped muscle with origins extending from the medial clavicle, the manubrium, the sternum, the anterior surfaces of the ribs 4 to 6, and some extension to the upper rectus abdominis fascia. The insertion is on the upper third of the humerus along the crest of the greater tubercle. Blood supply to the pectoralis major muscle is supplied by two arteries, the pectoralis branch of the thoracoacromial artery and the lateral thoracic artery. Both arteries arise from the axillary artery. Its blood supply, however, does not follow the fanning fibers of the muscle but inserts into the undersurface of the muscle, through the clavipectoral fascia.

The thoracoacromial artery runs deep to the middle third of the clavicle and usually has four branches, of which the pectoral branch pierces the clavipectoral fascia that surrounds the subclavian muscle and the pectoralis minor muscle. The pectoral branch then inserts on the underside of the pectoralis major muscle through its surrounding fascia with a vein and is readily visible on the undersurface of the muscle. The lateral pectoral nerve is usually near this vascular bundle and can also be seen inserting into the undersurface of the pectoralis major muscle. During flap elevation, both structures can be readily visualized and palpated to assist in their protection.

The pectoral branch of the thoracoacromial artery is usually the dominant blood supply to the muscle, but the lateral thoracic artery may give significant blood supply to both muscle and skin and should be preserved if possible. The lateral thoracic artery pierces the clavipectoral fascia laterally through the pectoralis minor muscle to enter the pectoralis major muscle. As noted, the lateral thoracic artery arises from the second portion of the axillary artery, but in 10% of patients, it may also arise as a branch off of the thoracoacromial artery.

An important consideration for the surgeon is the course of these two vessels. A line from the acromion to the xiphoid process is suggested as a landmark to grossly locate the course of the pectoral branch in the major muscle. However, the pectoral branch may have an arced rather than radial course in the pectoralis major muscle, prompting careful visualization of its course when dividing the pectoralis major muscle fibers for flap elevation. The lateral thoracic artery, traversing a more lateral route along the lateral border in the pectoralis minor muscle, may sometimes travel for several centimeters in that muscle before exiting the minor and entering the major muscle.

Generally, the pectoralis branch supplies the majority of the skin perforators overlying the pectoralis major muscle directly, while the lateral thoracic artery supplies the skin perforators beyond the border of the pectoralis major muscle laterally and inferiorly. For this reason, it is an important consideration to try to preserve the lateral thoracic artery, when possible, when evaluating the placement and design of the skin paddle. The needed arc of rotation of the PMMF may dictate the ability to save this lateral pedicle. Preservation of the lateral thoracic artery may limit the arc of flap rotation for the PMMF to the level of the tonsil fossa. Other vascular supplies to the pectoralis major that are necessarily sacrificed during flap harvesting include the superior thoracic artery and the intercostals and internal mammary perforating arteries.

The medial and lateral pectoral nerves innervate the pectoralis major muscle. They derive their motor roots C5-T1 through the brachial plexus as it courses under the pectoralis muscle through the axilla. The nerves are so named because the medial pectoral nerve arises from the medial cord of the brachial plexus and the lateral pectoral nerve arises from the lateral cord of the brachial plexus. Their courses to the pectoralis major muscle, however, give a different visual presentation to the surgeon. The lateral pectoral nerve is located more medially, in closer proximity to the vascular pedicle of the pectoral branch and vein. It is readily visible in this undersurface of the pectoralis major muscle and must be divided. This division is performed to reduce eventual bulk of the muscle flap through atrophy and also to release tethering tension to allow more arc of rotation and extension of the flap. It also must be divided to reduce the risk of strangulation of the pectoral branch of the artery after placement of the myocutaneous flap for the reconstruction. The lateral pectoral nerve would otherwise form a compressive band across the vascular pedicle that has just been rotated up and over the firm immovable clavicular bone. The medial pectoral nerve is also readily visible between the pectoralis minor and major muscles. Although named the medial pectoral nerve, as noted, it pierces through the pectoralis minor muscle more laterally, through the clavipectoral fascia and then into the undersurface of the pectoralis major muscle. It also must be sacrificed during mobilization of the flap for reconstruction.

A thorough understanding of the surgical anatomy will greatly improve the viability and success of the PMMF reconstruction (Fig. 10.1A and B).

Usually, the reconstruction of a defect in the lateral pharyngeal wall is performed immediately following the resection. Secondary reconstructions may be necessary to repair a fistula, radiation necrosis, or stricture or due to the medical stability of each patient. Prereconstruction clearance of surgical margins, meticulous hemostasis, and identification/preservation of important recipient bed neurovascular structures are important before embarking on the reconstruction.

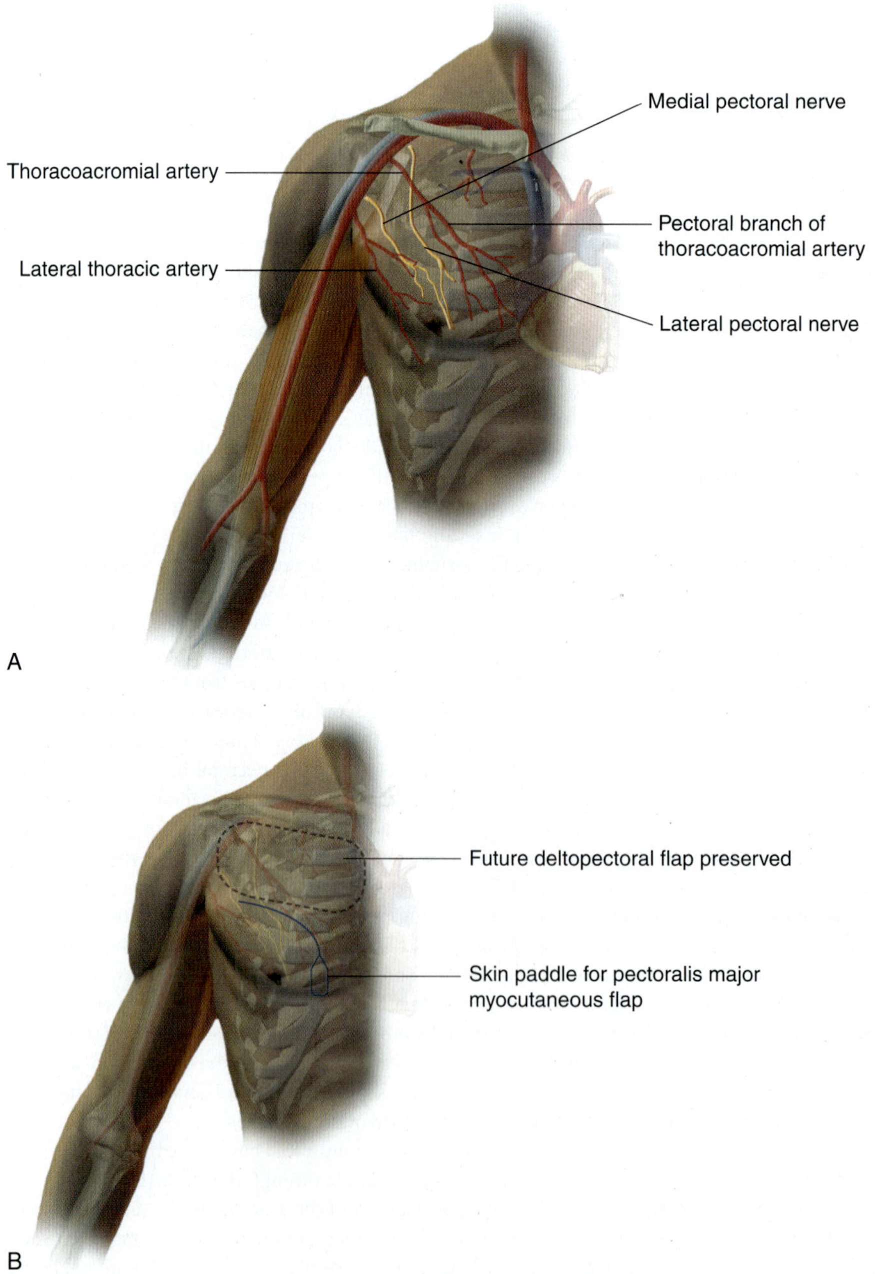

FIGURE 10.1
A. The pectoralis major muscle is supplied by the pectoral branch of the thoracoacromial artery. The vascular anatomy of the pectoralis major muscle is demonstrated here. **B.** Demonstrates the design of the skin paddle for the pectoralis flap (*blue*) and the preservation of the DP flap (*black dotted line*).

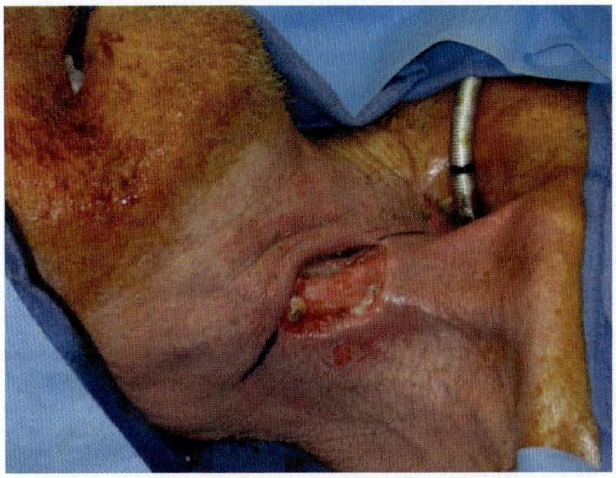

FIGURE 10.2
This photograph demonstrates a pharyngocutaneous fistula. Reconstruction of this defect is best accomplished with a pedicle flap of vascularized muscle and skin.

The chest is usually widely prepped and draped concurrent with the head and neck region. The use of barrier drapes can help separate any gastrostomy tube from the donor site. Until the harvest occurs, the area is usually covered with sterile towels and drapes to prevent contamination from the aerodigestive dissection superiorly as much as possible. Typically, during harvest, a separate OR table and instruments are used after the surgeon regowns to minimize contamination into the donor site or any tumor seeding potential. If the patient can be safely pharmacologically paralyzed during this aspect of the procedure, it is desirable to minimize muscular contraction during harvest.

For this example, a pectoralis flap is the best tissue to use to reconstruct an inferior lateral pharyngeal defect resulting from local recurrence and fistula formation after total laryngectomy (Figs. 10.2 and 10.3).

The representative case in the accompanying figures is a 68-year-old male with fistula formation of the right lateral pharynx after total laryngectomy with neck dissection and postoperative radiation therapy. After neck dissection and excision of nonviable tissue, the right lateral pharyngeal defect is measured.

Accurate assessment of the defect is the first important step in the reconstruction. Once the dimensions of the defect and its location and character are known, the size of the PMMF skin paddle needed can be determined. Proper placement of the skin paddle incisions is crucial. Finding the most inferior skin paddle margin is done first, in measuring the arc of rotation needed to reach the most superior edge of the defect without tension. This is accomplished by using either an unrolled 4 × 4 gauze or the umbilical tape that would have been used with the tracheotomy. The pivot point of the arc of rotation is located at the emergence of the vascular pedicle to the PMMF, at the middle third of the inferior border of the clavicle. This measurement is important to assure that the edge of the skin paddle will reach the superior aspect of the defect without tension, when the flap is rotated into position. It also alerts the surgeon as to the amount of skin paddle that may be needed beyond the pectoralis major muscle and thus may require inclusion of the rectus sheath for vascular perfusion.

The skin lying most medial and inferior on the pectoralis major has the fullest arc of rotation but often needs to be extended more inferiorly below the border of the pectoralis major muscle. The blood supply to this portion of most inferior skin is usually random but may have some supply from the lateral thoracic artery previously mentioned. It is important, however, to include the rectus fascia to capture as much random blood supply as possible. Knowing then the placement of the inferior edge of the skin paddle and the dimensions of the defect to be closed, a skin paddle is designed for the pedicled PMMF (Fig. 10.4).

Similar evaluation of the superior aspect of the skin paddle is tested using the gauze measurement technique to make sure that the superior aspect of the flap approaches the location of the inferior aspect of the

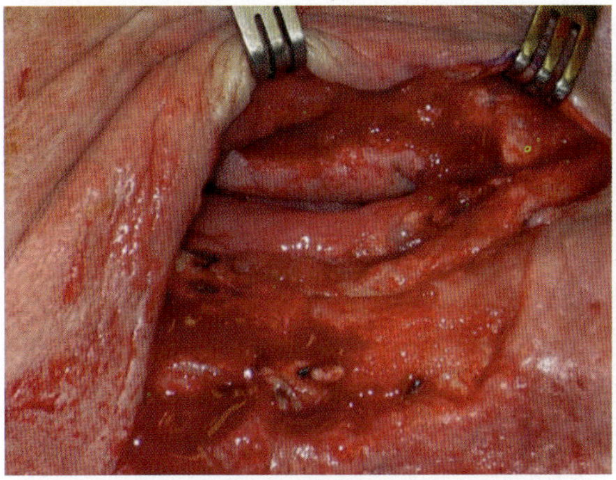

FIGURE 10.3
To reconstruct the defect, the edges of the fistula are prepared for reconstruction. An elliptical incision is made around the fistula to prepare for reconstruction.

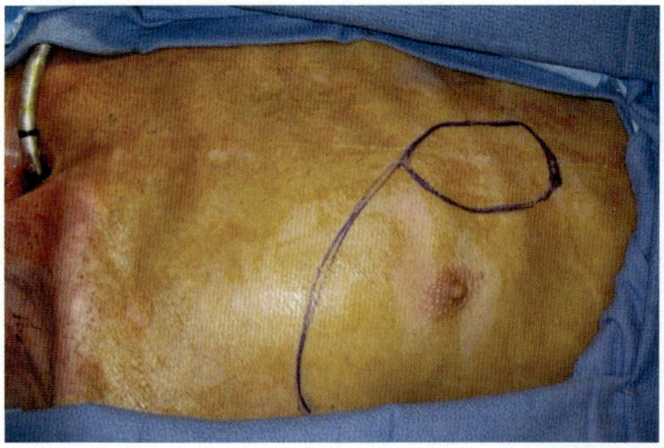

FIGURE 10.4
The appropriate skin paddle is designed on the chest wall to prepare for harvest of the flap.

defect. The center of the paddle is usually placed midline between the nipple and sternum but can extend to include both structures laterally and medially as needed. Too small a cutaneous paddle should not be drawn, as this will limit the number of cutaneous perforators to the paddle and compromise the entire cutaneous portion of the PMMF. Most skin paddles are drawn in a boat shape with the "pointy" bow of the boat being the superior aspect of the skin paddle and the "boxy" stern of the boat being the inferior aspect of the skin paddle. This paddle shape will help facilitate the closure of the chest wall defect. Elliptical-shaped paddles are also useful to help have an easier and more cosmetic donor site closure. As a general rule, the paddle should remain above the costal margin to ensure the best vascular supply to the distal portion of the PMMF.

The skin paddle is then drawn to size based on the accurate measurements of the defect. An oblique incision line from the superior lateral corner of the skin paddle to the anterior axilla is drawn. This incision line is important for two reasons. It helps to locate the lateral border of the pectoralis major muscle during flap harvest, thereby aiding in identifying the neurovascular boundaries rather than cutting across them with the skin incision. This incision is also placed, to avoid crossing into the region of the DP flap blood supply if this should be needed in a future surgery (Fig. 10.5).

The first incision made is from the anterior axilla to the superior apex of the skin paddle. This is then continued down the lateral portion of the skin paddle. These lateral incisions are made first to enable visualization of the lateral border of the pectoralis muscle, especially its most inferior extent. The inferior extent determines the extent of the cutaneous paddle that has the best axial blood supply. The remaining portion of the skin paddle beyond the inferior aspect of the pectoralis muscle is generally random in nature but usually reliable within limits. Determination of the inferior border of the pectoralis muscle may also allow further inferior placement of the skin paddle (redraw the paddle) as no other paddle incision have been made. This may result in less tension once the PMMF is rotated into a higher defect. It may also require more superior paddle harvest if the muscle is very short to ensure adequate blood supply to the inferior skin paddle.

Care is taken not to incise the pectoralis major fascia, while identifying the lateral border of the muscle. This also helps to avoid separating the fibers of the pectoralis major muscle and inadvertently injuring the lateral thoracic blood supply to the muscle. This also helps to distinguish the pectoralis muscles from the external oblique and serratus anterior muscles. The lateral incisions are subsequently undermined laterally enough in a plane superficial to the plane of the pectoralis fascia.

After the correct skin paddle location is again confirmed, the incisions are then continued circumferentially around the marked skin paddle, with care again not to incise the pectoralis major muscle fascia. The chest skin flap is medially dissected in the similar suprafascial plane toward the sternum and similarly for the inferior skin paddle incision toward the costal margin or below. Care is taken to not apply shearing forces on the skin

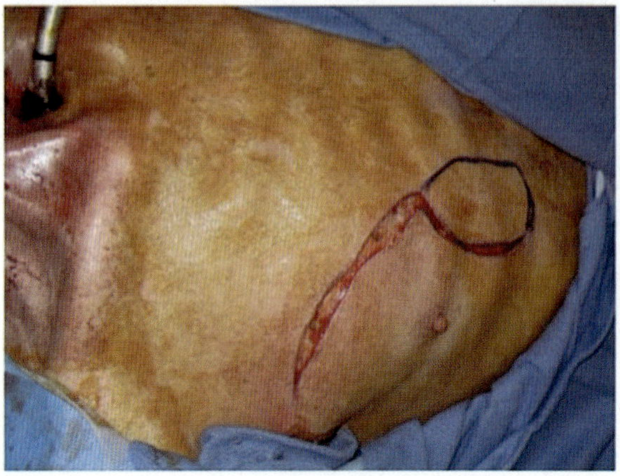

FIGURE 10.5
The incisions to harvest the pectoralis muscle are performed in such a way that the skin of the DP flap is left uninterrupted in the event that it is required for later reconstruction.

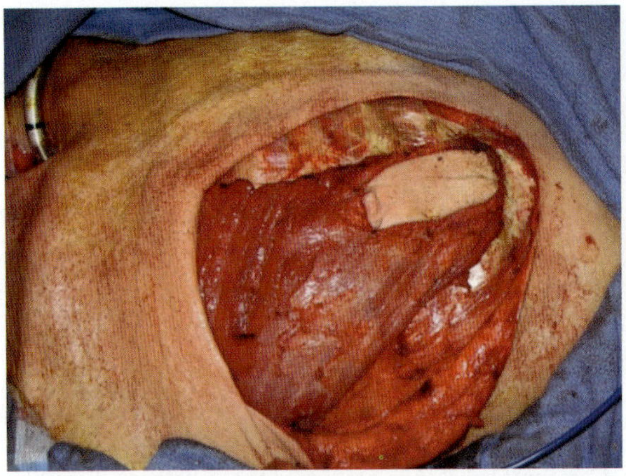

FIGURE 10.6
The skin paddle harvested on the pectoralis major muscle is sutured to the muscle to prevent stress and shear on the vascular perforators.

paddle, as it remains attached to the pectoralis muscle, that can hurt the perforating vessels, thus devascularizing the carefully designed skin paddle, bringing a disastrous effect to the final reconstruction. Absorbable 3-0 sutures are placed to anchor the skin paddle to the fascial surface of the pectoralis major muscle to reduce any shearing during flap harvest (Fig. 10.6).

The skin of the chest is then elevated superiorly and medially up to the clavicle to expose the pectoralis major muscle. Important considerations must be adhered to when elevating this chest skin flap. The dissection remains suprafascial to the pectoralis major until the line of the imaginary DP flap is traversed. The dissection then becomes subfascial to the pectoralis major fascia, in hopes of preserving the blood supply from the internal mammary perforators at the first four medial intercostal spaces to the DP region. This again helps preserve the blood supply of the DP flap should it be necessary in the future (Fig. 10.7). Attention is also needed when in the subfascial plane not to divide the pectoralis muscle fibers while approaching the clavicle. Care must be taken in the dissection since one could easily separate the clavicular head from the sternal head of the pectoralis major muscle and injure the pectoralis branch of the thoracoacromial artery. Subcutaneous dissection into the neck space is performed from both below and above. The tunnel should be of sufficient size to allow passage of the PMMF, without strangulation of its vascular pedicle. Usually, a four-finger width is sufficient. It is important to note that there are usually veins from the external jugular system that traverse over the clavicle medially and laterally to this tunnel and should be ligated to avoid postoperative hematoma formation. It is important to perform this elevation prior to incising and releasing the flap inferiorly. Once the PMMF is released from its costal attachments inferiorly, it bunches in the superior aspect due to the loss of tension and makes this superior chest skin flap dissection more technically difficult if not already performed.

The sternocostal insertions of the pectoralis major muscle are then separated from their attachments using Bovie cautery. This is approached widely and inferiorly, starting in a subfascial plane at the rectus fascia if the inferior margin of the skin paddle flap reaches to this level as needed for the reconstruction (Fig. 10.8). A wide base of the sternocostal margins of the pectoralis major muscle helps to protect the terminal branches of the pectoral artery. Taking a narrow strip of muscle may otherwise injure the vascular bundle from the

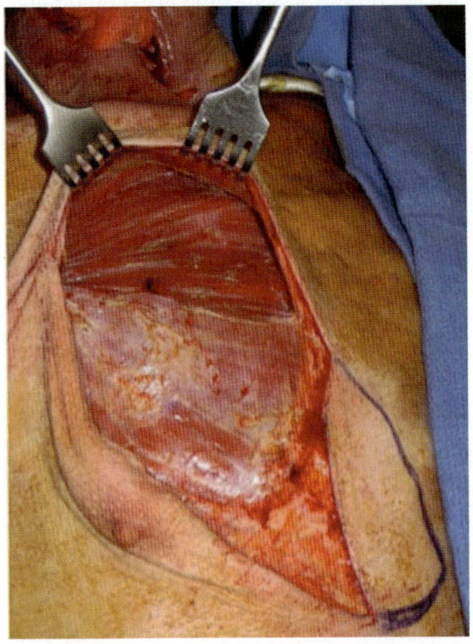

FIGURE 10.7
The dissection in this photo is subfascial to the pectoralis major fascia to preserve the blood supply from the internal mammary perforators at the first four medial intercostal spaces to the DP region. This again helps preserve the blood supply of the DP flap should it be necessary in the future.

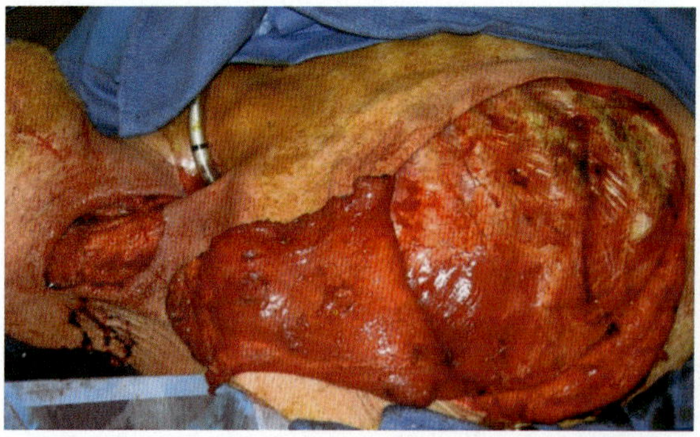

FIGURE 10.8
The dissection is performed in the subfascial plane at the rectus fascia if the inferior margin of the skin paddle flap reaches to this level as needed for the reconstruction.

thoracoacromial artery. The surgeon is reminded that the thoracoacromial artery may have a tortuous course to the inferior edge of the pectoralis major muscle. Care must be taken to not extend the cauterizing dissection deep to the level of the ribs and potentially penetrate the chest cavity.

The medial fibers of the pectoralis major muscle fibers are then divided from inferior near the xiphoid process in a superior line up to the medial third of the clavicle. It is important to stay lateral to the course of the internal mammary artery and its first four perforators superiorly, again, to avoid devascularizing the DP skin flap for the future if needed. In the inferior half of the medial flap harvest, intercostal arterial branches will be encountered and good hemostatic technique can help minimize subsequent hematoma formation.

The PMMF is now elevated from its costal insertions in an inferior to superior fashion. This usually requires cautery dissection in the inferior half of the flap harvest to separate the muscle from its costal attachments, but more superiorly, simple finger dissection in the plane between the pectoralis major and minor muscles can occur. The vascular bundle with the pectoral branch will be in full view within the pectoralis major fascia coming from superiorly. It is also readily palpable. The pectoralis minor muscle, with its origins on the costal rib attachments and clavipectoral fascia, are left intact. The lateral pectoral nerve will also be identified as it enters the undersurface of the pectoralis major and is divided (Fig. 10.9). Look for the lateral insertion course of the lateral thoracic artery and determine if it may also be preserved while maintaining adequate length for the rotation advancement of the PMMF, particularly if a random portion of the skin paddle is incorporated with the rectus fascia.

The PMMF is then gently rotated and guided through the tunnel, avoiding any twisting or tethering of the vascular pedicle or shearing of the skin paddle attached to the muscle (Fig. 10.10). If necessary, the flap can be rotated some to allow the skin paddle to be located externally to close a cutaneous defect, but this requires a larger tunnel and longer flap pedicle. Also, this type of defect may be better reconstructed with a skin graft on top of the pectoralis muscle rotated into position without twisting.

The skin paddle, which is fashioned slightly larger than the size of the defect, is sewn in one layer to the pharyngeal mucosa, incorporating the fascia, dermis, and skin. Usually, absorbable suture is used with adequate strength (3-0). Other layers of closure may also be added judiciously, and these may also help support the flap in position against gravitational forces (sewing muscle fascia to mandibular periosteum or to a locking reconstruction plate) (Fig. 10.11). As the PMMF pedicle now lies superficially on the surface of the PMMF in the neck, one must be careful in the placement of subsequent sutures and closure. Having the skin paddle slightly larger than the defect will avoid a tense skin surface at closure, which could also compromise the vascular flow to the skin flap.

During inset of the flap, the tension on the PMMF pedicle must be minimal or else further improvement in the rotation arc flap must be undertaken or the skin paddle repositioned. Improvement in the rotation of the arc

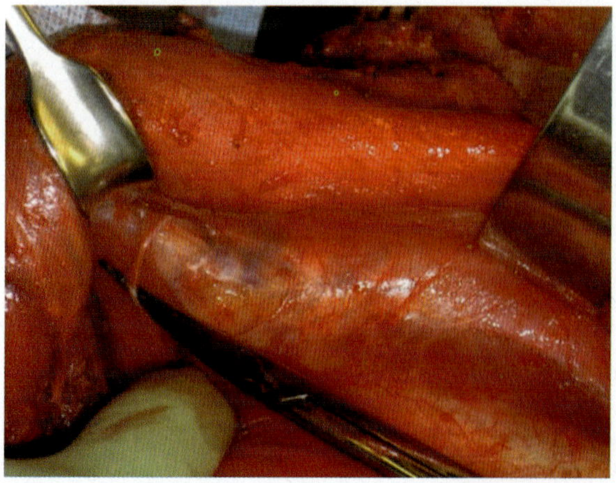

FIGURE 10.9
The lateral pectoral nerve should be identified as it enters the undersurface of the pectoralis major and is divided.

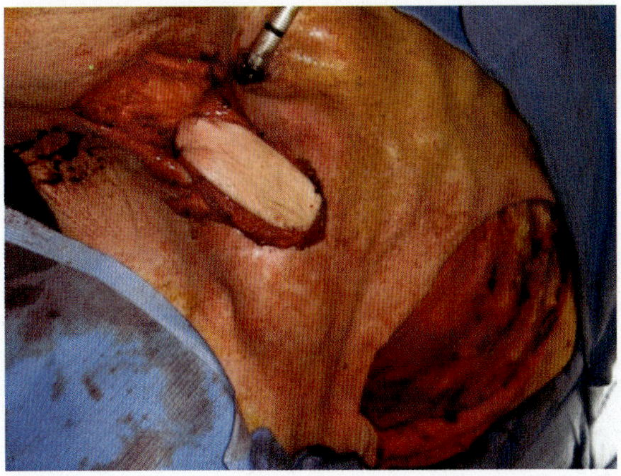

FIGURE 10.10
The PMMF is rotated and guided through the tunnel, avoiding any twisting or tethering of the vascular pedicle, or shearing of the skin paddle attached to the muscle.

can be obtained by releasing the humeral head of the PMMF, sacrifice of the lateral pedicle, and even takedown of a section of the clavicle bone. Flexing the neck can assist some but should not be relied upon as the sole remedy. The described temporary sutures holding the skin paddle to the muscle can be maintained or removed depending on the mobility of the skin paddle needed.

With the reconstruction complete, drains are placed in the neck wound. These should not be placed over the vascular pedicle. Attention is turned toward closure of the neck incision. The neck portion of the PMMF pedicle can be moved with some degree of freedom horizontally without causing tension. This can be advantageous to fill any dead space and cover any potential exposed neck vessels. Full closure of the neck incisions should occur only if there is no excessive tension on the flap. Sometimes, the bulk of the PMMF will prevent a tension-free or strangulation-free closure of the neck incision. If this is the case, then a split-thickness skin graft is placed over the exposed muscle belly of the pectoralis major and sutured to the skin edges of the neck incision in a loose tension-free closure (Fig. 10.12). At times, a vertical incision is also needed from the inferior neck incision toward the clavicle to release neck flap skin tunnel tightness over the PMMF pedicle. The exposed pedicle muscle can then be skin grafted as well. Usually, a simple overlying Xeroform gauze is all that is needed to keep the graft moist and facilitate adherence. A bolster may apply too much pressure on the PMMF pedicle. Cutaneously, the location of a palpable or dopplerable PMMF pedicle is marked with a suture to facilitate monitoring of the flap viability postoperatively.

The chest incision is usually closed primarily after wide undermining of the skin laterally and inferior medially. There is often an area of tension in this closure, but extensive undermining should be adequately done to make this tension as small as possible. Skin grafting at the donor site onto the chest wall is also an option (Fig. 10.13). For females, there is some distortion of the breast in the closure of this donor site, but this can be minimized with skin paddle design for the initial incisions. The use of some of the medial breast tissue can also provide bulk for the flap reconstruction if needed. Suction drains are inserted into the chest donor site per surgeon preference.

If a tracheostomy for maintenance of airway protection is required, it is sutured into position, and not tied, to avoid any circumferential ties and strangulation of the vascular PMMF pedicle. This can include compression from respiratory therapy ties to the tracheostomy mask or tight patient gowns.

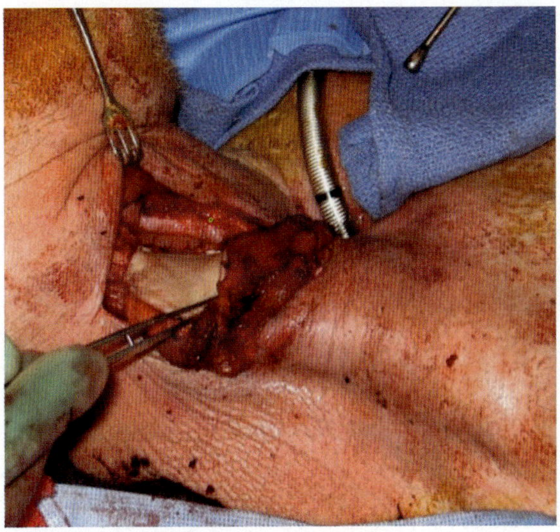

FIGURE 10.11
The layers of closure may also be added judiciously, and these may also help support the flap in position against gravitational forces (sewing muscle fascia to mandibular periosteum or to a locking reconstruction plate).

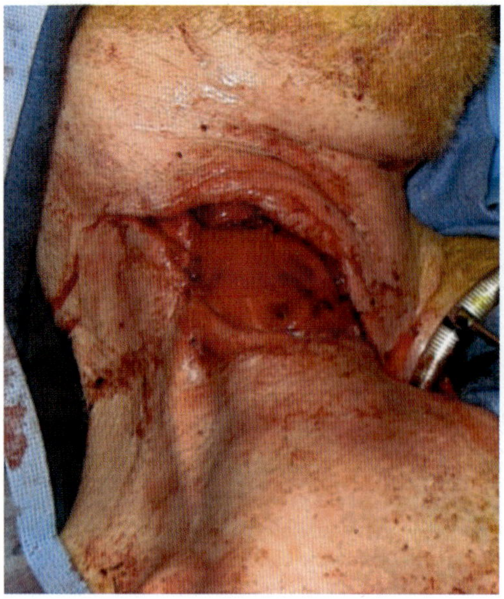

FIGURE 10.12
A split-thickness skin graft is placed over the exposed muscle of the pectoralis major and sutured to the skin edges of the neck incision in a loose tension-free closure.

POSTOPERATIVE MANAGEMENT

Postoperative management requires that the nonirradiated patients remains NPO for 7 days and radiated patients remain NPO for 14 days. I schedule a barium swallow before initiating an oral diet.

COMPLICATIONS

Complications may be related to the pectoralis donor site and the pharyngeal recipient site. Donor site complications are typically limited to wound breakdown because the pectoralis flap is straightforward to harvest and associated with very few significant neurovascular complications. The recipient site is at risk for fistula and infection. In turn, a salivary fistula may place the great vessels at risk. The muscle flap associated with the pectoralis donor site provides well-vascularized tissue in the event of a fistula.

RESULTS

In my experience, the results with this technique are excellent. The donor site is reliable, and the skin flap is ideal for pharyngeal reconstruction.

PEARLS

- Prepare with an optional reconstructive plan should the lateral pharyngeal defect involve more than 50% of the circumference of the pharynx or invade the base of the tongue or larynx.
- Include the rectus fascia when the skin paddle design length extends below the limits of the pectoralis major muscle border. Preservation of the lateral thoracic artery should also be desired for the survival of the extended skin paddle.

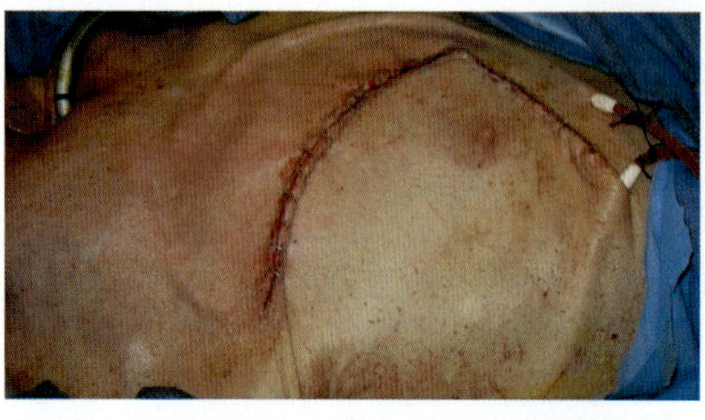

FIGURE 10.13
The donor site closure is usually achieved by rotating a large skin flap into the defect. Typically, this can be achieved with primary closure.

- The pectoral branch to the PMMF may be an arc rather than a straight line course through its length. Visualization during mobilization of the flap will avoid inadvertent injury to the vascular pedicle.
- Do not incise the pectoralis major fascia surrounding the skin paddle, with surrounding dissection being suprafascial to preserve perforating blood supply. This fascia provides strength to the inset sutures.
- Dissection superior to the DP flap inferior demarcation is subfascial to preserve the potential DP flap future reconstruction. Avoid injury of the internal mammary artery perforators of the first three intercostal spaces inferior to the clavicle.

PITFALLS

- Flap tension will lead to flap failure.
- Any dissection around the vascular pedicle or the investing clavipectoral fascia risks injury and failure of the pectoralis major flap. The clavicular and sternal attachments are divided for length instead.
- Division of the horizontal fibers of the pectoralis major muscle near its insertion to the humeral attachment for arc of rotation length improvement will avoid injury to the pectoral branch vessel but may of necessity divide the lateral thoracic artery branch. This later vessel division can be minimized, if done in a stepwise fashion, first through small increments of the horizontal muscle fibers, to titrate to the needed length of reach without tension.
- Failure to divide the lateral pectoral nerve may, strangulate the vascular pedicle of the pectoral branch if left intact for the rotation of the flap over the clavicle. Failure to divide the nerve will also reduce the length of the arc of rotation for the flap and allow persistent innervation of the muscle. This can yield bothersome voluntary contractions in the neck postoperatively, as well as prevent desirable muscle atrophy.
- Excessive undermining of the skin to the sternum superiorly above the fourth intercostal space will sacrifice the internal mammary artery perforators to a future DP flap.
- Suturing under tension a too-small skin paddle for the lateral pharyngeal defect may cause taut skin tension and compromise the perforating blood supply to the entire skin paddle.

INSTRUMENTS TO HAVE AVAILABLE

- Head and neck surgical tray

ACKNOWLEDGMENTS

I gratefully acknowledge the contributions of Mark J. Furin and Lisa Shnayder.

SUGGESTED READING

Ariyan S. The pectoralis major myocutaneous flap: a versatile flap for reconstruction in the head and neck. *Plast Reconstr Surg* 1979;63:73–81.

Magee WP Jr, McCraw JB, Horton CE, et al. Pectoralis "paddle" myocutaneous flaps: the workhorse of head and neck reconstruction. *Am J Surg* 1980;140:507–513.

Baek S, Lawson W, Biller HF. An analysis of 133 pectoralis major myocutaneous flaps. *Plast Reconstr Surg* 1982;69: 460–467.

Ossoff RH, Wurster CF, Berktold RE, et al. Complications after pectoralis major myocutaneous flap reconstruction of head and neck defects. *Arch Otolaryngol Head Neck Surg* 1983;109:812–814.

11 MANAGEMENT OF THE LATERAL PHARYNGEAL DEFECT: RADIAL FOREARM FLAP

Rod Rezaee

INTRODUCTION

Historically, defects of the pharynx have posed challenges to the head and neck reconstructive surgeon due to the complex nature of pharyngeal function from the standpoint of breathing and swallowing. The pharyngeal mucosa and musculature must generate pressure to assist with bolus transfer but additionally must maintain a patent airway. An intricate array of neuromuscular and sensory reflexes in addition to cognitive control allow for this to take place. Any interruption in this reflex arc poses the potential for aspiration and significant dysphagia. The presence of cancer, or the treatment of the cancer, either surgical or nonsurgical, can increase the challenge for the reconstructive surgeon in order to maintain a patient's basic function.

Total laryngopharyngectomy defects can be restored with a tubed flap design with no concern for aspiration and only concern for recreating a patent conduit connecting the tongue base to the esophagus. When the oncologic resection does not require removal of the larynx, the reconstructive challenge increases substantially. This is due to the added need not only to restore an intact watertight pharynx but to do so while preserving the ability to swallow and not impinge on the airway. To accomplish this goal, the reconstructive surgeon must carefully consider the needs of the patient as the decision is made on the donor site, design, and insetting of the flap.

The focus of this chapter is on reconstruction of the lateral pharyngeal defect using a free flap with an intact larynx.

HISTORY

It is critical to understand the patient's history to help determine the needs of the flap selected for restoration of the pharynx. Location of the cancer, prior surgery, radiation, chemotherapy, age, laboratory values (hematocrit, thyroid-stimulating hormone), medical history, and nutritional status (prealbumin) all factor into the decision algorithm. Discussion of surgical approaches should be undertaken preoperatively with the ablative and reconstructive surgeons to determine an optimal plan for safe and effective extirpation and reconstruction. Since a lateral pharyngeal lesion and defect may extend cephalocaudad to include the hypopharynx to nasopharynx, transmandibular versus transcervical approaches are possible and can add an additional challenge for flap reconstruction (Fig. 11.1). This may have implications for the type of flap chosen especially when the mandible is intact and there is a high lateral defect.

Although modern free flap teams can provide reconstruction very efficiently, there are certain patient situations when primary closure or pedicle flaps, either supraclavicular island or pectoralis major myocutaneous flaps, may be chosen to shorten operative times and reduce the risk of additional potential operations in the setting of a rare free flap compromise. For instance, patients of advanced age, those with cardiac conditions, or those

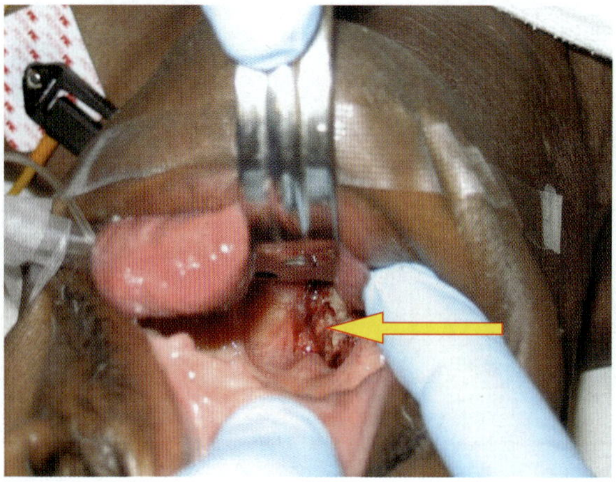

FIGURE 11.1
This figure is a transoral view of a carcinoma of the pharynx (*arrow*).

with aortic stenosis where added potential fluid shifts or operative time may increase the risk of perioperative events may be considered for regional tissue closure rather than free tissue repair. All patients benefit from a comprehensive multidisciplinary approach to designing a treatment plan. This also includes preoperative and postoperative assessment by the speech and swallowing team to achieve maximal functional outcomes.

PHYSICAL EXAMINATION

Physical examination requires attention to both the donor site and the recipient site. The donor site evaluation requires an Allen test on the upper extremity to ensure that there is an intact vascular palmar arch. Because the radial forearm free flap will be used for reconstruction, a careful examination of the volar surface of the forearm is important to ensure that there has not been trauma or prior surgery that may compromise the harvesting of the flap. It is important to plan the harvest of the forearm flap from the nondominant arm. The recipient site should be carefully evaluated to determine the size of the defect. This will help to determine the appropriate size of the skin flap reconstruction.

INDICATIONS

When I assess the lateral pharyngeal defect, I consider a number of factors in determining the need for a free flap. Prior radiation and surgery intuitively raises a concern about the quality and integrity of the local native tissues that I believe benefit from repair with vascularized grafts from a remote nonirradiated site (Fig. 11.2). If the defect connects to the neck, then flap reconstruction may be indicated especially if the defect is large or the quality of the tissue prevents a tension-free primary closure. Transoral defects from cancers removed in standard fashion or robotically that do not connect to the neck may be safely allowed to granulate or be closed with local flaps for carotid coverage. If there is communication with the neck and if there has been a radical neck dissection performed and I consider the carotid artery at risk either from wound breakdown externally or soilage from a potential salivary leak, free flap repair and regional coverage become important considerations. The carotid artery can become exposed internally or externally, and the risk of this must be assessed in the absence of the sternocleidomastoid muscle (SCM).

With an intact SCM, consideration can be given to pexing the medial aspect of the SCM to the prevertebral fascia when possible to potentially serve as a salivary diversion in the event of a fistula. Similarly, a flap can be designed such that a deepithelialized portion or additional soft tissue can be harvested to protect the carotid artery and provide a tissue barrier for protection between the pharyngeal reconstruction and the great vessels.

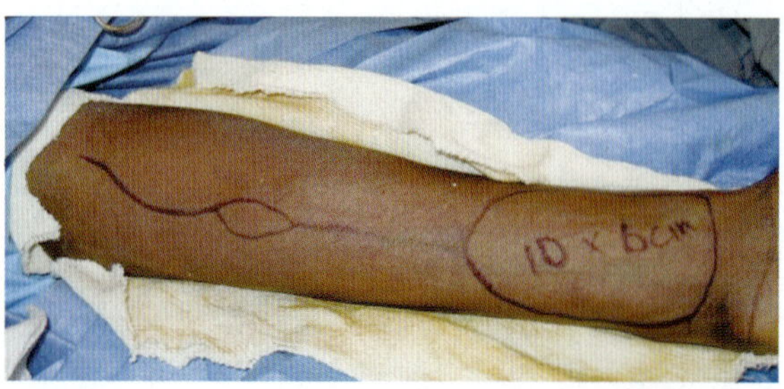

FIGURE 11.2
This photograph demonstrates the design for the radial forearm free flap. There is a cutaneous skin paddle for reconstruction of the pharynx and a second monitor skin paddle to evaluate the viability of the flap.

CONTRAINDICATIONS

There may be considerations in some settings where the radial forearm may not be ideal or feasible. For instance, I have had patients in whom rheumatologic conditions exist or severe Raynaud disease where the potential for added dexterity or vascular morbidity may not be reasonable. Additionally, a number of patients through the years have had the radial arteries harvested for prior cardiac surgery eliminating the radial forearm as a donor site. Prior free flaps or trauma may also preclude its use. In these patients, other potential fasciocutaneous sites must be considered, such as the lateral arm, rectus, anterolateral thigh (ALT), or scapula.

PREOPERATIVE PLANNING

My primary considerations in choosing a free tissue donor site include the size of the defect, rigidity of the cervical skin, donor vessel selection, and patient body habitus (Fig. 11.3). Secondary considerations are prior surgeries and prior oncologic treatments in addition to the patient's nutritional status. Ideally, I think of the best repair for a lateral pharyngeal defect to be a radial forearm flap for a number of reasons. Its thin pliable nature allows for an excellent tissue match for the lateral defect such that there is less difficulty aligning the thickness of the skin and mucosal anastomotic line, especially if it extends a distance onto the cervical spine region and posterior pharyngeal wall. While a thicker flap can certainly be used for closure, I have found that the thicker flaps can be the cause of airway and pharyngeal obstruction postoperatively that may later require attention to allow for decannulation and restoration of PO intake.

For example, if a bulkier flap is used, such as an ALT flap in a heavier-set individual and one in which there is a musculocutaneous perforator, it may be more difficult to close the neck if the native neck tissues are contracted from prior surgery or radiation. One can certainly consider a perforator ALT flap to minimize the need for harvest of the vastus lateralis or consider primary thinning of the subcutaneous adipose tissue, but the forearm gives such versatility with its inherent likeness to the pharyngeal mucosa and musculature in thickness that I believe it should be given first consideration for the lateral defect. A large proximal volume of skin and/or subcutaneous tissue may be included to be deepithelialized for carotid coverage and improved contour of the neck or externalized for a monitoring segment or repair of an external skin defect in a contracted neck. Additionally, its long vascular pedicle, ability to be neurotized, and potential use of the cephalic venous system give the reconstructive surgeon more options in both the vessel-replete and vessel-depleted necks. Its length allows for reach to the transverse cervical or contralateral neck, and the cephalic provides for a reasonable match for the external jugular vein when present. The paired venae comitantes can often be traced proximally in the arm to a unified larger vein or can be taken just distal to a bridging vein between them which may allow for a larger caliber anastamosis in those patients where the comitantes are small. The drawback through the years has been the donor site morbidity and need for a secondary surgical site to harvest the skin graft. I have not found the donor site morbidity and tendon exposure to be significant with meticulous attention to preservation of the paratenon during harvest and prevention of desiccation of the paratenon while awaiting skin graft repair. In many cachectic patients, the ALT flap resembles the forearm in thickness and quality and therefore may be the donor site of choice in those patients.

SURGICAL TECHNIQUE

Keys to successful reconstruction of the lateral pharyngeal wall involve having an intimate understanding and respect for the balance of providing a sealed pharyngeal conduit while minimizing the effect on maintaining a patent airway and ability to swallow without aspiration. Care must be taken to size the flap

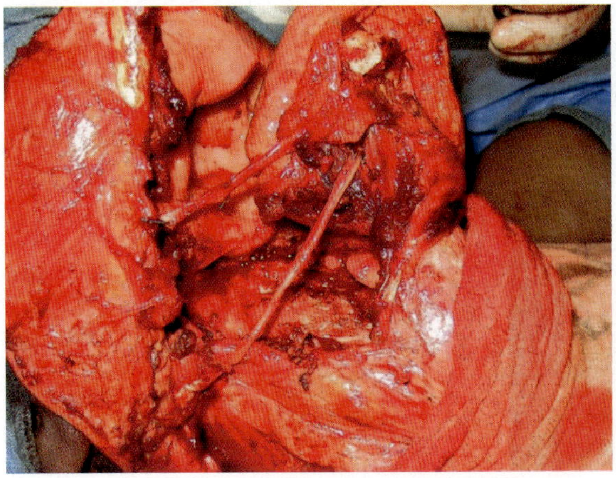

FIGURE 11.3
This photograph demonstrates a typical pharyngeal defect. Note that the cranial nerves have been preserved to assist with functional restoration.

appropriately not only in thickness but in overall dimensions. For instance, an oversized flap may produce redundancy that occludes the airway or obstructs the esophageal inlet. I keep in mind not only the primary size of the skin paddle but also potential edema that will occur for a period of time especially in those who have had radiation or those who will be going through radiation. Conversely, sizing a skin island too small may cause excess tension on the suture lines that could predispose to fistulization or flap and pharyngeal mucosal ischemia. My preferred suture is a 3-0 horizontal lubricated polyglactin suture to achieve a tension-free watertight closure. Over and undertying knots can lead to fistulization either by inducing ischemia along the suture line or by being too loose allowing for egress of saliva through an "air knot" or through sutures placed at too wide an interval. Although already precoated, I have the surgical scrub run the suture through a Xeroform gauze to minimize the friction as the suture is passed through the radiated tissue and ischemic flap. My thoughts are to minimize the chance of enlarging the size of the hole already created by the needle and the suture via a "sawing" mechanism akin to a Gigli saw used for cutting bone. While a theoretical advantage, I prefer the smooth feeling as I place and draw the suture through the tissue. Care must also be taken while making adjustments in suture length while tying the knot, making certain to keep the anastomotic line in a neutral plane while trying to prevent sudden repetitive bursts of force if the suture line is pulled upward or torqued in various directions while tying (often seen when tying is performed by a more junior level assistant). I also prefer polyglactin due to its absorption profile from a time standpoint (approximately 3 weeks) and hydrolysis degradation. This theoretically reduces the inflammatory response seen in sutures undergoing protein degradation and may allow for improved healing of the anastomotic line.

I begin the inset along the posterior pharyngeal wall and work cephalad toward any oro/nasopharyngeal component and caudad to transition to the esophageal inlet (Fig. 11.4). I periodically assess the length of the remaining pharynx and flap so as to make adjustments with length mismatch gradually over the course of many stitches, rather than having to reduce a large mismatch over the course of a few stitches. Care must be taken to prevent excess redundancy in the pyriform sinus in order to minimize the chance of a reservoir that could inhibit future swallowing and serve as a potential source of aspiration. Superiorly, one must work transcervically in those patients not opened with a mandibular split. I find it helpful to have an assistant retract the mandible and place the patient in slight Trendelenburg position to aid in reaching the highest point of the reconstruction. There are instances where the robot could be considered to aid in transoral repair and inset in a hybrid fashion in those patients not split or those whose tissues are rigid from prior therapy. The final line is the anterior aspect of the pharynx where I ultimately convert from a horizontal mattress with the knot directed into the lumen and on the flap side of the anastomosis to a modified Connell-type suture for the final centimeter of closure. The exact suture material and type of suture used are surgeon dependent but should be everting and tension distributing. If a mandibular swing is employed, care must be taken at the trifurcation point between the base of tongue/posterior floor of the mouth and superolateral pharyngeal wall, which is a natural watershed area that requires special attention. I use sutures that include all three walls of closure to allow for proper tissue coaptation at this site.

If the flap used is bulky or myocutaneous in nature, I usually consider using support sutures through the fascia or horizontal sutures through muscle to reduce the tension on the flap from the forces of gravity. In some instances, a large flap may allow for a second "bolstering" layer to the anastomotic lines. In other circumstances, it may preclude closure of the contracted neck skin, thus requiring thinning of the flap or split-thickness skin grafting. If thinning is performed, my preference is to do so while the flap is revascularized to minimize potential damage to primary or secondary perforators to the skin.

I prefer to inset the flap first when possible. In my opinion this minimizes trauma and movement of the flap pedicle while insetting. If ischemic time lengthens due to a difficult inset, I will revascularize and finish the inset after. I choose to neurotize flaps to allow for potential sensory input for the patient that may aid in detecting

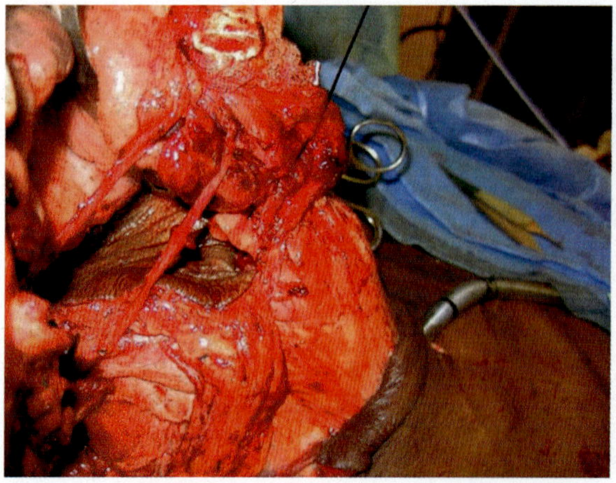

FIGURE 11.4
This photograph demonstrates the radial forearm free flap positioned into the defect. The adipose tissue lining the vascular pedicle of the radial forearm free flap is used to cover the great vessels during the healing process.

bolus or residual presence during swallow. A potential nerve donor is the local glossopharyngeal contribution. Vessel selection is a vast topic, but consideration may be given to allow for adequate draping of the pedicle to create a favorable geometry taking into consideration future neck movements that could predispose to a kink or obstruction of the vessels. Quality of vessels, size, location, and flap selected all play roles in the decision of which are chosen for recipient site. Please refer to those chapters dedicated to this subject as it is a critical part of the algorithm that has a direct impact on successful patient outcomes.

POSTOPERATIVE MANAGEMENT

The flap viability must be checked routinely. This may be performed with pinprick or Doppler evaluation. Postoperatively, the patient remains NPO for 7 days unless there has been prior radiotherapy in which case the patient remains NPO for 14 days. I prefer to perform a barium swallow evaluation prior to initiation of an oral diet. This ensures that there is no evidence of fistula or aspiration. The donor site is managed with a splint for 5 to 7 days. This helps to ensure that the skin graft used to reconstruct the donor site heals completely. After the skin graft is healed, I prefer to have the patient begin occupational therapy to ensure that strength and flexibility are regained in the donor site hand.

COMPLICATIONS

The main concern for a flap surgeon is vessel thrombosis leading to flap loss. Thankfully, with meticulous attention, success rates are in excess of 98% at my center and many high-volume major medical centers. Other concerns include fistula formation especially in those patients who have undergone prior radiotherapy. While present in some series in excess of 30%, if not recognized and managed appropriately, fistula formation can lead to flap compromise via inflammatory response, infection, external skin dehiscence, vessel exposure, and salivary contamination. Exposure and rupture of the carotid artery, either internal or externally, can occur, and one should be cognizant of the location of the great vessels in relationship to the fistula and skin breakdown. Hematoma formation, drug reaction, and perioperative cardiopulmonary complications must be identified and managed appropriately. The head and neck team must be vigilant with twice daily team rounds monitoring wounds and managing these complicated patients. Drains and flap checks must be done around the clock.

RESULTS

The radial forearm free flap provides an excellent method for reconstruction of the defect in the lateral pharyngeal wall. The pliable soft tissue associated with this donor site provides excellent restoration of the anatomy. The donor site is reliable and is associated with minimal donor site morbidity. In my experience, this donor site is a very popular approach for reconstruction of this defect. Although I have not used sensory innervation, this may improve the function, although there is a paucity of data to support this contention. The long vascular pedicle associated with this donor site is ideal for salvage surgery and for use in the vessel-depleted neck. I found that this donor site is my first choice for defects in the lateral pharyngeal wall.

PEARLS

- Thin pliable fasciocutaneous flaps such as the radial forearm or ALT (in thin individuals) are ideal donor sites for lateral pharyngeal reconstruction.
- Be mindful not to over or undersize the skin paddle.
- Consider the potential exposure of the carotid artery when insetting and draping the flap pedicle in the neck.
- Watertight closure is essential, paying careful attention to proper knot placement and tension.

PITFALLS

- Oversized flaps may inhibit functional outcomes for patients and may prevent decannulation and feeding tube removal.
- Lateral pharyngeal fistulization poses a risk to the carotid artery from contamination and exposure standpoint.
- Excess wound tension can predispose to fistula formation.

INSTRUMENTS TO HAVE AVAILABLE

- General head and neck surgical tray
- Microvascular surgical instrumentation

SUGGESTED READING

Sumer BD, Gastman BR, Nussenbaum B, et al. Microvascular flap reconstruction of major pharyngeal resections with the intent of laryngeal preservation. *Arch Otolaryngol Head Neck Surg* 2009;135(8):801–806.

De Almeida JR, Park RC, Genden EM. Reconstruction of transoral robotic surgery defects: principles and techniques. *J Reconstr Microsurg* 2012;28(7):465–472.

12 MANAGEMENT OF THE DEFECT OF THE BASE OF THE TONGUE

Eric J. Moore

INTRODUCTION

The base of the tongue (BOT) is a subsite of the oropharynx (OP). It consists of that portion of the tongue that lies posterior to the circumvallate papilla, and it extends to the vallecula at the base of the epiglottis posteriorly. The BOT contains squamous mucosal-covered lymphoid tissue (the lingual tonsil), skeletal muscle, and minor salivary glands and mucous glands. Squamous cell carcinoma and neoplasms of salivary gland origin frequently involve the BOT. Treatment of advanced cancer of the OP often involves removal of all or part of the BOT. The BOT plays a role in the oropharyngeal phase of swallowing. Its presence and function aid in formation of a food bolus and proper positioning of that bolus prior to the pharyngeal phase of swallowing. The BOT also aids in posterior displacement of the epiglottis and closure of the laryngeal inlet, thereby preventing aspiration of oral contents. Quality of life studies have demonstrated diminished swallowing function in patients undergoing treatment of oropharyngeal carcinoma. As the degree of the BOT involvement with cancer increases, the ability of the patient to develop an aspiration-free swallow is diminished.

Following resection of the BOT, the resulting defect can heal by second intention or be reconstructed with a local flap, a regional pedicle flap, or a microvascular free flap. While the first two options are often sufficient for subtotal defects in the BOT that involve less than 50% of that structure, more substantial subtotal and total defects of the BOT require major flap reconstruction to rehabilitate the patient. Pedicle flaps, such as the pectoralis major myocutaneous flap, have been used extensively for reconstruction of the BOT. They have as their major advantages ease of harvest, reliability, consistent anatomy, and minimal donor site morbidity. Pedicle flaps, however, have been associated with a higher rate of flap dehiscence, tissue necrosis, and fistula formation than microvascular flap reconstruction of the OP. The radial forearm free flap (RFFF) and the anterolateral thigh flap (ALTF) are the microvascular flaps employed most often in BOT reconstruction. They both provide vascularized soft tissue that can be folded and contoured to reconstruct the complicated three-dimensional geometry of the BOT and pharyngeal defect that is often created in resection of advanced OP tumors. While the RFFF has a longer history of use, the ALTF has been employed more often recently. The major advantage of the ALTF is the ability to close the donor site defect primarily. It provides a thicker amount of subcutaneous adipose tissue that can be an advantage or hindrance in flap design and contouring depending on the patient's body habitus.

HISTORY

When considering the ALTF donor site for reconstruction, I take not only a thorough general history but also a history focused on physical limitations related to the lower extremity including a history of prior injury or surgery that may preclude the ALTF donor site.

PHYSICAL EXAMINATION

In addition to a general physical examination, I also evaluate the lower extremity for scar, prior surgery, and muscular tone and evaluates the patient's gait. Because either leg can be used as a donor site, a history of knee instability, hip injury, or prior surgery may dictate which leg I use as a donor site. I also like to evaluate the thickness of the skin and the anatomy of the leg to determine whether the thigh is an appropriate donor site. If the tissue is too thick, I may consider an alternative such as the radial forearm flap. In contrast, if the thigh is too thin, I may consider a technique to add bulk to the flap or consider another donor site.

INDICATIONS

The indications for this technique include any BOT defect that requires bulk and epithelial lining. The ALTF was described in 1984 by Song et al., but it failed to gain popularity for some time, particularly in the Western literature and operating rooms. Two factors may have been responsible for this tempered enthusiasm: (1) The flap is associated with some variability in the vascular perforators and (2) the flap can be associated with extensive subcutaneous adipose tissue that can make contouring of the tissue difficult during the reconstruction of defects of the head and neck. Wei and others popularized the ALTF by clarifying the vascular anatomy, demonstrating the advantages of the long pedicle, and exploring the versatility of the generous cutaneous, fasciocutaneous, and myocutaneous tissue paddles that could be based on that pedicle.

Today, the ALTF is one of the most frequently employed microvascular flaps for BOT reconstruction. Adequate rehabilitation of a BOT defect requires maintenance of volume in the reconstructed tissue. While muscle and skin contract substantially in maturing flaps, subcutaneous adipose tissue is more reliably preserved. The abundance of subcutaneous adipose tissue in the ALTF allows the surgeon to design a flap of appropriate bulk and remain confident that the tissue volume will be preserved over the lifetime of the patient.

The ALTF is based on the descending branch of the lateral femoral circumflex artery, which arises from the profunda femoris artery. The artery is usually accompanied by two venae comitantes that occasionally join into one vein as they ascend. The vascular pedicle runs with the nerve to the vastus lateralis muscle in a space between the vastus lateralis and the rectus femoris muscles. The vascular pedicle supplies perforators to these muscles. The perforators to the anterolateral thigh skin can arise either as septocutaneous perforators (incidence approximately 15%) between the muscles or as musculocutaneous perforators (incidence approximately 85%) passing through the vastus lateralis muscle. In the case of septocutaneous perforators, the flap can easily be harvested as a thin septocutaneous tissue paddle. In the incidence of musculocutaneous perforators, the flap can be harvested as a musculocutaneous paddle by including a superolateral portion of the vastus lateralis muscle around the perforators or as a cutaneous perforator of the fasciocutaneous flap by meticulously dissecting the perforators through the vastus lateralis muscle.

The descending branch of the lateral femoral circumflex artery has a length between 8 and 16 cm in the adult patient. The arterial diameter is between 2 and 2.5 mm at its proximal portion, and the flap vein diameters are typically between 1.8 and 3 mm. These factors are favorable for most BOT reconstructions. The flap can be harvested as a sensate flap by including the anterior branch of the lateral cutaneous nerve of the thigh. Theoretically, the flap could be harvested as an innervated musculocutaneous flap by including the nerve to the vastus lateralis muscle.

Variability in the vascular anatomy of the ALTF has been studied, and this variability can make flap harvest difficult and, sometimes, not feasible. Shieh et al. described four variations in the skin perforators from the lateral circumflex femoral arterial system. The classic situation of vertical musculocutaneous perforators off the descending branch of the lateral circumflex femoral artery was observed in 56% of the patients. Variations included horizontal musculocutaneous perforators off the transverse branch of the lateral circumflex femoral artery (27%), septocutaneous perforators from the descending branch (10%), and horizontal septocutaneous perforators from the transverse branch (5%). Rarely, no suitable skin perforators can be found during elevation of ALTF, or the transverse branch will be of insufficient caliber or length to allow microvascular anastomosis. In these situations, the partially elevated flap is returned to the donor site and an alternative reconstructive flap will have to be elevated.

CONTRAINDICATIONS

Contraindications to reconstruction of the BOT include patient health factors, tumor factors, and donor site factors. As in all major ablative surgery of the head and neck and reconstruction, the length and extent of the procedure can put stress on the patient. Patients should have adequate cardiovascular and pulmonary function to tolerate this stress without the anticipation of major morbidity or mortality. Hypercoagulability conditions, extensive peripheral vascular disease, severe malnutrition, immunodeficiency, and surrounding tissue trauma from previous operative and nonoperative treatments can all complicate microvascular reconstruction. Previous surgery or trauma to the lower extremity needs investigation preoperatively to anticipate vascular or soft tissue damage that may preclude successful ALTF harvest.

PREOPERATIVE PLANNING

Preoperative planning includes assessment of fitness of the patient for a major surgical procedure, but this likely will have been done in consideration for tongue resection. No preoperative imaging studies or vascular studies need to be done, but the surgeon should ensure that the patient has not had a previous surgical procedure or any trauma on the lateral leg that would interrupt the vascular supply of the perforators from the lateral femoral circumflex artery.

SURGICAL TECHNIQUE

Study of swallowing function after subtotal and total glossectomy and microvascular reconstruction by Kamata et al. correlated improved function with protuberant tongue flaps that maintained their bulk. These reconstructive flaps were able to contact the posterior pharyngeal wall and obturate the oral space better than tongue reconstructions that were flat or depressed and of insufficient volume. I recommended designing a flap that was 30% wider than the resected soft tissue in order to ensure adequate postoperative volume. In design of the flap to reconstruct a BOT defect, I formed a template of the resected tissue that frequently forms an L shape owing to the fact that most BOT resections include a portion of the tonsillar fossa, lateral pharynx, and occasionally soft palate that also needs to be reconstructed. The height of the "L" is determined by measuring the most inferior aspect of the pharyngeal defect to the most superior aspect of the pharyngeal or palatal defect. The width of the widest portion of the "L" is determined by the width of the tongue base and pharyngeal wall defect. The width of the template at this level is increased by 25% to 30% to allow for anticipated flap contraction and atrophy (Figs. 12.1 to 12.3). The flap is typically 8 cm × 10 cm in the average base of tongue defect. With experience, the surgeon can estimate the extent of the defect and design a flap with generous proportions without waiting for a template, thereby harvesting the flap simultaneously with tumor extirpation by another team and decreasing the operative time. Excess flap tissue can be de-epithelialized and folded on itself for additional bulk or discarded as appropriate.

With the patient in the supine position, a line is drawn from the superolateral patella to the anterior superior iliac spine. A handheld Doppler is used to mark the position of the perforators. The perforators usually lie within a circle with a diameter of 5 cm from the midpoint of this line. The flap is designed as an oval centered on two to three of these perforators with the long axis of this oval parallel to the long axis of the thigh. The L-shaped tissue to be used is designed within this oval. The flap elevation begins with an incision of the medial side of the flap. Care should be taken to ensure that the initial incision is generously medial so as not to end up lateral to the perforators supplying the flap. Dissection is carried down to the fascia of the rectus femoris

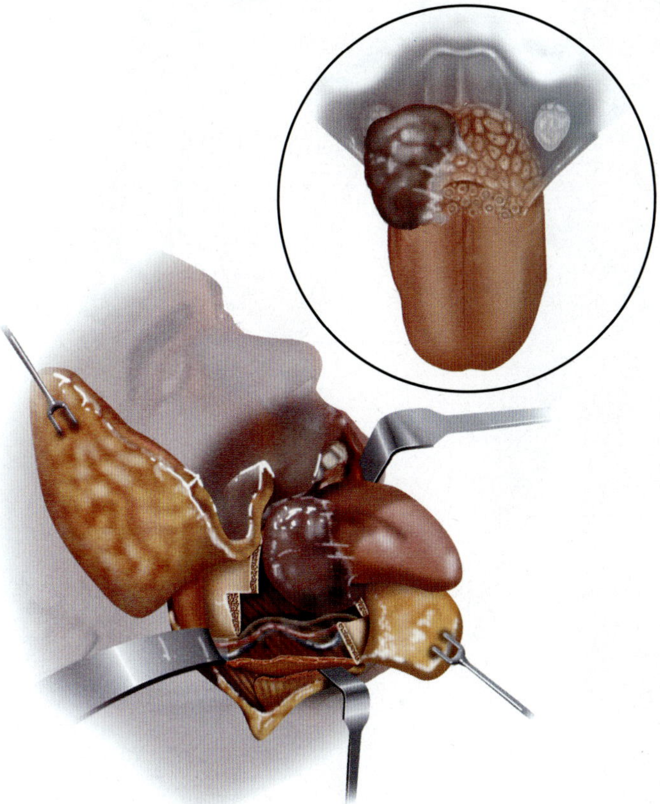

FIGURE 12.1
Base of tongue tumor exposure via mandibulotomy. Tumors can also be removed through transhyoid or transoral resection.

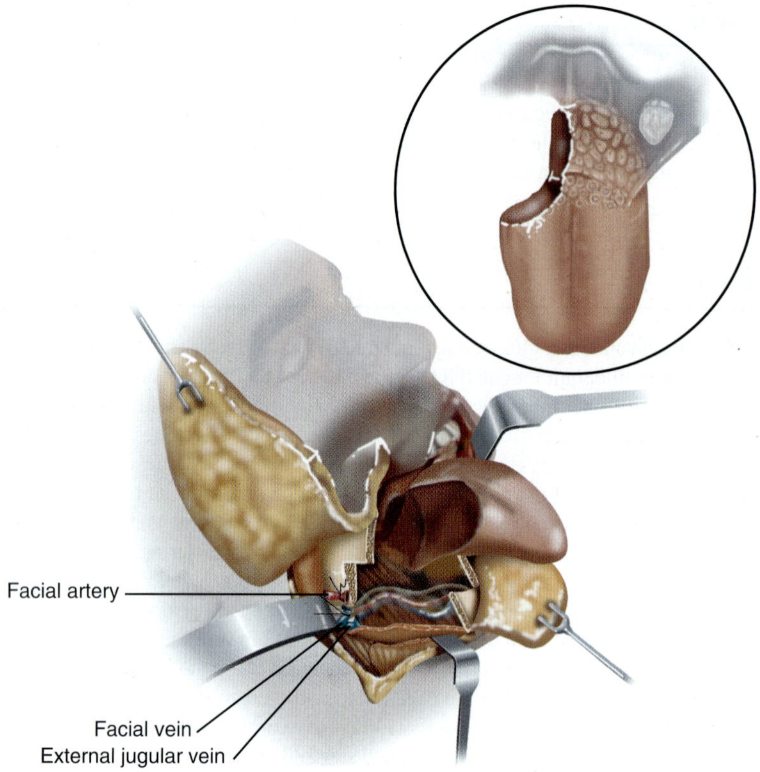

FIGURE 12.2
Resection of the tumor of the BOT. Flap design should be 30% wider than the width of the defect to provide adequate soft tissue bulk.

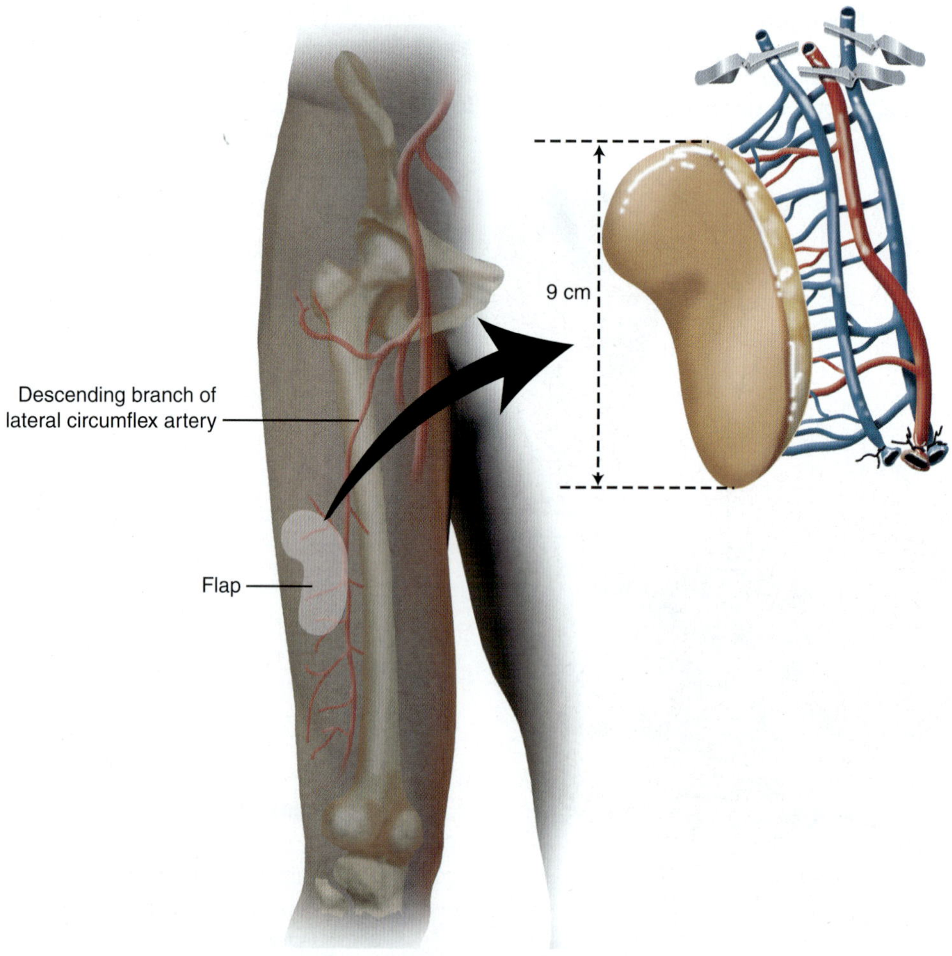

FIGURE 12.3
ALTF designed to include perforators from the descending branch of the lateral femoral circumflex artery.

muscle. Dissection can then proceed laterally in a suprafascial or subfascial plane depending on the surgeon's preference to harvest a fasciocutaneous or cutaneous flap. Dissection is carried meticulously laterally to identify either the septocutaneous perforators in the septum between the rectus femoris and the vastus lateralis or the musculocutaneous perforators piercing the vastus lateralis muscle lateral to the intermuscular septum. If the perforators are septocutaneous, the dissection proceeds easily along the medial side of the septum between the muscle bellies to identify the pedicle. If the perforators are musculocutaneous, the surgeon follows the septum to expose the pedicle, and then the medial side of these perforators is finely dissected through the muscle to their takeoff from the pedicle. Care is taken to preserve a thin cuff of muscle over the perforators to protect their integrity. Dissection of the perforators and the pedicle is easiest if it proceeds from distal to proximal. The perforators give off branches to the surrounding vastus lateralis on their lateral and posterior sides, and these branches must be clipped if the muscle is not to be included in the specimen. Alternatively, a cuff of vastus lateralis muscle can be harvested with the flap by incising the muscle lateral and posterior to the perforators after the circumferential incision of the skin flap.

After identification of the perforators and pedicle, the incision is completed around the skin paddle, and dissection is carried through the lateral vastus lateralis fascia. The distal continuation of the descending branch of the lateral circumflex femoral artery is clipped and divided. Dissection continues by freeing the perforators or muscle completely from their lateral and posterior attachments all the way to the pedicle, and then the pedicle is raised from distal to proximal with care to clip and divide the medial branches supplying the rectus femoris muscle. The flap elevation continues to the origin of the descending branch of the lateral femoral circumflex artery. Care should be taken to support the weight of the flap so as not to put tension on the pedicle during elevation. The flap can be left in situ without vessel division until the tumor extirpation is complete and the insetting for reconstruction can begin.

Prior to division of the flap pedicle, excessive subcutaneous adipose tissue can be trimmed away down to the level of the subcutaneous vascular plexus. Care should be taken not to thin the flap excessively around the perforators to prevent vascular compromise. The pedicle artery and veins are doubly clipped with microvascular clips for identification, and the flap is separated from the lower extremity and brought to the head table. Contouring is followed by insetting. The flap is inset with horizontal mattress 3-0 resorbable sutures with care to take large enough bites of native tissue to prevent the sutures from pulling through resulting in tissue dehiscence. The closure should be watertight (Fig. 12.4). If a mandibulotomy has not been performed, the surgeon may have to perform some of the insetting through the neck as well as the mouth, and an endoscope may be necessary to ensure adequate closure of the oral cavity and pharynx. The mouth should be flooded with saline at the completion of closure to ensure that no oropharyngeal leak occurs into the neck, as this can result in neck infection, vessel thrombosis, and flap failure.

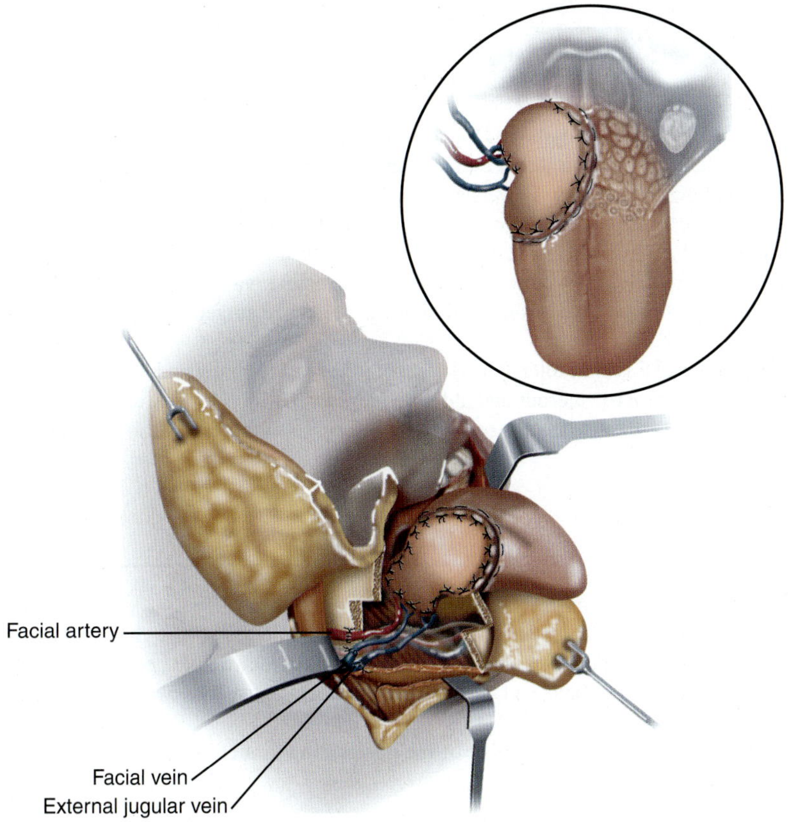

FIGURE 12.4
Flap inset for base of tongue reconstruction.

After complete flap inset, the vessels are draped into the neck with care to prevent tension or kinking. The reconstructive team should communicate with the resecting team regularly to ensure that adequate arterial and venous donor vessels are preserved for vascular anastomosis. The long pedicle of the ALTF gives the surgeon multiple options for vessel placement, but kinking can occur, and the geometry of the vessel placement in the neck deserves careful consideration. Both veins are anastomosed if possible to ensure adequate venous return. After vessel anastomosis, the neck is irrigated with sterile saline, and the neck wound is closed with adequate drainage. I prefer to monitor the flap with implantable Doppler placement, as the skin paddle of the OP reconstruction may be hard to visualize if a monitoring segment has not been externalized.

The donor site can nearly always be closed with skin undermining and primary closure with resorbable sutures over a drain. For reconstruction of the OP, the size of the skin paddle does not necessitate grafting of the donor site defect, but in the event of excessive donor site tension, the thigh wound could be reconstructed with a skin graft.

POSTOPERATIVE MANAGEMENT

The patient is monitored in the hospital with close surveillance of flap perfusion, wound drainage, and vital signs. Adequate nutrition is provided by a nasogastric feeding tube until oral intake can be initiated in 7 to 10 days. If enteral nutrition is needed past this point, then consideration should be given to placement of a gastrostomy tube. A tracheostomy tube is used until edema has resolved enough to allow the patient to breathe easily through the nose and mouth. Drains are removed from the neck and leg once their output decreases below 20 mL/d.

Early speech and swallowing physiotherapy and physical therapy are essential for maximal return to function both with OP function and ambulation. The patient should be encouraged to participate actively in speech and swallowing exercises. Motivated patients make more rapid progress than patients who are not encouraged.

COMPLICATIONS

Immediate postoperative complications such as hematoma in the donor site or recipient site, wound infection, flap partial or total necrosis, orocutaneous fistula, and wound dehiscence can occur. They are best managed by prevention, and this is best accomplished by careful preoperative patient selection and planning, meticulous execution, and attention to operative detail. Close postoperative management can identify problems when they first start to occur, and early recognition usually results in better management of complications. In the event of significant postoperative wound complications and flap failure, the surgeon may need to employ long-term use of antibiotics and chronic wound management, hyperbaric oxygen therapy, and revision surgery and flap design.

RESULTS

Patients who undergo greater than 50% resection of the BOT and reconstruction never achieve "normal" speech and swallowing, but they can expect to recover the ability to maintain nutrition with an oral diet and communicate effectively. The extent of swallowing recovery is inversely proportional to the amount of tongue resected, and it is loosely related to age, comorbidities, and baseline swallowing function before treatment.

Studies by Yanai et al. showed that 85% of patients undergoing total or near-total (>75%) resection of the BOT with laryngeal preservation were able to swallow an oral diet after tongue base reconstruction. With a carefully planned and executed ALTF tongue base reconstruction, the experienced surgeon can provide meaningful rehabilitation for the patient.

The donor site defect with the ALTF is well tolerated. The scar in the leg is lengthy and difficult to conceal, but the patient should expect to return to vigorous and unlimited leg activity after healing and a period of rehabilitation. Extensive resection of the vastus lateralis or injury to the nerve to the vastus can diminish leg strength and alter gait.

PEARLS

- Greater than 50% resection of the BOT requires reconstruction to preserve function.
- Maintenance of the bulk of the flap and the ability of the flap to contact the posterior pharyngeal wall and obturate the upper OP during swallowing improves function. The ALTF provides a long pedicle, adequate subcutaneous adipose tissue that maintains its bulk, and the ability to allow a simultaneous two-team approach to BOT resection and reconstruction.
- The ALTF is supplied by musculocutaneous perforators of the descending branch of the lateral femoral circumflex artery the majority of the time.

- The surgeon should consider a template of the defect and plan for some atrophy of the flap by designing the flap slightly wider than the defect.
- The flap should be meticulously inset in a watertight closure.
- Early speech and swallowing therapy and donor site physical therapy maximize function.

PITFALLS

- Failure to Doppler the perforators and begin the incision medial enough on the thigh may place the surgeon lateral to the perforators with the initial incision.
- Patients who require a skin graft for closure of the donor site have been shown to experience donor site morbidity.

INSTRUMENTS TO HAVE AVAILABLE

- Standard head and neck surgery set

SUGGESTED READING

Song YG, Chen GZ, Song YL. The free thigh flap: a new free flap concept based on the septocutaneous artery. *Br J Plast Surg* 1984;37:149.

Shieh SJ, Chiu HY, Yu JC, et al. Free anterolateral thigh flap for reconstruction of head and neck defects following cancer ablation. *Plast Reconstr Surg* 2000;105:2349–2357.

Wei FC, Jain V, Celik N, et al. Have we found an ideal soft- tissue flap? Experience with 672 Anterolateral thigh flaps. *Plast Reconstr Surg* 2002;109:2219–2226.

Yanai C, Kikutani T, et al. Functional outcome after total and subtotal glossectomy with free flap reconstruction. *Head Neck* 2008;30:909–918.

Chepeha DB, et al. Oropharygnoplasty with template based reconstruction of oropharyngeal defects. *Arch Otolarynglo Head Neck Surg* 2009;135(9):88.

13 MANAGEMENT OF THE COMPOSITE OROMANDIBULAR DEFECT: THE PECTORALIS MAJOR MYOCUTANEOUS FLAP AND RECONSTRUCTION PLATE

Derrick T. Lin

INTRODUCTION

Oral cavity defects including a segmental mandibulectomy can be a challenge for the reconstructive head and neck surgeon. Defects in this anatomical site may be due to oncologic resection, trauma, osteoradionecrosis, or infection/inflammation. To restore oral function, a composite graft consisting of both bone and soft tissue is ideal. The fibula, scapula, iliac crest, and osteocutaneous radial forearm are excellent donor sites for free tissue transfer. However, patient factors often play a role in decision making, such as unhealthy patients where limiting operative time and decreasing the risk of take back is essential, patients with extensive vascular disease, or patients with failed osteocutaneous free flap reconstruction. In these patients, placement of a reconstructive bar and a pectoralis major myocutaneous flap may be a safer option.

The goals of mandibular reconstruction are to reverse aesthetic deformity and functional loss. In general, lateral defects of the mandible left without reconstruction are better tolerated than are anterior defects. The use of a reconstruction bar and a pectoralis flap is usually considered in this setting. However, in the anterior mandibular defect, the use of a reconstruction plate and pectoralis flap often leads to extrusion of the plate with loss of structural support of the tongue, which results in functional deficits involving mastication and deglutition.

In the 1970s, the description of the myocutaneous circulation of the pectoralis flap led to its introduction in the use of head and neck reconstruction. The blood supply of this flap arises from the descending pectoral branch of the thoracoacromial artery. The consistency of this blood supply makes this reconstruction extremely reliable. The flap provides a large segment of skin and soft tissue, it is technically easy and efficient to harvest, it does not require a delay, and the donor site can be closed primarily. For decades, it has been the most popular flap for reconstruction after extensive resection of head and neck malignancies.

HISTORY

There are several options for managing a composite defect in the oral cavity. I find that a complete history is helpful in determining whether the patient is a candidate for free tissue transfer or reconstruction with a regional flap. Although free tissue transfer offers the optimal approach to reconstruction in select patients, regional flap reconstruction can offer an advantage. In patients with significant medical comorbidities, a surgical procedure that is less time intensive may be indicated. Other important aspects of the patient history relate to donor site availability. If the patient has had previous surgery or trauma that limit the donor site options, reconstruction with a regional flap may be indicated.

An important part of the history taking is exploring the patient's expectations. An understanding of these expectations can impact the reconstructive options. While some patients expect dental rehabilitation with osseointegrated implants, others are less motivated and will choose a less time-intensive surgery. A careful preoperative discussion and understanding of these expectations are essential in achieving a good result.

PHYSICAL EXAMINATION

Once the decision has been made to proceed with reconstruction using a regional flap, the physical examination is important in determining if the patient is fit for this approach. The physical examination will determine if the defect can be reconstructed with a regional flap. Prior chest wall surgery may preclude use of this donor site. Similarly, if a patient has a history of external beam radiotherapy to the head and neck, a reconstruction plate may not be ideal as it often extrudes over the course of time. Other important features of the physical examination are related to the type of defect. Through and through defects involving the cheek skin, the mandible, and the buccal mucosa typically require a free flap to achieve an adequate functional result.

INDICATIONS

In general, osteocutaneous free tissue reconstruction is preferred after composite resection with segmental mandibulectomy especially for the anterior defect. The choices include fibular, scapular, iliac crest, and osteocutaneous radial forearm free flaps. However, for patients with severe comorbidities, the reliability and the relatively shorter length of surgery with the pectoralis major flap should be considered.

There are, however, disadvantages in using the pectoralis major muscle for reconstruction. The harvest of the pectoralis myocutaneous flap often results in distortion of the chest, although the inframammary crease can be used for female patients. Additionally, some degree of shoulder dysfunction is to be expected since a major function of the pectoralis major muscle is to adduct and medially rotate the arm. With early physical therapy, this level of dysfunction is usually well tolerated.

CONTRAINDICATIONS

There are rare anatomic anomalies that would preclude the use of the pectoralis flap reconstruction. Congenital absence of the pectoralis major muscle occurs in 1 in 11,000 people. Poland also described the congenital absence of the sternocostal head of the pectoralis major muscle seen in conjunction with ipsilateral syndactyly.

The anterior segmental mandibulectomy defect is a relative contraindication for the use of a reconstruction bar and pectoralis flap. The use of the reconstruction plate as an anterior projection element leads almost uniformly to extrusion of the plate resulting in deprojection and loss of support of the tongue resulting in oral incompetence.

If the patient has preexisting severe trismus from either previous radiation therapy or tumor involvement of the pterygoid muscles, reconstruction of the defect with the pectoralis flap without the reconstruction plate should be considered. The placement of the plate may worsen the trismus and downgrade oral competence. By insetting the pectoralis flap alone and letting the mandible swing, the degree of trismus will often be improved. This is not a viable choice in anterior defect since it would result in oral incompetence.

PREOPERATIVE PLANNING

The donor site and defect must be carefully evaluated. Although major surgery or previous trauma to the pectoralis muscle would be a relative contraindication, previous sternotomy for cardiac or thoracic procedures spares traumatic injury to the pectoralis major muscle and is not a contraindication.

The skin overlying the pectoralis muscle should be evaluated for concerning lesions. The muscle should be palpated to ensure that the patient does not have one of the rare congenital abnormalities mentioned above.

Under anesthesia, the inferior aspect of the pectoralis major muscle should be palpated. In general, no more than 30% of the skin paddle should be distal to this point. The lateral and medial aspect of the proposed flap is then marked out and grasped to ensure that the donor site can be closed primarily. Using the clavicle as a hinge point, the proposed distal aspect of the flap should be able to reach the most distal aspect of the defect.

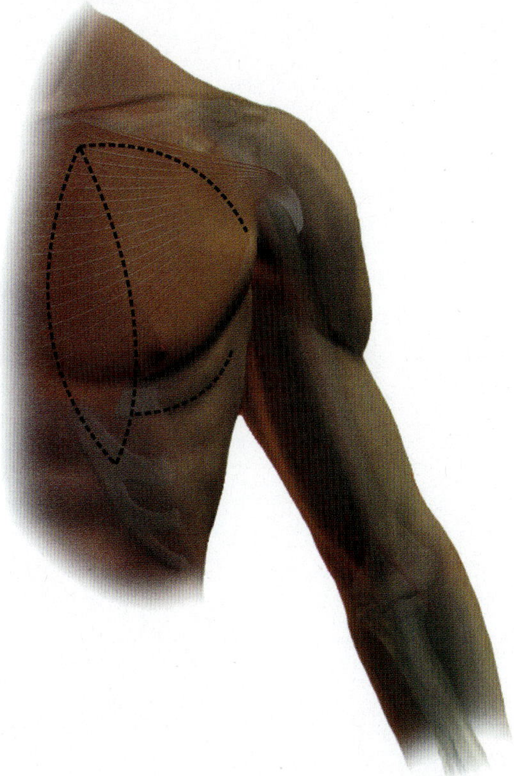

FIGURE 13.1
External markings on the left check for a pectoralis flap harvest.

SURGICAL TECHNIQUE

The skin is prepped from the clavicle down to the level of the umbilicus extending from the midline of the chest to the axilla. The skin flap is marked using a "pinch test" where the skin medial to the nipple to the midline chest is grasped, ensuring primary closure of the donor site. The superior aspect of the flap is usually marked out at the same horizontal plane as the axilla. The inferior aspect of the skin paddle is marked out with no more than one-third of the skin paddle distal to the inferior border of the pectoralis muscle (Fig. 13.1).

First, the incision is made on the lateral aspect of the proposed skin paddle. The lateral border of the pectoralis major muscle is identified, which allows me to refashion the skin paddle if a significant portion is not overlying the pectoralis muscle. Once the muscle is identified, the avascular plane between the pectoralis major and the pectoralis minor muscle is bluntly dissected. This allows identification of the descending pectoral branch of the thoracoacromial artery (Fig. 13.2). Two vascular pedicles are often identified. For mobilization purposes, the lateral pedicle can be sacrificed safely. Once the pedicle is identified, the medial skin incision is made at the level of the midline of the chest and carried down to the level of the pectoralis major muscle.

The skin paddle is tacked to the underlying pectoralis major muscles using 3-0 Vicryl sutures to avoid shearing during elevation of the flap. The pectoralis major muscle is then dissected off of the chest wall using electrocautery. Intercostal perforators must be carefully ligated or cauterized.

The medial attachments to the sternum are then transected to the level of the clavicle. Care must be taken to stay lateral to the internal mammary perforators in the second and third intercostal spaces. In a similar fashion laterally, the muscular attachments to the humeral head are divided up to the level of the clavicle, being careful not injure the cephalic vein.

The nerve of the pectoralis major muscle is identified intimately associated with the vascular pedicle. Prior to its transection, the pectoral nerve can be confirmed by stimulation. In my experience, it is important to divide this nerve to avoid constriction of the venous pedicle especially if the muscular portion of the flap needs to be rotated for reconstruction. The flap is then completely harvested, keeping the vascular pedicle in view (Fig. 13.3).

A tunnel is created in a subcutaneous plane approximately four finger breadths in size to allow rotation of the flap into the neck without constriction of the blood supply to the flap. The flap is then brought through this tunnel into the oral cavity defect.

A 2.4 locking reconstruction plate is used. Attempts are made to achieve appropriate occlusion especially in a dentulous patient. This can be accomplished by fashioning the plate prior to the mandibulectomy. If this cannot be done due to external erosion of the mandible by tumor, an external fixator may be used. Once the plate is in place, three screws are placed on both the proximal and distal aspects of the remaining bone (Fig. 13.4).

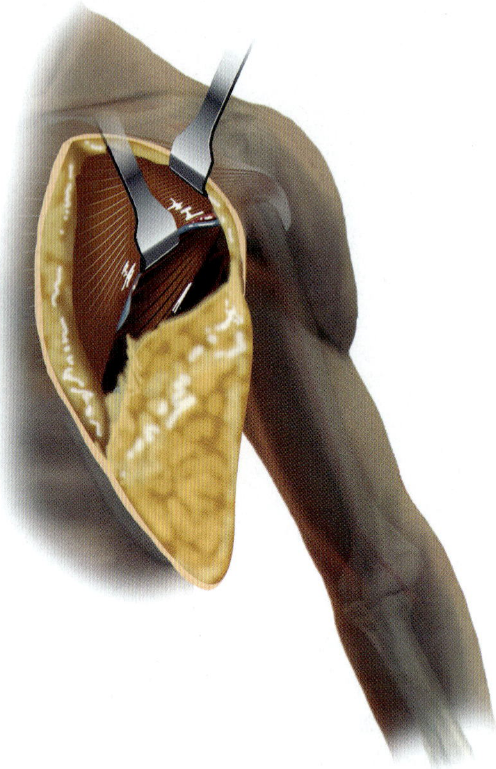

FIGURE 13.2
Pectoralis flap harvest. Vascular pedicle identified between pectoralis major and pectoralis minor muscles (*arrow*).

The flap is then brought medial to the reconstruction bar. Every attempt should be made to try to cover the reconstruction plate entirely with the pectoralis muscle flap.

Care must also be taken to orient the pedicle properly to prevent excessive twisting during its rotation into the head and neck region. The skin portion of the paddle is then inset from distal to proximal using 3-0 Vicryl horizontal mattress sutures (Fig. 13.5).

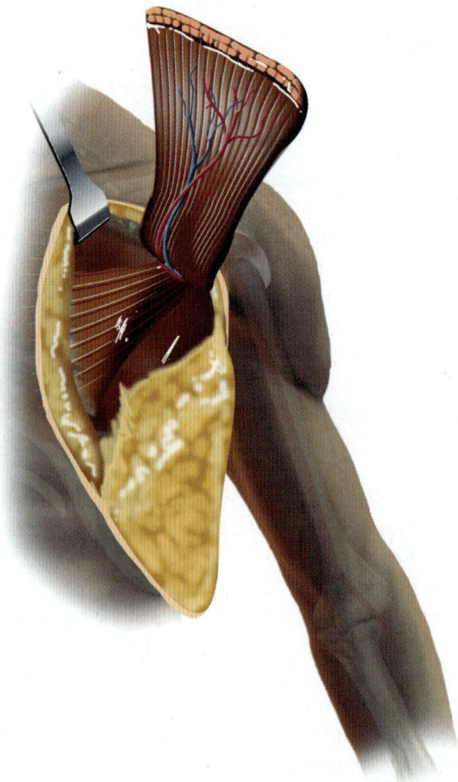

FIGURE 13.3
Complete flap harvest with vascular pedicle in view (*arrow*).

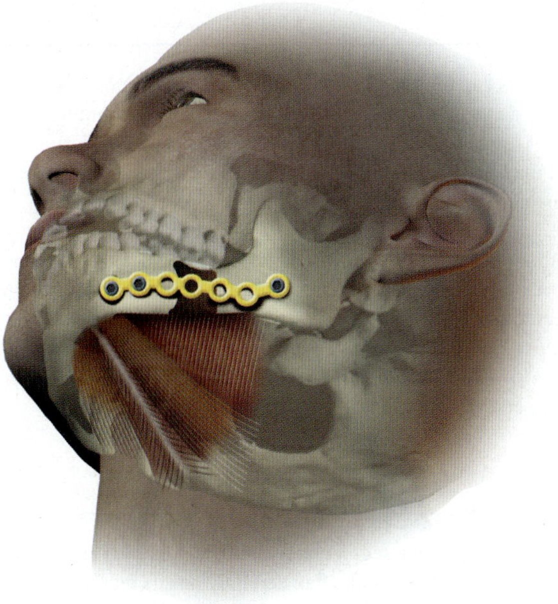

FIGURE 13.4
Lateral segmental mandibulectomy with reconstruction bar.

Prior to closure of the donor site, the remaining musculature at the humeral head is clamped and ligated to prevent bleeding from this area, which is a major cause of hematoma in the donor site. Two 19 French drains are placed in the chest. 2-0 Vicryl sutures are used for the deep layer closure, and a skin stapler is used to close the skin. Elevation of the skin flaps is often necessary to allow for tension-free closure.

POSTOPERATIVE MANAGEMENT

The flap must be carefully inspected for viability. Any change in arterial or venous supply requires exploration. Leeches may sometimes be required for venous congestion. Staples in the chest are typically removed on postoperative day 7.

Tracheostomy is generally required for approximately 7 days.

Nutrition is typically given through a nasogastric tube for a minimum of 7 days in nonradiated patients. In patients who have been radiated, I usually waits 2 weeks prior to initiating an oral soft diet.

I recommend an evaluation by a speech–language pathologist in these patients to help with regaining good swallowing function.

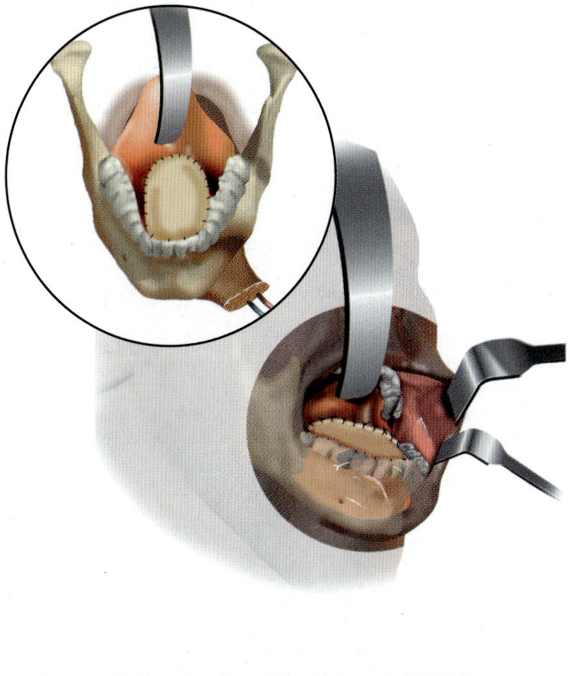

FIGURE 13.5
Skin paddle of the pectoralis flap inset into the defect in the oral cavity.

COMPLICATIONS

Complications are relatively rare in the use of a pectoralis flap for oral cavity reconstruction. The most common complication is a hematoma at the donor site. This is managed urgently with surgical exploration and ligation of any bleeding vessels.

Should a hematoma occur in the neck, the flap may be compromised due to pressure in the blood vessels from the collection of blood. This should also be managed with urgent surgical exploration and evacuation of the hematoma and gaining complete hemostasis.

Compromise of the vascular pedicle may sometimes occur. Arterial insufficiency can be detected at the time of harvest by carefully inspecting the skin to ensure viability. Venous insufficiency may occur due to constriction of the pedicle by the pectoral nerve if it has not been transected at the level of the subdermal tunnel. Leeches may be necessary when venous congestion occurs if exploration reveals no external compression of the pedicle.

Plate extrusion occurs at a rate of 20% to 30% for lateral mandibular defects and uniformly in anterior mandibular defects in my experience. This is usually seen anywhere from 6 to 24 months postoperatively.

RESULTS

Although the ideal reconstruction of the oromandibular complex for a segmental mandibulectomy is a composite graft incorporating bone, placement of a reconstruction plate and pectoralis flap certainly has its merits. For the unhealthy patient, the shorter operative time, hospital stay, and decreased risk of reexploration is of great benefit.

Extrusion of the plate continues to be a vexing problem. For the lateral defect, there is a 20% to 30% extrusion rate, while for the anterior defect, it is almost always expected. If this occurs, the plate must be removed and the mandible allowed to swing.

PEARLS

- The distal third of the flap may be random if necessary. Rectus fascia should be raised with the flap in this location.
- The muscular attachments to the humerus should be ligated to avoid a hematoma in the donor site.
- The donor site should be closed primarily.

PITFALLS

- The flap donor site can cause distortion of the breast in females that should be discussed preoperatively. If the defect is small, the skin paddle can be placed in the inframammary crease.
- If stay sutures are not used to secure the skin paddle on the muscle, shearing may occur.
- There is a high expected extrusion rate of the reconstruction plate with this procedure.

INSTRUMENTS TO HAVE AVAILABLE

- Standard head and neck surgery set
- Titanium mandibular reconstruction plates, drill, and reciprocating saw

SUGGESTED READING

Ariyan S. The pectoralis major myocutaneous flap. A versatile flap for the reconstruction in the head and neck. *Plast Reconstr Surg* 1979:63:73.

Gullane PJ, Havas TE, Holmes HH. Mandibular reconstruction with metal plate and myocutaneous flap. *Aust N Z J Surg* 1986;56:701–706.

Cordiero PG, Hildalgo DA. Soft tissue coverage of mandibular reconstructive plates. *Head Neck* 1994;16:112–115.

Kensuke K, Yoshiaki T, Yojiro I, et al. Reliable, minimally invasive oromandibular reconstruction using metal plate rolled with pectoralis major myocutaneous flap. *J Craniofac Surg* 2001;154:34–37.

El-Zohairy M, Mostafa A, Amin A, et al. Mandibular reconstruction using pectoralis major myocutaneous flap and titanium plates after ablative surgery for locally advanced tumors of the oral cavity. *J Egypt Natl Cancer Inst* 2009;21(4):299–307.

14 RECONSTRUCTION OF THE COMPOSITE OROMANDIBULAR DEFECT: FIBULAR FREE FLAP

Richard E. Hayden

INTRODUCTION

In 1973, Daniels and Taylor described the transfer of the first free skin flap, the groin flap pedicled on the superficial circumflex iliac artery (SCIA). Panje, Baker, et al. were the first to bring this free flap to head and neck surgery in 1975 when they used the free groin flap for tongue reconstruction. As a medical student, I worked with Rollin Daniels, MD at McGill University, performing microvascular reattachment of fingers. As a resident at the University of Toronto in the late 1970s, I studied under John Fredrickson, MD. Ostrup and Fredrickson had performed the first vascularized mandible reconstruction when they successfully transferred free vascularized rib for mandibular reconstruction in dogs in 1975. I worked with Fredrickson in 1977 using free groin flaps with attached iliac crest bone to repair oromandibular defects. The groin flap with bone was not successful as the SCIA reliably supplied the skin of the groin but not the iliac bone.

The modern history of oromandibular reconstruction using free flaps dates to 1978 when Taylor introduced the composite iliac crest flap pedicled on the deep circumflex iliac artery (DCIA). The DCIA not the SCIA supplied the iliac crest bone, and musculocutaneous perforators from the DCIA also supplied the skin overlying the iliac crest. His technique provided, for the first time, a reliable osseocutaneous flap with bone stock that could closely reduplicate the contours of the original mandible up to hemimandibular and angle-to-angle defects. An additional feature was that the bone stock was sufficient to easily accept osseointegrated implants. However, the soft tissue component was usually excessively bulky for most intraoral soft tissue reconstructions. It was comprised of a cuff of internal oblique, external oblique, and transversalis muscles with overlying adipose tissue and skin. The cutaneous branches of the DCIA coursed through this triad of abdominal muscles, medial to the iliac crest, to supply the overlying adipose tissue and skin. Therefore, a cuff of these muscles was required with the bone to protect the cutaneous blood supply. This, combined with the frequently slack abdominal wall and abdominal adipose tissue distribution found in many of these patients requiring oromandibular reconstruction, frequently led to an excessively bulky soft tissue component. This bulk was often a poor match for the intraoral soft tissue defect. Also, the requirement that this bulky soft tissue had to remain aligned with the adjacent iliac bone to avoid torsion or compression of the cutaneous blood supply led to a suboptimal intraoral soft tissue reconstruction.

Ramasastry identified the ascending branch of the DCIA as a separate vascular supply to the internal oblique muscle. Urken combined the findings of Taylor and Ramasastry to develop a composite flap that used the abundant reliable iliac bone covered intraorally with the equally reliable internal oblique muscle. He then externalized the excessively thick musculocutaneous component incorporating it as an external monitoring segment into the closure of the neck wound, ultimately discarding it at a later time. This solved the problems associated with attempting to close the intraoral defect with an excessively bulky muscle–adipose tissue–skin component. There remained, however, a geographic mandate wherein the size of the attached internal oblique muscle paddle limited the size of the intraoral soft tissue defect that could be reliably closed. Other issues that plagued the iliac crest flap were the relatively short vascular pedicle and the significant morbidity associated with the donor site. Nonetheless, it remained my first choice for oromandibular reconstruction from 1978 to 1985.

The radial forearm free flap was introduced to the West in 1981 and quickly became one of the most frequently used soft tissue free flaps for reconstruction of head and neck surgical defects for the next two decades. Harvest of a portion of the radius bone with this flap was popularized by Soutar in the early 1980s, but the small amount of available bone stock (one-third of the circumference of the radius) limited its application and therefore its popularity for oromandibular reconstruction. The potential morbidity associated with a pathologic fracture of the radius deterred many surgeons.

The free scapular skin flap was introduced by Dos Santos in 1980, and the free parascapular skin flap was introduced the following year by Nassif. Both flaps were vascularized by the cutaneous branches of the circumflex scapular artery. In 1985, Swartz and Banis developed the scapular composite osseocutaneous flap based on the circumflex scapular artery that they demonstrated supplied not only the two skin flaps but also the lateral border of the scapula. This flap provided a dramatic advance for oromandibular reconstruction. The skin paddle(s) could be huge, were usually relatively thin and pliable, and could be rotated 180 degrees on the axis of the bone. The skin paddle(s) could easily be contoured to intraoral or facial defects or to through-and-through defects. The lateral border of the scapula provided less bone stock than did the iliac crest but much more than did the radius. The average adult donor scapula could easily duplicate a hemimandible. The bone stock was inadequate for reliable osseointegration in the 1980s and 1990s although the smaller implants currently available make osseointegration in this setting modestly successful. The donor morbidity was less than that produced by the iliac crest flap and certainly much less than that associated with a potential pathologic fracture of the radius, an inherent risk with the radial forearm flap. The vascular pedicle was longer and of greater caliber than that of the iliac crest flap. The angular branch of the thoracodorsal system was identified as a separate vascular supply to the tip of the scapula by Coleman in 1992. This enhanced the options for contouring the bone segment of the scapular flap. The biggest negative associated with this flap for oromandibular reconstruction was the need for patient positioning to allow for flap harvest and head and neck surgical ablation. Synchronous two-team ablation and flap harvest can be done with the patient on a beanbag, in lateral 45-degree position, head turned on a neurosurgical headholder, but exposure is somewhat compromised for each team, and a synchronous contralateral neck dissection is extremely difficult. Asynchronous ablation and reconstruction demand a time-consuming turning of the patient during the case. Nonetheless, this was my absolute favorite flap for oromandibular reconstruction between 1985 and 1990.

Taylor had also introduced the free fibular flap in 1978 based on the peroneal artery and its venae comitantes. It was used primarily for long bone replacement until 1990 when Hidalgo demonstrated its utility for oromandibular reconstruction. It has been my preferred choice for oromandibular reconstruction since 1990 and by 2000 was unquestionably the gold standard of reconstructive surgeons worldwide.

The fibular flap provides up to 25 cm of vascularized bone, enough to reconstruct almost any defect of the mandible. It is important to maintain 6 cm of fibula and interosseous membrane proximally and distally to maintain the integrity of the knee and ankle joints. The bone is densely cortical, and I began placing osseointegrated implants at the primary surgery in 1990. Implant retention over decades has been excellent. The skin of the proximal lateral calf is often supplied by musculocutaneous perforators through the soleus muscles. The skin of the distal lateral calf is supplied by septocutaneous branches of the peroneal artery, which traverse the posterior crural septum between the peroneal musculature and the soleus muscle. These branches are more common in the lower half of the septum. Preoperative assessment of the cutaneous branches makes the harvest quicker and more reliable (see Preoperative Planning). Almost the entire surface of the lateral lower leg can be reliably harvested with rectangular skin paddles up to 20 × 10 cm. This is more than enough skin for almost all intraoral or through-and-through defects encountered. Multiple skin paddles are available depending on the number of cutaneous branches. In the patient with only a single cutaneous branch, large skin paddles are still possible and segmental deepithelialization of the paddle can produce multiple skin paddles for synchronous intraoral and extraoral coverage. The skin of the calf is usually thin and pliable but can be thick in obese patients; but this situation also applies to iliac crest and scapular flaps in these patients.

The quick and easy harvest is performed remote from the head and neck with the patient in the supine position. The donor morbidity is far less than either the iliac crest or scapula donor site. The vascular pedicle has large caliber vessels. The length of the vascular pedicle is somewhat relative. The absolute length of the peroneal pedicle from the proximal fibula is relatively short, but if distal fibula is to be used, which is most common, the proximal bone is discarded, lengthening the pedicle considerably. Conversely, when reconstructing an extensive mandibular defect, the bone is not shortened and the vascular pedicle goes directly to vessels in the ipsilateral neck while the proximal fibula replaces the ipsilateral mandible and the distal fibula replaces the anterior and contralateral mandible.

Contouring the fibula with its thick cortical bone requires ostectomies as "green stick" osteotomies are impossible. Preplanning (see Preoperative Planning) optimizes vascular pedicle length and its geometry with neck vessels. Elliptical skin paddles up to 6 cm wide and 20 cm long can usually be closed primarily leaving a vertical scar in the posterior lateral lower leg. Larger skin paddles require a skin graft.

The ease of harvest, reliability, huge skin and bone units available, adequate bone stock for predictable osseointegration, and low donor morbidity combine to make this the most useful and popular reconstructive option for oromandibular defects in the modern era.

HISTORY

When considering a fibula flap for reconstruction of an oromandibular defect, I take the usual thorough history, including coverage of issues that affect postoperative care and wound healing such as weight loss, diabetes, hypothyroidism, and substance abuse. It is also important to ask specifically about a history of previous fractures to the lower limbs, total knee replacement, or a history of deep venous thrombosis since this aspect of the medical history is frequently overlooked or forgotten by the patient. A history of diabetes or peripheral vascular disease is also important but I have found that the surprises that I have encountered are almost always associated with recanalized peroneal veins following deep vein thrombosis (known or unknown) or fracture. Any history of gait disturbance, unilateral ankle swelling, pain, or discomfort needs to be acknowledged, considered, and recorded.

PHYSICAL EXAMINATION

In addition to the usual complete physical examination, I pay close attention to the lower extremities. In particular, evidence of venous stasis or vascular insufficiency is noted. Significant varicosities can signal significant deep venous problems. Pedal temperature and pulses must be examined. Stigmata of previous surgery, trauma, or burns are significant. The symmetry of the calves and ankles, the thickness, and hair-bearing qualities of the lower leg skin are assessed. Most important, perhaps is an assessment of the vascular supply to each lower leg. There are rare anatomic vascular anomalies in which the ever-present peroneal artery may be dominant to the foot (peronea magna). This is the artery that will be harvested. Simple assessment of pedal pulses will not demonstrate these cases. I assess and record the skin supply and three-vessel runoff of each lower leg with objective, recorded Doppler and CT angiography. This is one of the deciding factors on choosing which fibula to harvest (see Preoperative Planning). This identifies any anatomic anomalies including arterial stenoses associated with peripheral vascular disease while also illustrating the cutaneous branches and their anatomic correlates.

INDICATIONS

With up to 200 cm^2 of skin and 25 cm of bone available, the fibula flap is indicated for almost all oromandibular reconstructions. The bone is sufficient in length to reconstruct almost total mandible defects and can be "double barreled" to provide mass sufficient to reduplicate the dentulous mandible for anterior and lateral defects. Before I started to harvest very large rectangular skin paddles, I treated through-and-through oral–facial–mandibular defects differently. For small intraoral combined with large extraoral defects, I would use the vascularized flexor hallucis longus (FHL) muscle attached to the fibula to fill the intraoral defect leaving the skin paddle to close the large extraoral facial defect. Intraoral mucosa, both buccal–labial and lingual, was sewn to the FHL muscle much as was done with the intraoral internal oblique muscle when it covered iliac crest bone replacing the mandible. These muscles quickly atrophy, leaving a tight mucosal surface over the intraoral neomandible. For defects that had large synchronous intraoral and facial soft tissue defects, I would use the scapula flap. Since I started harvesting very large skin paddles with the fibula, I find less use for the scapula flap and hardly ever use muscle only intraorally. The large skin paddles can be divided as separate perforator flaps when multiple cutaneous branches exist or a large skin paddle can simply be divided into separate skin surfaces by deepithelializing intervening segments. This allows for closure of large intraoral and facial defects with bone replacement. Very large intraoral defects such as subtotal or total glossectomy defects in concert with mandibular and facial skin defects are still repaired with scapular flaps incorporating very large scapular and parascapular skin paddles.

The osseocutaneous fibular flap as I now use it can easily replace hemitongue, symphysis-to-condyle mandibular defects even if they include the buccal mucosa. Equally easy to replace is the body-to-body mandibular defect with loss of the anterior half of the tongue even if the defect includes the chin. A lateral defect involving through-and-through cheek, facial defect, lateral mandible, floor of the mouth, and buccal lining is easy to replace, but as this defect extends more medial to include substantial amounts of mobile tongue, this technique loses its effectiveness since tongue tethering becomes a bigger factor. Intraoral defects can also include the oropharynx. The fibula composite flap can easily provide replacement of the tongue base, tonsil, or palate region along with the lateral and posterior mandible. Importantly, these defects rarely include an external facial defect. Also important is the need to preplan these reconstructions so that the distal fibula is at the condylar location, thereby allowing much more freedom with the orientation of the vascular pedicle (see Preoperative Planning). This technique also places the skin with the best blood supply (that of the distal leg) in the region of the soft tissue defect, thereby minimizing the risk of fistula formation. This is doubly important when reconstructing through-and-through defects. The most reliable skin paddle should always be used for the intraoral closure, thereby reducing the risk of fistula formation that could threaten the vascular anastomoses and thereby the entire reconstruction. Less reliable skin used for the external facial defect, if compromised, can be more easily replaced while preserving the microvascular anastomoses in the neck, the vascularized neomandible, and intraoral flap.

CONTRAINDICATIONS

Absolute:	Insufficient vascularity to the lower leg and foot
Relative:	Only one lower leg or foot
	Severe atherosclerotic changes on angiography
	History of deep venous thrombosis: noninvasive venography recommended
	History of trauma, fractures, or surgery on lower extremity: may choose contralateral leg, evaluate carefully

PREOPERATIVE PLANNING

Preoperative planning is more important with this flap than with most. The vascular supply to the potential flap is paramount, so if one leg is deficient and the other is not, the leg with the adequate blood supply is obviously chosen. In such cases, the issues reviewed below are still important although ideal design may have to be compromised.

In those patients who have adequate vascularity to both potential fibula flaps, there are important preoperative considerations required to maximize the utility of the flap. A fibula flap from either leg can be used to successfully reconstruct oromandibular defects. However, one side is always superior for each defect. There are constants and variables that need to be systematically assessed preoperatively in each case to determine the best choice of a flap.

The constants are as follows:

- The lateral aspect of the fibula is best for plate and screw application and should represent the external aspect of the neomandible.
- The peroneal vascular pedicle runs on the posteromedial aspect of the fibula so that this medial surface of the fibula should be avoided or protected from excessive manipulation or instrumentation and should never be the recipient of plates or screws.
- The cutaneous branches leave the peroneal vascular pedicle on the medial aspect of the fibula and course posterior to the bone toward the skin. In the proximal lower leg, they may perforate the soleus muscle on their way to the skin. In the more distal lower leg, most of these cutaneous branches run directly from the peroneal vessels into the posterior crural septum and on to the skin (septocutaneous). Some cutaneous branches can run into the intermuscular septum and then posteriorly through the lateral aspect of the soleus muscle to the skin (septomusculocutaneous).
- The anterior aspect of the fibula is the best location for placing osseointegrated implants especially at the time of primary reconstructive surgery. This approach minimizes risk to the vascular pedicle medial to the bone and to the cutaneous branches posteriorly. This means that the anterior aspect of the fibula is the ideal gingival aspect of the neomandible.
- The natural location of the skin paddle is posterolateral to the bone (Fig. 14.1).
- The distance between the peroneal pedicle on the medial aspect of the fibula and the skin, that is, the length of the cutaneous branches is finite. Therefore, rotation of the skin paddle anteriorly over the anterior aspect of the bone is also limited if one is to avoid excessive traction or compression of these cutaneous branches and subsequent vascular compromise of the skin paddle. There is usually sufficient arc of rotation available for the skin paddle to reconstruct intraoral defects from buccal sulcus to floor of the mouth, but lingual defects often put too much strain on the skin paddle brought from the lateral side (Fig. 14.2). Rotating the skin paddle posteriorly over the posterior aspect of the bone puts much less strain on the cutaneous branches since they are not draped over the lateral and anterior aspects of the fibula and is therefore useful for lingual and more medial defects. Therefore, for large intraoral soft tissue defects, the bone can be turned upside down so that the posterior aspect of the fibula now represents the gingival aspect of the neomandible, and this orientation gives much more latitude to the placement of the skin paddle especially for closing large intraoral defects involving the tongue. The posterior aspect of the fibula is less favorable for placing implants at the time of primary surgery but is equally good for delayed implant placement (Fig. 14.3).
- Skin paddles can be rotated 90 degrees on the axis of the fibula around their perforator(s) allowing for greater leeway in closing complex soft tissue defects. This is especially true for complex body–body mandibular defects with large anterior intraoral and extraoral soft tissue defects. It is critical, in such cases, to design the osteotomies so that the cutaneous supply, if there is only one, is geographically associated with the appropriate piece of fibula (usually the central segment) (Fig. 14.4).

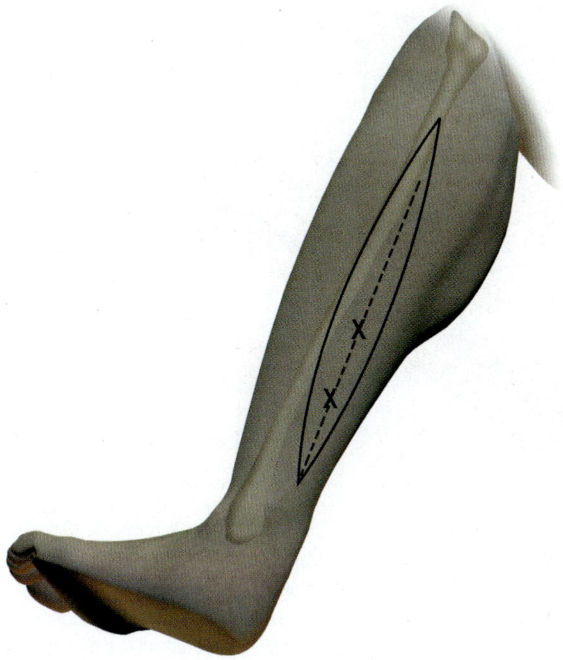

FIGURE 14.1
Leg flexed at the hip and knee illustrating flap harvest positioning. Note that the posterior crural septum starts near the junction of the proximal and middle thirds of the fibula and diverges posteriorly from the fibula as it runs to the distal leg. The most reliable cutaneous perforators traverse this septum, and any skin paddle should be oriented over the septum and not the fibula. Six centimeters of fibula should be preserved proximally and distally to ensure knee and ankle stability. The location of the peroneal nerve is indicated.

- The best cutaneous branches usually exit the intermuscular septum in the distal leg. Occasionally, the only cutaneous perforator is found about 6 cm proximal to the lateral malleolus, in other words, at the point where fibula bone harvest ends. It does not mean that the skin paddle harvest must end 6 cm above the lateral malleolus. In these cases, design the skin paddle to extend distally to incorporate this single perforator and be very careful when making the distal bone cut. This single septocutaneous branch can carry a very large skin paddle extending all the way to the proximal calf.
- The vascular pedicle is short before it joins the proximal bone.
- The nutrient vessel is less important for mandible reconstruction than it may be for long bone reconstruction since ostectomies are common for mandible reconstruction. The blood supply to the osteotomized bone is primarily periosteal and segmentally provided by the peroneal artery. This allows for sections of bone to be removed without compromising more distal bone. Though not imperative, when parts of the fibular bone are removed, I recommend preserving the intervening periosteum between bone segments, especially that along

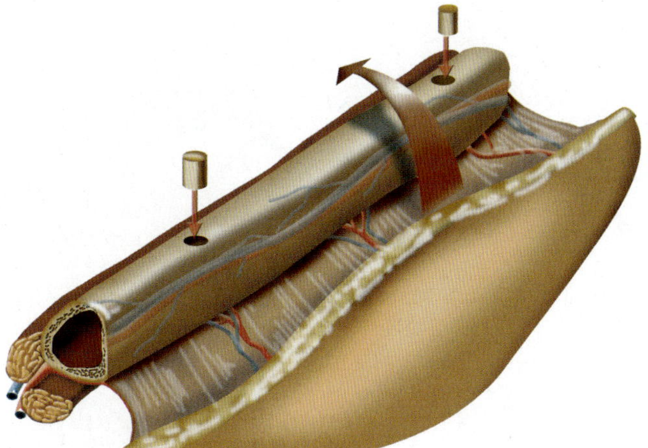

FIGURE 14.2 A right fibula osseocutaneous flap in its natural orientation illustrates the peroneal vascular pedicle from the proximal lower leg. The flat lateral border of the fibula is best suited for plate and screw fixation and therefore the best surface of the lateral aspect of the neomandible. The anterior aspect of the fibula is ideal for intraoperative placement of osseointegrated implants. The peroneal vascular pedicle can be seen coursing along the posteromedial aspect of the fibula between tibialis posterior and FHL muscle remnants. Cutaneous perforators can be seen traversing the intermuscular septum on the posterior aspect of the fibula. The *arrow* illustrates the limited arc of rotation of the skin paddle dictated by the length of the cutaneous perforators when the skin paddle is rotated anterior to the bone. This is not of concern when the soft tissue defect is extraoral or intraoral only to the floor of the mouth. More medial intraoral defects demand a better flap orientation.

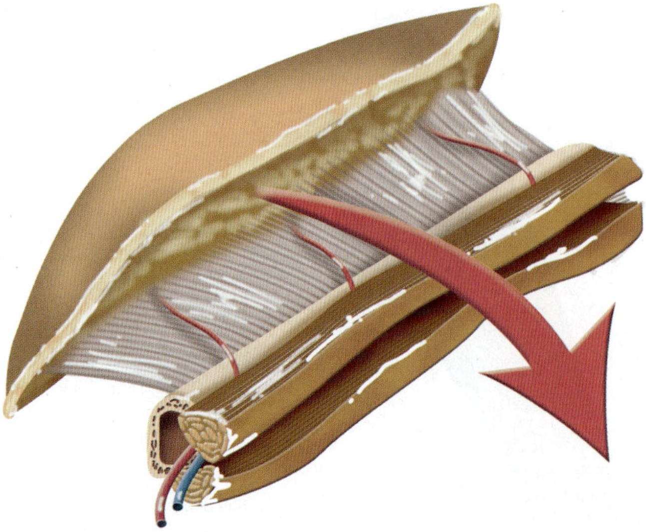

FIGURE 14.3 A right fibula osteocutaneous flap rotated 180 degrees along its long axis, still illustrating the peroneal vascular pedicle from the proximal lower leg. The lateral aspect of the right fibula (the lateral aspect of the neomandible) is now oriented toward the left, and the posterior aspect of the fibula is uppermost. Osseointegrated implants can be placed in the posterior aspect of the bone, but placement should be delayed. Intraoperative implant placement in the posterior bone increases the risk of vascular compromise to the flap. The *arrow* illustrates the much more generous arc of rotation of the skin paddle available when the skin paddle is rotated posterior to the bone. This rotation is better suited for reconstruction of more lingual (medial) defects. Figures 14.2 and 14.3 together illustrate only two of the four variables available within each leg during preoperative selection of which leg to harvest. These two variables, anterior surface of the fibula placed superior or inferior in the neomandible, are doubled when one turns the entire flap around end-to-end. Remember, depending on available recipient vessels, the vascular pedicle can exit the neomandible posterior or anterior in the neck and if anterior can be anastomosed to ipsilateral or contralateral neck vessels. These variables (options) are then doubled again if both legs have potential for a fibula flap.

the medial aspect of the fibula near the vascular pedicle (Fig. 14.5A). Try to avoid creating bone segments less than 2 cm in length as avascular segments within a viable flap have been reported. There would be some concern regarding the viability of the fibula proximal to the attachment of the peroneal vascular pedicle if a segment of periosteum were to be circumferentially removed. The proximal bone relies on the integrity of the periosteum associated with the peroneal vessels to survive.

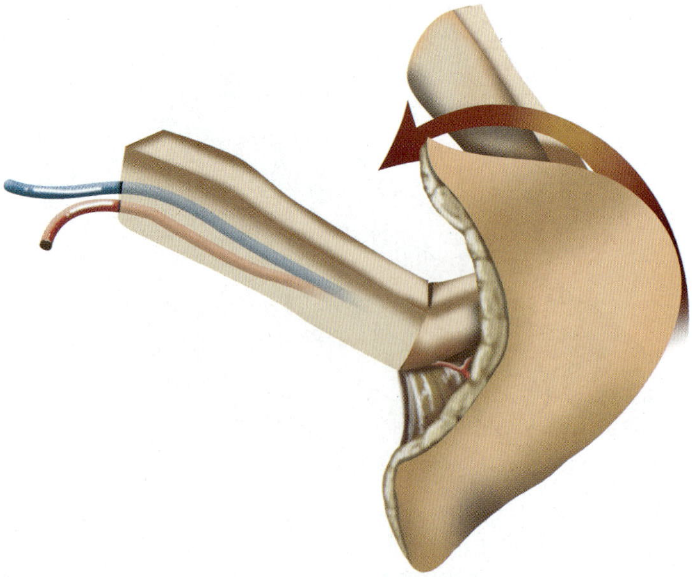

FIGURE 14.4 A right fibula osseocutaneous flap used to reconstruct an angle-to-angle mandibular defect, requiring significant soft tissue replacement of both intraoral and facial defects. The flap has been designed around a major cutaneous perforator that is associated with that portion of the fibula used to replace the anterior mandible. The intermuscular septum proximal and distal to that perforator has been sectioned allowing the skin paddle to rotate 90 degrees on the bone axis illustrated by the *arrows*. For large mandibular defects, requiring most of the fibula, the vascular pedicle always exits the neomandible posteriorly.

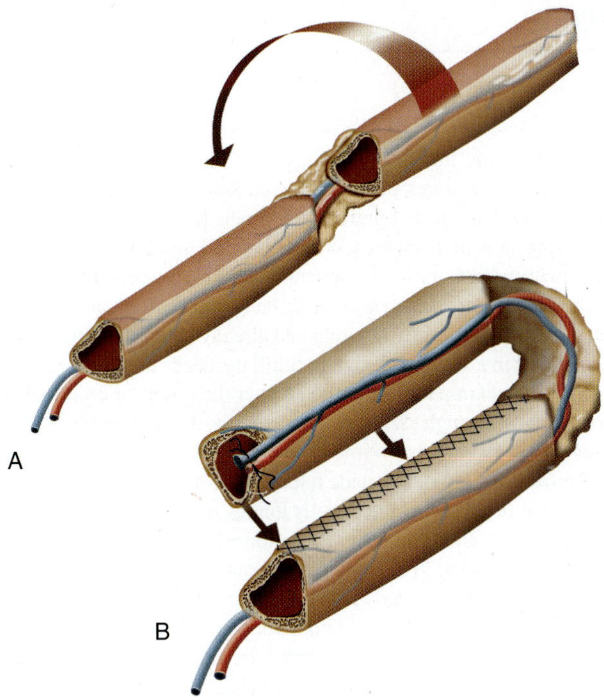

FIGURE 14.5 A. Illustration of a right fibula following ostectomy. Note the preserved periosteum and associated soft tissues with peroneal vessels supplying both the proximal and distal segments of bone. Note the flat lateral aspect of the fibula will be used as the lateral aspect of the neomandible. The *arrow* illustrates the intention to double barrel the fibula relocating the anterior aspect of each bone segment (*shaded*) into opposition. Ideally, the anterior aspect of each bone segment would have the periosteum incised longitudinally and reflected medially and laterally to expose the bone to be opposed. **B.** Illustration of the intended double-barrel procedure. *Arrow* illustrates the intended opposition of the denuded anterior surfaces of each fibula segment. Note that sufficient bone has been removed to allow repositioning of the segments without undue traction, torsion, or compression of the peroneal vascular pedicle connecting the two. Sufficient bone removal allows this soft tissue envelope containing the peroneal vascular pedicle to be positioned medial to the cut ends of both bone segments at the turn, avoiding potential compression at the interface between the double-barreled fibula and the native mandible.

- When employing the double-barrel technique, sufficient bone needs to be removed between the two “barrels” of fibula to allow the peroneal vascular pedicle to turn without torsion, kinking, or compression. Otherwise, the distal “barrel” might be devascularized (Fig. 14.5B).
- When using a double-barrel technique, be sure that the segment of fibula to be used for the gingival aspect of the neomandible is the “barrel” associated with the cutaneous branch. A segment (barrel) of fibula not associated with the cutaneous supply can be used for the basilar aspect of the neomandible.
- The left and right legs provide flaps with different geometry.

The Variables

- The bone defect: Is it a lateral, anterior, posterior, or combination of defects? How long is the defect? Will there be sufficient fibula for the double-barrel technique? Is there a defect that involves the condyle?
- The soft tissue defect: How large is the defect? Is it intraoral, facial, or through and through? Does the anterior soft tissue defect extend to both mandibular body segments? Is the oropharynx involved in the defect?
- Vessel availability in the neck: Ipsilateral, contralateral, or bilateral availability? What is the recipient vessel proximity to the neomandible? (Important in the vessel-depleted neck) Preoperative CT neck with contrast can be helpful.
- Cutaneous branch(es) of the flap. How many? Septocutaneous or musculocutaneous? Location (proximal, mid, or distal)? Is there more than one skin paddle available? Doppler or CT angiography of the legs can be helpful.
- Geometry of the flap: The peroneal vascular pedicle can be brought off the neomandible posteriorly, anteriorly, or go to the contralateral neck. This is the variable over which the surgeon has the greatest control and therefore will receive the most attention in preoperative planning. To best visualize this 3D plan, the beginning surgeon should make the templates as illustrated in (Figs. 14.2 and 14.3) (cut them out if helpful).
- Assessing the bone and soft tissue defects and keeping the constants always in mind, the variables can then be systematically assessed to determine the best leg from which to harvest the fibula flap.

SURGICAL TECHNIQUE

Flap Harvest

Minor variations in technique for the fibula flap harvest exist but represent inconsequential personal preferences in my opinion. The common features must include an anterior and posterior dissection, fibula section, and distraction and pedicle vessel dissection. I prefer the leg to be flexed at the hip and knee with a pressure pad protecting the heel. The dissection is done under tourniquet at 350 mm Hg.

The fibula is outlined with indicators for preservation of 6 cm of proximal and distal fibula. The posterior crural septum is marked for resident education, and the location of cutaneous perforators is identified by Doppler (even if location confirmed earlier by imaging and already marked on the skin). The flap is designed to include these cutaneous branches in a size and design to fulfill the needs of the reconstruction. Whether elliptical or rectangular, the long axis of the skin paddle is centered over the posterior crural septum, not over the fibula.

The anterior incision is made through skin and subcutaneous tissue. Even if the skin paddle is designed in the distal leg, the skin incision is extended proximally to the point where the proximal osteotomy cut is to be made (preserving 6 cm of proximal fibula). For wide flaps, the skin paddle is initially elevated from anterior to posterior in a suprafascial plane until over the peroneus longus muscle. This protects the superficial peroneal nerve in the lower leg. At that point, the fascia over the peroneal musculature is incised and the skin paddle is reflected posteriorly in a subfascial plane to demonstrate the anterior aspect of the posterior crural septum. For narrow flaps, the anterior skin incision is already over the peroneal muscles, so it can be extended through the skin, subcutaneous tissue, and fascia in one step. In both wide and narrow flaps, once the posterior crural septum is exposed, the septocutaneous branch(es) are evident. The delicate paratenon over the tendon of peroneus longus muscle should not be disturbed and should not be allowed to dessicate, as both insults will compromise potential skin grafting over the muscle. I like to reinforce the skin markings with the perforators in clear view since later in the case vasoconstriction can make them less obvious. The peroneal muscles are then dissected off the lateral fibula from posterior to anterior. Care must be taken near the septocutaneous perforators at the posterior margin of the bone as these can send branches anteriorly into the peroneal muscles. Control of these branches is best accomplished a few millimeters away from the septocutaneous vessels to avoid vasospasm. The periosteum of the fibula should be left undisturbed. Anterior reflection of the peroneal musculature for the entire length of the bone to be harvested reveals the anterior crural septum. This is incised close to the fibula over the entire length of the bone to be harvested. Hugging the bone, the muscles of the anterior compartment are released from the fibula, exposing the interosseous membrane on its medial aspect. This membrane is similarly incised close to the fibula over the entire length of the bone to be removed. Careful attention must be paid to any anterior retraction of the peroneal muscles in the proximal wound as the peroneal nerve can be damaged. The anterior dissection is now complete. Some surgeons like to cut and distract the fibula at this point, but I prefer to do the posterior dissection first.

The posterior skin incision is made and carried through the subcutaneous tissue and fascia with attention to preserve the sural nerve and saphenous vein intact if possible. The subfascial dissection then reflects the skin paddle anteriorly over the gastrosoleus muscle but not all the way to the posterior crural system. I prefer to now bluntly dissect into the avascular plane between the FHL and the soleus muscles in the distal wound. I then place a finger in this space directed proximally and separate the muscles carefully from distal to proximal looking for septomusculocutaneous perforators that might pierce the soleus muscle. If encountered, I reflect the skin paddle posteriorly and anteriorly, assessing the anterior and posterior aspects of the posterior crural system to get a clear picture of the septocutaneous branches. This allows me to determine if preservation of a small cuff of soleus muscle would provide more cutaneous blood supply. If so, a small cuff of soleus is excised around such perforators and left with the skin paddle. If no such perforators are found, the soleus is separated completely from the FHL and, more proximally, from the posterolateral aspect of the proximal fibula. Also in the proximal lower leg, if I am harvesting a skin paddle based on musculocutaneous perforators, these are dissected and preserved at this time. In either case, separation of the soleus from the proximal fibula exposes the posterior aspect of the proximal fibula. The peroneal vascular pedicle can be now seen as it courses distally disappearing under the most proximal fibular attachment of the FHL. I then incise the fascia on the posterior aspect of the FHL. This maneuver releases the posterior tibial neurovascular pedicle from its close association with the medial aspect of the FHL, reducing risk of inadvertent injury. The posterior dissection is now complete.

I now section the fibula proximally and distally leaving 6 cm of fibula and interosseous membrane undisturbed at each end. It is important, especially at the proximal osteotomy, to protect the peroneal vascular pedicle during osteotomy since it runs just deep to the bone. The fibula bone flap is now distracted laterally. It is being held in the leg by the tibialis posterior muscle on its medial surface and the FHL muscle on its posterior surface and by the peroneal vascular pedicle.

Blunt dissection through the anterior aspect of the tibialis posterior muscle at the distal bone cut reveals the peroneal artery and its venae comitantes. The vascular pedicle is ligated and sectioned in the distal leg. The tibialis posterior muscle is a pennate muscle and is now dissected from distal to proximal. Beginners should follow the middle of the chevron of the muscle to stay well medial to the vascular pedicle running along the posterior medial aspect of the fibula. More experienced surgeons may prefer to expose the vascular pedicle from distal to proximal. In either case, there are muscular branches of the peroneal vessels running to the tibialis posterior and the FHL muscles, which need to be controlled and severed. Once the tibialis posterior muscle has been incised proximally over a few centimeters, the FHL is exposed on its anterior aspect. (It had already been exposed on its posterior surface during the posterior dissection.) The desired amount of FHL to be harvested with the bone is now determined, and the incision of both muscles can be undertaken working from distal to proximal in the lower leg producing ever-increasing lateral distraction of flap. I prefer to use the harmonic scalpel for speed and reliable hemostasis. As the proximal origins of the FHL are approached, the peroneal vascular pedicle can be seen diverging medially from the fibula in the proximal wound. Incision of the deep fascia now exposes the posterior tibial neurovascular pedicle converging with the peroneal vascular pedicle in the proximal lower leg. Incision of the FHL muscle is completed at its proximal origin, but the posterior tibialis muscle needs to be incised all the way to the proximal bone cut. Dissection of the vascular pedicle can now begin. Often one or two muscular branches of the peroneal vessels to the soleus muscle need to be sacrificed to obtain maximal pedicle length. No vascular insufficiency to the soleus has been demonstrated secondary to this maneuver. The peroneal artery can be ligated and sectioned at the bifurcation with the posterior tibial artery, but the veins can be dissected even more proximally in the leg to attain greater length for the venous pedicle. The lateral venae comitantes of the posterior tibial artery can often be divided where it branches over to the medial venae comitantes of the peroneal artery. This produces a very large and long peroneal venous pedicle.

When pedicle vessel dissection is complete, bone wax is applied to the proximal and distal fibula stumps remaining in the leg and the tourniquet is released. Hemostasis is achieved and the flap replaced in the leg, which is wrapped in warm wet sponges and covered with an impermeable Mayo stand cover to maintain warmth.

The flap is not harvested until the ablative surgery and pathologic margin assessment are completed and recipient vessels have been prepared in the neck.

When the flap is harvested and the ischemia clock started, the pedicle vessels are sectioned and the leg wound is closed over a suction drain. If a skin graft is applied, a vacudrain or bolster dressing is placed and the lower leg placed in a posterior splint.

Flap Inset

Optimal flap orientation to facilitate inset (covered above) is a preoperative not an intraoperative concept. In fact, this concept would have been the primary preoperative consideration when choosing from which leg to harvest the fibula flap. One side is always superior, but either side can be made to work.

When the composite free fibula flap is delivered to the neck, the first thing that I do is to place the flap in its intended orientation over the mandibular defect. This allows me to measure the length of vascular pedicle required to comfortably reach the recipient vessels. This immediately dictates how much proximal fibula, if any, will need to be removed to produce optimal pedicle vessel geometry, and a quick check of the remaining fibula will demonstrate how much bone would remain to fill the rest of the mandibular defect. This is one area where preoperative 3D CT fibula ostectomy planning can be less reliable. This is especially true in those cases where much of the fibula is required for the mandibular defect and the recipient vessels are in question. It is never a problem when only distal fibula is required for the smaller defect and the neck vessels have not been disturbed by previous surgery.

The second important calculation to be made is the location of the cutaneous branch(es). The association of these branches with the bone is critical in choosing where to remove bone. Although careful removal of the periosteum from distal portions of the fibula does preserve the integrity of these cutaneous branches, they can be compromised by kinking, torsion, or traction. For this reason, I try to avoid sacrificing the bone immediately adjacent to septocutaneous perforators whenever possible. This bone–perforator relationship becomes more important in complex single skin paddle through-and-through soft tissue defects with large mandibular defects. It is also an important consideration if more than one skin paddle is employed irrespective if the size of the mandibular defect.

If proximal fibula needs to be sacrificed, I incise the periosteum along the lateral border of the proximal fibula and, using a large periosteal elevator, I elevate the periosteum off the entire proximal fibula to be removed.

Much is written about template construction for accurate fibula contouring. I employ a very inexpensive yet accurate method using 4-mm-thick Silastic sheeting. For anterior mandibular reconstruction, I make a 1-cm wide, 2D template of the basilar and of the gingival aspects of the mandible segment removed from the patient. If a single-barrel fibula replacement is planned, I use the gingival template to ensure a proper occlusal plane. If a double-barrel technique is planned, I use both templates. These templates have no curves but rather are angular to duplicate the defect with multiple straight segments comparable to the final contoured fibula. When I determine which portion of the fibula to contour, I measure the distance of the lateral aspect of each segment of the template. These measurements are accurately transferred to the lateral aspect of the fibula (Fig. 14.6). The angle required to duplicate the template is easily derived by cutting the 1-cm, 2D template from medial to lateral at each angle leaving only 1 mm of Silastic on the outer aspect of the template. The cut template is then opened and laid upon the anterior aspect of the fibula, where the triangle created by opening

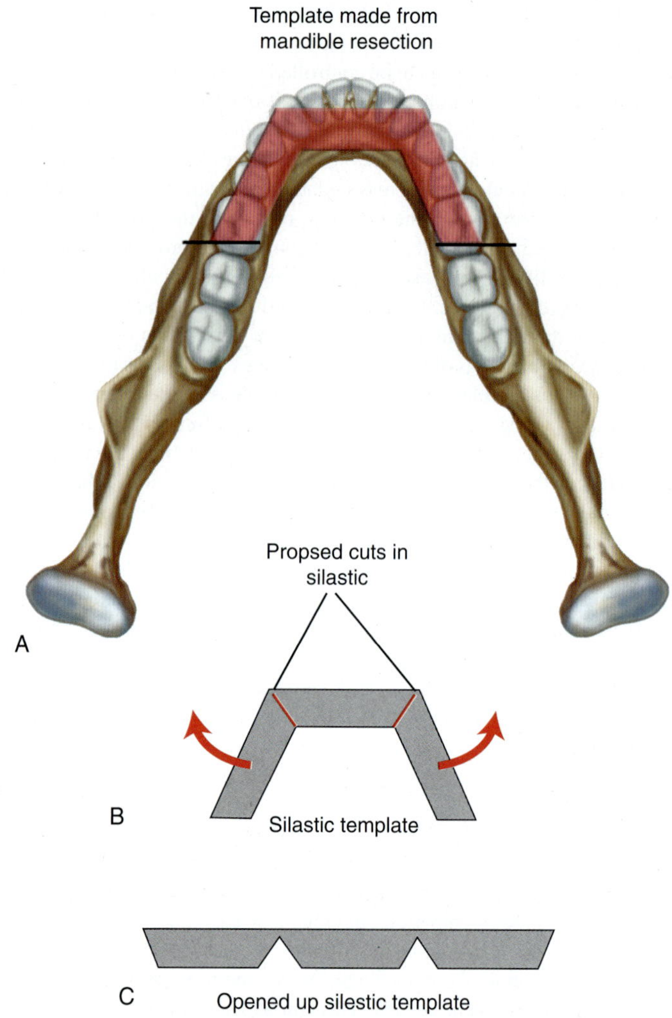

FIGURE 14.6 A. Illustration of a mandible from above with Silastic template (4-mm thick, 12-mm wide) overlaid on the gingival aspect of the anterior portion of the mandible that has been removed. Note that the central segment of the neomandible lies over the tooth roots, not the more anterior mentum. In this way, osseointegrated implants will be appropriately loaded in the occlusal plane. If the double-barreled technique is employed, a second template of the basilar aspect of the bone is made. Any double-barreled segments will therefore reside slightly more lateral and anterior in the neomandible. **B.** The Silastic template of the anterior mandible defect is cut from internal to external at the angles, leaving 1 mm of Silastic attached. This will allow outward rotation of the lateral segments illustrated by the *arrows*. **C.** When the lateral segments of the template are lined up with the central segment, the angles created accurately represent the triangular segments of fibula that need to be removed.

the template is marked on the bone with the apex on the lateral aspect of the fibula. With periosteal elevation and protection, a reciprocating saw is used to excise this wedge of fibula (Fig. 14.7) and the ostectomy "closed" on the medial aspect. Two miniplates are bent and secured with self-tapping screws to fix the new contour of the fibula before moving on to the next segment (Fig. 14.8). The same principle applies when reconstructing the angle and ascending ramus except that the Silastic template is cut from superior to inferior at the template angle (Fig. 14.9). When opened, this template is applied to the lateral aspect of the fibula and the apex of the wedge of bone to be removed is on the inferior aspect of the fibula (neomandible). That ostectomy is therefore "closed" along the superior aspect of the fibula (neomandible) (Fig. 14.10).

I have employed much more sophisticated (and expensive) techniques including preoperative modeling to include bone-cutting jigs. This can save time but at some considerable expense (often not covered by insurance), and the final result, in my hands, is no different.

For simple straight line defects of the body of the mandible in the dentulous patient, no template is required if a reconstructive bone plate has been preapplied. Simple measurement of the bone defect (both gingival and basilar if a double barrel is to be used) will suffice. Always use a saw to fine-tune the cut ends to maximize bone-to-bone contact.

When multiple ostectomies are needed for the mandible reconstruction, I measure, cut and contour the fibula from proximal to distal. I plate and screw fixate each contour of the neomandible before cutting the next. The reason for this is to insure maximal bone contact for rapid, reliable bone healing.

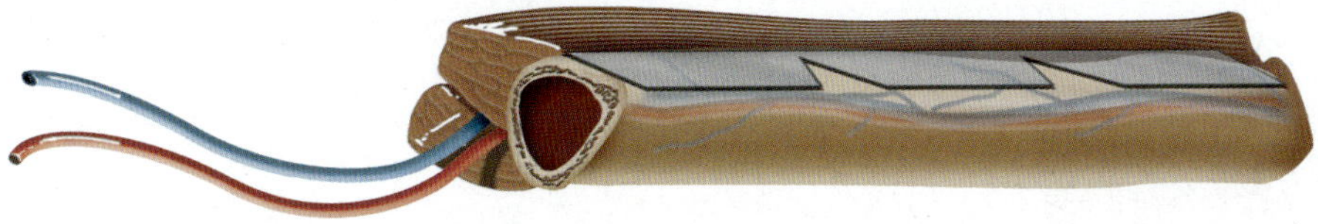

FIGURE 14.7 The straightened template is laid on the anterior surface of the fibula. The periosteum over the intended ostectomies is incised and reflected. A small malleable ribbon retractor is insinuated around the fibula to protect the peroneal vessels and the ostectomies marked and removed with an oscillating saw. The fibula segments are then closed at each ostectomy site and secured with two miniplates using monocortical screw at each ostectomy site.

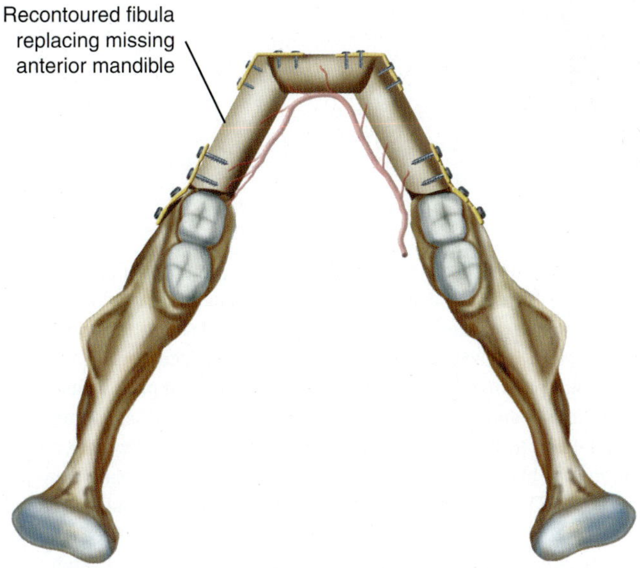

FIGURE 14.8
The recontoured neomandible is illustrated fixed to the native mandible with mandibular plates and screws. Due to the paucity of forces on the neomandible and the thickness of fibula cortex, monocortical screws are sufficient for fixation. If intraoperative placement of osseointegrated implants is intended, this should be carried out after the neomandible is firmly fixed in its new location. This will allow maximized orientation of the implants in the occlusal plane, thereby minimizing potential cantilever forces on the implants with attendant failure rates.

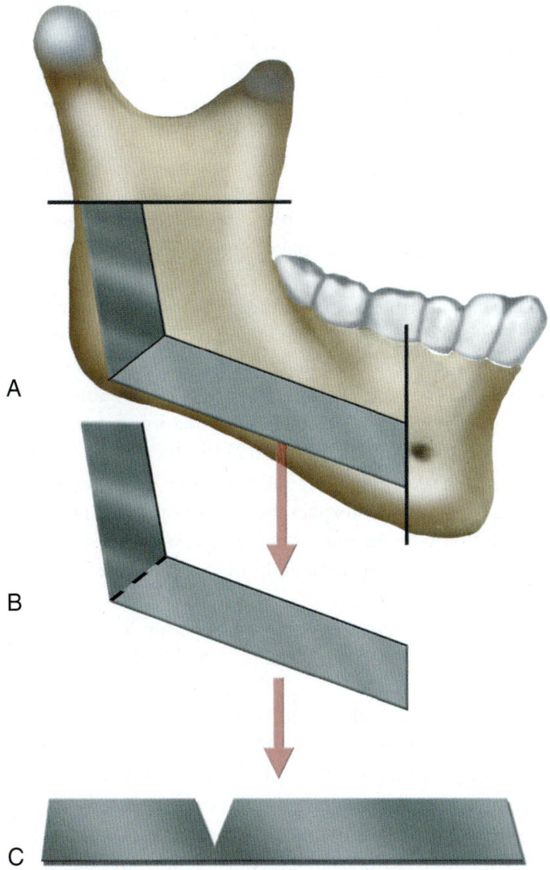

FIGURE 14.9
A. Illustration of a right lateral mandible defect of body and ramus with the Silastic template replicating the intended neomandible. Note the importance of reconstructing the angle of the mandible. The anterior aspect of the reconstruction need not be at the basilar aspect of the mandible. **B.** The template illustrating the intended cut from superior to inferior at the angle preserving 1 mm of Silastic. **C.** The template opened to illustrate the exact dimensions of the intended ostectomy of the fibula required to duplicate the neomandible. This time, the template is opened, straightened, and laid on the lateral surface of the fibula, such that the apex of the triangular ostectomy is at the posterior border of the fibula. As in Figure 14.7, the periosteum at the intended ostectomy site is incised and reflected. A small malleable ribbon retractor protects the peroneal vessels during the ostectomy with an oscillating saw. The fibula segments are closed at the ostectomy sites and plated.

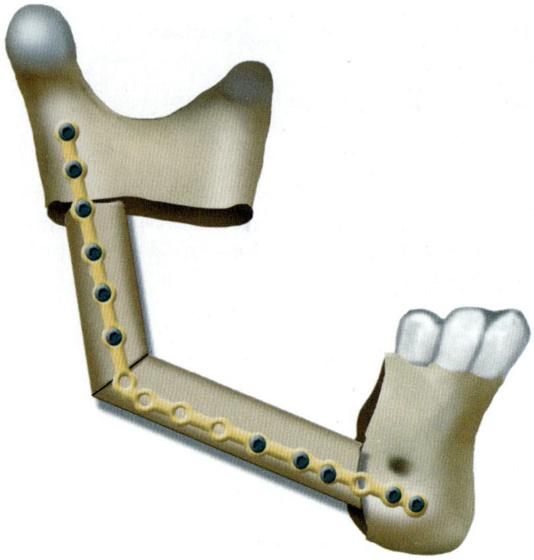

FIGURE 14.10
Illustrates neomandible reconstruction of a right mandible defect with fibula bone.

This brings up the perennial discussion regarding miniplate versus reconstructive plate fixation. My prejudice for over 20 years has been for dual miniplate fixation at each fibula–fibula ostectomy site with heavier reconstructive plates used to secure the fibula to the native mandible. Increasing literature seems to support this notion that the stress shielding provided by one-piece reconstructive plates over vascularized bone may result in more fibula atrophy over time. For large edentulous mandibular defects (e.g., angle-to-angle), I match the fibula neomandible to the upper arch with a template and direct approximation. The anterior ostectomy sites will be fixed with miniplates and the fibula attached to the mandibular ramus remnants with separate reconstructive plates. For smaller defects in the dentulous mandible, I contour a single reconstructive plate from the mandible prior to resection or from a preoperative 3D mold. This is used to maintain occlusion and, for lateral mandibular defects, will be left in place. For defects that include the anterior mandible, I use it to maintain occlusion while I contour the neomandible. After the neomandible is fixed in place, I cut out the symphyseal aspect of the reconstructive plate leaving its proximal and distal portions to fix fibula to mandibular remnants. This is done for two reasons. First, the single reconstructive plate contoured to the mental protuberance fails to represent the occlusal plane of the neomandible but rather is too far forward. If the fibula was contoured to this plate, the patient would experience a pronounced underbite following dental rehabilitation. Second, if the fibula neomandible is contoured in its proper occlusal alignment, a significant space exists between anterior neomandible and the reconstructive plate. This can cause significant pressure on the deep aspect of the mental soft tissues with no apparent benefit. For these reasons, I remove the anterior aspect of the reconstructive plate after the neomandible is in place. An alternative for those dentulous patients with only the anterior mandible sacrificed is maxillomandibular fixation to maintain occlusion. The neomandible is then contoured to match the occlusal plane, fibula–fibula segments secured with miniplates, and larger plates used to secure fibula–mandible segments.

Attention to this anterior–posterior differential in location of the mandibular gingival versus the mental protuberance is important for optimal functional dental rehabilitation of the neomandible. Also important to remember is the medial–lateral differential associated with the mandibular body where the occlusal surface (gingival) is medial to the basilar aspect of the mandible. This is an equally important consideration often overlooked when surgeons attach a fibular segment to a reconstructive plate oriented along the inferior aspect of the mandibular body. Osseointegrated implants placed vertically in a fibula segment at this location will fail to duplicate the occlusal relationships with the maxillary dentition seen in the original mandible. For optimal dental rehabilitation, the fibula segments, both anterior and lateral, need to respect the occlusal plane. Anteriorly, this is accomplished by establishing the neomandible posterior to the mental prominence. For isolated anterior mandible defects, I have used double-barrel fibula to duplicate the vertical height of the mandible and even triple-barrel fibula to restore both mandibular height and mental protrusion.

For lateral (body) defects, I prefer the double-barrel technique but remember the superior "barrel" of the fibula (replacing the gingiva) must be located slightly medial to the inferior "barrel," which will be replacing the basilar bone.

When very large mandibular defects are reconstructed, there is inadequate fibula length for double-barrel techniques. Other techniques have worked well. For example, placement of the fibula in a more superior position within the mandible (not along the inferior border) allows for more successful dental rehabilitation. At the same time, in these patients, a large deepithelialized skin paddle placed along the inferior mandibular aspect (with or without a bone plate for support) provides facial contouring approximating the original mandible. The height of the fibula can also be augmented secondarily with bone grafts or by osseodistraction. Of course, for the longtime edentulous patient with an atrophic mandible and no interest in or plans for dental rehabilitation, all these considerations become theoretical.

As mentioned above, when the double-barrel technique is employed, it is important to orient the superior (gingival) barrel and the intraoral skin paddle first. Any compromise of this portion of the reconstruction could lead to salivary leakage and even flap loss. The inferior (basilar) barrel should be positioned after the more important superior barrel and intraoral skin are secure and uncompromised, since the role of the inferior barrel is more aesthetic than functional. For this reason, I always choose the portion of the fibula to be used for the gingival barrel that has the best association with a cutaneous perforator. It is important to remember that successful bone union between fibula and mandible or fibular segments can be compromised by inadvertent inclusion of any soft tissues between the bony surfaces.

Common surgical sense must prevail for determining the order in which to inset skin paddle(s) and fibula bone into the oromandibular defect. In any case, I like to have the bone fixated before starting the microvascular surgery. For wide open defects with excellent exposure, that means that I revascularize the flap before insetting the skin paddle. This allows for easy evaluation and control of any previously controlled subcutaneous bleeding sites before the wound is closed. There are few things more frustrating than encountering an inaccessible bleeder after bone fixation. This is another reason for establishing excellent hemostasis on the flap while it is still vascularized in the leg.

For many through-and-through defects, intraoral exposure may be severely limited after bone fixation; therefore, the intraoral soft tissue defect needs to be reconstructed first, the bone fixated second, and the flap revascularized third before external defects are closed. This still allows for more limited assessment and hemostasis after the flap is revascularized and before the face and neck are closed.

POSTOPERATIVE MANAGEMENT

The leg is kept in a posterior splint for 5 days during which the patient is ambulated with assistance and without weight bearing. The splint is removed after 5 days and the patient encouraged to ambulate with slowly graduated weight bearing.

If a skin graft has been placed, the bolster dressing or vacudrain is removed after 8 days.

Suction drain of the lower leg is removed when drainage meets criteria.

A nasogastric tube is placed and the patient kept NPO for at least 10 days if no radiation has preceded the surgery and for 14 days if radiation has occurred.

Peridex mouth rinses.

Hourly flap check for the first 72 hours.

COMPLICATIONS

- Pressure trauma to the heel. Avoid by placing the patient's foot in a foam pad and limiting the time of leg elevation.
- Instability of the knee or ankle may occur if insufficient proximal or distal fibula (interosseous membrane) is preserved.
- Nerve damage. Exercise prudent avoidance of the posterior tibial neurovascular pedicle and be careful with placement of the retractors on the proximal peroneal muscles.
- Hematoma: Avoid by exercising judicious hemostasis after flap harvest and tourniquet release and by applying bone wax to the stumps of the fibula.
- Poor skin graft take. Can be minimized by careful preservation of the paratenon over the peroneal tendon to include avoidance of desiccation of this paratenon during harvest.
- Vascular compromise of bone segments. Can be avoided by minimizing periosteal elevation and by maintaining a 2-cm minimal length on bone segments.
- Vascular compromise of the skin paddle through excessive torsion, traction, or compression of the cutaneous perforator(s) during flap inset can be avoided with proper preplanning and careful flap manipulation during inset.

RESULTS

In 378 consecutive fibula osseocutaneous free flaps which I have performed over 22 years, 3 flaps were lost to pedicle vessel compromise for a success rate of 99.2% for the osseous flap. In addition, six patients, who had well-vascularized bone flaps, suffered skin flap necrosis (two total and four partial but sufficient to require additional surgery). Each case could be attributed to excessive torsion or traction of the cutaneous perforators. This leaves a success rate of 97.6% for the cutaneous flap.

Three cases in which the fibula was used to reconstruct osseoradionecrosis defects suffered delayed recipient artery rupture 7 to 10 days postoperatively. In no case was the fibula bone or skin paddle lost. Each case was attributed to the poor vascularity of the wall of the recipient artery from the excessive radiation resulting in a delayed pseudoaneurysm and rupture.

Nonunion at the mandibular reconstruction site occurred in five cases and was corrected surgically by open reduction, freshening of the bone edges, and internal fixation. Each case was felt to be related to unintentional inadvertent inclusion of soft tissue between bone surfaces at the time of reconstruction. One patient suffered what appeared to be avascular necrosis of a 1.5-cm central segment of fibula in a multiosteotomized, 3D reconstruction of a very large oromandibular defect including ramus, body, symphysis, and contralateral mandibular body. All of the fibula, proximal and distal to this segment, and the overlying skin paddle remained viable over 9 years, and no further surgery was required. It was felt that the bone contouring had been overly aggressive, leaving inadequate periosteal blood supply to this small fibula segment.

No patient suffered significant functional loss in the leg or foot. All patients experienced some swelling in the operated lower leg lasting for weeks to months.

One patient required surgical evacuation of a significant hematoma in the lower leg.

For those patients who required skin grafts to the donor site, approximately 10% experienced delayed wound healing of at least some portion of the grafted site most frequently over the peroneus longus tendon. All of these wounds ultimately epithelialized with conservative management.

PEARLS

- Preoperative evaluation of the vascularity of the lower leg including identification of the cutaneous branches is important. Use CT angiography but do not forget the venous system. If there is a history of deep vein thrombosis, may need venogram as well.
- Preoperative evaluation of vascularity in the neck is especially important in the vessel-depleted neck.
- Using the defect requirements, the recipient vessel availability, and the constants associated with each potential fibula flap, determine preoperatively the leg that provides the superior fibula flap.
- Maximize bone-to-bone contact.
- Maximize pedicle vessel geometry.
- Optimize the relationships of the skin paddle(s) and their perforators with the bone segment(s) to be used.

PITFALLS

- Remember to align the neomandible with the upper arch. The fibula segment does not have to be placed at the inferior rim of the mandible. Double-barrel techniques are available.
- Smooth the angles created in the anterior neomandible.
- Secure and maintain the chin pad in natural position on the neosymphysis after body-to-body mandibular reconstruction or the lip–chin complex may slip inferiorly during healing. Be wary of pressure dressings over the neosymphysis to avoid pressure necrosis of the chin pad.
- Do not tolerate postoperative seromas or hematomas in the vicinity of the vessel anastomoses.

INSTRUMENTS TO HAVE AVAILABLE

- Head and neck surgery tray
- Reciprocating saw

SUGGESTED READING

Virgin FW, Iseli TA, Iseli CE, et al. Functional outcomes of fibula and osteocutaneous forearm free flap reconstruction for segmental mandibular defects. *Laryngoscope* 2010;120(4):663–667.

Baumann DP, Yu P, Hanasono MM, et al. Free flap reconstruction of osteoradionecrosis of the mandible: a 10-year review and defect classification. *Head Neck* 2011;33(6):800–807.

Cannon TY, Strub GM, Yawn RJ, et al. Oromandibular reconstruction. *Clin Anat* 2012;25(1):108–119. doi: 10.1002/ca.22019.

15 RECONSTRUCTION OF THE TEMPOROMANDIBULAR JOINT

Brett A. Miles

INTRODUCTION

The temporomandibular joint (TMJ) is unique among the joints of the human skeleton (Fig. 15.1). It is a critical component of the craniomandibular articulation and functions quite uniquely when compared to other skeletal articulations in the human body. The primary function of the TMJ is to support mastication and articulation of the dentition, a complex biomechanical process that is beyond the scope of this chapter. The TMJ also plays a critical role in speaking and swallowing and is central to all mandibular functions.

Reconstruction of the TMJ, regardless of the indication, attempts to preserve the function of the mandible as well as to maintain facial symmetry. Duplication of the complex functional properties of the TMJ is impossible with current techniques; however, maintaining adequate opening, functional occlusion, and acceptable facial aesthetics are the requirements of appropriate reconstruction. The surgeon must keep these goals in mind when planning reconstructive surgery involving the TMJ.

HISTORY

Patients will often have pain in the preauricular region, pressure sensations, or occlusal disturbances when presenting with processes involving the TMJ. Patients may report other symptoms such as ear pain, clicking/grinding noises, and rarely inability to open the mouth.

PHYSICAL EXAMINATION

Often the necessity for TMJ reconstruction can be predicted by evaluating the underlying disease. The physical examination of the TMJ requiring reconstruction may range from a completely normal examination in the case where joint resection is necessary for oncologic margins to a severely abnormal examination with complete inability to open the mouth. The patient may exhibit varying levels of trismus, progressive malocclusion, and pain within the joint. Hyperplastic conditions of the condyle may result in shifting of the mandible toward the unaffected side. Conversely, destructive processes may result in mandibular shifting toward the affected side. Occlusal and mandibular excursive mobility should be evaluated and abnormalities such as midline shifts, asymmetry, or other abnormalities of function documented.

The maximum interincisal opening distance should be measured and documented (distance between the upper and lower incisor edges with maximal opening, mm). Examination of the external auditory meatus on the affected side is critical to assess for invasive disease into the meatus or erosion of the tympanic plate of the temporal bone.

Facial nerve function as well as regional sensory disturbances should be evaluated and appropriately documented as the frontal branch of the facial nerve, greater auricular nerve, and auriculotemporal nerve may be involved with pathologic processes in this area. The chest and rib cage in particular should be examined for evidence of previous surgery or trauma.

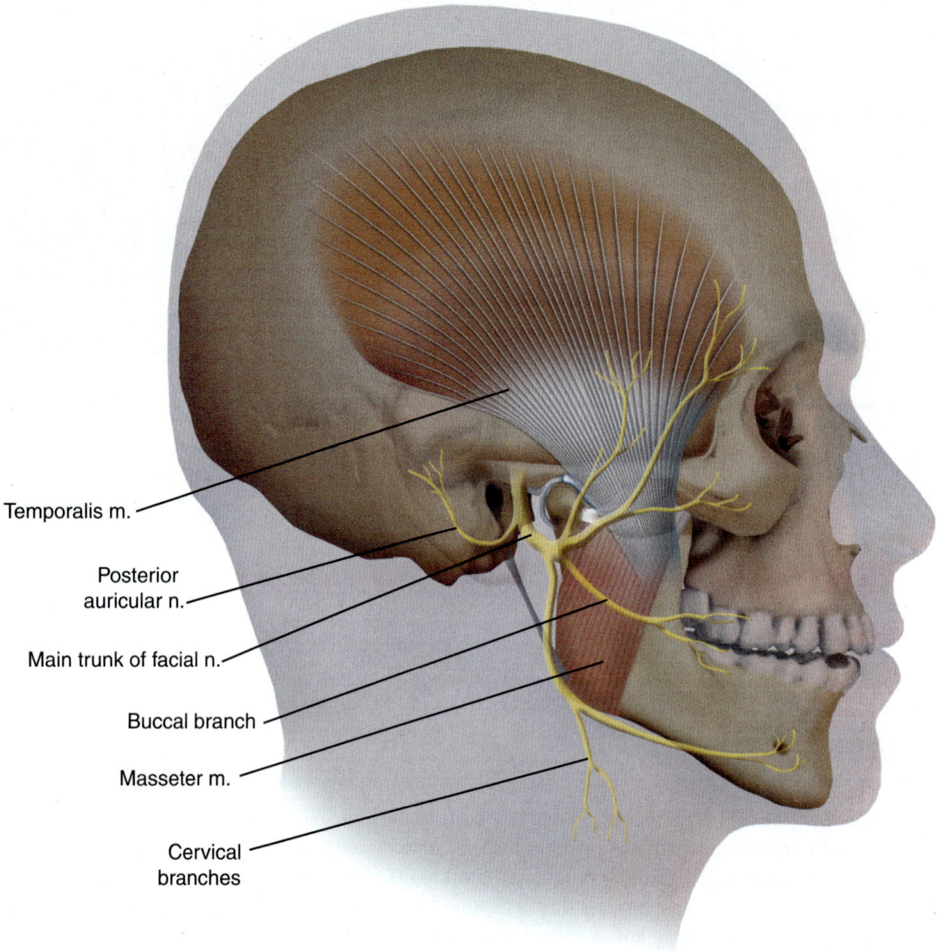

FIGURE 15.1
The temporomandibular joint region, muscles, and facial nerve location.

INDICATIONS

Common indications for reconstruction include benign and malignant processes of the TMJ, or malignant lesions involving the region. Sequelae from adjuvant radiotherapy or bisphosphonate therapy may require resection and reconstruction of the TMJ. Malignant lesions of the temporal bone may also rarely result in the necessity of resection and reconstruction of the TMJ. Malignant processes of the overlying soft tissues such as squamous cell carcinoma or cancer of the parotid gland may invade the temporomandibular region and require ablative procedures to the TMJ. Benign lesions of the mandibular condyle such as condylar hyperplasia, or severe osteoarthritis as well as malignant lesions such as chondrosarcoma or osteosarcoma are also indications for TMJ reconstruction. While osteonecrosis of the TMJ is rare, extensive radiation damage or trauma to the area may also be an indication for reconstruction.

Indications for TMJ reconstruction are summarized below:

- Benign condylar conditions (condylar hyperplasia, severe arthritis)
- Odontogenic tumors (ameloblastoma, myxoma)
- Malignant tumor of the TMJ/condyle (osteosarcoma, chondrosarcoma)
- Malignant tumor in the TMJ region (squamous cell carcinoma, cancer of the parotid gland, sarcoma)
- Severe traumatic injuries (gunshot wounds)
- Osteonecrosis (osteoradionecrosis [ORN], bisphosphonate related osteonecrosis of the jaws [BRONJ])

CONTRAINDICATIONS

There are no specific contraindications to reconstruction of the TMJ. In some cases, reconstruction of the condyle of the mandible must also be accompanied by reconstruction of the glenoid fossa to avoid middle cranial fossa complications (i.e., extensive temporal bone resections). It should also be noted that reconstruction of the TMJ may not be necessary in selected cases and that reasonable function and occlusion may be maintained with appropriate rehabilitation, even in the absence of articulation of the mandible with the skull base.

PREOPERATIVE PLANNING

Anatomy

The TMJ is unique in the human skeleton as it is classified as a ginglymoarthrodial joint, that is it functions as both a rotational hinge as well as providing gliding movements during wide excursions. The condyle of the mandible articulates with the glenoid fossa of the temporal bone, separated by the articular disc. This disc is composed of dense fibrocartilage, unlike the hyaline cartilage found in most other joints in the skeleton. The TMJ and its associated articular disc are supported by several ligaments that connect the condyle to the base of skull including the temporomandibular ligament and the capsular ligament, as well as the stylomandibular and sphenomandibular ligament. The muscles of mastication, namely the temporalis and masseter muscles, as well as the lateral and medial pterygoid muscles further support and provide movement of the joint. It is the anatomic arrangement of these ligaments and muscles that allow for the complexity of mandibular function. Other anatomical considerations in the region include the parotid gland, which lies directly on the capsular ligament of the TMJ directly below the zygomatic arch. The temporal branches of the facial nerve traverse the zygomatic arch in this region and are the motor nerves most commonly at risk during joint reconstruction (Fig. 15.1). In addition, sensory branches of the auriculotemporal nerve pass on the posterior–medial aspect of the condyle and supply the skin of the temporal area as well as portions of the auricle and external auditory canal. The superficial temporal artery and vein are adjacent to the auriculotemporal nerve branches and may be encountered during dissection of the condyle in this region. Medial to the glenoid fossa at the level of the skull base, the middle meningeal artery passes intracranial via the foramen spinosum. Care must be taken when resecting the condyle to avoid aggressive dissection in this area. Additionally, the external carotid artery lies posterior and medial to the mandibular ramus (as well as the maxillary branch medial to the condylar neck) and should be identified if dissection in this area is indicated. Reconstructive surgery of the TMJ requires an understanding of both the anatomy of the craniomandibular articulation as well as the surrounding structures to provide for functional reconstruction while avoiding iatrogenic sequelae.

Imaging Studies

There are no specific imaging studies required for reconstruction of the TMJ; however, CT with contrast enhancement is relatively standard for evaluation of this area. In addition, panoramic radiographs may be useful to evaluate the extent of odontogenic tumors and cysts as well as other pathologic processes involving the mandible. Occasionally, MRI may be indicated to evaluate the soft tissue surrounding the TMJ as well as the articular disc for pathologic involvement. The pathologic process rather than the planned reconstruction primarily drives the appropriate imaging modality, unless custom TMJ prostheses are planned.

SURGICAL TECHNIQUE

A wide variety of reconstructive techniques have been used to restore the form and function of the TMJ and are listed below.

- Autogenous graft (costochondral, sternoclavicular) (Figs. 15.2 and 15.3)
- Free tissue transfer (fibula, metatarsal) (Fig. 15.4)
- Stock alloplastic reconstruction (titanium, silicone, acrylic, condylar prostheses)
- Custom alloplastic reconstruction (total joint prosthesis) (Fig. 15.5)

Reconstruction of the joint with alloplastic materials is beyond the scope of this chapter; however, advantages such as avoiding donor site morbidity, and a wide variety of options have led to the adoption of this technology for many indications. Problems with material wear and prosthetic failure have been reported and are the disadvantages of alloplastic materials.

Autogenous grafting is also widely used with the costochondral graft being the most commonly used graft. Advantages of the costochondral graft include growth potential in pediatric applications as well as providing autologous tissue with low donor site morbidity and relative ease of harvest. Other options such as the sternoclavicular joint and free metatarsal grafts may be useful in selected situations.

Another indication for autogenous grafting is in the reconstruction following resection of malignant tumors requiring radiotherapy, and in general, alloplastic materials should be avoided if radiotherapy is planned. An exception to this would be in the case of reconstruction in the pediatric age group in which case radiotherapy to autogenous grafts may result in severe ankylosis and in some cases osseous union to the temporal bone. In this situation, alloplastic materials may be used until the completion of therapy and the autologous grafting may be staged if desired. In cases of severe tissue injury and previous radiation where vascular supply is in question, free tissue transfer techniques should be considered.

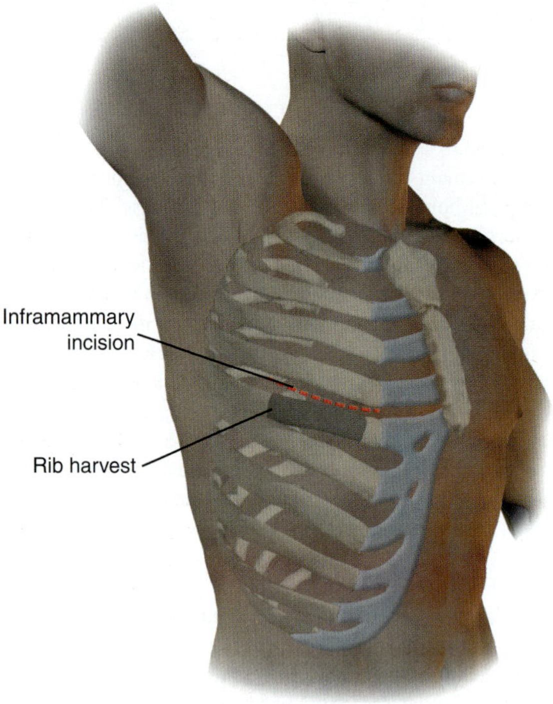

FIGURE 15.2
Inframammary incision design for rib graft harvest.

Transcervical Approach

The transcervical approach to resection of the condyle has been well described. The ramus of the mandible is stripped free from the surrounding soft tissue in a subperiosteal plane, and the planned resection is performed, delivering the mandibular ramus and condyle inferiorly through the neck. The coronoid process is sectioned or stripped to release the mandible from the temporalis muscle, and the condylar attachments are released with electrocautery and periosteal dissection. The remaining ramus is then prepared, and the previously harvested costochondral graft (see Technique below) is then seated into the glenoid fossa and fixated to the native mandible with titanium plates and screws. The soft tissue attachments of the pterygomasseteric sling are then reapproximated to the ramus/condyle construct with permanent sutures to support the mandibular ramus.

Regardless of transcervical or transfacial approach, the condyle should be secured to the glenoid fossa to prevent postoperative migration. This can be achieved with a variety of techniques including circumzygomatic prolene sutures (using a passing awl) or suspension sutures secured to titanium miniplates placed on the zygomatic arch via a small preauricular incision (Fig. 15.3).

The costochondral graft offers the advantage of a cartilaginous surface opposing the glenoid fossa; however, several interpositional materials may be used to replace the TMJ/disc including auricular cartilage, temporalis muscle, tensor fascia, or alloplastic materials (if alloplastic materials or osseous grafts are used for reconstruction) (Figs. 15.4 and 15.5). Ideally, the temporomandibular disc can be left in situ to support the reconstruction.

Transfacial/Preauricular Approach

Often during the course of tumor ablative surgery or due to anatomical considerations, the lateral ramus and condylar resection proceeds via a combined transcervical and preauricular approach. In these situations,

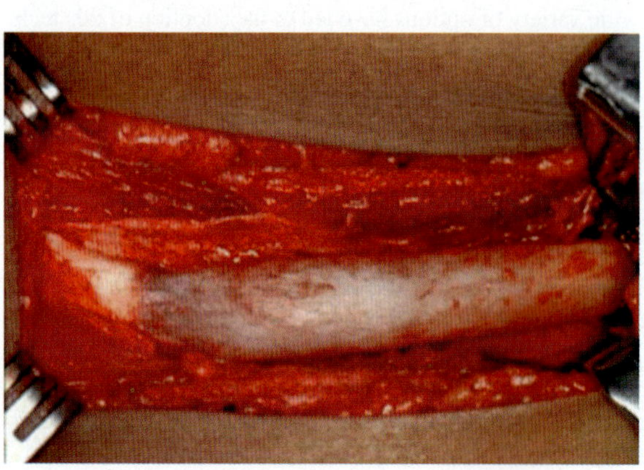

FIGURE 15.3
Costochondral rib harvest and graft inset for condylar reconstruction.

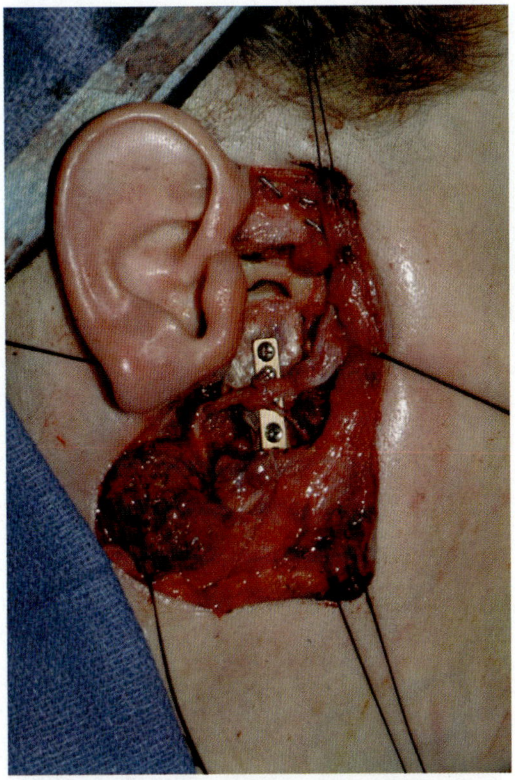

FIGURE 15.4
Fibular free tissue transfer for condylar reconstruction, in situ (via combined preauricular and transcervical approach). Facial nerve preservation was possible in this situation.

identification and preservation of the facial nerve is required. Cases in which oncologic principles require sacrifice of the facial nerve are obviously less problematic during reconstruction of the condyle. In the event that exposure of the condyle is required with preservation of the facial nerve, there are two possible approaches. A parotidectomy may be performed to identify the branches of the facial nerve at risk and to expose the ramus of the mandible and condyle. This is often required during ablative procedures. Alternatively, a preauricular approach proximal to the cartilage of the external auditory canal may be performed to the level of the temporalis fascia. The temporalis fascia may then be divided revealing the temporal adipose tissue pad, and dissection may proceed to the level of the root of the zygomatic arch. Subperiosteal dissection anteriorly will allow for retraction of the superficial temporal vessels, auriculotemporal nerves, and temporal branch of the facial nerve, which are superficial to this level of dissection. In some situations, formal facial nerve dissection is required (Fig. 15.4). The capsule of the TMJ may then be exposed and incised allowing for access to the mandibular condyle for completion of the resection. The ligamentous attachments and pterygoid muscles may be isolated and tagged at the time of resection of the ramus or condyle and reattached with permanent suture to the condylar reconstruction.

Costochondral Harvest

The technique of rib harvest has been well described. An inframammary incision is designed overlying the appropriate rib for harvest (Fig. 15.2). Generally, the sixth, seventh, and eighth ribs offer sufficient osseous and cartilaginous grafting material for reconstruction of the condyle.

Dissection with electrocautery through the fibers of the pectoralis major/minor muscles and the serratus anterior muscle posteriorly is performed to expose the anterior surface of the rib. Subperiosteal dissection of the rib is performed to allow for sectioning of the graft, which can be accomplished with a reciprocating saw or rib rongeur. The neurovascular bundle located inferiorly is avoided with careful dissection. Periosteal elevators should be used to protect the pleura during rib sectioning. Inadvertent violation of the pleural cavity requires underwater closure of the pleural space with maximal lung inflation to avoid significant pneumothorax. The graft is then cut to length, and the cartilaginous portion of the graft is trimmed with a scalpel, so that approximately 5 mm of cartilage remains on the condylar surface of the graft. Large amounts of cartilage are unnecessary and prone to fracture. A chest radiograph should be obtained after costochondral harvest.

POSTOPERATIVE MANAGEMENT

Perhaps the most important aspect of temporomandibular reconstruction is the postoperative rehabilitation. Disarticulation of the condyle and reconstruction separates the muscles of mastication from the mandible, and postoperative physical therapy must be employed during the first 6 to 12 weeks of healing to avoid permanent

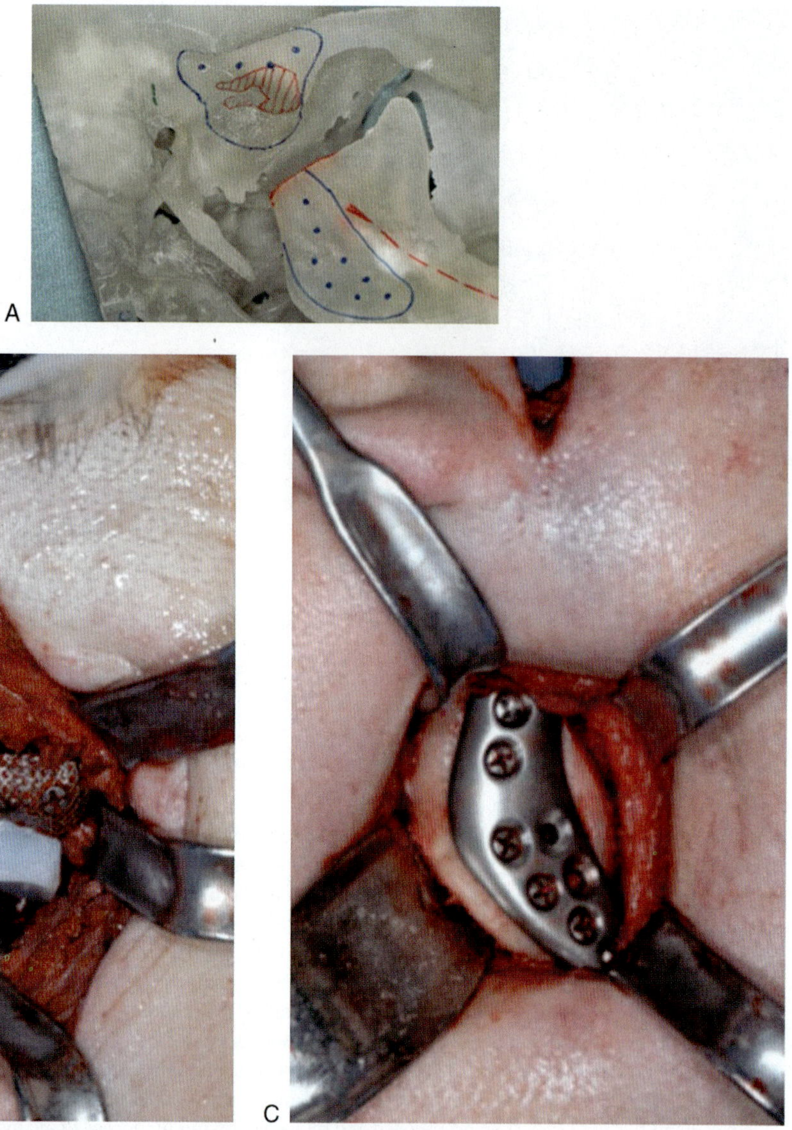

FIGURE 15.5 A–C. Total custom joint prosthesis with stereolithographic surgical model. Note combined preauricular and retromandibular approach to allow for placement of the condylar and fossa components of the prosthesis.

facial deformity, malocclusion, and poor functional results. In addition to the technical aspects mentioned above, dentate patients should have the occlusion supported with arch bars and guiding elastics to maintain the occlusion during healing. Maximal opening and excursive movements should be initiated 1 week after surgery and continued for several weeks to prevent postoperative trismus and malocclusion. The importance of maintaining the maximum opening possible cannot be overstated. This is especially important if radiotherapy or radiotherapy is planned postoperatively. Inappropriate postoperative rehabilitation resulting in severely limited opening is not easily addressed in the majority of cases.

COMPLICATIONS

Complications of reconstruction of the condyle include injury to sensory and motor nerves, infection, and perforation of the external auditory meatus. Donor site complications such as pneumothorax are managed in the standard fashion. A small, stable pneumothorax may be observed, but a chest tube is indicated for a large or expanding pneumothorax.

Long-term complications such as graft migration, graft resorption, and the resulting malocclusion can be avoided by employing condylar suspension techniques, arch bars with guiding elastics, and elastic jaw support straps. Rigorous physiotherapy and monitoring are required in the postoperative period to avoid occlusal disturbances and the associated functional consequences.

RESULTS

Functional results, in general, are quite good with condylar reconstruction. Some mild limitation of excursive and opening movements is to be expected. The majority of patients will tolerate a normal diet when healing is complete. Postoperative trismus related to adjuvant therapy and surgery remains problematic for patients with extensive malignant tumors.

PEARLS

- Reconstruction of the ramus and/or condyle can be performed with autogenous or alloplastic techniques, the selection of which is driven by a variety of considerations including diagnosis, age, and reconstructive goals.
- Coronoidectomy should be performed in the majority of cases to prevent postoperative trismus.
- Interpositional grafts should be considered if the temporomandibular disc is resected.
- Cartilage of costochondral grafts (sixth, seventh, and eighth ribs) should be trimmed to approximately 5-mm thickness.
- Postoperative rehabilitation is the single most important factor in the long-term success after reconstruction of the condyle.
- Correction of unfavorable results is extremely challenging once 6 to 8 weeks of healing has elapsed.

PITFALLS

- Prosthesis hardware failure continues to be a challenge long term.
- Patients undergoing radiotherapy postoperatively are at increased risk of exposure of hardware, osteonecrosis, and graft resorption.
- Autogenous grafts are prone to osteoneogenesis and ankylosis in patients in the pediatric age group, and rehabilitation is critical.
- Injury of the temporal branch of the facial nerve can be avoided by meticulous surgical technique
- Damage to the middle meningeal artery medial to the mandibular condyle must be avoided.
- Inappropriate postoperative physiotherapy may result in inadequate mouth opening and malocclusion, which is extremely difficult to correct.

INSTRUMENTS TO HAVE AVAILABLE

- Standard head and neck reconstruction tray
- Steven tenotomy scissors, curved 15 cm 6 inches
- Baby Metzenbaum scissors 14 cm 5 ¼ inch
- DeBakey straight 1.5 mm tip
- Rib harvest set

SUGGESTED READING

Saeed N, Hensher R, McLeod N, et al. Reconstruction of the temporomandibular joint autogenous compared with alloplastic. *Br J Oral Maxillofac Surg* 2002;40(4):296–299.

Khariwala SS, Chan J, Blackwell KE, et al. Temporomandibular joint reconstruction using a vascularized bone graft with Alloderm. *J Reconstr Microsurg* 2007;23(1):25–30.

Marx RE, Cillo JE Jr, Broumand V, et al. Outcome analysis of mandibular condylar replacements in tumor and trauma reconstruction: a prospective analysis of 131 cases with long-term follow-up. *J Oral Maxillofac Surg* 2008;66(12):2515–2523.

Driemel O, Braun S, Müller-Richter UD, et al. Historical development of alloplastic temporomandibular joint replacement after 1945 and state of the art. *Int J Oral Maxillofac Surg* 2009;38(9):909–920.

Singh V, Verma A, Kumar I, et al. Reconstruction of ankylosed temporomandibular joint: Sternoclavicular grafting as an approach to management. *Int J Oral Maxillofac Surg* 2011;40(3):260–265.

16 MANAGEMENT OF THE ISOLATED CONDYLAR DEFECT

Neal D. Futran

INTRODUCTION

The need for surgical reconstruction of an isolated defect of the condyle and ramus of the oromandibular complex is usually the result of resection of a neoplasm involving the temporomandibular joint (TMJ). This entity is uncommon and can arise as a primary mass of the TMJ, as an extension of a neoplasm from surrounding tissue, or from metastases from a distant site. A detailed history, clinical examination, imaging studies, and tissue diagnosis are paramount in surgical planning.

Surgical resection of tumors of the TMJ is challenging as a result of various factors including preservation of the facial nerve, need for skull base resection, and/or necessity of lateral temporal bone resection. Reconstruction of these defects is also challenging, as functionally the TMJ plays a key role in jaw movement, mastication, and facial contour.

Resection of tumors involving the TMJ results in various defects, with most resulting in resection of the condyle of the mandible, and possibly the meniscus and glenoid fossa. The decision-making process and various reconstructive options for defects of the condyle are discussed; however, this chapter focuses on the reconstruction of the isolated condylar defect using the fibula free flap.

HISTORY

Primary lesions of the TMJ in a variety of ways often mimic much more common disorders of the TMJ. Patients may give a history of unilateral facial swelling or asymmetry, obstruction of the external auditory meatus, middle ear effusion, malocclusion, chronic dysfunction of the TMJ, pain, or aural fullness. Patients less commonly may describe hypesthesia in the distribution of the mandibular branch of Cranial Nerve V. This variability often results in a delay in diagnosis with patients often receiving an initial diagnosis of TMJ, or in fewer patients a diagnosis of parotitis. Table 16.1 lists a differential diagnosis of masses involving the TMJ.

Patients presenting with a malignant tumor originating from surrounding structures with secondary involvement of the TMJ may present with features similar to primary masses in the TMJ. More commonly, however, they will present with features of malignancy such as significant pain, otalgia, dysphagia, trismus, facial weakness, or infiltration of the skin.

Each patient's past medical and surgical history should be reviewed in detail. The patient's general health and his or her ability to tolerate a general anesthesia should be evaluated. Special attention should be given to any conditions that might compromise wound healing, such as diabetes or malnutrition. A history of peripheral vascular disease should also be investigated, as this may be pertinent in any patient in whom free tissue transfer is being considered.

TABLE 16.1 A Differential Diagnosis of Masses Involving the Temporomandibular Joint. Benign and Malignant Masses of the TMJ

Benign	Malignant	Metastasis from Distant Sites	Locoregional Spread from:
Chondroma	Chondrosarcoma	Breast	Oral cavity
Condylar hyperplasia	Fibrosarcoma	Lung	Parotid
Osteoblastoma	Multiple myeloma	Oral cavity	
Osteochondroma	Osteosarcoma	Prostate	
Osteoma	Synovial cell sarcoma		
Tophaceous pseudogout			

PHYSICAL EXAMINATION

Any mass involving the head and neck requires a thorough evaluation. Suspicion of a mass involving the posterior mandible and TMJ may not be obvious. Attention to facial symmetry or unilateral facial swelling may reveal an underlying mass. The parotid gland should be palpated for discrete masses or lesions (Fig. 16.1). The TMJ should be assessed, noting dysfunction of the joint (clicking, locking, crepitus) or trismus. The skin should be examined for any suspicious cutaneous lesions. Examination of the ears should be performed with evaluation for unilateral middle ear effusion or decreased hearing. Any finding of unilateral effusion warrants assessment with flexible nasopharyngoscopy. The oral cavity and oropharynx should be examined looking for any suspicious lesions. Any residual dentition should also be evaluated. In addition, the oropharynx should be examined for deviation of the tonsil or lateral pharyngeal wall, as this may represent a mass arising from the parapharyngeal space. Evaluation of the cranial nerves should be performed as their involvement may indicate malignancy, perineural spread, or involvement of the skull base. Special attention should be given to the facial nerve and any weakness should be docu-

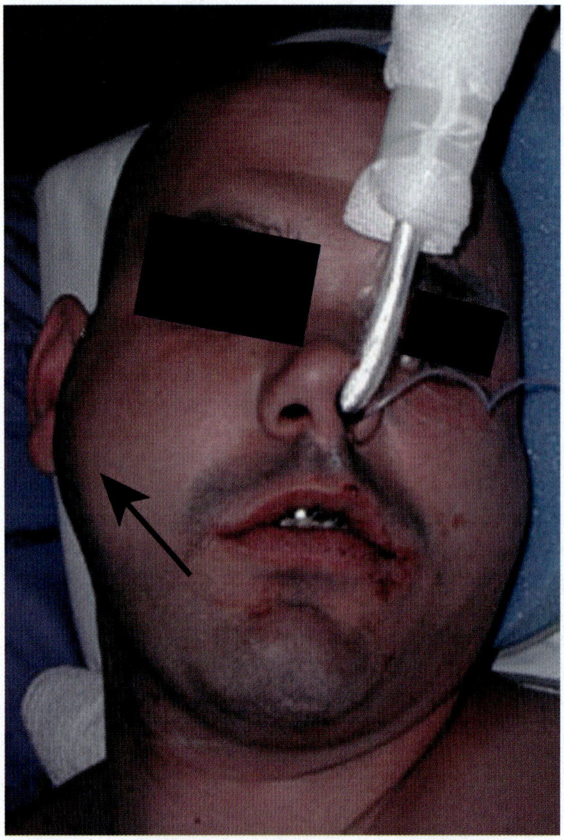

FIGURE 16.1
This figure demonstrates a tumor involving the parotid gland and TMJ (*arrow*).

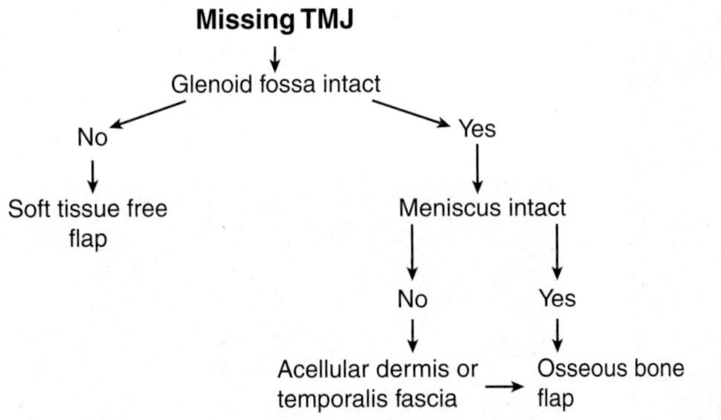

FIGURE 16.2
An algorithm for reconstruction of the TMJ.

mented as this may alter surgical planning. Fixation of the skin to the mass or considerable pain suggest a malignant tumor.

INDICATIONS

Although multiple options exist for reconstruction of the TMJ, an understanding of when to use certain reconstructive techniques is critical to surgical success and patient outcome (Fig. 16.2). Perhaps most important in the decision-making process is assessment of the glenoid fossa. This can usually be evaluated preoperatively with the use of imaging studies but should also be assessed intraoperatively. If the glenoid fossa remains intact after completion of surgical ablation and confirmation of surgical margins, an osseous microvascular free flap can be used for reconstruction. Prior to inset of the free flap, the capsule of the glenoid fossa should be assessed, and if intact, the free flap may be inset. However, if no meniscus is present, soft tissue should be placed in the glenoid fossa. Multiple types of soft tissue have been used, all with some degree of success. Some examples include acellular dermis, free fascia, periosteum, or temporalis muscle. Absence of soft tissue between the end of an osseous free flap and the glenoid fossa results in bone on bone reconstruction, possibly resulting in ankylosis and subsequent trismus.

If surgical ablation to clear surgical margins requires resection of the lateral skull base, glenoid fossa, and condyle, reconstruction with an osseous microvascular flap is contraindicated. Instead, a soft tissue flap should be used to protect the brain from a prosthetic or bony condylar reconstruction. As described below, a flap of adequate bulk should be used to restore appropriate facial contour, and maxillomandibular fixation (MMF) will be required with gradual use of guiding elastics to allow occlusal guidance.

CONTRAINDICATIONS

There are no contraindications to reconstruction of the condyle using the fibula donor site unless the donor site lacks the three-vessel distal runoff required to harvest the flap.

PREOPERATIVE PLANNING

Any lesion of the head and neck found on clinical examination and in agreement with the patient's history should be biopsied appropriately.

Since primary tumors of the TMJ are rare, the head and neck surgeon more commonly encounters tumors involving the TMJ as a result of locoregional spread. These tumors may originate from the parotid gland, skin, or oral cavity. Imaging starts with a CT scan of the neck with contrast (Fig. 16.3) as this provides good soft tissue detail and excellent detail regarding bony involvement. MRI may also be necessary to provide improved soft tissue detail, to demonstrate potential neural involvement, and to provide additional information regarding skull base involvement. If involvement of the lateral temporal bone is suggested on initial CT scan of the neck, a dedicated temporal bone CT with and without contrast should be ordered. In patients with residual dentition, a Panorex may be beneficial to assess the quality of the remaining teeth. Establishing a histopathologic diagnosis is critical in providing the correct treatment plan. Tumors of the oral cavity, parotid gland, or skin can often be directly evaluated and biopsied in the clinic. If not directly accessible, histopathologic evaluation can be obtained through fine needle aspiration biopsy (FNAB), with or without the aid of imaging modalities. If the diagnosis is still in question, open biopsy may be necessary.

Primary tumors of the TMJ are less accessible to biopsy than are tumors of the parotid, oral cavity, or skin. These tumors are typically benign hyperplastic lesions of the TMJ or malignancy of some tissue derivative of the TMJ. Given the anatomic location, imaging is the least invasive method of evaluating these neoplasms. A review of the literature by Shintaku et al. suggests that a panoramic radiograph is a good screening study

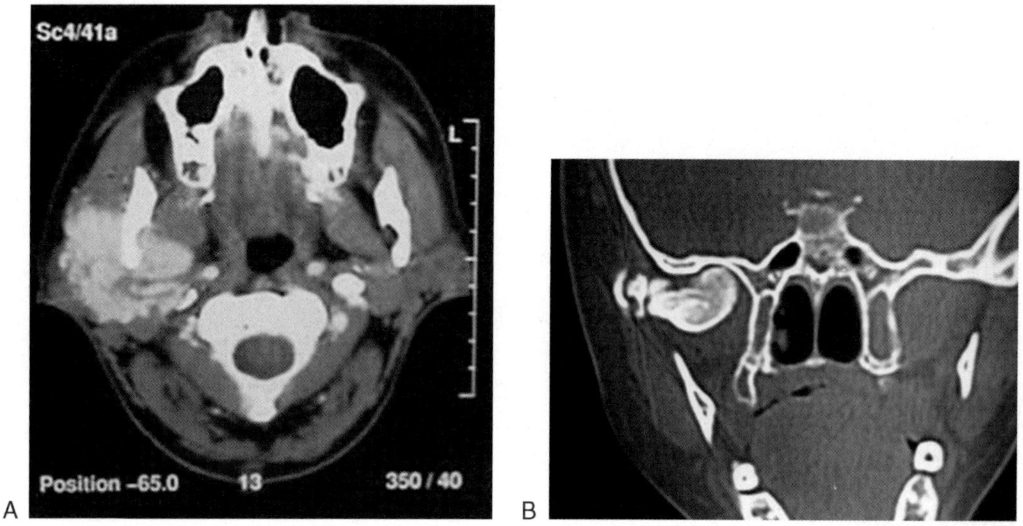

FIGURE 16.3
A. CT scan demonstrating a mass in the right parotid involving the TMJ. **B.** CT scan demonstrating a primary tumor of the TMJ.

for hyperplastic lesions of the TMJ being 97% sensitive and 45% specific. CT imaging is 70% sensitive and 100% specific in defining bony abnormalities. MRI is useful in evaluating TMJ lesions as it also assesses the surrounding soft tissue and is able to differentiate benign and malignant bony TMJ tumors with 44% sensitivity and 95% specificity. Imaging modalities combining functional and morphologic modalities, such as single positron emission CT and positron emission tomography, demonstrate improved sensitivity in assessing hyperplastic conditions of the TMJ. Single positron emission CT has demonstrated 100% sensitivity and specificity when assessing a hyperplastic condyle. Although these imaging modalities aid in treatment planning, histopathologic evaluation may also be necessary. Given the anatomic location of the TMJ and lack of access, FNAB with the aid of CT may be employed, or open biopsy may be required.

The peroneal artery and its paired venae comitantes supply the fibula flap and its overlying skin paddle. Routinely, these vessels are ligated during flap harvest. In some patients, perfusion to the donor extremity is dependent on the integrity of these vessels. Peripheral arterial occlusive disease (PAOD) of the lower extremity may prevent the use of the fibula flap due to inadequate collateral circulation to the donor extremity and also render the pedicle vessels unusable. Vascular anomalies have also been reported whereby sacrifice of the peroneal vessels would result in ischemia in the donor leg, as the peroneal vessels are always present. Assessment of the vasculature of the lower extremity should be performed preoperatively to prevent possible complications in the donor site.

Previously, lower extremity angiography was the "gold standard" for peripheral vascular assessment of the lower extremities. Although accurate, angiography is expensive, is invasive, and carries the risk of complications including embolus, hemorrhage, vessel injury, thrombosis, and contrast reaction. Magnetic resonance angiography and CT angiography have also been used to assess lower extremity vasculature. Although accurate and noninvasive, these studies are expensive and unable to determine the presence and quantity of cutaneous perforators. Color flow Doppler (CFD), an inexpensive, noninvasive ultrasound examination, uses both brightness node (B-mode) ultrasound and Doppler signal measurements to evaluate both quantity of blood flow and blood vessel patency in vessels as small as 1 mm in diameter. When compared to angiography, CFD is as sensitive and specific for vascular anatomy and PAOD. Examination of lower extremity vasculature using CFD in patients considered for fibula free tissue transfer is accurate in evaluating the vasculature of the lower extremity, diagnosing PAOD, and confirming patency of the flap pedicle vessel and donor site viability. Moreover, accurate identification and marking of cutaneous perforators from the peroneal artery can be achieved, allowing the surgeon to anticipate the viability of the skin paddle.

Resection of the mandible usually is a result of advanced stage squamous cell carcinoma or cancer of the parotid gland. More typical malignancies of the oral cavity rarely involve the TMJ, which may be explained by exit of the neurovascular bundle below the condyle or due to limited lymphatics in this region. Surgical resection of the typical cancer of the oral cavity involves osteotomies made inferior to the muscle attachments to the condyle with resection to obtain clear margins involving the body of the mandible, angle, and lower ramus (Fig. 16.4). The lateral pterygoid muscle and capsular attachments are preserved, and usually, a reconstruction plate can be fixed to the remnant of the condyle.

The necessity of resecting the TMJ to achieve appropriate tumor margins for an advanced cancer of the oral cavity or parotid gland or primary tumor of the TMJ results in a challenging defect for the reconstructive surgeon. The TMJ is a diarthrodial joint playing a key functional role in jaw movement, mastication, and mandibular form. Unique to the TMJ is its ability in jaw opening to perform rotational movement followed by gliding motion, thereby allowing for maximal divergence. The condyle of the mandible, with its lateral pterygoid attachments, is separated from the glenoid fossa by the joint capsule and meniscus. Disruption of the condyle or meniscus can result in incapacitating instability of the joint, trismus, and chronic pain. Reconstruction of the TMJ provides a complex challenge to the surgeon to restore TMJ function, facial symmetry, occlusion, and mastication. A variety of reconstructive techniques to address defects of the TMJ and/or the condyle have been described in the literature.

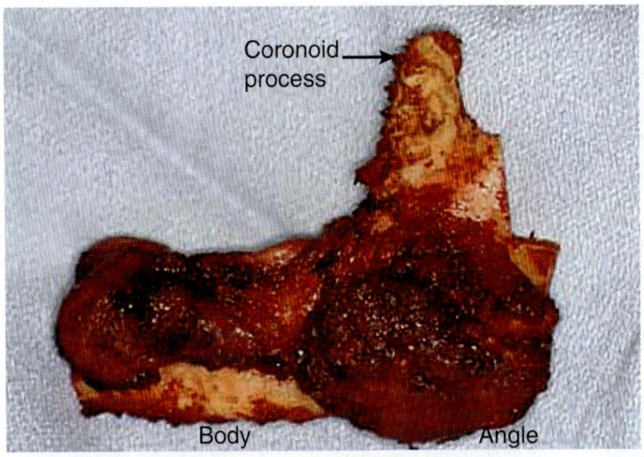

FIGURE 16.4
A surgical specimen demonstrating complete resection of the tumor of the oral cavity and the adjacent mandible.

Prosthetic Implants

Prosthetic implants have been used to replace the missing condyle. Although the use of a prosthetic implant is technically feasible, and may be considered for patients who are free flap candidates, it has fallen out of favor. Both titanium and stainless steel implants have been associated with complications including fracture of the plate or erosion of the skull base, heterotopic bone formation, intracranial perforation, and facial paralysis. Other alloplastic materials, such as Proplast-Teflon TMJ implants, have also been associated with implant migration, implant fracture, local erosion, middle cranial fossa perforation, and foreign body reaction. The use of alloplastic implants is generally limited to defects of the condyle and ramus and not the large mandibular defects common to head and neck cancer.

Soft Tissue Reconstruction

Although vascularized bone is now accepted as the standard tissue for reconstruction of the mandible, there are certain circumstances, which may preclude the use of these methods.

Patients with significant comorbidities and poor overall prognosis may benefit from less complex reconstruction allowing for more rapid recovery and less morbidity. Also, as described above, osseous reconstruction is contraindicated in patients requiring resection of the glenoid fossa. In contrast to defects of the anterior mandible, where rigid reconstruction using bone is of paramount importance to achieve optimal functional and aesthetic outcome, lateral defects are associated with significantly less morbidity; in fact most of the morbidity associated with these defects results from inadequate soft tissue lining and bulk, not lack of bone. Use of the rectus abdominis free flap (RAFF) to reconstruct defects of the posterior mandible and condyle has been described (Fig. 16.5). The anterolateral thigh flap has similar characteristics of bulk and minimal donor site morbidity, and other vascularized soft tissue flaps (both free and pedicled) may also be considered.

Although this type of reconstruction has demonstrated good outcomes regarding speech and swallowing, disadvantages include worsened cosmesis due to blunting of the mandibular angle and varying degrees of malocclusion in dentate patients. Blunting of the mandibular angle can be addressed by secondary procedures addressing soft tissue fullness in the neck. Malocclusion, although difficult to eliminate, can be minimized with use of guiding elastics.

Fibula Free Flap

The fibula free flap has become the most popular tissue for reconstruction of the mandible providing up to 25 cm of bone if needed. This flap, based on the peroneal artery, and its associated venae comitantes, can be used as an osseous or osteocutaneous flap. The skin paddle is reliable and is based on septo- or musculocutaneous perforators. The fibula is dense cortical bone that can tolerate multiple osteotomies allowing precise contouring of the neomandible. Its successful use in reconstruction of the TMJ and condyle is well documented. Preoperative assessment, harvest, and inset of this flap for the isolated defect of the condyle are described in detail below.

Morbidity of the donor site of the fibula free flap is minimal. Closure of the donor site can usually be performed primarily; however, a split-thickness skin graft may be necessary as tight closure can result in compartment syndrome. Postoperatively, patients remain in a splint for the first 4 to 5 days and then are encouraged to ambulate with assistance. In general, most patients are able to resume full activity within a few weeks. The iliac crest is another choice when considering a vascularized bone flap and is most commonly used when significant atherosclerotic and peripheral vascular disease preclude use of a fibula free flap, as the deep circumflex iliac vessels supplying the iliac crest are likely to be patent. The description of this flap is beyond the scope of this chapter.

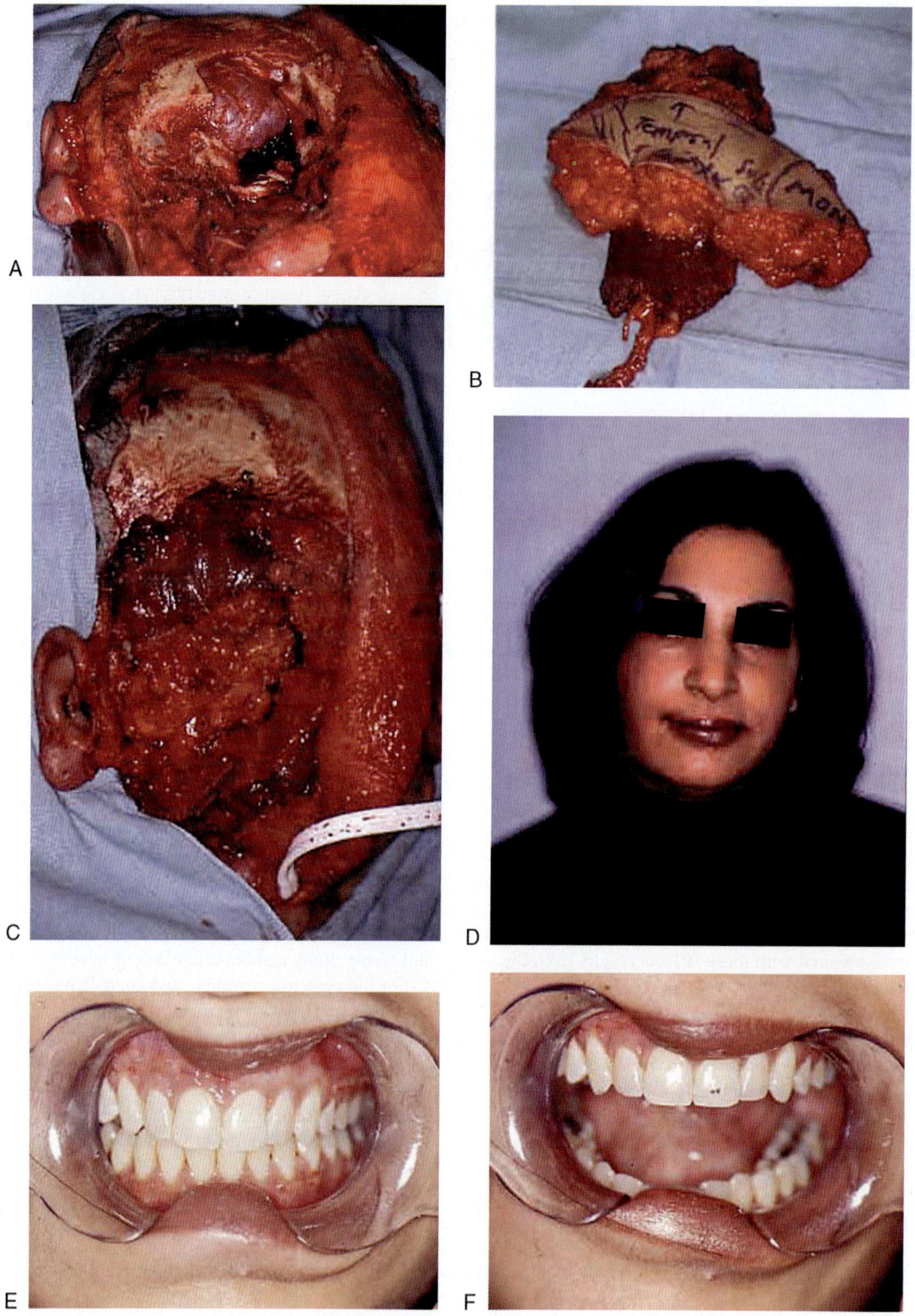

FIGURE 16.5
A. Surgical defect with condyle, ramus, and glenoid fossa absent. Temporal lobe of brain exposed. **B.** Harvested RAFF. **C.** Flap with majority of flap skin deepitheliazed. **D.** Postoperative result at 1 year. **E.** Postoperative occlusion at 1 year. **F.** Postoperative interincisal opening at 1 year.

SURGICAL TECHNIQUE

Usually, the leg ipsilateral to the defect is selected for flap harvest. This allows for the vascular pedicle to exit at the angle or body of the mandible for anastomosis to the vessels in the neck. It also presents the lateral aspect of the fibula for placement of fixation screws. Prior to harvest, approximation of the intermuscular septum is performed by assessment of the topographical anatomy and identifying the fibular head superiorly and the lateral epicondyle of the ankle inferiorly. A line is then drawn connecting these two anatomical landmarks. An elliptical fibular free flap skin paddle is designed over the distal two-thirds of the intermuscular septum, as the dominant septocutaneous perforators are located in this region. Flap harvest is then performed with a tourniquet pressure of 350 mm Hg. Incision of the anterior limb of the skin paddle is performed, carrying the incision through the skin and subcutaneous tissue. The peroneus longus is identified, and the fascia over this muscle is incised. Subfascial dissection is then performed from anterior to posterior allowing identification of the intermuscular septum and any septocutaneous perforators, which may be present. Care is taken not to violate the intermuscular septum as this may compromise the viability of the skin paddle. After leaving a cuff of muscle, the peroneus longus, peroneus brevis, and extensor hallucis longus are elevated off of the fibula allowing identification of the contents of the anterior compartment: the deep peroneal nerve, anterior tibial artery, and anterior tibial vein. With further medial dissection, the interosseus septum is identified. The interosseus septum is then incised proximally and distally along its length. The fibula is then divided with a bone cutting saw leaving at least 7 cm of proximal and distal fibula bone in place. Preservation of 7 cm of proximal and distal fibula bone ensures stability of the knee and ankle joint, respectively. Division of the fibula allows lateral retraction of the bone facilitating the remainder of the flap harvest. Division of the tibialis posterior muscle is performed along its entirety exposing the peroneal artery and venae comitantes. The distal peroneal artery and venae comitantes are ligated distally. Care should be taken to remain in the middle of the chevron oriented fibers of the tibialis posterior as dissection too close to the medial surface of the fibula may result in damage to the peroneal artery and venae comitantes. Incision of the posterior limb of the skin paddle is now performed with the incision carried through the skin and subcutaneous tissue allowing identification of the soleus muscle. The fascia of the soleus muscle is incised and a cuff of soleus muscle taken to protect any musculocutaneous perforators, which may perfuse the skin paddle. The fibula flap remains attached in the leg by the flexor hallucis longus. Moving from distal to proximal, the flexor hallucis longus is divided leaving a cuff of muscle attached to the flap. At this point, the flap remains attached by the proximal peroneal artery and venae comitantes. Prior to division of the pedicle, the tourniquet is released, flap perfusion assessed, and hemostasis achieved. The proximal pedicle is then divided and the graft used for reconstruction.

Exposure is performed though either a lip-splitting or cervical incision. After completion of the resection, exploration of the neck is performed and recipient vessels are identified in the neck (Fig. 16.6A). Recipient

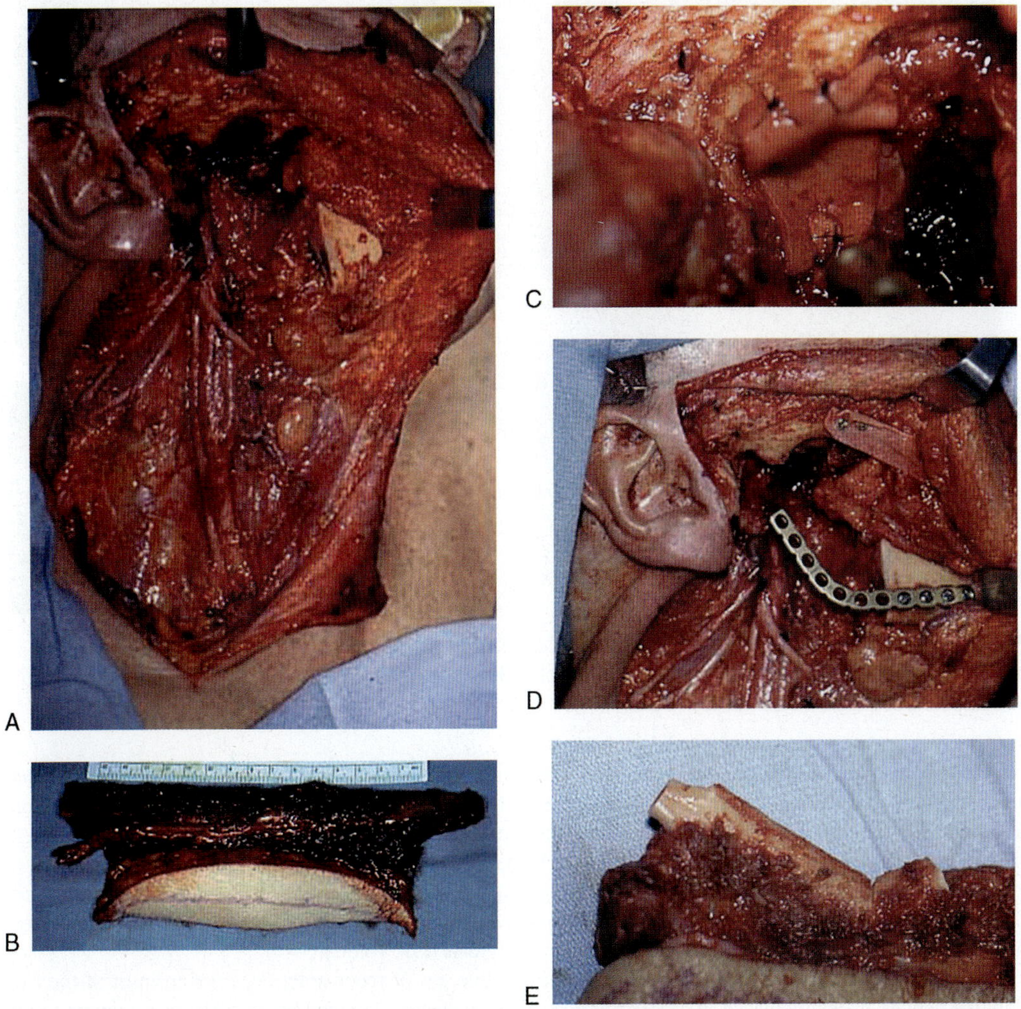

FIGURE 16.6 A. Surgical defect with the glenoid fossa intact. **B.** Harvested fibula free flap. **C.** Placement of acellular dermis in the glenoid fossa to replace the TMJ meniscus. **D.** Placement of the reconstruction plate. **E.** Contouring of the fibula flap to neocondyle.

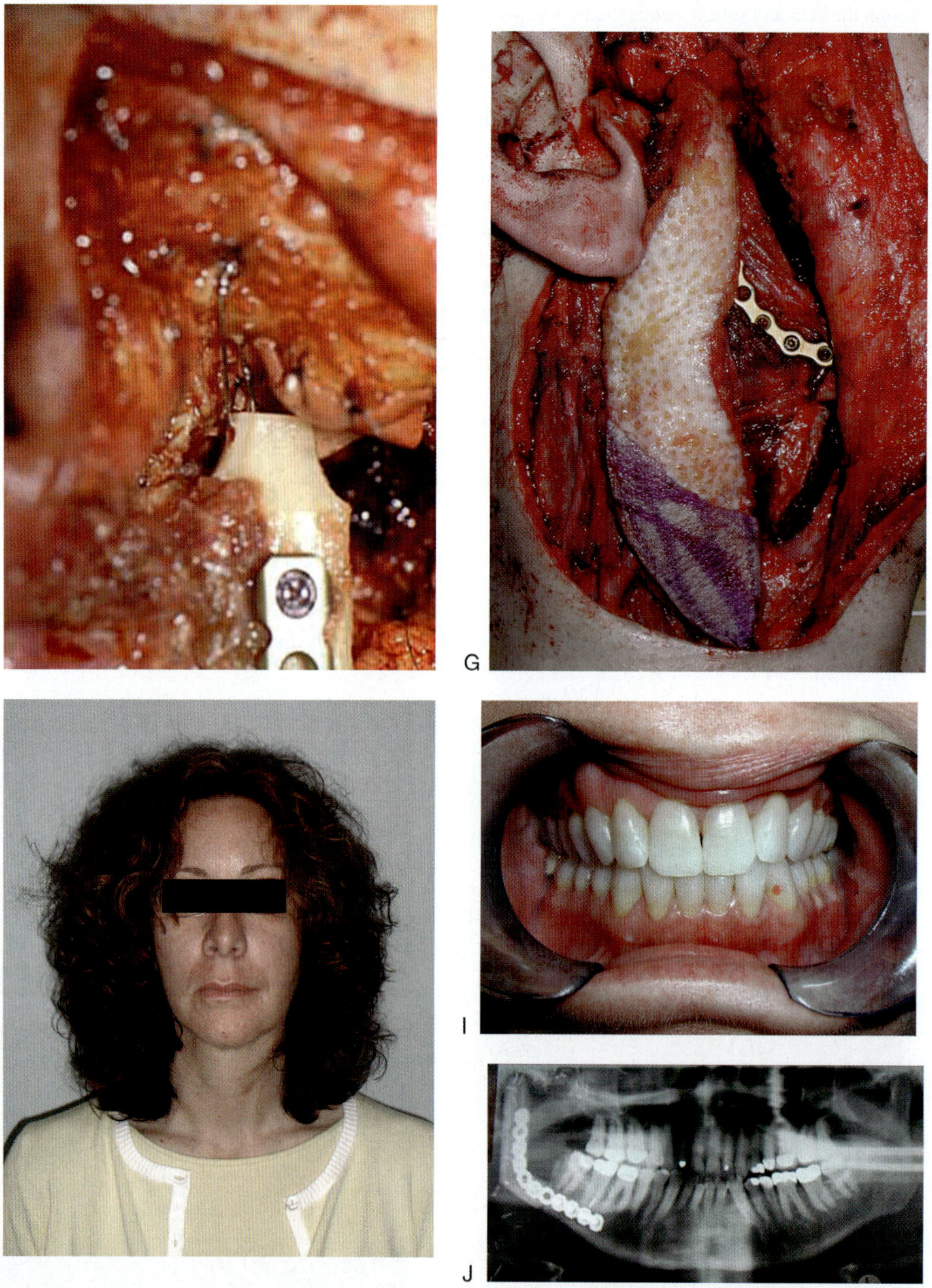

FIGURE 16.6 (*Continued*) **F.** Wiring of neocondyle into the root of the zygomatic arch. **G.** Flap deepithelialized for cheek bulk. Small portion is left intact inferiorly to act as flap monitor. **H.** Postoperative result at 1 year. **I.** Occlusion with maximum intercuspation. **J.** Panoramic radiograph at 1 year.

vessels may also be identified during neck dissection. Once recipient vessels have been identified in the neck and cleared of surrounding tissue, the proximal peroneal artery and paired venae comitantes of the fibula free flap are divided (Fig. 16.6B). The flap is transferred to the defect in the head and neck. As previously discussed, the use of a microvascular osseous flap should only be performed if the glenoid fossa is intact.

Prior to insetting the free flap, the glenoid fossa capsule must be assessed. If absent, placement of soft tissue, such as a free fascial graft, temporalis flap, or acellular dermis, is required to prevent scar or callus formation within the reconstructed joint and subsequent ankylosis (Fig. 16.6C).

Maintenance of occlusion is critical to the ultimate success of reconstruction. Prior to inset of the free flap, the dentate patient is placed in MMF. For edentulous patients, the mandible is positioned midline to the maxilla. If feasible, reconstruction plates may be fashioned from the native mandible prior to resection, thereby obviating the need for intraoperative MMF.

A pear-shaped burr is used to smooth the outer cortex of the residual native mandible facilitating maximal contact of mandible to the reconstruction plate. A locking reconstruction plate is bent to the contour of the mandible, restoring occlusion after inset of the fibula flap. If desired, a prefabricated plate may also be used. The reconstruction plate is secured to the native mandible using appropriately sized bicortical screws (Fig. 16.6D).

The length of the total bone defect is measured and marked on the distal portion of the fibula. Measurement of the distance from the superior aspect of the condyle to the inferior aspect of the angle of the mandible ensures correct mandibular height. Prior to removing excess proximal fibula, the periosteum is cleaned from the proximal portion of the fibula, thereby freeing the pedicle. The excess fibula is then removed. Osteotomies are performed carefully to provide correct width, projection, and mandibular height. The distal portion of the fibula fitting into the glenoid fossa is contoured with a cutting burr to a condylar shape (Fig. 16.6E). The distal fibula bone is maintained superior to the reconstruction plate to facilitate its fitting into the joint. The fibula is secured to the reconstruction plate with nonlocking monocortical screws. If possible, each segment of fibula should be secured with two screws. Once in place, the neocondyle is secured in the joint space. Holes are drilled through the anterior lip of the glenoid fossa and through the neocondyle, and a 24-gauge wire is used to secure the two in place (Fig. 16.6F). A heavy nonabsorbable suture may also be used if preferred. The soft tissue paddle is then inset and deepithelialized as necessary (Fig. 16.6G). The microvascular anastomoses are then performed in the usual fashion. Figure 16.6H–J demonstrates the postoperative result at 1 year.

Condyle Transplant

When oncologically safe, reconstruction of the TMJ using an osseous microvascular flap with a nonvascularized condylar transplant has also been described. At the time of reconstruction, the condyle, which has been removed with the resected specimen, is attached to the free flap with miniplates. This technique allows precise positioning of the osseous microvascular flap into its native position in the glenoid fossa. Facial symmetry is improved due to accurate graft length, proper positioning of the angle of the mandible, and subsequent restoration of preoperative posterior facial height. Dual joint function of the mandible may be preserved, allowing potential maintenance of preoperative occlusion. Partial resorption of the condylar transplant occurs in some patients; however, this has not been associated with a decrease in function, interincisal opening, position of the mandible, or abnormal symptoms such pain, trismus, or ankylosis. The degree of postoperative interincisal opening achieved is inversely proportional to use of radiation therapy and the amount of soft tissue resected, particularly in the infratemporal fossa.

POSTOPERATIVE MANAGEMENT

Postoperatively, patients are maintained on a soft diet for 3 months to allow for the appropriate healing. I use elastic bands to guide occlusion when necessary. In the event of malocclusion, I typically manage this aggressively with orthognathic guidance using either arch bars with elastic bands or a retainer. The donor site is typically managed with conservative wound care.

COMPLICATIONS

A retrospective case series of 518 consecutive mandibular reconstructions performed at our institution identified 44 patients requiring TMJ resection and reconstruction. Flap selection was performed according to the algorithm described above. Perioperative complications were assessed. Of the 44 patients, there were no flap failures. Malocclusion occurred in 3/7 dentate patients reconstructed with soft tissue and in 2/24 dentate patients reconstructed with bone. Patients were treated with guiding elastics for a mean of 23 days. Other perioperative complications included two cases of temporary facial nerve paralysis and three instances of wound infection.

Other reported complications during free flap reconstruction of the TMJ include cerebrovascular accident, myocardial infarction, hypoperfusion of the free flap due to venous thrombosis of the microvascular anastomosis, and hematoma in the neck.

RESULTS

Functional outcomes after TMJ reconstruction with microvascular reconstruction are poorly documented. The same retrospective case series performed at our institution also assessed functional results after free flap reconstruction of the TMJ in regard to diet, speech, and maximal interincisal distance. Overall, 93% of patients resumed an oral diet. Thirty-eight percent of patients (16 dentate and 1 edentulous) achieved a regular diet, 54% (14 dentate and 10 edentulous) achieved a soft diet, and 3 patients remained PEG dependent. All 44 patients were intelligible over the phone. Maximal interincisal distance ranged from 2 to 4.5 cm with a mean of 3.6 cm. Patients who received radiation therapy experienced an average loss of 1.1 cm of interincisal opening. No statistical differences were found in any variable in patients undergoing fibula reconstruction with or without condyle autotransplantation.

PEARLS

- TMJ replacement with osseous free tissue transfer is reliable, is reproducible, and restores function. Optimal results rely on the new condyle being properly seated and maintained in the glenoid fossa.
- Soft tissue flaps are successful in situations not suitable for bony reconstruction of the condyle.

PITFALLS

- Malocclusion may result if guiding elastics in dentate patients are not used to achieve a stable occlusion.
- Postoperative radiotherapy, though necessary in many cases, is a critical factor that limits joint function in this group of patients.

INSTRUMENTS TO HAVE AVAILABLE

- Standard head and neck surgical set
- Reciprocating saw

ACKNOWLEDGMENT

I gratefully acknowledge the contributions of Thomas J. Gernon, MD.

SUGGESTED READING

Lindqvist C. Erosion and heterotopic bone formation after alloplastic temporomandibular joint reconstruction. *J Oral Maxillofac Surg* 1992;50:942–949; discussion 950.

Lindqvist C. Rigid reconstruction plates for immediate reconstruction following mandibular resection for malignant tumors. *J Oral Maxillofac Surg* 1992;50:1158–1163.

Kroll SS. Reconstruction of posterior mandibular defects with soft tissue using the rectus abdominis free flap. *Br J Plast Surg* 1998;51:503–507.

Wax MK, Winslow CP, Hansen J, et al. A retrospective analysis of temporomandibular joint reconstruction with free fibula microvascular flap. *Laryngoscope* 2000;110:977–981.

Abramowicz S, Dolwick MF, Lewis SB, et al. Temporomandibular joint reconstruction after failed teflon-proplast implant: case report and literature review. *Int J Oral Maxillofac Surg* 2008;37:763–767.

17

MANAGEMENT OF THE TOTAL MANDIBULAR DEFECT

Peter C. Neligan

INTRODUCTION

The indications for total mandibular reconstruction are relatively rare. However, it is important to understand the principles involved so that the various segments of the mandible can be reconstructed optimally. In addition, it is relatively rare that the mandible needs to be reconstructed in isolation. Far more common is the setting in which bone reconstruction is required in combination with replacement of intraoral lining, reconstruction of the external skin envelope, or both. The most common requirement for reconstruction is that of the segmental defect, and there are principles that apply depending on which segment is involved. Boyd classified mandibular defects based on the segment of mandible involved together with the soft tissue requirement, either mucosa (m) or skin (s). This is helpful when planning reconstructions.

Mandibular reconstruction has evolved over the past three decades from a complex and often not very successful venture to a very reliable, if still complex, technique. The main reason for this advance has been the incorporation of microsurgical techniques and the development of reliable flaps for reconstruction. Of these developments, the most significant has probably been the description of the fibula as a suitable bone to achieve mandibular reconstruction. For while there are other flaps that can be used, and there are specific indications where some of these may be better, the fibula has emerged as the gold standard for mandibular reconstruction. The concept of maintaining quality of life has become particularly important in the overall care and treatment of cancer patients. Thus, even patients with a very limited life expectancy are routinely reconstructed if it is expected that their quality of remaining life would be significantly enhanced. The high success rate of head and neck reconstructive procedures has allowed for significant improvement in both functional and aesthetic results and has completely changed the conceptual approach to mandibular reconstruction. Only patients who are medically unfit to tolerate a long operation or have a grave prognosis are excluded as candidates for resection and immediate reconstruction.

HISTORY

Because the fibular free flap donor site is the most common donor site used for total mandibular reconstruction, the history is centered around factors that may limit the use of this donor site. Prior injury to the lower leg, peripheral vascular disease, or disturbance in gait are all issues that need to be considered in taking history from a patient who requires a total mandibular reconstruction. Prior injury to the lower leg may limit the use of the fibula bone or may have left the patient with significant gait disturbance that could become functionally devastating following a fibula harvest. Significant peripheral vascular disease commonly afflicts the lower extremities. Patients with a history of lower extremity claudication, vascular insufficiency, or poor lower extremity circulation should be carefully evaluated using lower extremity vascular imaging. Because the fibular donor site is the only bony donor site that provides the length of bone necessary for complete mandibular reconstruction, there are few alternative choices.

PHYSICAL EXAMINATION

Reconstruction of the total mandibular defect can be performed primarily or secondarily. Arguably, the latter represents a more significant challenge than does the former because one needs to contend with the scar contractures and limited soft tissue envelope. In both cases, a careful physical examination will determine if there are remaining condyles, dentition, and an appropriate soft tissue to accommodate the vascularized bone reconstruction. In cases where the condyles are present, the design of the flap can be altered to use the remaining bone. In contrast, if the examination reveals that the condyles are not present, the distal aspects of the fibula will need to be designed to recreate the joint. The examination of the dentition is important to determine if the patient will require dental occlusal management during surgery to maintain the appropriate dental occlusion following surgery. Finally, a careful assessment of the soft tissue is important in determining if a skin paddle should be included in the design of the flap. All aspects of the examination are important; however, these issues are the most important when considering total mandibular reconstruction.

INDICATIONS

While it is true that some defects do not necessarily require reconstruction with bone, my personal bias is to reconstruct all mandibular defects with a bone flap unless there are specific patient factors that preclude that. Fortunately, this situation is rare.

The lateral mandibular defect can be reconstructed with a plate and soft tissue flap. However, if the plate fractures (and, over time, this is more likely to happen), the patient will require a further reconstruction, probably with bone. So from my perspective, it is easier to use a bone flap in the first place and avoid this problem altogether. Central mandibular defects, however, require reconstruction with bone. Use of a plate and soft tissue flap invariably results in exposure of the plate over time. This is totally avoidable if a bone flap is used and is the one situation in which use of a bone flap is mandatory.

The third area to be considered when thinking about total mandibular reconstruction is the condyle and the temporomandibular joint. Various techniques have been proposed to reconstruct the condyle. These include use of a reconstruction plate incorporating a condylar head, grafting of the existing condyle onto the bone flap used for the reconstruction, use of a costochondral graft to replace the mandibular neck and condyle, or the use of soft tissue interposition between the bony construct and the condylar fossa. My personal preference is to use interposition of soft tissue. I have used periosteum for this purpose with good results.

While there are several bone flap options for mandibular reconstruction, there is general consensus that the fibular flap is the gold standard. It combines good bone stock, adequate length, as well as soft tissue that is very suitable for most applications within the oral cavity. The length of fibula that can be harvested approaches 25 cm, sufficient length to reconstruct almost all defects. The bone stock is such that it accommodates osseointegrated dental rehabilitation. One criticism, however, is that the bone height is less than that of the mandible. This can be important for fitting osseointegrated teeth. There are a number of potential solutions to this. One is to fudge the inset of the fibula so that, instead of matching the fibula with the inferior border of the mandible, the bone is inset a little higher to minimize the discrepancy between the alveolar border of the mandible and the fibula. Harvesting a cuff of flexor hallucis longus (FHL) with the bone helps to soften the interface between the mandibular border and the fibula and hides the potential step between the inferior border of the mandible and the inferior border of the fibula. Another strategy is to double barrel the fibula, stacking one segment on top of the other. This technique can be used for shorter mandibular defects, but for larger defects, it is less applicable as it uses up too much bone length. A final strategy is to vertically distract the fibula.

The mandible is an arch, while the fibula is a straight bone. In order to make an arch, multiple osteotomies may be required. The blood supply of the fibula is both endosteal and periosteal, a fact that renders it most amenable to multisegmental osteotomies and precise shaping. However, it has been shown that the more bone segments in the construct, the greater the risk of devascularization. Finally, the donor defect following fibular harvest is very acceptable despite the fact that it has been shown that there is a significant deleterious effect on foot and ankle function.

CONTRAINDICATIONS

If the preoperative evaluation does not demonstrate three-vessel perfusion, the fibula is contraindicated.

PREOPERATIVE PLANNING

The reliability of the fibular skin paddle has been controversial. Initially, there was a sense that the skin paddle was not universally reliable though there is excellent evidence that this is not the case. In the early days, it was common practice to get an angiogram of the lower limb to determine the patency of the peroneal vessels, a practice that most people abandoned. However, more recently, as our knowledge of the perfusion of the integument has improved, interest in mapping the blood supply of our flaps has undergone a renewal. The use of CT angiography has become popular in determining the blood supply of flaps. This has come from the development of perforator flaps and is a very useful tool. While it is most widely used in autologous breast reconstruction, it is equally applicable to all flaps. The CT angiogram not only can depict where the vessels are but also maps their course, their relationship to the musculature, and so on. It shows anatomic variability where, in the past, it was discovered during the dissection and while it is not necessary to have a CT angiogram in order to raise a fibular flap, it takes the guesswork out of the dissection and makes it more predictable, quicker, and probably safer. It is particularly relevant to the placement and dissection of the skin paddle. Another very useful tool in determining flap perfusion is the use of indocyanine green dye. This is a fluorescent dye that when injected intravenously can be detected using a laser light source that excites the fluorescence and near-infrared fluoroscopy that detects it. This technology is widely available. In the United States, the system is called SPY and is marketed by LifeCell Corporation (Branchburg, NJ). While this is not necessary in order to safely raise a fibular osseocutaneous flap, it is a useful tool in predicting flap viability and avoiding problems. This is particularly the case if there is any doubt as to the viability of the skin paddle.

SURGICAL TECHNIQUE

One of the first things surgeons are concerned about is whether it matters which fibula to take for a given defect. The short answer is that for most defects it does not matter. However, there are some important things to remember. The orientations of the skin paddle and of the pedicle are the two major determining factors. The optimal relationship of the skin paddle to the bone is as it appears in the leg. So if a right-sided mandibular defect with a need for intraoral lining is being reconstructed, an ipsilateral fibula will work well and the pedicle will be at the angle of the mandible. If it is better for the pedicle to come out anterior, then a contralateral flap would work better.

It is important to mark the fibular head and the lateral malleolus and to measure back from these two points. A length of about 6 cm at either end will protect the ankle mortice distally and the peroneal nerve proximally. While it is not necessary to harvest all the intervening bone, it is easiest to do so, even if all the bone is not required. The unwanted bone can be discarded making dissection of the pedicle easier. As long as the distal and proximal 6 cm of bone are preserved, morbidity will not be a major issue.

It is important to realize that the blood supply to the skin passes in the posterior crural septum, and this structure is approximately 2 cm behind the axis of the fibula. In a thin individual, it can be appreciated on the surface of the limb. It is also important to realize that the blood supply of the peroneal skin compartment is musculocutaneous proximally and septocutaneous distally. For that reason, a skin paddle more distally placed will be more likely to have a septocutaneous blood supply. Consequently, I plan the skin paddle in the distal third (Fig. 17.1). If a second skin paddle is required, it can be dissected based on one of the more proximal musculocutaneous perforators. This is a situation where a preoperative CT angiogram is particularly useful. These vessels can also be detected with a handheld Doppler prior to beginning the dissection. However, while the Doppler will give good information on the position of the perforator, the CT angiogram gives additional information on the course of the perforator, its relationship to the musculature, and its relationship to the peroneal vessels.

Regardless of the type of fibular flap being harvested, osseocutaneous or bone-only flap, my preference is to harvest the fibula through a lateral approach. Figure 17.2 demonstrates the incision lines and their relationship to the various structures in the leg. The anterior incision of the skin flap is made, and the incision is carried through the subcutaneous tissue down to the fascia. The superficial peroneal nerve (SPN)

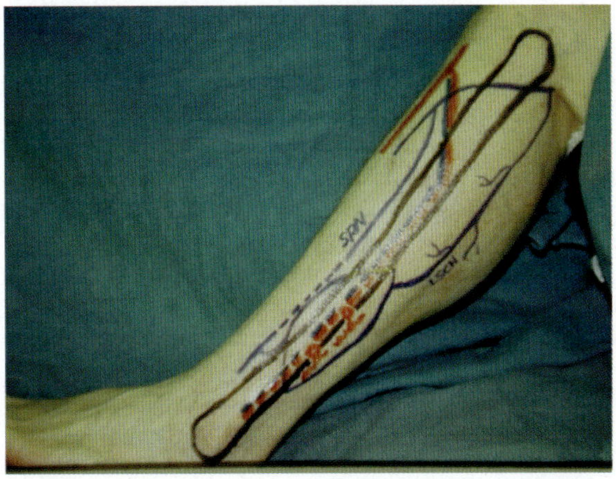

FIGURE 17.1
The skin paddle is placed in the distal third to take advantage of the septocutaneous perforators. More proximal perforators are musculocutaneous. Note that this skin paddle has a dual sensory nerve supply, from a recurrent branch of the superficial peroneal nerve (SPN), and from the lateral sural cutaneous nerve (LSCN).

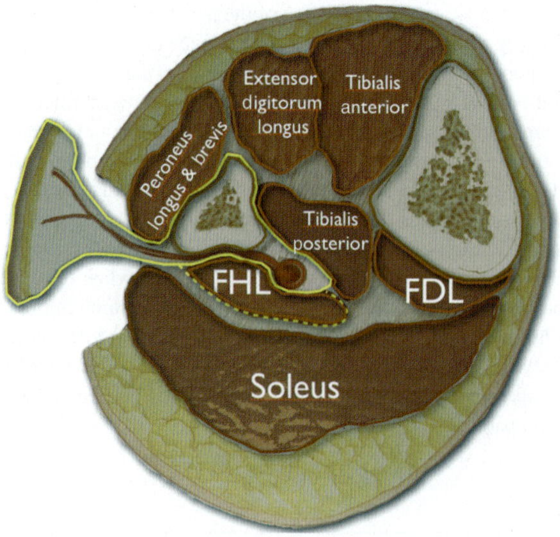

FIGURE 17.2
This schematic diagram of the cross-sectional anatomy of the lower limb shows the relationship of the various structures and incorporating the peroneal artery with the skin perforators traversing the posterior crural septum. The standard incisions are marked in *yellow* showing the structures harvested with the flap. *Dotted yellow line* indicates that Flexor Hallucis Longus (FHL) can be harvested with the flap if desired. (FDL, flexor digitorum longus.)

can be seen deep to the fascia and is preserved by incising the fascia just posterior to it. The fascia can then be swept off the underlying muscle with a finger, and this reveals the anterior leaf of the posterior crural septum. I generally keep all of my dissection anterior, only making the posterior skin flap incision when most of the dissection is complete. The proximal skin incision is also made at this time in continuity with the incision already described. The fibula is now approached from the lateral aspect, along the anterior leaf of the posterior crural septum, leaving some muscle fibers on the bone in order to protect the periosteum, since the fibula, aside from its endosteal supply, also has a robust periosteal blood supply. It is this periosteal supply that I mostly rely upon in maintaining viability of the bone. As soon as the lateral border of the fibula is reached, dissection then proceeds anteriorly, hugging the bone and taking care not to breach the periosteum. The next structure encountered is the anterior crural septum, and this is divided along the length of the fibula. This gives access to the anterior compartment. It is important to be aware of the fact that the anterior tibial vessels are in relatively close proximity to the dissection at this point and can potentially be damaged if care is not taken. The easiest way to avoid this is to hug the bone during the dissection. Retracting the muscles of the anterior compartment, dissection now proceeds around the fibula. The next structure encountered is the interosseous membrane, which is a very strong structure. Prior to dividing it, I like to carry out the osteotomies on the fibula. Care must be taken to preserve at least 6 cm of fibula at either end in order to protect the ankle mortice distally and the peroneal nerve proximally. Bone levers are placed behind the bone, once again, hugging the bone. I use Hohmann bone levers. The narrow end of the lever is convex, and this facilitates placing it around the bone and in close proximity to it. Then, using an oscillating saw, the osteotomies are done proximally and distally, cutting down on the bone lever in order to avoid injury to the underlying structures, and, most particularly, avoiding injury to the pedicle. Bone clamps are then applied to the fibula, and the bone is rotated laterally. This allows visualization of the interosseous membrane. This is now divided, and as it is incised, the surgeon can feel the fibula move laterally and the space between tibia and fibula open up. Next, the peroneal vessels are identified distally and are divided. The vessels lie behind the tibialis posterior muscle, and this is now split over the pedicle so that the pedicle comes into direct view, lying on the flexor hallucis longus muscle. Various muscular branches are divided as the dissection proceeds. The pedicle runs along the length of the bone, but proximally, it can be seen to deviate medially toward the tibia. Further dissection will reveal its origin, branching from the posterior tibial artery. This completes the pedicle dissection.

The length of bone that is required is now determined. The mandibular defect is carefully measured. It is important when translating this measurement to the fibula to remember that the mandible is curved bone and the fibula is a straight one. Osteotomies will need to be made in order to convert it to a curved bone. In general, these osteotomies are closing osteotomies. This implies that a wedge of bone has to be excised in order to create the curve, and, if a significant length of mandible needs to be replaced, multiple osteotomies may be required. To add greater complexity to total mandibular defects, these osteotomies are multiplanar and three-dimensional. Not only must the curve of the mandible be reproduced but the angle of the mandible also needs to be replicated.

There are many ways to plan the osteotomies that need to be performed in order to accurately replicate the shape of the mandible. These range from free-hand guesswork (not recommended) to stereolithographic modeling and plate prebending. My personal preference is to use the native mandible as a template. The ablative team bends a reconstruction plate to the mandible prior to mandibular resection. This plate is also predrilled to the mandibular remnants. In this way, when the plate is replaced on the mandible after resection, the lateral elements of the mandible will maintain their relationship to the maxilla. Maintenance of this biarched relationship is key to successful mandibular reconstruction. In total mandibular reconstruction, simply prebending the

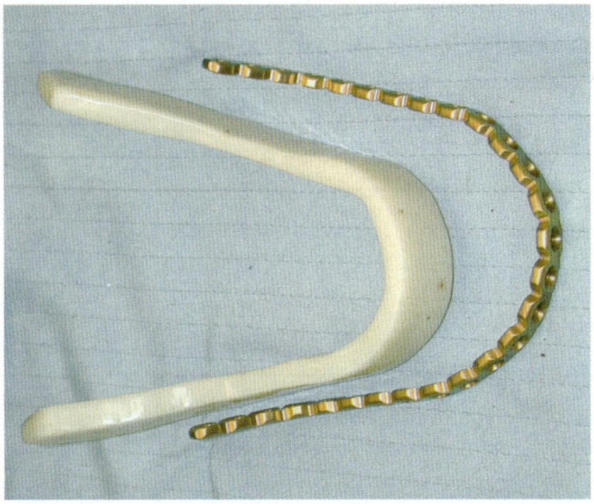

FIGURE 17.3
This is a methyl methacrylate template made from patient CT scans. The plate can be prebent to this template. Stereolithographic representations can also be manufactured from CT images.

plate will not work. In these cases, some sort of preoperative modeling is required. Stereolithographic modeling is expensive but very accurate. A model is made of the mandible from a three-dimensional CT scan. A plate is bent to this model to ensure maximal accuracy. Alternatively, a different version can be created with methyl methacrylate based on a CT scan (Fig. 17.3). This is probably less accurate, but, nevertheless, it is arguable whether these reconstructions are so unforgiving as to demand absolute precision. My personal opinion is that absolute precision is not completely necessary. This is because of the improved technology of locking plates that do not demand absolute apposition of plate to bone along the entire length of the plate, unlike nonlocking plates. What is necessary is that the arch be reasonably accurately reproduced and, probably more importantly, that the relationship of the reconstructed mandible to the maxilla replicates the relationship that existed before the resection.

My personal technique involves determining the osteotomies based on the dimensions of the prebent plate, that is, the plate that has been bent to the existing mandible prior to resection. I try to keep my osteotomies to a minimum, reducing the number required by "rounding off" the ends of each osteotomy segment (Fig. 17.4). Once the osteotomies have been completed and assuming there is some remnant of mandible to which I am attaching my construct, I leave the bone ends on the fibula a little longer than measured so that I can make the final adjustments as I inset the fibula to the mandible. This allows for a press fit and ensures maximal apposition of the bone.

From a practical point of view, I like to inset the soft tissues first, assuming that I am replacing intraoral lining. This allows easier access for once the bone is inset, access to the oral cavity is reduced. Once

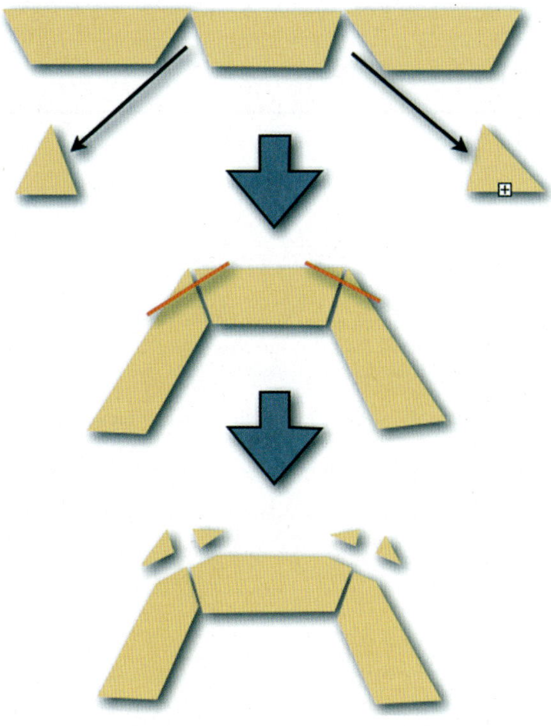

FIGURE 17.4
A closing wedge osteotomy is designed to create a curve in the fibula. Two wedge osteotomies are shown. This curve can be further enhanced by resecting the apices of the bone cuts as shown.

the soft tissue is inset, the bone fit is performed following which the microvascular anastomosis is carried out. If the flap is providing external skin cover, then this part of the inset is done last, after intraoral reconstruction and bony fit.

POSTOPERATIVE MANAGEMENT

The patient is required to wear a lower leg donor side split for 7 days. The patient is restricted to a soft diet for 6 weeks to allow the fibular bone flap to heal.

COMPLICATIONS

There are many potential complications that include malunion of the bone graft, necrosis of the fibular skin paddle, and donor site morbidity including skin sloughing, foot drop, and instability of the ankle.

RESULTS

Mandibular reconstruction has reached a level of reliability, reproducibility, and aesthetic and functional acceptability that could not have been imagined 30 years ago. Nevertheless, it remains a complex procedure that demands attention to detail and meticulousness in its execution.

PEARLS

- Determine what is being resected and plan accordingly.
- Determine which fibula is most advantageous to use.
- Position skin paddle distally.
- If in doubt, do a preoperative CT angiogram.
- "Round off" osteotomies.

PITFALLS

- When determining bone length, do not forget to take into account that the wedge osteotomies will be discarded so a greater length of bone is required.
- Determine beforehand the optimal positioning of the skin paddle relative to the bone. Remember the best relationship is what is in the leg.

INSTRUMENTS TO HAVE AVAILABLE

- Standard head and neck surgical set
- Reciprocating saw

SUGGESTED READING

Hidalgo DA. Fibula free flap: a new method of mandible reconstruction. *Plast Reconstr Surg* 1989;84(1):71–79.

Boyd JB, Gullane PJ, Rotstein LE, et al. Classification of mandibular defects. *Plast Reconstr Surg* 1993;92(7):1266–1275.

Boyd JB, Morris S, Rosen IB, et al. The through-and-through oromandibular defect: rationale for aggressive reconstruction. *Plast Reconstr Surg* 1994;93(1):44–53.

Schliephake H, Neukam FW, Schmelzeisen R, et al. Long-term quality of life after ablative intraoral tumour surgery. *J Craniomaxillofac Surg* 1995;23(4):243–249.

Wilson KM, Rizk NM, Armstrong SL, et al. Effects of hemimandibulectomy on quality of life. *Laryngoscope* 1998;108(10):1574–1577.

Ko EW, Huang CS, Chen YR. Temporomandibular joint reconstruction in children using costochondral grafts. *J Oral Maxillofac Surg* 1999;57(7):789–798; discussion 99–800.

18 MANAGEMENT OF THE COMPOSITE THROUGH-AND-THROUGH DEFECT: SCAPULAR FREE FLAP

Brian B. Burkey

INTRODUCTION

Large composite defects of the head and neck produced by extensive surgical ablation or trauma can pose a distinct challenge for the reconstructive surgeon. In particular, the three-dimensional reestablishment of juxtaposed skin, soft tissue, and bone requires careful tissue importation and realignment to ensure an appropriate return of form and function.

Multiple methods of reconstruction are available for large composite tissue defects. Previously, soft tissue muscular regional flaps, such as the pectoralis major myocutaneous flap, trapezius flap, sternocleidomastoid flap, latissimus dorsi flap, and platysma flap, were used to repair the soft tissue defect, and the mandible was repaired with a plate or left to "swing." However, over the last 25 years, the vascularized transfer of both bone and soft tissue (osteocutaneous and osteomyocutaneous free flaps) has become a widely used and successful means for single-stage reconstruction of the composite tissue defect. Urken et al. reported a high success rate of 96% for oromandibular microvascular reconstruction. Vascularized bone reconstruction yields optimal results for several reasons: (1) Reconstruction of an osseous defect with similar tissue provides the most ideal construct to retain its three-dimensional form; (2) vascularized bone is able to sustain the inherent mechanical forces and structural demands required; and (3) vascularized bone has a greater ability to survive in the bacteria-rich environment of the head and neck.

The osteocutaneous and osteomyocutaneous free flaps most often used by head and neck reconstructive surgeons for composite tissue reconstruction are the iliac crest–internal oblique flap, scapula flap, and fibula flap. Among these, the scapula flap provides a substantial amount of skin, muscle, and bone, which are able to be harvested and are uniquely oriented to fill large defects. For this reason, the scapula flap is ideal for reconstruction of large composite defects and is the most versatile of the bone-containing flaps.

The scapular flap, based on branches of the circumflex scapular vessels, and its use in free tissue transfer were first described by dos Santos in 1980. Shortly thereafter, Swartz and Sullivan described the use of this flap in nearly 60 patients for both maxillary and mandibular reconstruction, establishing its role in reconstruction of various defects in the head and neck.

Anatomy

The vasculature of the scapular and parascapular fascia and skin, latissimus dorsi muscle, and medial, lateral, and tip segments of the scapula bone emanate from the subscapular arterial arcade. The axillary artery branches into the subscapular artery and then to a posterior branch called the circumflex scapular artery (CSA). However, in 3% of cadaver dissections, the CSA originates directly from the axillary artery. The subscapular artery further branches into a descending branch called the thoracodorsal artery (TDA), which supplies the latissimus dorsi muscle, with several branches extending to the serratus anterior muscle, allowing for use of both muscles on the same pedicle.

The CSA is found at the midlateral border of the scapula, passing posteriorly and under the subscapularis muscle. The artery curves around the lateral aspect of the scapula and emerges at the omotricipital space, a triangle created by the long head of the triceps muscle, the teres major muscle, and the teres minor muscle. This triangle can frequently be palpated as a depression just lateral to the scapular bone near its midpoint. By this point, the artery has provided branches to the subscapularis, teres major and minor, and infraspinatus muscles. The artery projects through the triangle and sends a branch to vascularize the lateral corticocancellous scapular bone prior to emerging from this space. These branches supply the periosteum of the scapula. Two main fasciocutaneous branches then extend to form the scapular (transverse) and parascapular (descending) vessels. The horizontal scapular artery runs about 2 cm inferior to the spine of the scapula toward the spine. The descending branch runs approximately 2 cm medial and parallel to the lateral scapula border toward the scapula tip. These vessels define the two large fasciocutaneous paddles that may be harvested with the circumflex scapular system. These paddles may be harvested either separately or together and may incorporate the skin overlying the latissimus dorsi muscle.

The CSA averages 4 mm wide at its origin and may range between 2 and 6 mm in diameter. The artery is accompanied by two venae comitantes that usually converge before draining into the axillary vein, but the venous drainage may be variable in position and pattern. The length of the pedicle from the lateral border of the scapula is approximately 6 cm. About 2 to 3 cm of pedicle length exists between the scapular border and the fasciocutaneous segment. This allows the skin segment independent maneuverability from the bone, which is the defining characteristic of this flap and the advantage it has over all of the other osseous flaps.

The skin segments are classified as fasciocutaneous flaps that are supplied by vertical perforators from the fascial layer deep to the subcutaneous adipose tissue. A subcutaneous vascular plexus additionally supplies the skin. Therefore, the flap may be peripherally debulked of subcutaneous adipose tissue and fascia, although care must be taken when doing this to protect any dominant perforators. Additionally, the fasciocutaneous segment may be divided into separate skin islands based on the dominant perforators.

The lateral aspect of the scapular bone is harvested with the lateral circumflex system, starting just inferior to the glenohumeral fossa. Typically, the bone is 1.5 cm thick, 3 cm wide (as the bone is cut at this distance from the lateral edge), and 10 to 14 cm long. The bone is thinnest at the midpoint of the scapula, which may pose a significant drawback to this flap. The tip of the scapula is supplied by the angular branch of the TDA and may be confidently harvested with the inclusion of this vascular branch. The tip can then be left attached to the lateral border of the scapular bone or can be detached on its own pedicle, the latter allowing for a second piece of bone with this flap that can be placed well distant (>10 cm) from the primary bone segment.

Finally, the latissimus muscle or muscle and overlying skin, and/or the serratus muscle, can be harvested with this flap with the inclusion of the TDA, by taking the flap vessels at the subscapular artery and vein (the "megaflap"). This muscle and additional soft tissue may then be used to fill large soft tissue defects in the parapharyngeal space and neck, all with tissue from one harvest and on one vascular system demonstrating the unique ability of this versatile flap and vascular system.

HISTORY

Patients typically present with complex tumors, benign and malignant, or trauma involving the head and neck. The scapula free flap is ideal for large, composite tissue reconstruction. Typically, these patients have through-and-through defects or anticipated defects involving the maxilla and/or the mandible (requiring skin, bone, and mucosal reconstruction). This flap is ideal in these circumstances because it affords the ability for osseous reconstruction coupled with simultaneous fasciocutaneous coverage by two large cutaneous paddles, which may be placed distant from the bone.

A history of prior shoulder surgery should be investigated, including rotator cuff surgery, as this may damage the vasculature of the flap. Also, inquiries about prior neck surgery may give clues to preexisting damage to neck recipient vessels or to cranial nerve (CN) XI. The latter may cause significant shoulder dysfunction prior to and after harvest of the scapular flap and is a relative contraindication to the ipsilateral use of this flap.

PHYSICAL EXAMINATION

A thorough examination of the defect site is required, along with necessary imaging to determine the extent of the defect. Preoperative shoulder function should also be evaluated. Detachment of the teres major muscle during harvest may hinder a preoperatively weak shoulder girdle. As previously noted, patients should be identified who have had a previous ipsilateral radical neck dissection with sacrifice of the spinal accessory nerve or other surgery or trauma to the scapular area.

INDICATIONS

The benefit of this flap is its great versatility. The flap affords the advantages of a variety of different muscle, bone, and skin paddle components that may be customized to reconstruct a large composite defect. Additionally, there is a relative maneuverability of these segments allowing added ability to inset tissues as needed, without undue tension on individual segments.

In my practice, this flap has four specific uses. First, patients with through-and-through defects of the oromandibular complex, and/or with facial skin defects extending superior to the oral commissure, will require extensive intraoral and extraoral soft tissue reconstruction that is not possible with any other osseocutaneous flap. In these defects, the dual skin paddles are particularly useful with one skin paddle being used to line the intraoral mucosal defect, while the other can be used for soft tissue or skin reconstruction of the extraoral defect. Obviously, simultaneous bone reconstruction may also be achieved by the same flap should the defect involve a segmental mandibulectomy. The cheek area superior to the oral commissure can be repaired without tension due to the freedom of the skin paddle from the bone segment.

Second, I use this flap in patients who require osseous reconstruction but have severe lower extremity atherosclerotic disease and/or diabetic sequelae preventing the use of a fibula free flap. If preoperative vascular imaging (such as by magnetic resonance angiography) finds significant bilateral lower extremity vascular disease that puts the fibula flap or the lower leg at risk of insufficiency, my flap of choice is the scapula free flap. The iliac crest–internal oblique donor site can be quite morbid due to gait changes and hernia, and the skin component is often quite thick in Western populations and therefore I prefer the scapula flap over the iliac crest flap despite the inability of a two-team approach.

Third, patients who may need a "megaflap" for an abundance of skin and soft tissue required for adequate reconstruction along with bone are good candidates for this flap. The scapula free flap allows the unique ability to harvest the scapular (transverse) and parascapular (descending) skin paddle systems, along with the thoracodorsal system, as a single unit. The thoracodorsal system may be simultaneously harvested to create a "megaflap" that provides latissimus dorsi and serratus anterior muscles and overlying skin for reconstructing massive soft tissue defects. Generally, the harvest site is able to be closed primarily given the laxity of the skin of the back.

Finally, I prefer this option in patients who have extensive maxillectomy defects, which require reconstruction of the orbital floor, skull base, palate, and cheek soft tissue/skin. The thinner bone of the tip of the scapula is ideal for reconstruction of the orbital floor, while the thicker bone can be used for the reconstruction of the maxilla, malar eminence, alveolus, medial buttress, or lateral buttress. The dual skin paddles are useful as one paddle may be deepithelialized for soft tissue filling while the other is used for lining of the palate or replacement of the skin of the cheek depending on the exact requirements of the defect.

CONTRAINDICATIONS

The versatility of the scapula flap is afforded by providing two large skin paddles and bone. However, there is no innervation or nerve graft accompanied with the scapula flap. Therefore, this flap cannot be used where reinnervation is planned. The flap harvest may add additional morbidity to an individual who has ipsilateral preexisting shoulder compromise from prior shoulder surgery or CN XI sacrifice. In this situation, the contralateral side or a different flap may be better choices. It should be noted that harvesting the scapula flap in patients without this history has no long-term effect on shoulder function or mobility.

Due to the relative short width and bulk of the harvested bone (2 to 3 cm), dental rehabilitation with implants will probably not be achievable. Additionally, if the amount of bone length required is greater than 14 cm (i.e., greater than angle-to-angle reconstruction), then the scapula may not provide enough bone length. In these situations, the fibula free flap may offer greater cortical bone thickness for implant placement and bone length for reconstruction of a very large bone segment.

PREOPERATIVE PLANNING

A thorough preoperative medical evaluation should be pursued in patients who are potential candidates for this flap, particularly patients with cancer of the head and neck as they are at high risk for perioperative and postoperative complications including pulmonary embolism, alcohol withdrawal, stroke, pulmonary insufficiency, pneumonia, myocardial infarction, and deep vein thrombosis. Ideally, malnutrition and hypothyroidism should be corrected preoperatively to aid in healing.

Patients who have undergone previous significant head and neck surgery should obtain preoperative imaging with computed tomography angiography to determine the patency of recipient vessels. In particular, in patients who have had neck dissection with resection of the internal jugular vein, the contralateral neck should ideally be used for recipient vessels. Preoperative imaging of the subscapular vascular system is not necessary.

In my experience, these vessels are rarely affected by atherosclerotic disease or congenital anomalies, and the vessels are well suited for anastomosis to recipient vessels in the neck.

Importantly, surgical planning must include a discussion among the entire ablative and reconstructive surgical teams regarding intraoperative positioning of the patient and the sequence of surgical procedures. Although it is possible to perform some of the harvest during the tumor resection, this requires cordial interaction among the surgeons so that typically the harvest is performed at the conclusion of the tumor resection and vessel preparation in the neck. This lack of a simultaneous two-team approach is the *major* disadvantage of the scapular system of flaps.

A physical therapy evaluation should be obtained preoperatively to document shoulder girdle function, range of motion, and strength. Physical therapy exercises should be maintained in the postoperative period.

SURGICAL TECHNIQUE

The operating bed is equipped with a bean bag, prior to the patient arriving in the operating room. The patient is placed in the supine position, and general anesthesia is accomplished. The patient is then rolled into a lateral decubitus position to expose the axilla and the midline spine. The ipsilateral arm is left free of IVs and other attachments to allow its full sterile prep in the field. A clothed 1-L bag of IV solution is then placed under the side of the patient, approximately 12 cm inferior to the axilla, to avoid compression of the brachial plexus during the case. The bean bag is deflated to maintain the patient in this position, and the sterile prep is then carried out to include the entire head and neck and back within a single surgical field. Drapes are placed and the patient is allowed to roll back into the supine position, and the oromandibular resection is carried out by the extirpative team. The patient is then rolled back into the lateral decubitus position and the bean bag used to maintain the patient in this position, as before.

The scapula osteocutaneous flap is usually harvested with a single segment of bone from the lateral border and two skin paddles. This description focuses on that procedure, with small comments made for other flap variations. The lateral border and tip of the scapula are outlined and the ipsilateral arm extended (Fig. 18.1A) The omotricipital triangle is palpated, and the presumed site of the artery is marked. The superior border of the skin incision is marked approximately 2 cm inferior to the scapular spine and extending as far medial as necessary for size and is extended laterally just beyond the tip of the omotricipital triangle. Larger skin paddles are encouraged until the surgeon is experienced, in order to accommodate all of the major skin perforators. The medial skin incision is drawn from the lateral tip of the previous incision and extending inferiorly approximately 4 cm lateral to the lateral border of the scapula, again as far as is necessary for the reconstruction. Curvilinear borders to the individual skin paddles are then drawn and allowed to connect over the body of the scapula, so that the skin paddles are harvested as one unit and only divided once the harvest is complete and the requirements for the inset determined (Fig. 18.1B).

The skin and subcutaneous tissues are then incised down to muscle or the fascia of the infraspinatus, as appropriate, and elevated in this plane from medial to lateral. Of note, I leave the very lateral edge of the skin intact initially to avoid inadvertent disruption of the skin segment. The skin is elevated to the lateral border of the scapula and then stopped to avoid disruption of the cutaneous pedicle. Usually, these pedicles can be identified on the underside of the flap during elevation. Likewise, the skin is elevated off of the deltoid, latissimus, and teres muscles and the latissimus muscle retracted inferiorly (Fig. 18.2). If a latissimus myocutaneous flap is to be harvested as part of a "megaflap," the skin segment should be outlined and the

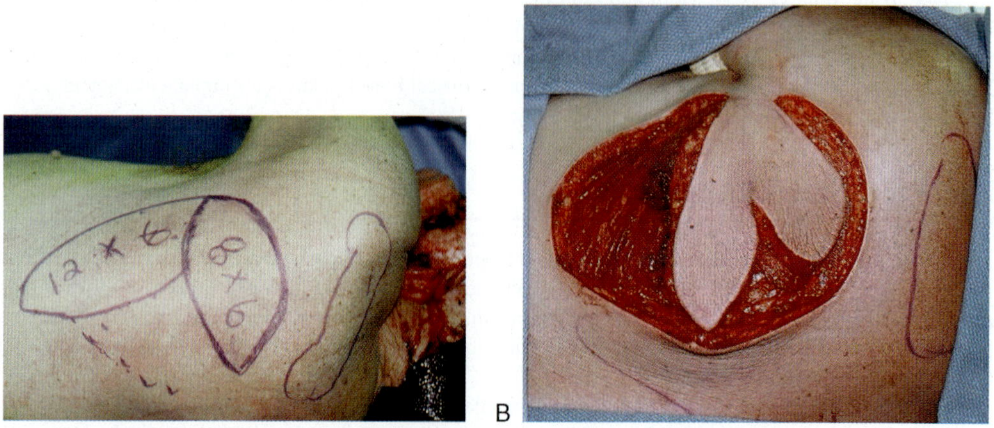

A B

FIGURE 18.1 Skin paddle design and elevation. **A.** Design of scapular and parascapular skin paddles over the left scapula. Note the outline of the scapular spine and the scapular tip. **B.** The skin paddles have been incised to expose the underlying soft tissue, but the skin connection is maintained laterally.

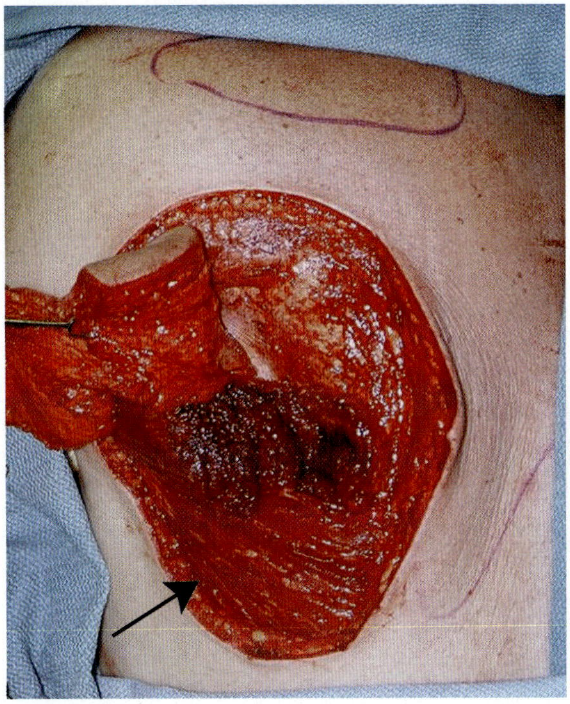

FIGURE 18.2
Skin paddle elevation is completed with the delineation of the latissimus muscle (*arrow*) inferiorly and the teres major muscle superiorly.

latissimus flap can be harvested to the edges of the scapula at this time, with final connections made at the conclusion of the scapular harvest.

The teres major muscle is now isolated in 360-degree fashion near its insertion on the lateral scapular border and divided with care not to injure underlying vessels. The muscle can then be retracted with a Deaver retractor. The arm is retracted laterally and rotated internally, thus exposing the contents of the axilla. The proximal CSA can now be identified with its venae comitantes, running laterally into the axilla from the lateral border of the scapula. Fascial attachments can be divided over the vessels and the vessels followed into the axilla. The branches to the teres major must be divided to allow further dissection. I prefer small and medium clips to control these vessels. The TDA can be identified at this point going inferiorly, along with its branch to the scapular tip. If the harvest of the scapular tip and/or the latissimus flap is desired, the TDA is left intact. Likewise, if I feel that the length and caliber of the vessel are sufficient with the harvest of just the CSA, further dissection of the vessel is not necessary. Otherwise, the TDA pedicle is divided, and the artery and venae comitantes are followed to the subscapular vessels. Again, usually the venae comitantes form one vein, which may then divide prior to entering the axillary vein. Meticulous dissection and hemostasis are critical at this point to allow identification of all anatomic structures and avoid injury to the vessel. Blunt dissection is discouraged, and hemostasis can be aided by the use of bipolar cautery.

Once the vessels are identified and freed in 360-degree fashion from the axillary vessels to the lateral border of the scapula, the harvest of the bone can begin. The glenohumeral joint is palpated, and the superior border of the bone harvest is defined 1 to 2 cm inferior to this landmark. The required length of bone is then measured, with some leeway, and marked. If the tip is to be included, it is best to preserve the angular vessels and so dissect these free from the tip to the proximal pedicle. A bone width of 3 cm is then measured from the lateral border, and incisions are now carried through the infraspinatus muscle to isolate the bone margins, with division of the periosteum. This area is relatively vascular, and the patience of the surgeon is necessary to gain complete control of periosteal vessels. The superior bone margin has several large vessels nearby, and these are near the vascular pedicle, so careful control in this area is especially important. Once defined, osteotomies are carried out with a sagittal bone saw, with care not to injure the vascular pedicle, which should be protected with small retractors during this maneuver. Finally, the bone is released, and now incisions are carried just deep to the bone, through the subscapularis muscle, again with care to visualize and not to injure the vascular pedicle. Once the bone is released, bleeding is controlled and final soft tissue attachments at the skin/adjacent flaps are divided, and any further dissection required on the proximal pedicle is completed. The flap is now ready for harvest with the transection of the CSA or subscapular vessels. The donor vessels should be controlled with permanent 2-0 silk sutures.

Meticulous hemostasis is assured, and closure of the incision is begun. Small drill holes are placed in the new lateral border of the scapula approximately 2 cm apart, and the teres major muscle is now approximated with 2-0 absorbable sutures (PDS or Vicryl). The skin is widely undermined and closed in layers over flexible drains, which are placed to bulb suction. The patient is now rotated into the supine position for reconstruction. A sterile dressing can be applied now or at the conclusion of the case. The surgical defect is now inspected (Fig. 18.3).

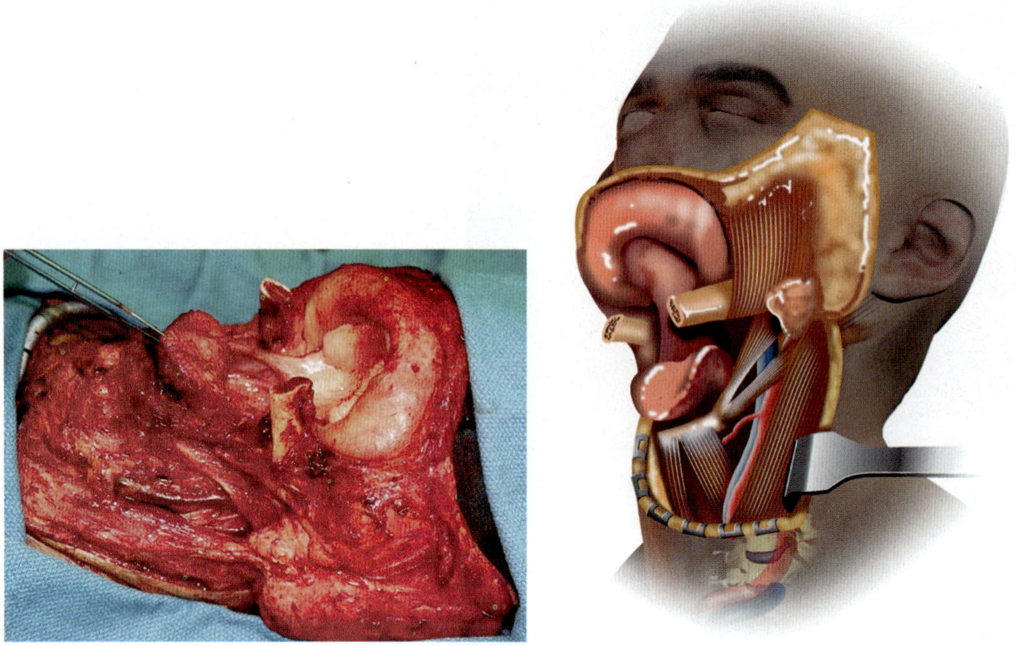

FIGURE 18.3 A through-and-through composite defect of the anterior oromandibular region, as viewed from inferiorly. Note the remaining lateral mandibular segments and the small remnant of the base of the tongue.

An osteotomy may be necessary during plating of the scapular bone (Fig. 18.4). The blood supply of the bone is primarily through the periosteum, and therefore, at the site of a closing ostectomy, the periosteum should be carefully conserved and osteotomies made with a saw or Rongeur biting forceps. The superior bone is the thickest and will require a saw, but the more inferior bone can occasionally be divided with the biting forceps. It should be noted that the pedicle to the bone usually enters at the more superior location. If the angular artery to the tip is preserved, this section of the bone may be completely detached from the remainder of the bone and moved on its separate vascular pedicle.

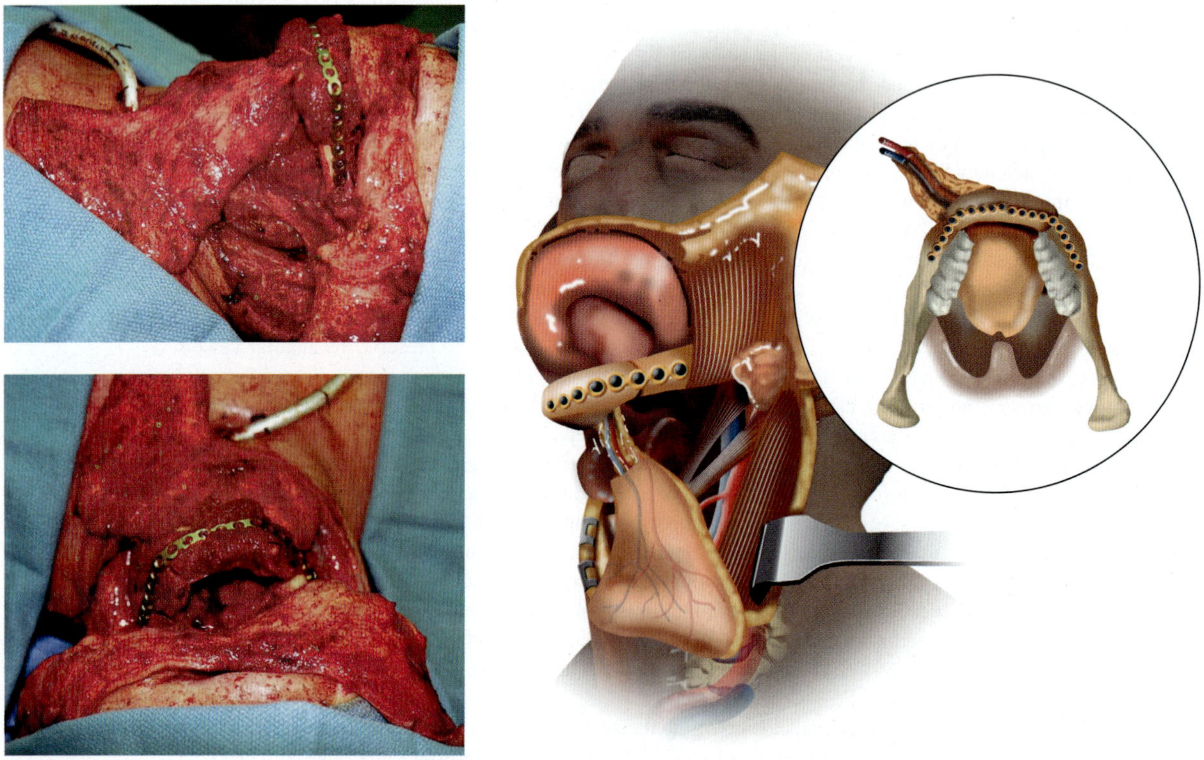

A

B

FIGURE 18.4 The osseous reconstruction of the composite defect. **A.** The composite defect with a reconstruction plate and the scapular bone in place, viewed from laterally. Note the connected skin paddles suspended and draped inferiorly. **B.** The same view from above, after closing ostectomies were performed and plating of the scapula bone segments.

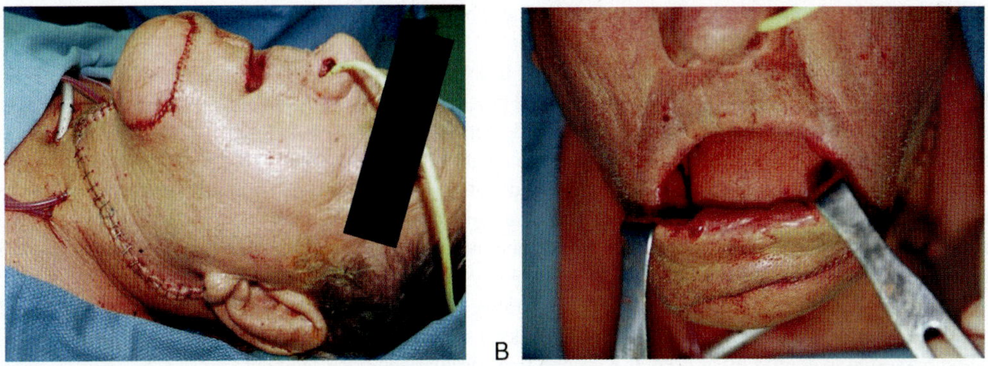

A B

FIGURE 18.5 The cutaneous reconstruction of the composite defect. **A.** The skin paddles have been separated and one placed externally, in the area of the mentum, as seen from this lateral view. **B.** The other skin paddle is placed intraorally to reconstruct the anterior tongue defect.

Once the bone is in place in the recipient site, the vessels are anastomosed and the flap is revascularized. This is generally relatively easy given the large caliber and excellent quality of the flap pedicle. The skin paddles can now be divided into the sizes required by the reconstruction (Fig. 18.5). The pedicle to the skin paddles can be identified visually or with Doppler, and incisions are made appropriately. The skin and soft tissue can be divided down to the deep fascia as this is the layer with the blood supply. This allows for mobilization of the skin paddles from each other and from the bone segment of the flap, allowing for complex three-dimensional reconstructions, as noted previously.

POSTOPERATIVE MANAGEMENT

Postoperative flap monitoring is particularly important to observe for warning signs of venous congestion and arterial insufficiency. This is most commonly accomplished by continuous monitoring with a handheld Doppler and physical examination of the visible skin paddle. Hematoma, infection, or dehiscence of the incision may compromise the flap, which mandates surgical exploration. If vascular compromise is evident, the flap pedicle and anastomosis should be explored in an effort to salvage the flap. The drain is removed when output is less than 30 mL per 8-hour period, for 3 consecutive periods.

In the initial postoperative recovery, the ipsilateral arm should be positioned anteriorly and medially, usually supported on the patient's abdomen by a pillow. Once the patient is ambulating, the arm is supported by a shoulder sling, which supports the elbow and prevents inferior drift of the arm. Inpatient physical therapy is initiated once the patient is mobile. A postoperative physical therapy regimen is established with the patient to be maintained after hospital discharge. The sling is used for 2 to 3 weeks and physical therapy maintained until postoperative function is optimized, usually 4 to 6 weeks.

Patients are typically discharged from the hospital 5 to 10 days after surgery, depending on their postoperative course and comorbidities. Close outpatient follow-up after discharge is recommended for evaluation of surgical sites.

COMPLICATIONS

There are few complications related to this approach; however, the most important aspect of the scapular reconstruction is related to the vascular anatomy. When planning a flap that requires both a bone graft and a latissimus muscle, the subscapular system must give rise to the thoracodorsal vascular system. If the thoracodorsal system has a separate takeoff (from the axillary vessels), then the combined flap (megaflap) cannot be harvested as a single flap. This will require two separate microvascular anastomoses. This vascular anomaly can only be determined with certainty at the time of surgery.

RESULTS

Multiple authors in their published series of cases have demonstrated excellent success using the scapula osteocutaneous free flap. Swartz et al. demonstrated the application of this flap in 26 patients with large defects secondary to cancer surgery or severe trauma. Five patients underwent reconstruction for maxillectomy defects and 21 for complex composite oromandibular defects. Their report described the multiple and versatile flap orientations to reestablish these complex three-dimensional defects, while having no flap failures. Osteotomies performed did not adversely affect the vascularity of the bone as long as the periosteum was maintained intact.

Only two patients in their series developed difficulties with shoulder motion due to noncompliance with postoperative range of motion physical therapy exercises.

Sullivan et al. described the use of the scapular free flap in 36 patients. Three patients suffered flap failure due to arterial insufficiency, venous thrombosis, and gross contamination of the neck due to fistula. They demonstrated osseous reconstruction of angle-to-angle defects of up to 14.5 cm in length in two patients; however, in most patients, the upper limit of harvestable bone length is 14 cm. Multiple skin paddles were used in many of the reconstructions. Six months postoperatively, all patients stated that their shoulder was functional but half had mild to moderate shoulder limitations, particularly in abduction and external rotation. The authors found that noncompliance with physical therapy and preoperative accessory nerve function was important as a predictor of postoperative shoulder dysfunction.

Coleman and Sultan further advanced the versatility of the scapula free flap by defining the angular vascular pedicle that supplies the inferior aspect of the lateral scapula. This allows the distal tip of the scapula to be safely harvested in continuity or used as a second free vascularized bone segment.

In my experience, the scapula osteocutaneous free flap is an ideal choice for the reconstruction of complex osseous and soft tissue defects. Its versatility is due to its dual soft tissue skin paddles and ample bone to reconstruct complex oromandibular, maxillary, and lateral skull base defects. Because of this versatility and its minimal harvest site comorbidities, the scapula free flap became used more commonly than other methods of osseous free tissue transfer in my practice.

In my series, the mean bone length that was harvested was 8.4 cm (range 6 to 12 cm), and the mean cutaneous area harvested was 109 cm^2 (range 48 to 240 cm^2). Compared to the iliac crest and fibula free flaps, the scapula free flap provided similar bone length while supplying significantly larger skin and soft tissue paddles (up to double in overall area) that were further able to be divided into separate vascularized islands. The ability to harvest multiple and maneuverable skin paddles gives this flap a distinct advantage over other osteocutaneous reconstructive options. Among 24 scapula free flaps, I have experienced one flap failure, and all donor sites were able to be successfully closed primarily. An objective study of shoulder limitations postoperatively (average 17.6 months) showed only minimal reductions in strength and range of motion. Subjectively, most patients stated that their activities of daily living were limited minimally or not at all.

Given the above described experiences, the scapula free flap is a superb choice for vascularized osteocutaneous reconstruction of complex defects. It bears significant reconstructive potential with minimal postoperative morbidity. In particular, the flap is ideal for the reconstruction of complex oromandibular and maxillectomy defects.

PEARLS

- Maintaining meticulous hemostasis and excellent visualization during the flap harvest is critical to the success of this operation. Retraction with a large retractor (e.g., Deaver) in the axilla is encouraged, as is adequate personnel to provide this retraction.
- The scapula osteocutaneous free flap is a versatile flap based on branches of the circumflex scapular vessels.
- A wide reconstructive potential is available due to this flap's large dual skin paddles and bone component. Particularly, the skin islands and bone have separate vascular pedicles, allowing for variable orientations.
- The flap may be harvested in conjunction with the latissimus dorsi musculocutaneous flap with the incorporation of the thoracodorsal vessels ("megaflap"). In this case, the proximal pedicle is the subscapular vessels.
- The flap is ideal for reconstruction of (1) through-and-through composite defects of the oromandibular complex, involving resection of the mandible and intraoral and extraoral soft tissue/skin/mucosa and (2) complex and extensive maxillectomy defects that require reconstruction of the orbital floor, skull base, palate, and cheek soft tissue/skin.
- The scapula osteocutaneous flap is most useful where the soft tissue needs of the reconstruction surpass the capabilities of the radial forearm osteocutaneous and/or fibula osteocutaneous flaps. In this situation, the time to harvest the scapula flap outweighs both the harvest of a second flap and the potential complications that accompany trying to put an inadequate flap under tension in the oromandibular region.
- This flap should be considered in patients requiring osseous reconstruction but who have significant lower extremity atherosclerotic disease preventing the use of the fibula free flap.
- The use of postoperative physical therapy is *essential* for maintaining shoulder mobility and range of motion.

PITFALLS

- Previous surgery in the axilla or shoulder may have caused injury or scarring to the flap vessels and may increase the risk of flap loss. In general, avoid harvest on the side of previous neck dissection.
- The risk of dissection in the axilla during harvest of the scapula flap should not be underestimated. Large vessels and/or the brachial plexus are in the field, and the surgeon should only undertake this operation after previous experience, best obtained in the cadaver lab.

- The bone stock that can be obtained with this flap is a relative disadvantage in those few patients where the future use of implant-borne dentures or other prostheses is likely. The iliac crest–internal oblique flap may be the best option in some of these cases.
- A major drawback of this flap is the need for intraoperative repositioning that is required for harvesting the flap.

INSTRUMENTS TO HAVE AVAILABLE

- Standard head and neck surgery set
- Reciprocating saw
- Mandibular plating set
- Rongeur biting forceps

ACKNOWLEDGMENT

I gratefully acknowledge the assistance of Rahul Seth, MD, during the preparation of this manuscript. His effort and expertise made the completion of this work possible.

SUGGESTED READING

Rowsell AR, Davies DM, Eisenberg N, et al. The anatomy of the subscapular-thoracodorsal arterial system: study of 100 cadaver dissections. *Br J Plast Surg* 1984;37(4):574–576.

Swartz WM, Banis JC, Newton ED, et al. The osteocutaneous scapular flap for mandibular and maxillary reconstruction. *Plast Reconstr Surg* 1986;77(4):530–545.

Sullivan MJ, Baker SR, Crompton R, et al. Free scapular osteocutaneous flap for mandibular reconstruction. *Arch Otolaryngol Head Neck Surg* 1989;115(11):1334–1340.

Sullivan MJ, Carroll WR, Baker SR, et al. The free scapular flap for head and neck reconstruction. *Am J Otolaryngol* 1990;11(5):318–327.

Burkey BB, Coleman JR Jr. Current concepts in oromandibular reconstruction. *Otolaryngol Clin North Am* 1997;30(4): 607–630.

Coleman SC, Burkey BB, Day TA, et al. Increasing use of the scapula osteocutaneous free flap. *Laryngoscope* 2000;110(9):1419–1424.

19 THE SUBTOTAL MAXILLARY DEFECT: TEMPORALIS MUSCLE FLAP

Peter D. Costantino

INTRODUCTION

Acquired palatomaxillary defects always present a challenge for the head and neck reconstructive surgeon. Maxillectomy defects can have a negative impact on deglutition and nutrition, speech, and communication, in addition to self-image and social acceptability. The lack of a uniform classification of these defects has limited prospective multicentered studies for assessment of the ideal method of reconstruction. Obturators/dental prostheses, local tissue flaps, pedicled myocutaneous flaps, myofascial flaps, and free bone/tissue transfer have all been employed successfully over the years. In my experience, midfacial and specifically palatomaxillary reconstruction can be achieved safely, effectively, and with minimal risk by implementing local pedicled tissue transfer from the lateral side of the head through a hemicoronal or bicoronal approach, using the temporalis muscle flap (TMF) and/or temporoparietal fascia flap (TPFF). The latter can also be harvested with calvarial bone attached as a composite flap. Both flaps can also be used in combination with any type of hardware prosthesis for both primary and secondary reconstruction of the palate with excellent functional and aesthetic results.

Previously, when direct visual surveillance was the way we monitored cancer recurrence, resection cavities were left open and the obturator was the only measure used to achieve a better functional outcome after ablative surgery. The use of a prosthesis is no longer the standard for many of these patients who are part of the working, socially active population. Obturators are imperfect and can still result in oronasal leakage, hypernasality, and reflux of liquids into the nasal cavity. Scarring and healing may also necessitate multiple revisions and fitting procedures. In addition, patients commonly feel the burden of frequent cleaning and the requirement for adhesive anchoring, as well as the need for wearing obturators whenever they need to speak or drink, which can be inconvenient. With advances in radiologic surveillance tools and the evolution of surgical techniques, tissue reconstruction has become the standard of care. This concept was confirmed in a study of palatal defects in which a group of 10 radial forearm free flap patients was compared to a group of 10 patients wearing obturators. Both groups had similar mastication, taste, and appearance satisfaction; however, patients with flap reconstruction had better scores in speech, comfort, and social interaction.

There have been alternative local tissue flaps that have become historical footnotes and are no longer used. The laterally based forehead flap was soon rejected due to the resulting facial deformity. The functional deficits of swallowing and lingual function have eliminated the tongue flap. The masseter flap provided limited pedicle length and resulted in contracture and atrophy. Palatal island flaps are still used but are not recommended in radiated patients.

The TMF, vascularized by the deep temporal arteries, was first mentioned in 1872 for temporomandibular joint reconstruction and then several years later for reconstruction of middle fossa skull base defects. Gillies and Konig, in the1920s, were the first to use the TMF for maxillary reconstruction and posttumor reconstruction, respectively. Campbell in 1948 was the first to use it for palatal defects. Sheehan then advanced the harvesting technique by removing the zygomatic arch to allow for improved mobilization and rotation toward the palatomaxillary complex. Wise and Baker took this further by detaching the muscle from the mandibular condyle. Bakamjian also contributed by describing the condylectomy for attaining additional flap length as well as using the temporalis reconstruction for isolated palatal defects. It was then Demas and Sotereanos who described the current technique of transposition through the posterolateral wall of the maxillary sinus. Over the past two decades, the TMF has been thoroughly described for palatal defects in multiple large series. These studies have confirmed the safety and efficacy and versatility of the flap for the reconstruction of maxillectomy and palatectomy defects following tumor resection.

The temporoparietal fascial flap also has a long history dating back to the late 19th century. Monks and Brown, independently from different sides of the Atlantic, described the use of the TPFF that was nourished by the superficial temporal vessels for the reconstruction of eyelid and auricular defects. It took about 80 years for this flap to begin to gain further popularity for oral cavity reconstruction. Recently, however, the TPFF has been employed for many types of oral, maxillary, and palatal defects as both a fascial and osteofascial flap. The harvest technique has varied little over time.

HISTORY

When considering a temporal muscle flap for reconstruction of the subtotal maxillary defect, both general and local issues must be considered. The general issues affecting wound healing such as weight loss, diabetes, hypothyroidism, and substance abuse must be sought in the history. A history of trauma to the temporal region is of course of great importance since this scarring or loss of blood supply may interfere with the development of temporalis flap. Similarly, a history of radiation to this area would interfere with healing. Since inevitably a concavity will remain in the area of the temporalis muscle donor site, a query should be made to the patients about their occupation and whether they have specific cosmetic issues in which a defect in this area may interfere with their livelihood. In this case, plans should be made for reconstructing the donor site or selecting an alternative one.

PHYSICAL EXAMINATION

Cosmetic deformities resulting from palatomaxillary resection include a wide variety of defects from facial asymmetry and eye malposition to skin defects and cavity formation. Reestablishment of a scaffold-like phenomenon is crucial taking into consideration vertical and horizontal parts of the palatomaxillary complex. Functionality is also to be taken into consideration in reconstructing a palatomaxillary defect. The primary goal is to achieve a complete separation between the nasal and oral cavities that will facilitate normal speech, swallowing, and mastication.

The physical examination is important with regard to the anatomy and viability of the flaps as well as with size and precise location of the tumor in the context of a postablation reconstruction. In order to provide the most appropriate reconstruction and the best functional outcome, the surgeon must have a complete understanding of the postablation defect, or in other words, the total extent of the tumor. The examination is important with regard to the involved surrounding structures, the size of the tumor, and the necessary extent of bone and tooth removal. In theory, one would like to implement one of the previously described classification systems of palatomaxillary defects in their evaluation (although none are completely effective).

Examination of the donor site should reveal any previous incisions, trauma, or radiation changes, in addition to an adequate pulse for the TPFF. The strength and/or atrophy of the temporalis muscle is crucial in the examination and can further be emphasized while having the patient clench the teeth. The integrity of all the cranial nerves, specifically CN V and VII, should be thoroughly evaluated. Any deficit could provide information regarding extent of tumor involvement. Nasal endoscopy, examination of the orbit and extraocular movements and loss of sensation in the infraorbital nerve distribution, and the presence of loose teeth give relevant information regarding the extent of the tumor.

INDICATIONS

Maxillary defects often involve soft tissue, bone, and even skin. Sometimes, reconstruction has to take into consideration each part separately. After Ohngren's first classification for maxillectomy defects in 1933, several classifications came out later and were mainly oriented toward safe oncologic boundaries disregarding resumption of normal function. The medical literature had to wait many decades to see reports describing classifications oriented toward reconstruction. The goal of these classifications is to try to achieve uniform data usable to devise a standard reconstruction algorithm. Spiro et al. in 1997 suggested a classification based on the number of maxillary walls involved, divided into limited, subtotal, and total defects. Soon thereafter, based on their experience in 108 patients, Davison et al. proposed a reconstruction algorithm involving prosthetic obturation, nonvascularized bone grafts, local or regional flaps, and microvascular free tissue transfer. He divided the defects into "complete" and "partial." Most recently, Brown and Shaw presented their 15-year experience that implemented a classification system in which classes 1 to 5 describe the increasing extent of maxillary defect in its vertical dimension, with a focus on the functional aspect of the loss. Out of their 147 patients, only one stage 3 and three stage 5 patients had a TMF or TPFF flaps, whereas all the rest had either soft tissue or composite free flaps (see Chapter 22).

Both temporalis and temporoparietal pedicled flaps are generally preferred to free flap reconstruction in many cases because they are reliable, versatile, pedicled flaps that are regionally located and carry minimal morbidity and minimal functional deficit after their harvest. Complex donor sites, prolonged anesthesia time, as well as financial costs can be avoided by implementation of these flaps. Additionally, they are employed in place of appropriate microvascular transfers when there are limitations at the flap harvest site and the recipient vessels in the neck, as well as medical comorbidities that requires shorter anesthesia time. These flaps can be the primary flap for reconstruction in the edentulous patient and are also very reliable and stable in the face of radiation treatment. In general, local flaps are especially necessary when the technology and expertise required for free flap reconstruction are unavailable.

The TMF and TPFF are often my preferred method of reconstruction for the less complex defects, that is, those defects that are partial maxillary defects and involve the lateral maxilla, alveolus, and the palate. Both flaps, especially the temporalis flap, have proven to be reliable in their harvest and effective in their reconstruction. The TMF due to its reliable vascularity provides adequate bulk and proximity to the larger defects, while the TPFF, the thinnest flap in the human body, is pliable and durable and has been appropriate for smaller defects less than 2 cm. Only the TPFF is implemented for anterior palatal defects that include the alveolus due to its malleability and lack of bulk when placed in the premaxillary region. The TPFF is also preferred for centrally located palatal defects. The temporalis muscle can be used for subtotal palatal defects and can be harvested bilaterally for total palatal defects.

CONTRAINDICATIONS

The contraindications to the TMF or TPFF are related to any previous trauma, surgery, or radiation to the temporal scalp and temporal fossa region. Any planned sacrifice of the lateral internal maxillary artery where the deep temporal arteries exit would compromise the TMF. Similarly, if there is no detectable pulse either by palpation or by Doppler evaluation of the superficial temporal artery, then the TPFF cannot be employed. Most importantly, as discussed above, the indications for the flap must be fulfilled and the patient must counseled appropriately on what to expect from this type of reconstruction and the need for delayed dental restoration.

PREOPERATIVE PLANNING

The two primary components of the preoperative evaluation are the extent of tumor involvement and the availability and appropriateness of the TMF and TPFF for reconstruction. In addition to the physical examination outlined above, radiologic imaging including computed tomography scan and magnetic resonance imaging, or both, is required preoperatively. Due to the lack of direct visualization and ability to fully characterize tumors in the palatomaxillary complex, the radiologic imaging provides integral information that determines the extent of the tumor resection and, therefore, helps in the determination of which reconstructive flap is most suitable to the situation. Specifically, the size of the defect, its specific location in the palate—anterior, midline, and posterior—and the extent of the resection must be estimated prior to the operation (Table 19.1). Pathologic diagnosis also determines the aggressiveness of the surgery, the need for immediate reconstruction, and the likelihood of postoperative radiation. The physical examination and imaging also confirm that vascular supply to the muscle and the fascia will be available once the resection has been performed. From a practical setup standpoint, the temporal and infratemporal fossa can easily be prepared in the surgical site and do not require any specialized instrumentation or complex technology.

Before discussing the surgical technique for harvesting either of these flaps, the surgeon must have a full understanding of the layers of the scalp and the anatomy of the temporal fossa. Because of the variety of terms applied to the layers of this area, the following is a description using their preferred terminology.

The scalp is a five-layered structure. The most superficial layer is the skin with its hair follicles and sebaceous and sweat glands. The skin is firmly adherent to the underlying subcutaneous tissue that consists of strong collagen bundles and the superficial vessels of the scalp. In the temporal scalp, just deep to this layer is the temporoparietal fascia. Then comes a layer of loose areolar tissue and the superficial layer of the deep temporal fascia, the temporalis muscle, and the deep layer of the deep temporal fascia that is continuous with the pericranium in that region (Fig. 19.1).

More specifically, immediately deep to the skin and the subcutaneous tissue, just beneath the hair follicles and adipose tissue exists the temporoparietal fascia (sometimes called superficial temporal fascia). This layer is contiguous with the superficial musculoaponeurotic system as it passes over the zygomatic arch into the

TABLE 19.1 Indications for Different Palatal Defects of TMF Versus TPFF

Defect	TMF	TPFF
>2 cm	X	
≤2 cm		X
Anterior alveolar		X
Central palatal		X
Includes anterior maxillary wall and/or orbit	X	
Bilateral/subtotal	X	

midface inferiorly. The fascia is contiguous with the galea aponeurotica above the temporal line superiorly and the occipitalis posteriorly. The fascia ranges from 2 to 4 mm in thickness and can be harvested in dimensions up to 17 × 14 cm. Deep to the temporoparietal fascia is a loose areolar and avascular tissue layer that separates the fascia from the temporalis muscular fascia. This areolar layer allows the superficial scalp to move freely over the deeper structures, that is, the more fixed temporalis muscular fascia, that is, the superficial layer of the deep temporal fascia. The temporalis muscle and pericranium are then deep to these fascial layers. Confusing the issue further is the division of the temporalis muscular fascia as it splits into a superficial and deep layer (of the superficial deep temporal fascia) surrounding a pad of adipose tissue at the temporal line of fusion, at about 2 cm above the zygomatic arch (Fig. 19.1). The temporalis muscle fascia is contiguous with the pericranium above the superior temporal line and is contiguous with the masseter muscle fascia deep to the arch of the zygoma.

In the lateral aspect of the scalp, the blood supply is by way of the superficial temporal artery, a terminal branch of the external carotid artery that ascends posterior to the ramus of the mandible and becomes superficial 4 to 5 mm anterior to the tragus as it emerges from the parotid tissue. The vasculature fans out in an axial pattern from the inferior aspect of the temporoparietal fascia, giving off the middle temporal artery. Approximately 3 cm above the zygomatic arch, it divides into the terminal frontal and parietal branches (Fig. 19.2). The superficial temporal vein generally runs superficial to and with the artery, but variability, including branching or

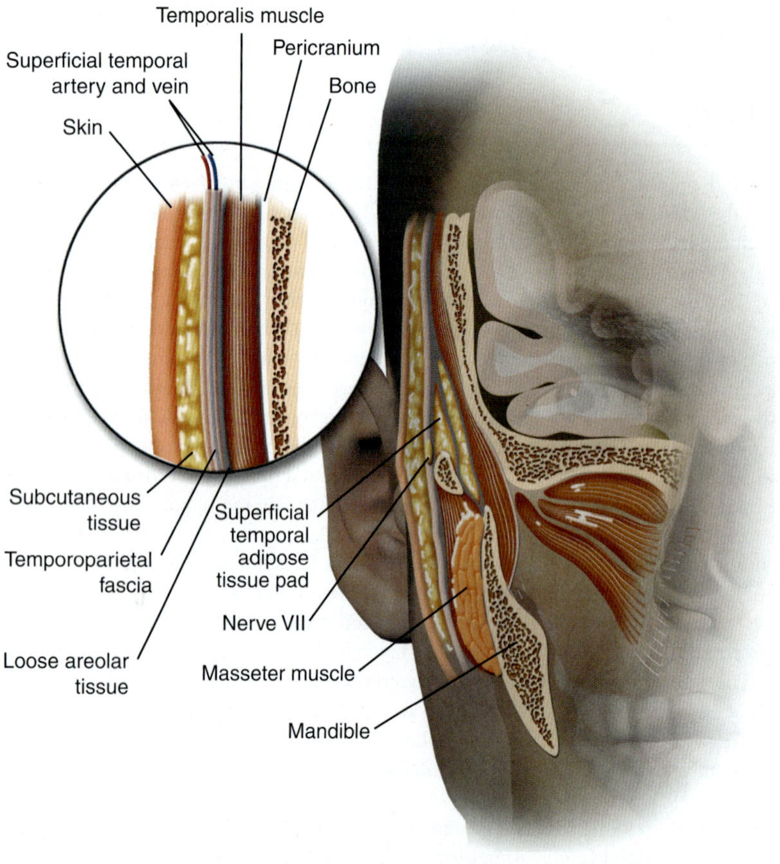

FIGURE 19.1
Anatomy of the layers of the scalp superior to the superior temporal line.

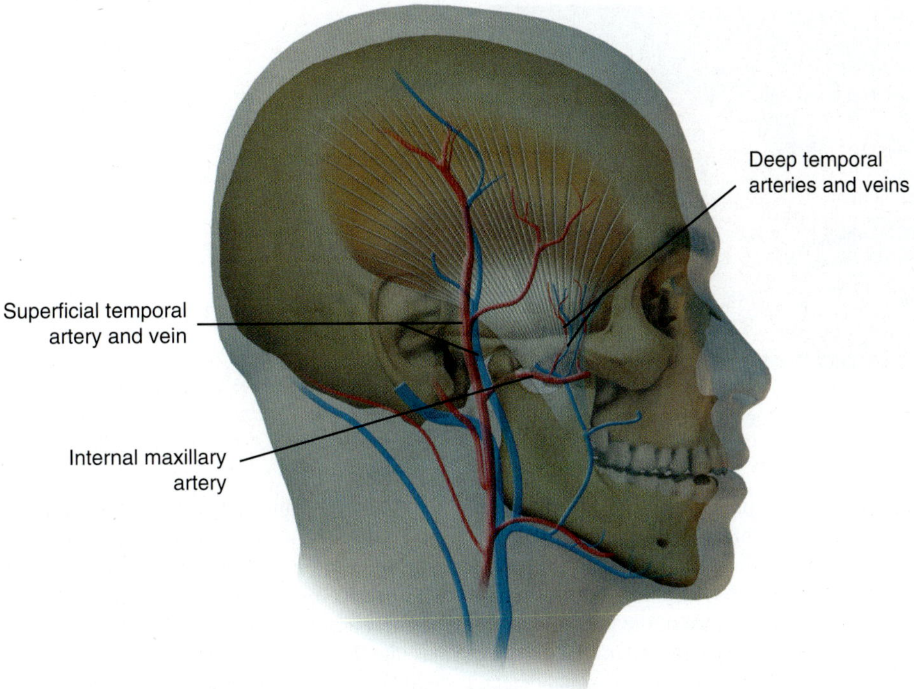

FIGURE 19.2 Gross vascular anatomy of the TPFF and TMF.

a posterior course, may be encountered. The auriculotemporal nerve, a sensory branch of the mandibular nerve, lies posterior to the superficial temporal artery within the temporoparietal fascia. The frontal branch of the facial nerve traverses an oblique course over the zygomatic arch, which can be estimated by a line connecting a point 0.5 cm inferior to the tragus to a point 1.5 cm lateral to the superior brow. This nerve also lies within the temporoparietal fascia, and elevation of the flap anterior to the frontal branch of the superficial temporal artery should proceed with caution to avoid injuring this nerve.

SURGICAL TECHNIQUE

Prior to making the incision, a facial nerve monitor is placed in the medial brow to provide continuous monitoring of the frontal branch of the facial nerve. It is secured with a 5-0 silk suture. The incision is then designed as described below. Shaving the hair is avoided by braiding in such a fashion that the incision is clearly demarcated. The patient is then prepped and draped with the patient supine with the head in a lateral position.

Exposure is obtained through a bicoronal incision over the vertex of the cranium in the case of men with hair loss. In women, a curvilinear incision is created beginning from off midline anteriorly on the forehead and then curving in a C-shaped fashion first posteriorly and then anteriorly to the pretragal crease or posttragal region. Inferior extension of the incision is performed as needed. A coronal incision sweeping anteriorly within the hairline is created over a length of approximately 15 cm. (A T-shaped incision over the parietal region has also been described.) A superior–posterior flap just deep to the subcutaneous adipose tissue of the scalp through the dense connective tissue is then elevated. Visualizing and preserving the hair follicles and subcutaneous adipose tissue superficially and the superficial temporal vessels in the flap deep is necessary to prevent alopecia and to maintain the vascular integrity of the scalp and hair follicles as well as those of the flap. One series reported a vessel injury rate of 22.6%. This dissection can be quite tedious. Upon elevation of the scalp, the pericranium is left attached to the lateral skull superiorly in a fan-shaped fashion. The anterior flap is elevated in the same subfollicular plane until the suspected location of the frontal branch of the facial nerve. The location can be estimated by a line from the tragus to the lateral aspect of the eyebrow or by the temporal hairline. The nerve stimulator may be used to assist and to confirm the location of the facial nerve.

The frontal branch of the superficial temporal artery is now ligated, the anterior flap is divided, and the dissection is carried deep to the temporal adipose tissue pad to the superficial layer of the deep temporal fascia. A separate posteroinferior flap is similarly elevated, thereby exposing the temporoparietal fascia over the entire right temporoparietal region. The length of the flap can then be elevated by incising the temporoparietal fascia in a paddle-like fashion that can be up to 17 cm in length and 14 cm in width. The TPFF is then sequentially elevated and dissected from the superficial layer of the deep temporal fascia along with the deeper loose areolar tissue and the superficial temporal artery and vein pedicle down below the zygomatic arch to the level of the auditory canal. The pedicle can be narrowed to approximately 2 cm (Fig. 19.3). The preauricular crease

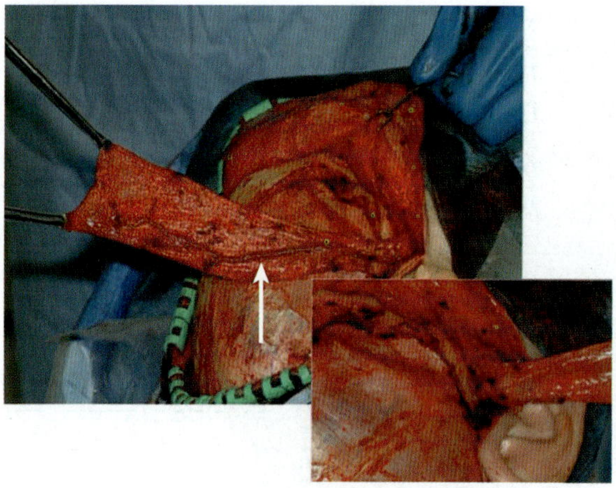

FIGURE 19.3
Harvest of large TPFF. Note the primary vascular pedicle running centrally through the flap (*arrow*). **Inset.** narrowing of the pedicle to less than 2 cm, thereby allowing for maximum extension and rotation.

is dissected so that maximal rotation of the flap is possible. The zygomatic arch is then exposed posteriorly, and the superolateral orbit is exposed anteriorly. The layers of the anterior scalp and the temporal region are retracted in a more anterior direction to expose the lateral edge of the orbit and the anterior border of the temporalis muscle. The temporalis fascia insertion at the lateral edge of the orbit is incised, and using blunt dissection, a tract is made over the surface of the temporalis muscle but deep to the zygomatic malar eminence medial to the coronoid process to the lateral wall of the maxillary sinus into the infratemporal fossa. A wide tunnel is then created into the maxillary sinus and the palatal defect. It should be large enough to accommodate for postoperative edema of the flap and prevent strangulation of the pedicle. The pedicle is then transposed into the defect through the created tunnel. One must be careful not to torque or twist the flap nor put it under tension in order to preserve maximal flow. In the case of centrally located defects, a Caldwell-Luc approach should be added to ensure that the posterior maxillary defect is adequate and that there are no restrictions or sharp bony edges in the nasal cavity. The palatal defect must be prepared and demucosalized if this is a secondary procedure. The flap is then sutured circumferentially into the defect. The wound is then closed over a drain with a single layer of staples superiorly and in a multilayered fashion inferiorly in the tragal region. A sterile compression dressing is then applied.

Temporalis Muscle Flap

Surgical Anatomy

The temporalis muscle resides in the temporal fossa at the lateral portion of the skull deep to the TPFF. The muscle origin is the temporal line and can be palpated in most patients. The tendinous insertion is on the coronoid process and along the anterior ramus of the mandible. The temporalis flap can be approximately 11 × 12 cm in length and width and 1 cm in thickness at its maximum (Fig. 19.4A). The arterial supply is from the external carotid artery by two routes. The first more superficial one is immediately above the zygomatic arch. Here the superficial temporal artery gives off the middle temporal artery that is directed to the temporalis muscle. The principal arterial supply of the flap is the deep temporal arteries that branch off the internal maxillary artery. The temporalis muscle gets its vascular supply from the deep temporal artery entering the muscle at the level of the TMJ medially, often described as being medial to the level of the coronoid process of the mandible. The anterior and posterior deep temporal vessels course along the undersurface of the muscle.

The muscle bulk of the TMF allows for a sturdy reconstruction of the palatal defect (Fig. 19.4B). The muscle is easily manipulated, rotated, and overturned in its placement depending on the defect and the necessary arc of rotation. It can easily be incorporated with other reconstructive materials for large palatomaxillary defects. Harvesting the temporalis muscle involves dissecting the superficial temporal fascia and the deep pericranium in continuity with the flap. Doing so reserves all of the neurovascular integrity of the flap. If the additional length is needed, the zygomatic arch can be temporarily removed and replaced after rotation of the flap. A coronoidectomy can also be performed to lessen tension on the muscle and to add additional length.

Technique

The patient is positioned and prepped, and an incision is created in a similar fashion to the TPFF. For the temporalis harvest, the incision is made and carried down through the skin, subcutaneous tissue, and galea, down to periosteum centrally extending laterally to preserve the temporalis muscle. More inferior–lateral the incision is carried down to the deep temporal fascia extending to the preauricular sulcus in posttragal fashion.

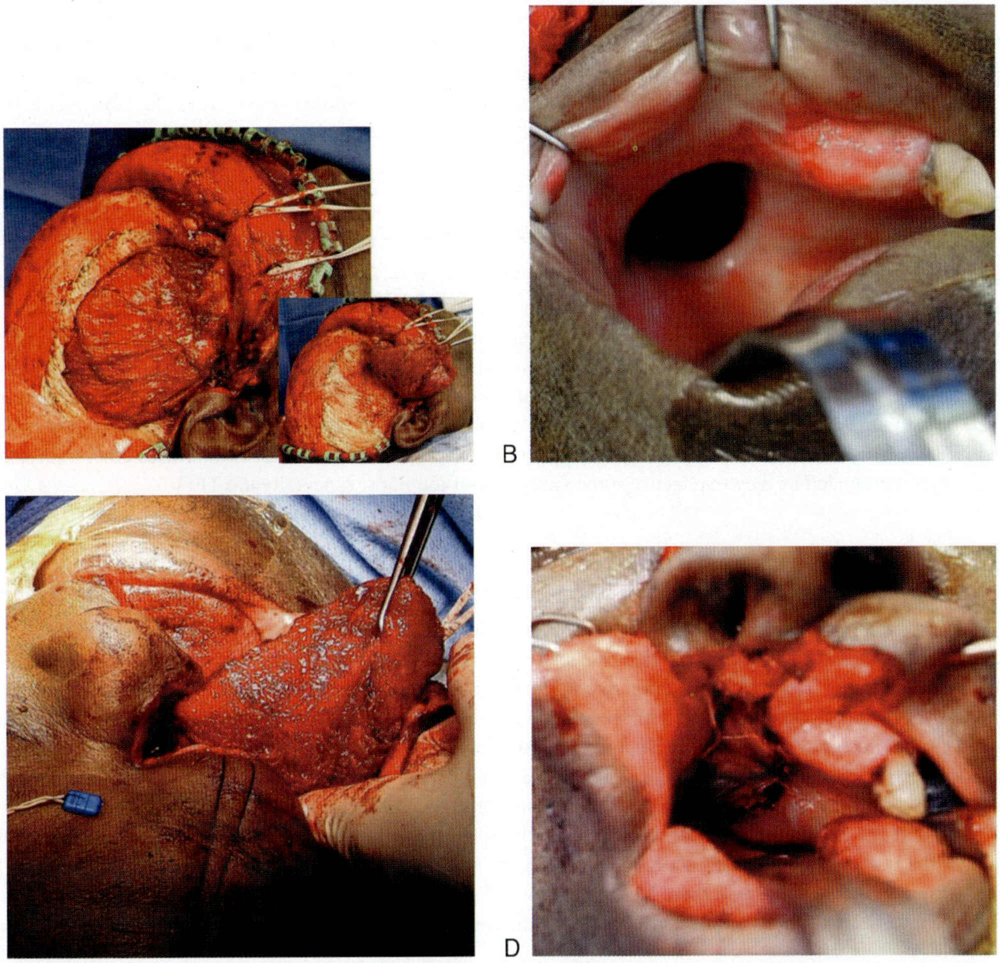

A B C D

FIGURE 19.4 A. Harvested TMF with elevation of the temporal adipose tissue pad along with the scalp. Preservation of the facial nerve was elevated along with the flap. The superolateral orbital rim and zygomatic arch is exposed (**inset**). The full extent of the muscle elevation is demonstrated. **B.** Right palatal defect greater than 2 cm in a patient with previous maxillectomy and chemoradiation treatment of a squamous cell carcinoma. **C.** The TMF is tunneled through the posterior wall of the maxillary sinus into the defect. **D.** The flap is inset and circumferentially sutured with a watertight closure into the defect previously shown in Figure 19.4B.

A subperiosteal elevator is used to elevate flaps anteriorly and posteriorly. Rainey clips can be applied to assist with scalp hemostasis. Subperiosteal scalp flap elevation is performed superiorly. Elevation of the flap over the layer of the superficial deep temporal fascia is continued anteriorly until the lateral margin of the orbit. The temporal pad of adipose tissue is now entered, and further elevation is performed protecting the frontal branch of the facial nerve. Once the zygomatic arch is reached, care is taken to elevate the remaining soft tissue in the subperiosteal layer of the arch to protect the zygomatic branch of the facial nerve. Upon complete exposure of the zygomatic arch, zygomatic or orbitozygomatic osteotomies can be performed to allow for additional extension and rotation of the flap and improved exposure of the infratemporal fossa. The coronoid process can also be dissected and removed at the sigmoid notch to add even more rotation and extension.

The TMF is now elevated using Bovie cautery within the confines of the temporal fossa. The flap is elevated inferiorly to the zygomatic arch. The temporalis muscle is then released from the undersurface of the zygomatic arch to free the entire temporalis muscle for transposition into the palatomaxillary defect. Similarly to the TPFF, a wide tunnel is then created into the maxillary sinus. It should be large enough to accommodate for postoperative edema of the flap and prevent strangulation of the pedicle. Blood pressure can be dropped below 65 mm Hg to temporarily shrink the muscle bulk. The pedicle is then transposed into the defect through the created tunnel. The muscle can be transposed with either the superficial fascia facing into the defect of the deep surface of the muscle or with inversion of the muscle (Fig. 19.4C). One must be careful not to torque or twist the flap nor put it under tension in order to preserve maximal flow. The flap is otherwise sutured circumferentially into the defect (Fig. 19.4D). The muscle flap can also be divided into an anterior and posterior flap. When this occurs, the anterior flap is used for the defect reconstruction and the posterior flap is left in the temporal fossa and brought anteriorly to fill in the donor site soft tissue defect.

Prior to closure, the donor site defect can either be left alone or the temporal fossa can be filled with a variety of materials. I prefer adipose tissue grafts for tissue replacement over alloplastic materials due to the surgical communication with the oral cavity and the theoretical risk of infection of an implant. Once adipose tissue is placed and secured to the surrounding tissue, the wound is closed in a two-layered fashion over a drain and then dressed with a compression dressing over the adipose tissue graft.

POSTOPERATIVE MANAGEMENT

The patient is admitted for observation after both TMF and TPFF reconstruction. The Hemovac drain is kept until there is less than 10 cc of output over a 24-hour period. This is especially important when there is an autologous adipose tissue graft for fear of seroma and subsequent infection. The patient is also observed for hematoma and flap viability. The patient is placed on a clear diet for 24 hours and then advanced to full liquids for 5 to 7 days postoperatively. When the flap appears to be viable at a week, the patient may advance to a soft diet. As an outpatient, the patient must continue to be followed for the presence of any fluid collection or flap dehiscence. Mucosalization of the flaps is usually complete within 4 to 8 weeks. Mouth rinses other than saline are not recommended as they may cause some sloughing of the flaps, especially the TPFF.

COMPLICATIONS

Complications that are common to both procedures include hematoma, temporary or permanent facial nerve paralysis, flap dehiscence and/or flap necrosis leading to fistula, and flap contracture. Postoperative alopecia is more common after TPFF reconstruction due to the subfollicular dissection. Temporal hollowing and changes in mastication are more common in TMF reconstruction especially in the cases when the entire muscle is used and a coronoidectomy is performed. Hyponasality and temporary nasal obstruction may occur if the muscle is also transposed into the nasal cavity. Occasionally, a second-stage tissue augmentation is needed after TMF for a persistent concavity of the donor site. The literature reports a 13% incidence of flap loss, 19% facial nerve paresis, and 3% facial nerve paralysis for the TMF. Specific studies propose that the larger the defect, the greater the risk of complications especially with regard to chewing difficulty and flap dehiscence. Due to the thin scalp flap in TPFF harvest, there have been reports of scalp epidermolysis. There have been no complications such as necrosis or fistula formation after irradiation of these flaps reported in the literature.

RESULTS

In my experience, both the TMF and TPFF have exceeded expectations with regard to palatal reconstruction. Postoperatively, patients have minimal short-term problems, but there have been no long-term complications and almost all patients have had excellent results with regard to functional and aesthetic outcome. While some revisions were necessary for fistula formation, there has been no incidence of permanent facial nerve paralysis or total flap loss. On one occasion, a TPFF was used in a patient who had previously undergone chemoradiation and had a significant enough dehiscence that a TMF was used as an adjunct. Experiences such as these have helped to shape my approach and indications for each of these flaps. More recently, these flaps, especially the TPFF, have been employed endoscopically for a variety of skull base defects. They continue to demonstrate flexibility and a broad spectrum of use.

PEARLS

- The surgeon should have an understanding of the indications for local versus free flap reconstruction of the palate as well as the contraindications for both.
- Preoperative evaluation must include a comprehensive understanding of the postablative defect. A complete physical examination and appropriate radiologic imaging must be performed prior to surgery to demonstrate the complete extent of the tumor.
- Prior to the operation, the donor site must be examined carefully. Signs of trauma, previous surgery, and/or radiation must be noted. The muscle strength and bulk of the temporalis muscle should be confirmed. Palpation or Doppler of the superficial temporal artery is imperative prior to TPFF harvest.
- The surgical anatomy of the scalp and underlying layers of the temporal fossa must be completely understood including the location of the vascular supply of each flap, that is, the deep temporal arteries and superficial temporal artery, in addition to the location of the frontal branch of the facial nerve.

PITFALLS

- The surgeon should be aware of the methods to extend and prolong the length of each flap—specifically, removal of the zygomatic arch and coronoidectomy for the TMF and the dissection of the superficial temporal pedicle for the TPFF.
- The tunnels through which the flaps are transposed must be large enough to accommodate the expected flap edema in the immediate postoperative period to avoid strangulation of the flap.
- Close follow-up in the postoperative period with regard to wound care and the appropriate advancement of diet is important for long-term success of the flap reconstruction.

INSTRUMENTS TO HAVE AVAILABLE

- Standard head and neck surgical tray
- Soft tissue elevators

SUGGESTED READING

Brown WJ. Extraordinary case of horse bite: the external ear completely bitten off and replaced. *Lancet* 1898;1:1533.

Bakamjian V. A technique for primary reconstruction of the palate after radical maxillectomy for cancer. *Plast Reconstr Surg* 1963;31:103–117.

Demas PN, Sotereanos GC. Transmaxillary temporalis transfer for reconstruction of a large palatal defect: report of a case. *J Oral Maxillofac Surg* 1989;47:197–202.

Panje WR, Morris MR. The temporoparietal fascial flap in head and neck reconstruction. *Ear Nose Throat J* 1991;70:311–317.

Genden EM, Wallace DI, Okay D, et al. Reconstruction of the hard palate using the radial forearm free flap: indications and outcomes. *Head Neck* 2004;26(9):808–814.

20 THE SUBTOTAL HARD PALATE DEFECT: RADIAL FOREARM FREE FLAP

Mark A. Varvares

INTRODUCTION

The major goals of palatomaxillary reconstruction include both restoration of function and an acceptable cosmetic outcome. The functional considerations include maintenance of a functional oral cavity of appropriate dimensions, the separation of the oral and nasal cavities to prevent nasal regurgitation and hypernasality, a framework to allow masticatory function, and an osseous structure to which to anchor a dental prosthesis and to provide the structural foundation for the nasal base.

Through-and-through defects of the oral cavity to the nasal cavity traditionally have been managed with oromaxillofacial obturators. The advantages of this approach include achievement of acceptable functional outcome without additional surgery, the ability to monitor the cavity for recurrent tumor, and the ability to restore functional dentition mounted on the obturator. Disadvantages include the extreme problems with hypernasality when the obturator is removed for cleaning, the hygienic issues related to obturator and cavity maintenance, and difficulty retaining the prosthesis in the edentulous patient.

The radial forearm free flap (RFFF) is useful as a fasciocutaneous flap for the reconstruction of defects involving the central palate without involvement of the alveolar ridge or for defects involving the central palate and the alveolar ridge posterior to the canine. Such defects are classified using the classification outlined by Okay et al (2001) as class Ia and class Ib defects, respectively (Fig. 20.1) Such defects do not involve loss of premaxillary bone and soft tissue, and therefore, the reconstructive demands related to nasal support and premaxillary projection are avoided. More extensive defects involving a larger area of the hard palate and including the alveolar ridge anterior to the canine and the premaxilla would be difficult to repair using a RFFF unless it contained an osseous component (radial forearm osseofasciocutaneous flap) or other osseous components are included in the reconstruction.

HISTORY

I am careful to ask whether the patient has a history of prior surgery or injury to the forearm donor site since this could compromise the blood supply to the skin paddle. Additionally, I always determine the dominant hand so that I can plan to harvest from the nondominant hand to limit the potential impact on the patient's quality of life.

PHYSICAL EXAMINATION

A physical examination should always include an evaluation of the forearm donor site to establish if there has been injury or prior surgery that may preclude use of this donor site. An Allen test should also be performed to determine if there is an intact vascular palmar arch. The dimensions of the tumor to be excised as well as the anatomic sites to be removed should be recorded. Photographs of the defect should be made to incorporate into the medical record.

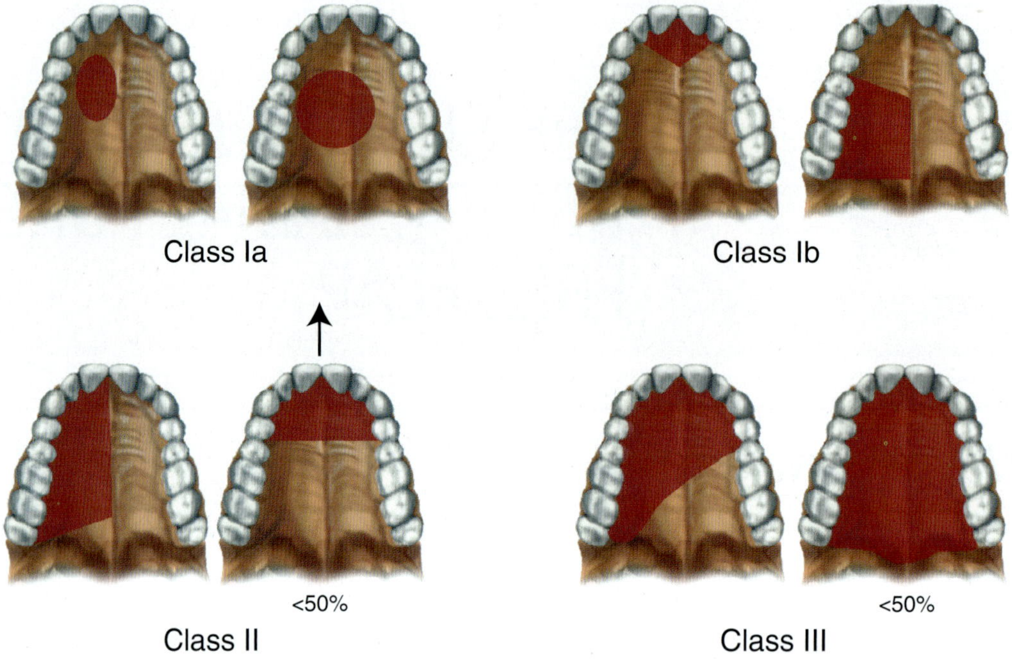

FIGURE 20.1 The Mount Sinai classification of palate defects. Class Ia defects involve any portion of the hard palate but not the tooth-bearing maxillary alveolus. Class Ib defects involve premaxilla or any portion of the maxillary alveolus and dentition posterior to the canines. Class II defects involve any portion of the hard palate and tooth-bearing maxillary alveolus and only one canine. The anterior margin of the defect lies within the premaxilla. This class includes transverse palatectomy defects that involve less than 50% of the hard palate. Class III defects involve any portion of the hard palate and tooth-bearing maxillary alveolus including both canines. This class includes total and transverse palatectomy defects that involve more than 50% of the hard palate. (Redrawn from Okay DJ, Genden E, et al. Prosthodontic guidelines for surgical reconstruction of the maxilla: a classification system of defects. *J Prosthet Dent* 2001;86:352–363.)

INDICATIONS

The RFFF has been the most frequently used flap for head and neck reconstruction since the 1980s. It has been used for nearly every head and neck soft tissue defect that one can encounter. This flap is widely employed due to its ease of harvest, large blood vessels, low donor site morbidity, and potential for simultaneous two-team surgery and for the quality and quantity of tissue available. This donor site has also recently gained popularity as an osseofasciocutaneous flap, useful for reconstruction of composite defects with a small bone component. It has also been previously reported as being useful for reconstruction of subtotal defects of the palate.

Genden et al. (2004) recently described a series of patients with class Ia and Ib defects who were reconstructed using a RFFF. As part of this study, they performed a functional and quality of life comparison with a similarly matched group of patients who used an obturator. They found improved function and quality of life in those patients who had undergone flap reconstruction. The major goal of the soft tissue reconstruction was to provide oral–nasal separation and improve the overall quality of life of the patient. In their series, patients who achieved dental rehabilitation did so by using a dental prosthesis anchored on remaining dentition or osseointegrated implants in the bone of the native palate.

The RFFF is a fasciocutaneous flap best used in the reconstruction of the subtotal palate defect when the defect is classified as class Ia or Ib. In addition, it is possible to use the RFFF as an osseofasciocutaneous flap with the transfer of vascularized bone when the defect requires it. This donor site can also be used in combination with nonvascularized bone grafts. An example of the use of the RFFF as an osseofasciocutaneous flap is in the reconstruction of a premaxillary defect when it is desirable to restore the premaxilla.

CONTRAINDICATIONS

Defects that require extensive bone replacement which is a demand not met by this donor site are contraindications to this technique, as are previous trauma or surgery to the forearm donor site and a negative Allen test.

PREOPERATIVE PLANNING

Prior to harvest of the RFFF, it is important to note that the patient has an intact palmar arch. A clinical Allen test can be done that reliably demonstrates the safety of harvest of the radial artery. It is also possible to obtain a more objective test such as a Doppler Allen test in a vascular laboratory. Typically, this is done only if the clinical Allen test leaves any doubt as to the findings.

SURGICAL TECHNIQUE

The majority of palate reconstructions using a RFFF can be performed using a transoral approach with a neck incision for vascular access for recipient vessel isolation. The pedicle of the RFFF is usually one that easily allows inset of the soft tissue and bony components in the oral cavity with adequate length of the vessels to reach the recipient vessels in the neck.

Prior to harvesting the RFFF, it is important to note that the patient has an intact palmar arch. A clinical Allen test can be done that can reliably show the safety of harvest of the radial artery. It is also possible to obtain a more objective test such as a Doppler Allen test in a vascular laboratory. Typically, this is done only if the clinical Allen test leaves any doubt as to the findings.

The flap is harvested based on the dimensions of the defect of the recipient site. The skin paddle is outlined centered over the radial artery in the distal forearm just proximal to the skin crease of the wrist. The flap can be extended over on to the dorsal surface of the forearm, particularly if one is interested in capturing the distal portion of the cephalic vein in the skin paddle. This ensures that if the caliber of the cephalic vein is adequate proximal in the antecubital fossa, the flap will be adequately drained using the cephalic vein alone (Fig. 20.2).

The arm is exsanguinated using an Ace wrap after the outline of the flap is made in the distal forearm and a curvilinear incision is drawn from the proximal portion of the skin paddle to the anterior cubital fossa. A tourniquet, which has had previously been placed above the elbow, is inflated to 90 mm Hg greater than the patient's resting systolic blood pressure. Skin incisions are then made circumferentially. Dissection starts either medially or laterally depending on the surgeon's preference. If dissection starts laterally, the skin and subcutaneous tissues are dissected off of the brachioradialis muscle and tendon. The cutaneous branch of the radial nerve is identified, as it exits deep to the brachioradialis tendon. Care is taken to mobilize the cephalic vein along with the skin paddle as the flap is mobilized from lateral to medial. Once the brachioradialis tendon is exposed, care is taken to leave paratenon overlying this tendon (and all the tendons in the forearm). The radial artery can be visualized in the groove between the brachioradialis and flexor carpi radialis. The flap is then mobilized medially, and dissection is carried out from medial to lateral, again carefully leaving paratenon overlying the tendons of the flexor carpi ulnaris, palmaris longus, and flexor carpi radialis. Once the flexor carpi radialis muscle tendon is identified and the flap mobilized lateral to this tendon, the radial artery distally in the forearm at the level of the distal portion of the skin paddle can be dissected and ligated using a 2-0 silk suture.

The flap is then mobilized from distal to proximal by mobilizing the radial artery out of the groove between the brachioradialis and flexor carpi radialis tendons. On the deep surface of this plane of dissection, there is a transverse layer of fascia that can be identified reliably and indicates that the dissection is proceeding in the appropriate level. Once the dissection and mobilization reach the proximal portion of the skin paddle, the skin flaps of the forearm proximal to the skin paddle are elevated at a level of dissection above the muscle fascia. Care must be taken to be certain that the cephalic vein is not injured in this elevation of soft tissue from the proximal forearm. Dissection continues along the vascular pedicle proximally by separating the brachioradialis and the flexor carpi radialis muscles and mobilizing the radial artery and its venae comitantes from this space. Dissection continues toward the antecubital fossa until adequate length of the pedicle has been achieved. Of note, it is important not to carry the dissection of the radial artery

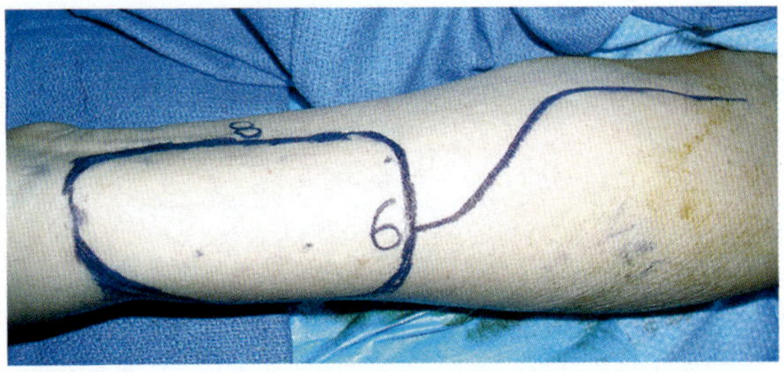

FIGURE 20.2
Typical outline of the fasciocutaneous RFFF on the left arm, with placement of the paddle laterally to capture the cephalic vein as well as the radial artery.

proximal to the radial recurrent vessel in the proximal forearm. I dissect proximal enough into the antecubital fossa to find the communicating vein between the confluence of the venae comitantes of the radial artery and cephalic vein. This allows a single venous outflow draining both the superficial and deep systems of the flap. It is not essential for this connecting vessel to be mobilized as the flap may be adequately drained using either of the superficial or the deep systems. There may be cases, however, where one of the two systems may not appear as robust. Harvesting the flap vein in this manner may avoid a problem of inadequate venous outflow. Once this stage of the dissection is completed, the tourniquet may be released, the flap and the arm perfused, and hemostasis obtained both on the flap and it's pedicle and the donor site. Once the recipient site is ready for flap inset, the arteries and veins are clamped at their takeoff in the antecubital fossa and the vessels ligated.

When harvesting the radial forearm osseofasciocutaneous free flap, the procedure is modified such that as the dissection is done distally in the forearm from the lateral aspect, the radial artery is not separated from the radius. The distal portion of the radius is identified, and the periosteum is scored using a Bovie cautery. The radius is then measured, and a harvest of approximately one-third of the thickness of the medial aspect of the distal radius is made. A boat-shaped ostectomy is outlined and incised using a sagittal saw (Fig. 20.3). Care is taken to preserve the soft tissue attachments between the radial artery medially and the radius.

If an osseofasciocutaneous flap is harvested, the Orthopedic Service is asked to place a heavy fracture plate along the lateral aspect of the distal radius to prevent a pathologic fracture. The donor site is then closed as any other RFFF donor site. A split-thickness skin graft of 0.018 inch is harvested from the thigh. This is used to cover the portion of the defect that corresponds to the skin paddle. The proximal portion of the flap harvest is drained with a closed suction drain, and the skin is closed in multiple layers, usually a subcutaneous layer of absorbable suture followed by a skin layer of either staples or nylon or fast-absorbing chromic sutures.

Prior to flap transfer and inset, recipient vessels must be isolated and a connection must be made between the area of vessel exposure in the neck and the flap inset site. An appropriate vessel in the setting of palate reconstruction is the facial artery and vein with the external jugular vein as a possible recipient vessel as well. If a neck dissection has not been done, an incision consistent with that used for excision of the submandibular gland is made. Excision of the submandibular gland will help to locate the facial artery and vein and create some working room to allow the microvascular anastomosis to be performed. The main trunk of the facial artery can be preserved when excising the submandibular gland if care is taken only to divide the glandular branches of the facial artery and not to be quick to divide the main trunk of the facial artery as is frequently done in excision of the submandibular gland (Fig. 20.4).

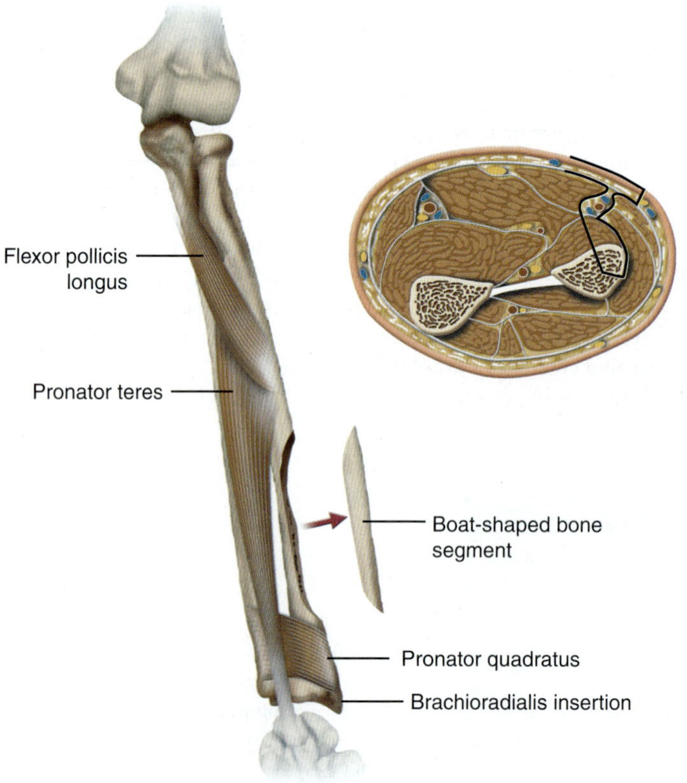

FIGURE 20.3
Schematic showing the area of harvest of the distal radius and the relationships to the pronator teres insertion and pronator quadratus.

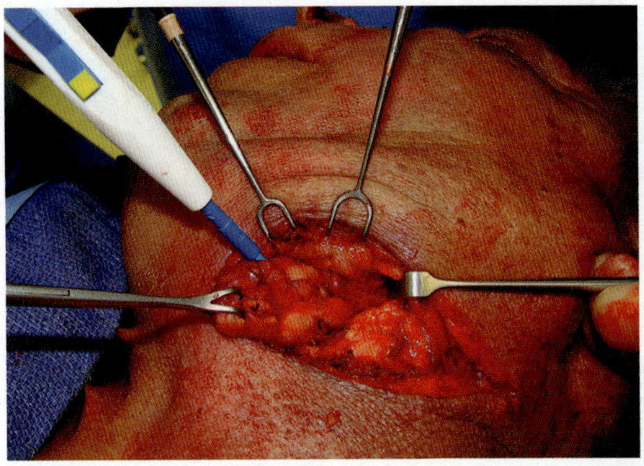

FIGURE 20.4
Removal of the submandibular gland with maintenance of the facial artery in continuity to allow a greater vessel length as a recipient vessel for midface and palate reconstruction.

Once the vessels are isolated, a connection is created from the neck to the ablative site. There are two different anatomical levels that can be used. In most cases, I prefer a subcutaneous tunnel. This dissection proceeds from the neck incision used for vascular access by dissecting in a supraplatysmal plane from the neck to the midface. The advantage of this approach is that the supraplatysmal plane protects the marginal mandibular nerve and, as dissection proceeds more cephalad, all of the distal branches of the facial nerve. Once dissection of this tunnel is extended cephalad to be adjacent to the defect, it is connected with the recipient site of the midface. This does require dissection through the superficial musculoaponeurotic system (SMAS) into the oral cavity. This is done bluntly by spreading the tissues in the direction of the branches of the facial nerve. The tunnel must be wide enough to allow the flap to be pulled from the neck into the midface or allow the vessels to be passed from the defect into the neck. Typically, a tunnel three or four fingers breadth wide will be adequate. It is important to obtain meticulous hemostasis during creation of the tunnel to prevent postoperative bleeding that could lead to a hematoma and flap compromise.

The second option for creating the tunnel connecting the neck to the midface is to use a deeper plane of dissection. This would require a subplatysmal dissection extending superiorly directly overlying the periosteum of the mandible and masseter muscle. This is a layer of dissection deep to the branches of the facial nerve, thereby preventing the potential injury to these nerves. An advantage of this plane of dissection is that it brings me right into the appropriate plane of the maxillary defect, usually by passing through the buccal space and its pad of adipose tissue.

Once the vessels are isolated and the tunnel is created, the flap is brought into the inset position. I typically prefer to pull the flap from the neck through the tunnel into the recipient site in the oral cavity. This allows me to know that there is not been any twisting of the vascular pedicle in the tunnel while the flap has been positioned. Retrograde placement of the vessels into the neck from the mouth by floating them through a prepositioned Penrose drain is another useful technique.

Once the flap has been brought through the tunnel into the oral cavity, it is inset into the defect and sewn to the mucosal edges using an absorbable Vicryl suture. This must be a watertight closure. Nasal secretions will be exposed to the deep surface of the flap where the vascular structures are located. This typically is not a problem and has not resulted in a higher risk of flap failure. Once inset is completed, revascularization is performed.

In patients who are undergoing reconstruction with an osseofasciocutaneous flap, the bone component of the forearm flap is plated into position followed by soft tissue inset.

Once the flaps are vascularized, the wound is irrigated and suction drains are placed, and then the wound is closed in layers.

Case report: This patient presents with a premaxillary defect that extends from the second premolar on one side to its corresponding premolar on the other. There was a through-and-through defect into the nasal cavity, with loss of premaxillary support. The patient was not interested in osseointegrated implants into the reconstructed bone and desired not to have an obturator. Nasal and premaxillary projection was achieved by placement of an arch-shaped split calvarial bone graft (Fig. 20.5). This was covered with a RFFF (Fig. 20.6). At 3 months, the reconstruction is well healed intraorally (Fig. 20.7), and the patient has excellent anterior nasal support.

POSTOPERATIVE MANAGEMENT

The RFFF donor site is rather easy to manage postoperatively. The donor site is splinted with the hand slightly extended. The arm is dressed using Xeroform gauze followed by web roll and Kerlix followed by a ventral splint and then ACE wrap. The splint is left in place for 7 days, at which point it is removed and the skin graft evaluated. Therapy is started once the splint is off to help with mobilization of the writs.

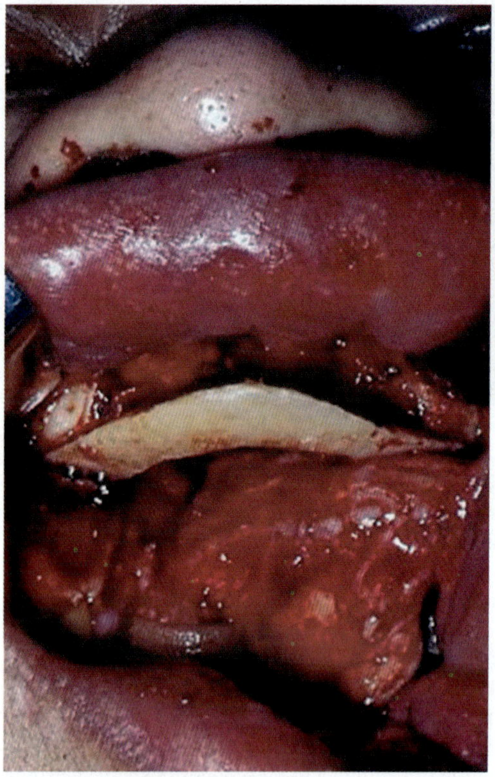

FIGURE 20.5
Defect of anterior palate, premaxilla, and floor of the nose with a calvarial bone graft in place just prior to wrapping the radial forearm free flap to cover the nasal surface, necessary because of the nonvascular nature of the bone graft.

COMPLICATIONS

The most significant complication that occurs using a RFFF for palate reconstruction is flap failure. A hematoma in the tunnel leading to flap compromise is a possible cause of flap failure. It is important to secure excellent hemostasis of the tunnel at the time of its development to prevent bleeding postoperatively. In addition, it is extremely important during flap harvest to be certain that all the small vessels off the pedicle are

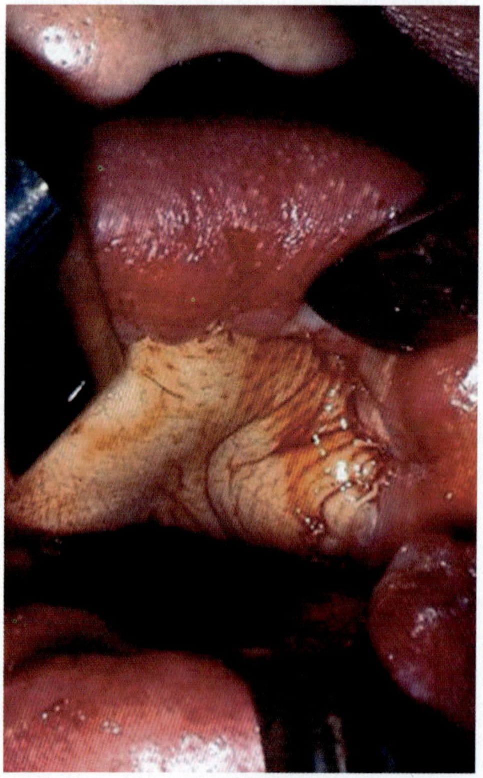

FIGURE 20.6
Radial forearm free flap in position at the end of the procedure.

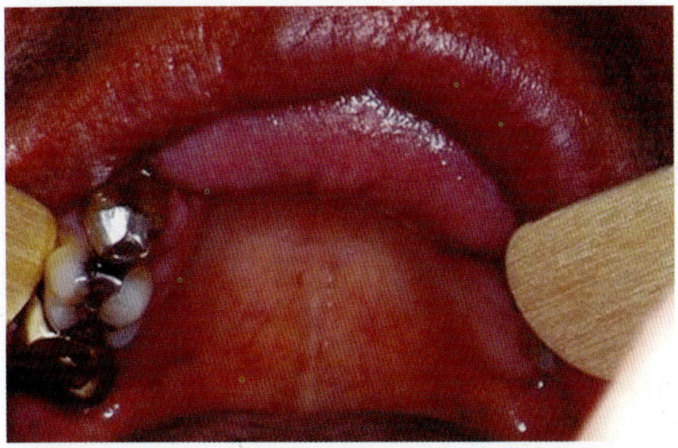

FIGURE 20.7
Results at 6 weeks, flap well healed in the anterior palate region.

clipped or coagulated so as not to allow bleeding once the flap is revascularized and inset into the recipient site. It would make it very difficult to isolate and locate the bleeding vessels on the pedicle once the flap is inset.

RESULTS

The RFFF has been shown to be a very reliable technique for reconstruction of multiple head and neck defects. In properly selected patients, the RFFF can reliably improve function and quality of life of the patients with subtotal palate defects.

PEARLS

- Proper patient selection is the key to success as in all reconstructive techniques. The reconstructive technique described is best suited to patients with Okay defect class 1a and 1b.
- Patients with large defects involving the premaxillary area are best reconstructed with a flap that has an osseous component. This could include the radial forearm osseofasciocutaneous flap or another donor site such as the fibula or scapula.
- All patients who undergo reconstruction of major defects in the palate who desire eventually to have full dental restoration must be counseled as to the expense and time that is typically invested to be able to achieve this goal.

PITFALLS

- Usually, the dental component of the rehabilitation is not covered by insurance and is an out-of-pocket expense for the patient.

INSTRUMENTS TO HAVE AVAILABLE

- Standard neck dissection tray
- Tourniquet of appropriate circumference
- Midface rigid fixation plating system

SUGGESTED READING

Yang G, Chen B, Gao Y, et al. Forearm free skin flap transplantation. *Natl Med J China* 1981;61:139.

Okay DJ, Genden E, Buchbinder D, et al. Prosthodontic guidelines for surgical reconstruction of the maxilla: a classification system of defects. *J Prosthet Dent* 2001;86:352–363.

Genden E, Wallace DI, Okay DJ, et al. Reconstruction of the hard palate using the radial forearm free flap: indications and outcomes. *Head Neck* 2004;26:808–814.

Kim JH, Rosenthal EL, Ellis T, et al. Radial forearm osteocutaneous free flap in maxillofacial and oromandibular reconstructions. *Laryngoscope* 2005;115(9):1697–1701.

Karamanoukian R, Gupta R, Evans GR. A novel technique for the prophylactic plating of the osteocutaneous radial forearm flap donor site. *Ann Plast Surg* 2006;56(2):200–204.

21 THE TOTAL HARD PALATE DEFECT: RECTUS ABDOMINIS FREE FLAP

Mark A. Varvares

INTRODUCTION

Restoration of function and acceptable cosmetic outcome are the two major goals of palatomaxillary reconstruction. The functional considerations include maintenance of an oral cavity of appropriate dimensions, the separation of the oral and nasal cavity to prevent nasal regurgitation and hypernasality, providing a framework to allow masticatory function, an osseous structure on which a prosthesis can be anchored and dental rehabilitation, and a structural foundation of the nasal base. The cosmetic implications related to this last point are obvious, to appropriately maintain the proper position of the midfacial structures including nasal support, premaxillary structure, and more superiorly and laterally structures related to midface skeletal contour. Ideally, total reconstruction of the palate would best be accomplished using a composite flap of soft tissue and bone.

Potential donor sites include the scapular osseofasciocutaneous flap, the fibular osseocutaneous flap, the radial forearm osseocutaneous flap, and the iliac crest osseomyocutaneous flap. The use of these sites would allow both the restoration of skeletal structure onto which one could build midfacial support and secure implants for dental rehabilitation as well as a soft tissue component to cover the transferred bone. However, in some patients, it may not be possible to reconstruct with a bone-containing flap. Such examples would be patients with severe medical comorbidities, not allowing the lengthier operative procedure usually required with the osseous flaps, or patients in whom the osseous donor sites are not available for whatever reason. For instance, patients with severe peripheral vascular disease, which would prohibit the use of a fibular osteocutaneous flap would be one example. A morbidly obese patient with an unavailable scapular donor site would be another example. In such cases, a soft tissue flap donor site may be the best option. Also, patients with palate defects that include a massive facial or periorbital component may be best served by transferring a soft tissue flap with an abundant quantity of tissue of different components (muscle and cutaneous tissue) to allow the successful reconstruction of a complex defect with multiple reconstructive requirements (palate, orbit, and facial skin). This chapter discusses the role of the rectus abdominis free flap for reconstruction of the entire palate.

HISTORY

The patient history is important in determining if there are any contraindications to harvesting from the rectus donor site. Prior abdominal surgery is the most common restriction. Other considerations include a history of an abdominal hernia that may preclude the use of this donor site.

PHYSICAL EXAMINATION

The physical examination entails an examination of the defect and the abdominal donor site. When using the rectus abdominis donor site to reconstruct a total palatal defect, the donor tissue may not be ideal if the patient is obese. Depending on the body habitus, the donor site may provide a flap that is too thick to comfortably reconstruct a palatal defect. In obese patients, the skin paddle can be removed to reduce the thickness of the flap and a skin graft can be placed over the vascularized muscle or the muscle can be left exposed in the oral cavity and be allowed to mucosalize. The physical examination is the only way to determine if the rectus is an appropriate donor site.

INDICATIONS

The rectus abdominis flap is indicated when a subtotal or total hard palate defect is anticipated and when osseous flap donor sites are not available. Other indications would include when a large volume of tissue is required for repair of a complex three-dimensional midface defect that may include the hard palate, orbital contents, and facial skin.

CONTRAINDICATIONS

Contraindications to this flap include patients who are morbidly obese, patients who have had previous abdominal surgery, or patients in whom previous inguinal hernia repair may have rendered the deep inferior epigastric vessels unusable.

PREOPERATIVE PLANNING

Preoperatively, it is important to measure the defect and determine the dimensions of the skin paddle required to reline the oral defect. In most cases of total palate reconstruction without a complicated midfacial defect such as orbital exenteration and midface resection, it is preferred to use the rectus abdominis free flap as a muscle-only flap. This prevents problems related to what in nearly all patients can be a very thick subcutaneous layer. A myocutaneous flap is used with more extensive facial and orbital defects when the abdominal wall subcutaneous tissues are of manageable thickness.

SURGICAL TECHNIQUE

Whether the flap is taken as a muscle-only flap or as a myocutaneous flap, some basic anatomical landmarks need to be noted. The key anatomical landmarks for harvest of the rectus abdominis flap are the linea alba, the linea semilunaris, and the arcuate line (Fig. 21.1). The linea alba is the midline condensation of the rectus sheath. The linea semilunaris marks the lateral border of the rectus sheath, which contains the rectus muscle. The rectus sheath is composed of the aponeuroses of the three major muscles of the anterior abdominal wall: The external oblique, internal oblique, and transverses abdominis. At the horizontally oriented arcuate line, which is located halfway between the symphysis pubis and the umbilicus, the layers of the rectus sheath transition. Superior to the arcuate line, the anterior layer of the rectus sheath is composed of the entire aponeuroses of the external oblique and the split aponeurosis of the internal oblique. The posterior layer is composed of the posterior leaf of the aponeurosis of the internal oblique and the aponeurosis of the transversus abdominis. Deep to this is the transversalis fascia. Inferior to the arcuate line, all three muscle aponeuroses create the anterior layer of the rectus sheath, and the posterior layer is made up entirely of transversalis fascia (Fig. 21.2). This anatomical point of distinction that occurs at the arcuate line is important because any myocutaneous flap that will include in the harvest the anterior layer of the rectus sheath below the arcuate line requires that the anterior rectus sheath defect be reconstructed with mesh; otherwise the patient is at significant risk for formation of a hernia.

It is important to palpate the femoral pulse prior to harvesting the flap. Just proximal to the femoral pulse will be the external iliac artery and vein. The deep inferior epigastric artery and vein take origin from the external iliac artery and vein to run on the deep surface of the rectus abdominis muscle. These vessels run the entire vertical length of the muscle and anastomose with the superior epigastric vessels, which are the terminal branches of the internal mammary artery.

The major musculocutaneous perforators that supply the skin overlying the rectus abdominis muscle are found in the periumbilical area. They radiate from the umbilical area, but the dominant vessels run in a posterior, lateral and superior direction toward the ipsilateral tip of the scapula. Any rectus musculocutaneous free flap must be harvested with preservation of these perforating vessels remaining in continuity as they pass out from the muscle through the anterior rectus sheath to supply the overlying skin and subcutaneous tissues (Fig. 21.3).

When harvesting the rectus abdominis free flap as a musculocutaneous flap, the flap elevation proceeds as follows: The desired dimensions of the cutaneous paddle are outlined again in the area of the densest musculocutaneous perforators in the periumbilical area (Fig. 21.3A–F). The skin paddle may be used to replace palatal

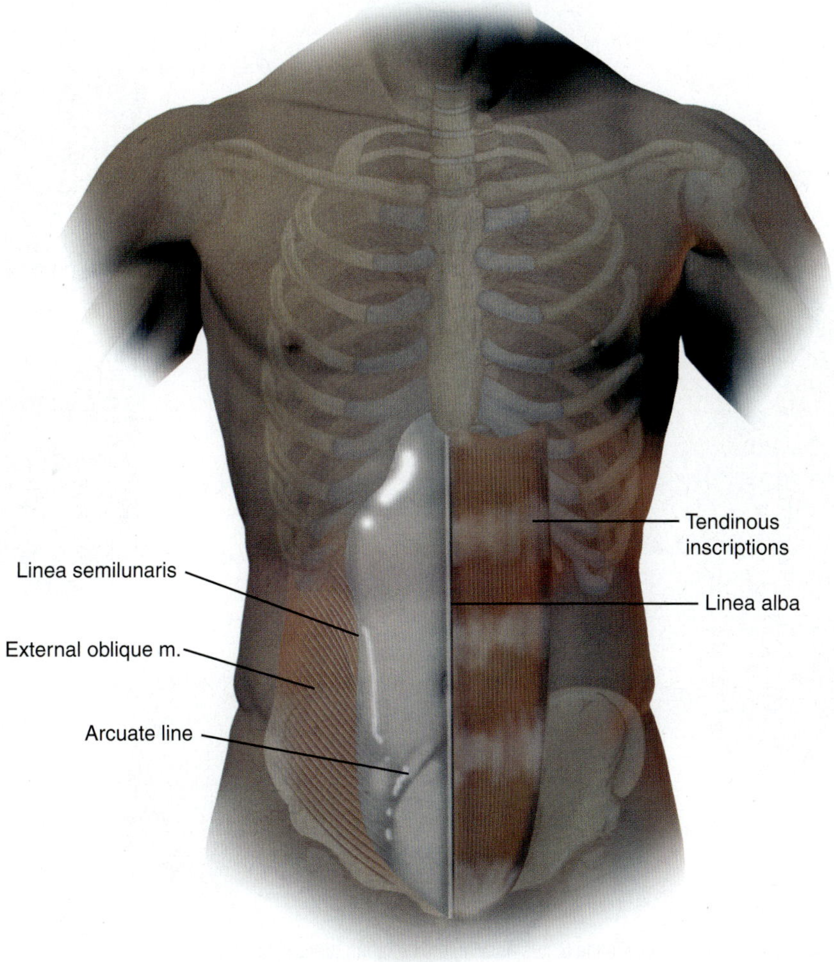

FIGURE 21.1 Schematic showing the key landmarks of the anterior abdominal wall and boundaries of the rectus sheath; the linea alba, the linea semilunaris, and the arcuate line.

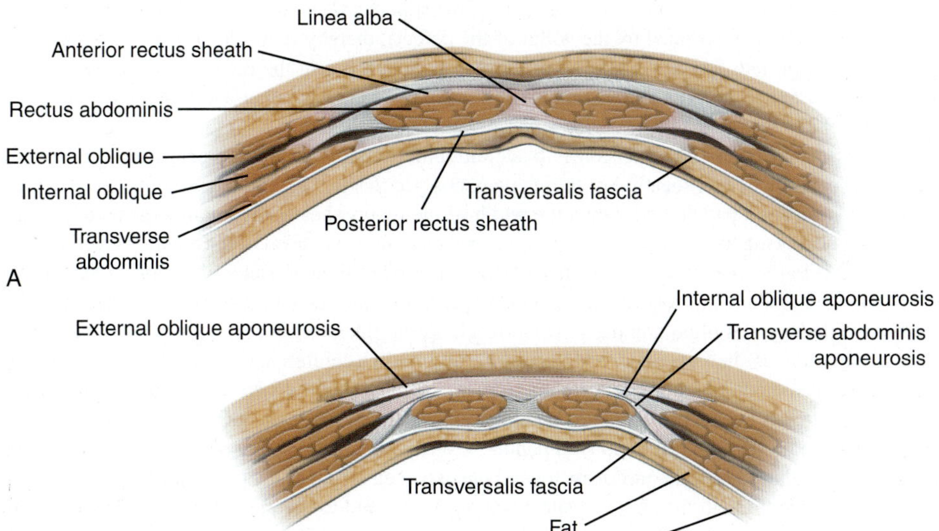

FIGURE 21.2 Diagram showing the contents of the rectus sheath and the layers of the sheath above and below the arcuate line. **A.** Relationships of the aponeuroses of the muscles of the anterior abdominal wall above the arcuate line. Note that the middle layer splits to surround the rectus muscles. **B.** The anatomy of the rectus sheath below the arcuate line. Note that all 3 aponeuroses pass anterior to the rectus muscles and only the travsversalis fascia is found posterior to the rectus muscles.

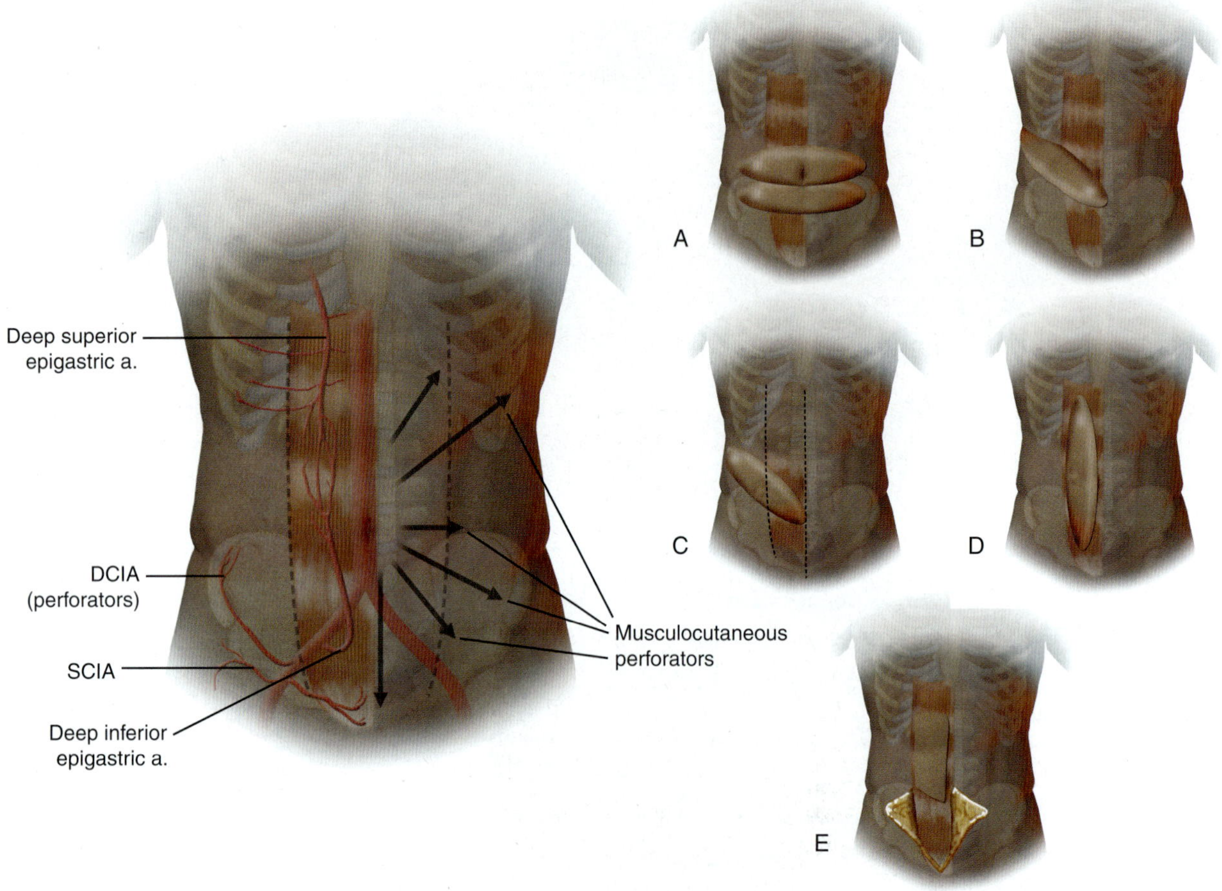

FIGURE 21.3 **A.** Diagram showing the primary vascular supply to the rectus muscle, the radiating periumbilical perforators, with the dominant vessels traveling in a trajectory toward the ipsilateral tip of the scapula. **B–F.** Options for the design of the skin paddle of the rectus abdominis myocutaneous flap.

mucosa or facial skin or obliterate the orbit. Often, multiple cutaneous paddles may be created to reconstruct different aspects of the defect. If a desired dimension of the skin paddle is such that its length exceeds the width of the rectus muscle (as determined by the width of the defect), thereby requiring a portion of the flap that is not directly overlying muscle, this extension of the flap is drawn out in the direction of the vector from the umbilicus to the scapular tip. This allows capture of the axial vessels that penetrate through the anterior rectus sheath and travel in a plexus in this posterior, superior, and lateral direction.

As the dissection begins, the incision is made circumferentially around the skin paddle to the level of the anterior layer of the rectus sheath. For those cutaneous paddles that extend lateral to the linea semilunaris because of the need for a paddle wider than the width of the rectus sheath, the initial incision to the depth of the deep fascia begins medial to the linea semilunaris and extends to the level of the anterior layer of the rectus sheath and lateral to this line, to the aponeurosis of the external oblique muscle. Elevation of the most lateral portion of the component can proceed from lateral to medial taking the cutaneous portion directly off of the aponeurosis of the external oblique muscle. Upon reaching the linea semilunaris, the anterior layer of rectus sheath that will support the cutaneous paddle can be outlined circumferentially and incised. Laterally, this incision is made just medial to the linea semilunaris. This requires that the fasciocutaneous extension that was mobilized lateral to this line be dissected just medial to this lateral anterior sheath incision. Following the anterior sheath incision around the proposed skin paddle, a vertical incision can be made from the midportion of the inferior edge of the skin paddle inferiorly toward the expected origin of the deep inferior epigastric vessels. This incision is made through the skin and subcutaneous tissue and to the anterior layer of the rectus sheath. The anterior layer of the rectus sheath is incised and opened exposing the entire rectus muscle on the ipsilateral side. The rectus muscle superior to the skin paddle can be identified through this opening in the anterior rectus sheath. The muscle at this point superiorly can be transected, and the muscle and attached skin paddle can then be mobilized out of the rectus sheath from superior to inferior.

As dissection proceeds inferiorly, it is important to take the entire muscle when the flap is harvested in this manner. At about the umbilicus, the deep inferior epigastric artery and vein will be visible on the posterior aspect of the rectus sheath. This dissection then continues inferiorly until the vessels can be dissected to the origin off of the external iliac vessels. The more inferiorly the dissection proceeds, the more lateral in relation to the rectus muscle the vessels become. To facilitate dissection at this point, it helps to divide the origin of the rectus abdominis muscle just above the symphysis pubis. This must be done with full knowledge and visualization of where the nutrient pedicle is located. This step improves the exposure and allows dissection of the inferior epigastric vessels fully to origin off the external iliac vessels. In most cases, this full pedicle dissection will result in the ability to harvest the deep inferior epigastric vein proximal to the point at which the two venae comitantes join to form a single vessel, which then empties into the external iliac vein. This larger caliber vein (3.5 mm) will facilitate an easier venous anastomosis.

Once the recipient site is ready, the flap can be harvested in the usual fashion with clamping of the artery first, then the vein, and then suture ligation of the origin of these vessels off of the external iliac vessels.

If a muscle-only flap is to be taken, a vertical incision is made paralleling the ipsilateral rectus muscle. This is carried down through skin and subcutaneous tissue down to the anterior layer of the rectus sheath. The rectus sheath can then be opened, the muscle transected superiorly and then mobilized out of the sheath, and the harvest completed, as described above.

Meticulous attention to closure of the donor site is important. In most cases, the anterior layer of the rectus sheath defect taken above the arcuate line can be closed directly with permanent Prolene sutures. If this cannot be accomplished, then typically one may repair this defect using Marlex mesh. The incisions in the anterior layer of the remaining rectus sheath then are closed directly using prolene suture. Suction drains are placed, and the subcutaneous and cutaneous tissues are closed.

Flap Inset

Usually adequate exposure of the palatal defect has been created by the ablative team. If a neck dissection has not been performed, the neck must be explored and the vessels isolated with recipient vessels identified for the microvascular anastomoses. An optimal vessel pair in the setting of palate reconstruction is the facial artery and vein, with the external jugular vein as a possible recipient vessel if necessary. An incision similar to what would be used for an excision of the submandibular gland may be used. Excision of the submandibular gland is usually done along with isolating the vessels, as it will help not only to isolate the facial artery and vein but also to create some working room, improving exposure to allow the microvascular anastomosis to be performed more easily. The main trunk of the facial artery can be preserved when excising the submandibular gland if care is taken only to divide the glandular branches of the facial artery as the main trunk passes over the superior portion of the gland. This will help to provide a longer recipient artery, keeping the anastomosis from being performed with the inferior border of the body of the mandible obstructing the view of the vessels through the microscope. For this reason, when the facial artery is used as a recipient vessel, the surgeon should not to be quick to divide the main trunk of the facial artery as it passes over the posterior belly of the digastric muscle as is frequently done in excision of the submandibular gland.

Once the vessels are isolated, a connection is created from the neck to the defect. In many cases that include resection of palate, facial skin, and orbit, only the inferior aspect of the tunnel need be created, as the resection has completed the most distal portion of the connection. There are essentially two different planes that can be used. In most cases, I prefer the subcutaneous tunnel. This dissection would proceed from the neck by dissecting in a supraplatysmal plane to the level of the midface. An advantage with this approach is that this supraplatysmal plane protects the marginal mandibular nerve and, as dissection proceeds more cephalad, all distal branches of the facial nerve. Once this dissection is adjacent to the defect, the tunnel must be connected with the recipient site of the midface, and typically, this does require a blunt dissection through the superficial musculoaponeurotic system into the oral cavity. This is done bluntly by spreading the tissue in the same direction as the branches of the facial nerve. The tunnel must be wide enough to allow the flap to be pulled from the neck into the midface or allow the vessels to be passed from the defect into the neck. Typically, a width equal to four fingerbreadths will be adequate. It is important to obtain meticulous hemostasis during creation of the tunnel to prevent bleeding into the tunnel postoperatively that could lead to a hematoma and flap compromise.

The second option for creating the tunnel connecting from the neck to the midface would be to use a deeper plane of dissection. This would require a subplatysmal dissection extending superiorly directly overlying the periosteum of the mandible and masseter muscle. This is a deeper layer of dissection and is deep to the branches of the facial nerve, thereby preventing potential injury to the nerve. Once the vessels are isolated and the tunnel is created, the flap is brought into the inset position. I prefer to pull the flap from the neck through the tunnel into the recipient site in the oral cavity. This approach allows certainty that there is not been any twisting of the vascular pedicle in the tunnel while the flap was being positioned. Retrograde placement of the vessels into the neck from the mouth by using a Penrose drain filled with normal saline is another approach.

This technique requires first passing the large Penrose drain from the defect into the neck, then clamping the drain inferiorly. The drain is then filled with normal saline, and the vascular pedicle is fed retrograde into the saline-filled drain. The drain with the pedicle contained in it is then slid through the tunnel

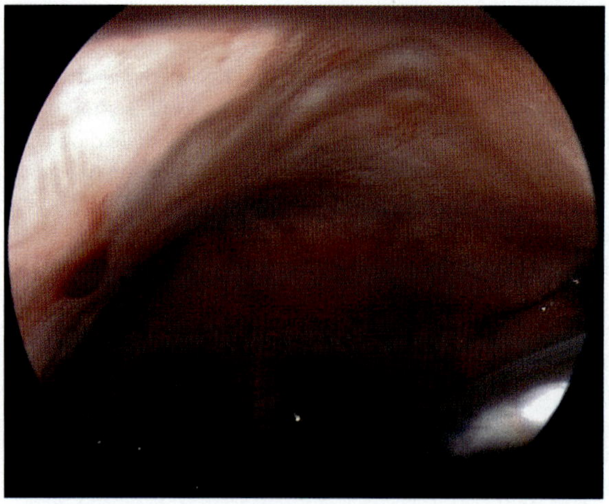

FIGURE 21.4 Appearance of right palate reconstructed with rectus muscle 18 months postoperatively.

into the defect. This technique is particularly useful if the distal component of the flap is too bulky to pass from the neck through the tunnel and into the defect, as can occur with some rectus abdominis myocutaneous flaps.

Vein grafts are rarely needed if the anastomosis is to be performed in the ipsilateral neck, given the considerable length of the rectus muscle that allows ample pedicle length. In cases in which there has been previous sacrifice of potential recipient vessels in the ipsilateral neck, a vein graft may be necessary to allow the anastomosis to be carried out in the contralateral neck.

In some cases, the superficial temporal vessels may be a very appropriate set of recipient vessels, depending on their caliber, which vessels remain available in the neck (such as in revision cases) and the exact details of the defect. Although the bigger the recipient vessels (as long as there is no size mismatch) the better, these vessels should be considered prior to using a vein graft to the contralateral neck.

The inset is relatively simple with suturing of the skin or muscle to the surrounding mucosal margins. This needs to be performed without redundancy to prevent prolapse or the muscle sagging into the oral cavity (Fig. 21.4). Attention should be paid to the point of the inset where the flap pedicle enters the defect such that a watertight repair is completed, decreasing the likelihood that saliva will enter the tunnel and result in an infection that could cause thrombosis at the anastomotic site that can rarely be salvaged in the setting of infection.

In cases where there is a large midface or orbital defect, the cutaneous paddle is to be used to obliterate the orbit and the midface, and the muscle proximal to the skin paddle is the component that is used to repair the palate defect (Fig. 21.5A and B). Once the flaps are vascularized, hemostasis is obtained and neck closure can proceed as well as closure of the facial skin.

POSTOPERATIVE MANAGEMENT

The donor site requires relatively little care. Suction drains are placed both into the donor site and into the deck, which are left in place until the output is less than 10 mL over 10-hour shift. I find the use of an abdominal binder to be helpful in early mobilization of the patient to help manage the pain at the donor site. Monitoring of the flap should be done in accordance with the operating surgeon's regimen. Most recently,

A

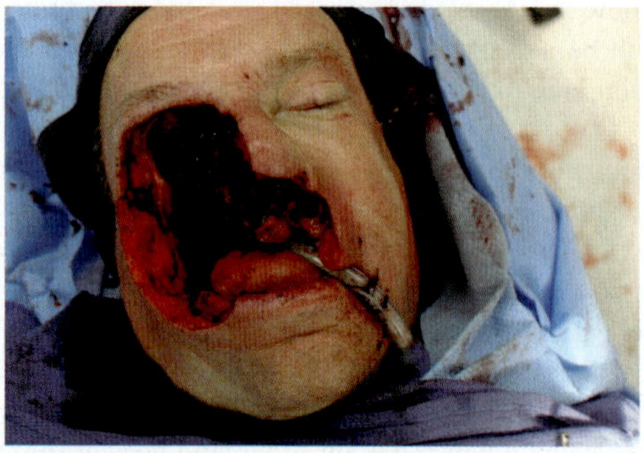

B

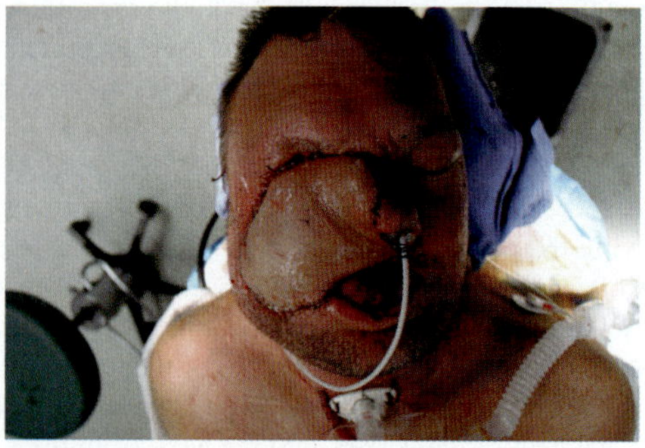

FIGURE 21.5 **A.** A patient with recurrent squamous cell carcinoma of the palate and maxilla. The lesion involves the infraorbital and eyelid skin and the entire maxillary sinus and palate. Defect involving orbit, facial skin, and entire right hard palate. **B.** Rectus abdominis myocutaneous flap obliterates the entire orbit and replaces resected infraorbital skin and provides lining for the ipsilateral hard palate.

I have incorporated the Synovis implantable venous Doppler, which is attached to one of the two rings of the venous coupler. This allows monitoring using a more objective signal and does not require the nursing staff (which does most of our flap monitoring) to go hunting for a signal using a handheld Doppler probe even when the flap vessel is marked with a suture. Monitoring is usually discontinued after 5 days, and the Doppler wire is removed at the bedside.

Patients are fed via a nasogastric tube and should be NPO for at least 5 to 7 days depending on the defect, the health of the recipient bed, and the confidence the team has in the healing at the flap/recipient site interface.

COMPLICATIONS

The two most significant complications related to this procedure are the development of a hernia at the donor site and flap compromise related to hematoma developing in the tunnel connecting the neck and the recipient site.

Hernias can be prevented by meticulous closure of all defects involving the anterior layer of the rectus sheath. It is also important to avoid using the anterior layer of the rectus sheath below the arcuate line as the posterior layer of the rectus sheath is significantly weaker and the risk of hernia at that location is greater. To prevent hematoma in the connecting tunnel, it is very important that hemostasis be obtained during creation of this tunnel and during flap harvest.

RESULTS

Typically, the use of rectus abdominis free flap achieves the desired goal of reconstructing the palate and separating the oral cavity from the nasal cavity. For more extensive ablations that include the palate and other midface components, it provides abundant soft tissue that can be useful for not only reconstructing the palate but also reconstructing the other related defects. This nonosseous flap is not the optimal reconstruction for defects in this area, but typically, the patients who undergo this reconstruction are unlikely to go on to full dental rehabilitation with an implant-borne dental prosthesis.

PEARLS

- Appropriate flap design is the most important point to keep in mind when using the rectus abdominis free flap for this specific defect.
- For patients who require reconstruction of the palate only and who do not necessarily require reconstruction of the midface or orbit, a muscle-only flap is ideal. This provides very well-vascularized muscle that will beautifully and reliably reconstruct the palatal defect.

PITFALLS

- Donor site morbidity can be significant if there is a breakdown at the donor site, so careful attention to the closure of the donor site is important to avoid donor site morbidity.
- It is critical to be certain that the tunnel is appropriately placed and that appropriate hemostasis is obtained.

INSTRUMENTS TO HAVE AVAILABLE

- Standard head and neck surgical set
- General surgery tray
- Marlex mesh

SUGGESTED READING

Pennington DG, Pelly AD. The rectus abdominis myocutaneous free flap. *Br J Plast Surg* 1980;33:277–282.

Chicarilli ZN, Davey LM. Rectus abdominis myocutaneous free-flap reconstruction following a cranio-orbital-maxillary resection for neurofibrosarcoma. *Plast Reconstr Surg* 1987;80:726–731.

Urken ML, Turk JB, Weinberg H, et al. The rectus abdominis free flap in head and neck reconstruction. *Arch Otolaryngol Head Neck Surg* 1991;117(9):1031.

Nakatsuka T, Harii K, Yamada A, et al. Versatility of a free inferior rectus abdominis flap for head and neck reconstruction: analysis of 200 cases. *Plast Reconstr Surg* 1994;93(4):762–769.

Yokoo S, Komori T, Furudoi S, et al. Indications for vascularized free rectus abdominis musculocutaneous flap in oromandibular region in terms of efficiency of anterior rectus sheath. *Microsurgery* 2003;23:96–102.

22 THE TOTAL HARD PALATE DEFECT: ILIAC CREST WITH INTERNAL OBLIQUE FREE FLAP

James S. Brown

INTRODUCTION

There is a reluctance to use the iliac crest donor site for free tissue transfer because of the perceived donor site morbidity, although the site remains popular for nonvascularized grafts. There are publications, however, that have compared this site to the fibula, and both can cause problems. Reconstruction of the maxilla, including the maxillary alveolus, hard palate, maxillary buttress, orbital floor, or orbit itself, results in a varied defect that has been classified (Fig. 22.1), and this is regularly referred to in this chapter.

Low maxillectomy defects not resulting in loss of alar support can be adequately reconstructed with a fibula flap which has been well described, or adequately obturated especially with implant-retained prostheses. If the resection involves the orbital floor (Class III) or the removal of the eye (Class IV), then obturation can give poor results especially after radiotherapy, and reconstruction of the defect is generally preferred. The main methods of free tissue transfer described involve the iliac crest (deep circumflex iliac artery [DCIA]), fibula (peroneal artery), and scapula (circumflex scapula or thoracodorsal angular artery [TDAA]). This chapter describes the use of the DCIA with internal oblique for the reconstruction of Class II-IVb-d defects.

HISTORY

A history of prior surgery or injury in the area of the donor site should be sought. When considering the DCIA flap for maxillary reconstruction, it is important to determine if the patient has a history of gait disturbance or deep vein thrombosis.

PHYSICAL EXAMINATION

The physical examination should focus on identifying evidence of prior surgery or injury in the area of the donor site. Not uncommonly, male patients may have undergone repair of an inguinal hernia. Prior surgery or injury to this region may compromise the reliability of the flap, and an alternate donor site should be considered.

INDICATIONS

The DCIA with internal oblique can provide a high-quality reconstruction of the maxillary bone for all the defects (Class I-IV), and the internal oblique muscle provides an ideal lining for the oral cavity and nasal passage. This flap is superior to the others, especially in the Class III defect when the orbital floor is removed but the orbit retained. The flap can be harvested as a tripartite perforator flap with a vascularized bone graft, muscle flap, and skin paddle.

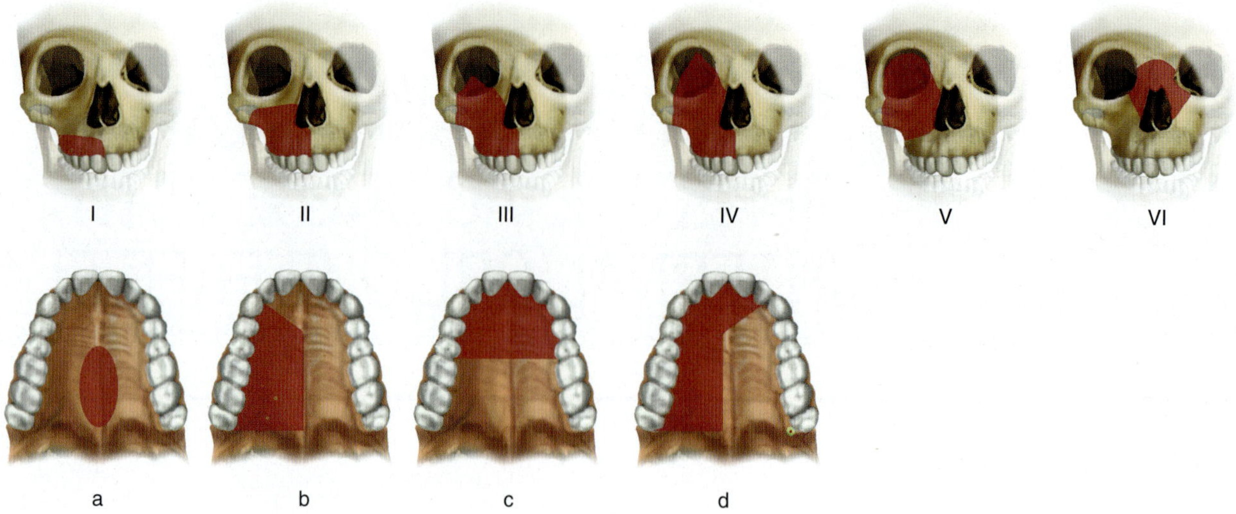

FIGURE 22.1 Classification of palatal, maxillary, and midface defects.

CONTRAINDICATIONS

The vascular pedicle is short, and the flap harvest requires care, making use of the flap less popular. The advantage of the flap is the size of the bone and ability to shape it to the defect (nasal and orbital), as well as the use of muscle to line the nasal cavity and sinus and provide a very natural result for palatal reconstruction. However, when the neck is depleted of vessels, an alternative donor site with a longer vascular pedicle should be considered, or vein grafts should be prepared.

PREOPERATIVE PLANNING

Preparing the Recipient Site

The principle of selective neck dissection and postoperative radiotherapy in controlling regional recurrence is well established, and as a result, the facial artery and vein can be retained in continuity when preparing recipient vessels in the neck. In general, the pedicle will not reach below the inferior border of the mandible, and so the anastomoses are usually performed above the inferior border being careful to protect the mandibular branch of the facial nerve. I have used superficial temporal vessels occasionally, but it is sometimes possible to divide the retromandibular vein and bring that forward for the venous anastomosis. For either of these options, it is essential to preserve the facial vein to allow drainage through the internal jugular vein. In my experience, the majority of vein grafts have been used for inadequate arterial flow through the facial artery. Papaverine can be used to treat vessel spasm, and if this is not successful, the arterial anastomosis is redone and then an IV bolus of 5,000 units of heparin is given just prior to the release of clamps, after completion of the redo anastomosis. Using these measures has negated the need for vein grafts in the arterial system for the last 5 years.

SURGICAL TECHNIQUE

The skin markings include the pubic tubercle medially, the iliac vessels, anterior superior iliac spine (ASIS), iliac crest, costal margin, proposed osteotomies and internal oblique muscle, and the incision (Fig. 22.2). It is possible to place the anterior osteotomy as much as 40 mm posterior to the ASIS for a Class II-IVb defect as the length of the bone is not a factor. This may not be possible for Class II-IVd defects crossing the midline as the reconstruction needs to span from the zygomatic buttress to the premolar region controlaterally. If raising a skin perforator flap, then the perforators are situated 74 mm (range 50 to 105) posteriorly from the ASIS and 8 mm (range 1 to 35) above the iliac crest and can be identified with a handheld Doppler. It is perfectly reasonable to raise skin or adipose tissue as a perforator component to the internal oblique muscle and the iliac crest to replace loss of facial skin. The incision runs about 20 mm above the line of the iliac crest from the iliacs to posterior to the planned posterior osteotomy. As with all incisions, this can be extended if better exposure is required. If including a perforator skin island, then plan this island around the likely perforator following Doppler identification.

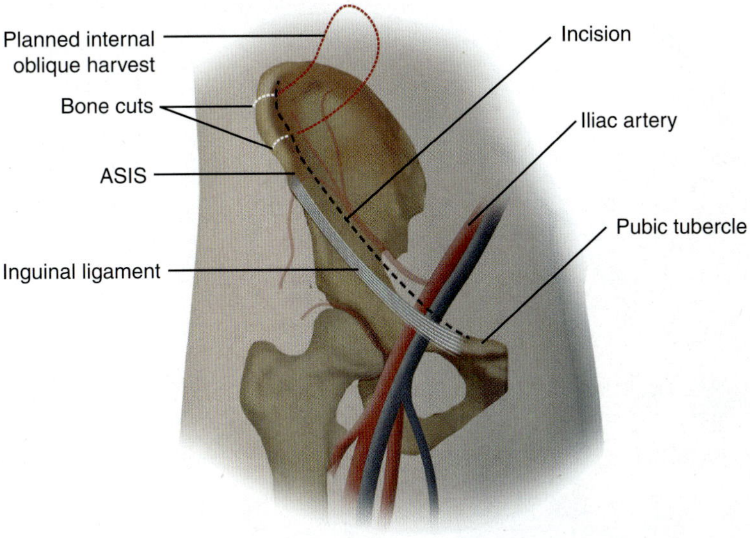

FIGURE 22.2
Exposure of the vascular pedicle can be accomplished with an incision along the iliac crest axis.

Incise the skin, and if raising a perforator flap, identify the perforator before exposing the external oblique muscle with its fibers running in a line from the costal margin to the pubic tubercle. At this point, dissect out the perforator vessel to where it should enter the DCIA and vein just anterior to the ASIS. Next incise the external oblique muscle about 20 mm above the iliac crest from the iliacs to the posterior osteotomy. This plane between the external and internal oblique is easy to separate as there is only a thin layer of adipose tissue. It is best to have access to the internal oblique muscle as far as the costal margin posterosuperiorly and the rectus sheath anteriorly. Next, outline the muscle to be harvested (Fig. 22.3) and begin to incise the fibers of the internal oblique muscle running in the opposite direction to the external oblique muscle where the muscle is thickest about 40 mm above the iliac crest posteriorly. This dissection is best done sharply with a scalpel to avoid damage to the ascending branch of the DCIA that lies in the fascia between the muscles. For this reason, it is essential to keep the fascia with the internal oblique muscle to leave fresh-looking muscle, which is the transversalis (fibers running horizontally) exposed. In most cases, it is easy to see the ascending branch on the undersurface of the internal oblique muscle. The posterior incision goes all the way to the iliac crest, but the anterior incision stops about 20 mm above the ASIS and can then be continued toward the iliac vessels. The DCI vessels lie in the transversalis fascia between the ASIS and the iliacs, but it is best to follow the ascending branch that takes you to the DCIA. It is not necessary to disrupt the attachments to the ASIS or the inguinal ligament as the vessels are accessed from the abdominal side. The pedicle dissection to the iliacus can now be completed, noting that the DCIV often descends just as it enters the iliac vein, before going back to the iliac crest and incising transversalis to reveal iliacus lying more inferiorly.

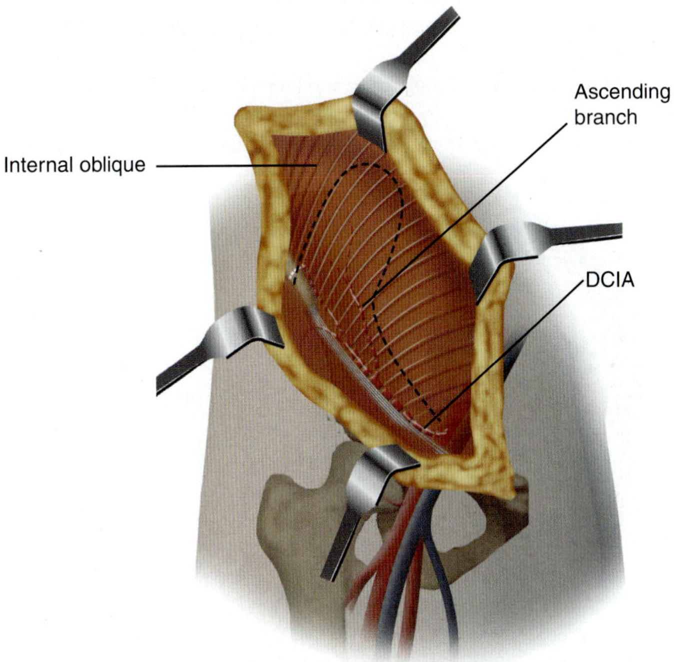

FIGURE 22.3
The DCIA and ascending branch shown lie under the internal oblique but can be easily dissected once the muscle has been incised as shown.

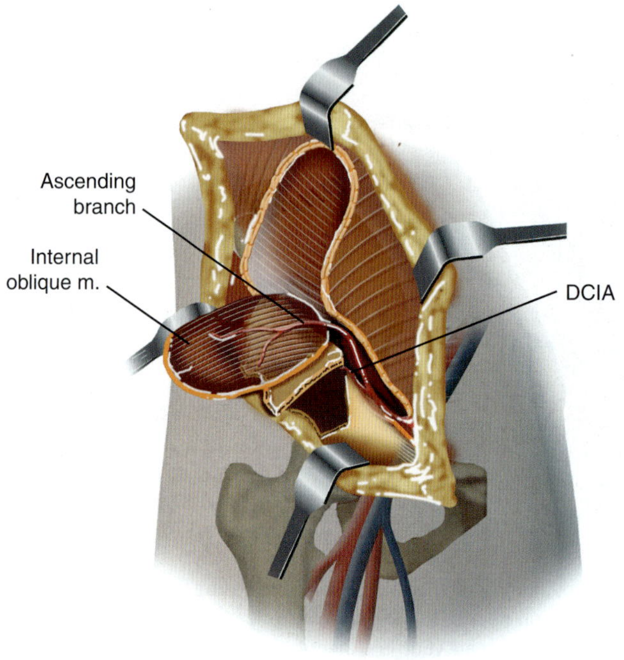

FIGURE 22.4
Once raised, the flap can be left pedicled until the time of inset.

The anterior osteotomy has to be done from the lateral side of the iliac crest. It is better to pass an instrument down the abdominal side of the iliac crest to ensure protection of the pedicle prior to this anterior vertical osteotomy. Then make the posterior osteotomy to the depth required. At this point, the iliacus muscle can be incised at the planned depth of the osteotomy from the abdominal side. It is often easier to make the osteotomy from the abdominal side especially for longer bone spans such as reconstructing the mandible. Make sure you can see the anterior and posterior osteotomies at their depth prior to making the osteotomy to release the bone toward the abdomen and the side of the pedicle. At this point, the flap is raised and can be left on the pedicle prior to transfer to the head and neck (Fig. 22.4).

The ipsilateral iliac crest is raised so that the pedicle lies posteriorly and the lateral side of the bone is also lateral in the reconstructive site. This ensures that the crest of the ridge replaces the alveolus and the deeper part of the iliac bone can be fashioned to reconstruct the piriform aperture of the nose, lateral nasal bones, and the orbital floor to articulate with the buttress of the zygoma. The muscle then lies in the region of the hard palate, and there is sufficient bulk to obturate the sinus defect, form a neopalate, and reline the nasal cavity (Fig. 22.5). Horizontal placement of the bone means there is insufficient bone to support the alar region and there is little room for the muscle that is best used to reform the palate and obturate the dead space. A miniplate placed at the maxillary alveolus and the zygomatic buttress will provide sufficient fixation. If there is a need for reconstruction of the nasal bones or orbital floor, then nonvascularized bone can be used from the donor site although titanium mesh is often preferred for the orbital floor.

In complex defects, it is an advantage to prepare a sterolithographic model so that templates can be prepared to help especially with reconstruction of the orbit. The microvascular anastomoses can be carried out at this point. Some surgeons are concerned that the vessels pass on the lateral surface of the mandible and

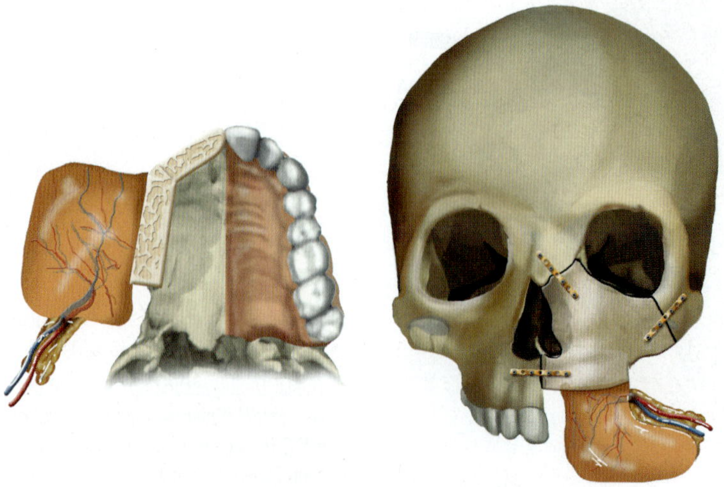

FIGURE 22.5
Vertical orientation of the graft for defects of the vertical maxilla.

TABLE 22.1 Comparison of Suitability for Composite Free Flaps to Reconstruct and Provide Rehabilitation for Maxillary Defects

Class of Defect	Fibula	Scapula (Circumflex Scapula Artery)	Scapula (TDAA)	Iliac Crest (DCIA)
Class IIb-d	Best option if alar support not required	No real advantage for this option		Best if poor alar support
Class IIIb	Can be used if inserted using Rodriguez's technique	There is reasonable height but poor muscle option	Good option but implant-retained dental rehabilitation unlikely	Best option as good height of bone and adequate width for oral rehabilitation
Class IIId	Very difficult to cross midline and support the orbit and nasal region	Reasonable but less chance of oral rehabilitation and poor muscle option	Unlikely that sufficient length of bone will span across the midline	Sufficient height and length to span the defect and support the orbit and nasal region
Class IVb	Difficult to plan skin islands and poor muscle bulk	May be useful if facial skin requires reconstruction	Good option especially if facial skin required but dental rehabilitation difficult	Good option with high chance of implant-retained oral rehabilitation
Class IVd	Not possible to include span	Reasonable bone length and good option if facial skin is required	Insufficient bone length	Sufficient bone and muscle but less good if facial skin is required

therefore potentially can be compressed against the bone. In our experience, this has not been a problem. The last two failures with this flap for maxillary reconstruction were in April and June 2004 both for vein grafts, which were inadequate in size for the vein in one case and a severe kink in the arterial system in the other.

In the management of these patients, it is essential to involve the prosthodontist who will be advising the patient on both dental and facial rehabilitation. Patients will wish to know whether it is possible to have their dentition restored and in Class IV cases, the chance of an orbital prosthesis. The composite flap options of fibula, scapula, and iliac crest are well known, and in Table 22.1, I have tried to indicate the various defects and how they can best be reconstructed.

The DCIA is still not a first choice in many units even for the Class IIIb,d type defects for which I think it is ideal. The morbidity of the donor site is often stated as a reason not to consider this option, but it is probably because the flap harvest is not straightforward, and the reconstructive surgeon may not be familiar with this option. In Europe, the DCIA has been used extensively for reconstruction of the mandible, and so adapting the technique for the maxilla is less of a problem. I routinely incorporate the internal oblique muscle in the reconstruction to ensure a dual blood supply of the graft and to use the muscle as a marker in case of flap compromise. If the aim of the reconstruction is to restore form and function, then this donor site provides the best bone option in terms of height and width. The ability to raise the internal oblique muscle and use the skin as a perforator flap adds to the versatility of the flap.

In my own unit, we generally keep the DCIA option for those cases in which dental rehabilitation is a primary aim and for Class III defects when we think it is the best option for orbital support, as well as easy articulation with the nasal region and the zygomatic buttress. The muscle is ideally placed to obturate the sinus region, line the nasal cavity, and provide a very natural healed hard palate. There are reports of using the TDAA scapula tip option, but the bone is thin, and although the face and orbit can be addressed, there is little chance of implant-retained dental rehabilitation. The main reason for the popularity of this option is the long pedicle, which makes the flap easier to insert and potentially more reliable. I have lost two bone elements of the flap, which is supplied both by the angular branch of the thoracodorsal as well as by the circumflex scapula arteries. Extending the bone harvest beyond the area of angular artery supply indicated by Senerivatne may be risky, and similarly, osteotomies to shape the bone may compromise the blood supply. Rodriguez has described an ingenious method of insetting the fibula for this defect, but this requires favorable perforators to plan the skin islands and considerable ability with this flap.

Closure of the donor site is an essential part of the operation and, in my view, poor closure is the main reason for excess donor site morbidity if the attachments of the ASIS have been kept intact. Using PDS, suture the transversalis muscle to the iliacus, being careful not to pierce the peritoneum. There is then a defect of the internal oblique muscle that must be reinforced with mersilene mesh and secured with Prolene (Fig 22.6). Small holes are prepared in the cut region of the iliac crest, and the mesh sutured securely to the bone and residual muscle to close the defect. A suction drain can be placed over the mesh prior to closing the internal oblique and then the skin in a four-layered closure.

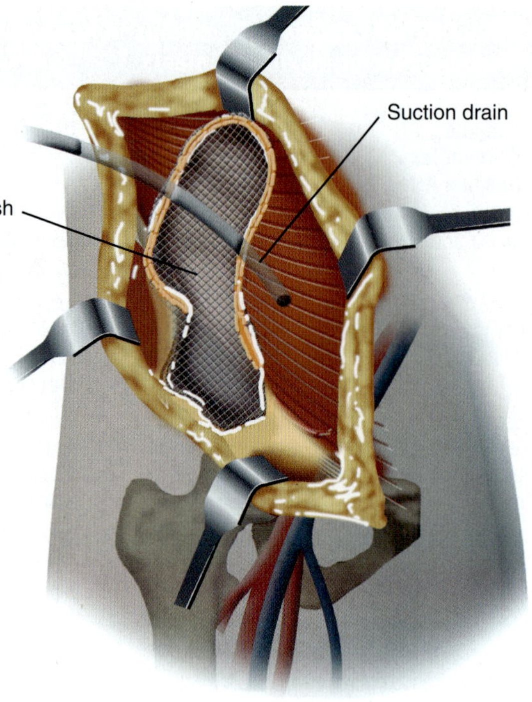

FIGURE 22.6
Typically mesh is not required; however if necessary it can be used to aid the closure.

POSTOPERATIVE MANAGEMENT

There are no special measures to take postoperatively, but as the muscle can be difficult to monitor, I often use an implantable Doppler to aid flap surveillance. It is important to make sure that bowel sounds return after a short ileus and that there is a soft abdomen on palpation.

COMPLICATIONS

Complications are related to the reconstruction itself or the donor site. The short pedicle is responsible for most complications because revascularization of the flap in the vessel-depleted neck can be a challenge. Whenever we use this donor site for maxillary reconstruction, a heightened sense of vigilance and awareness is required because of the technical challenges related to placing the bone graft into position, orienting the muscle flap, and ensuring that the vascular pedicle is in an appropriate position to allow for revascularization.

RESULTS

The bone graft stock is excellent for accommodating osseointegrated implants, and the extensive bone graft will also serve to reconstruct extensive maxillary defects that involve the orbit, zygoma, and/or the alveolus. There has been no comparative data to other options of reconstruction, and so no claims can be made with robust data. The claims in this article are based on opinion, but if the technique is used successfully, the results will not disappoint.

PEARLS

- Ipsilateral iliac crest to the defect for an ideal curvature of the bone and the best part of the bone (crest) for replacement of the alveolus
- DCIA with internal oblique muscle is probably the best option for Class IIIb,d defects requiring dental rehabilitation.
- The use of muscle to line the nasal cavity and restore the hard palate is ideal for a natural-looking palate and implant–bone interface.
- Retain the facial vessels in continuity when preparing the recipient site.
- The anterior osteotomy can be made 40 cm posterior to the ASIS to ensure a longer pedicle without compromising the vascularity of the flap and the muscle quality.

- Close cooperation with a maxillofacial prosthodontist is essential.
- This surgery is very complex and specialist units with multiple reconstructive options and experience would best serve such cases.

PITFALLS

- Vein grafting of the arterial system may be required if the flap cannot be perfused with pharmacologic assistance.
- Donor site morbidity will be increased if the attachments of the ASIS are disrupted and there is poor attention to detail and failure to reinforce the internal oblique muscle on closure.
- Attention to hemostasis is even more important than in standard surgery, and so take your time and maintain a dry field while harvesting the flap.

INSTRUMENTS TO HAVE AVAILABLE

- Standard head and neck surgical set
- Reciprocating saw
- Miniplating system
- Marlex mesh

SUGGESTED READING

Triana RJ, Uglesic V, Virag M, et al. Microvascular free flap reconstruction in patients with partial and total maxillectomy defects. *Arch Facial Plast Surg* 2000;2:91–101.

Brown JS, Jones DC, Summerwill A, et al. Vascularised iliac crest with internal oblique muscle for immediate reconstruction after maxillectomy. *Br J Oral Maxillofac Surg* 2002;40:183–190.

Rodriguez ED, Martin M, Bluebond-Langner R, et al. Microsurgical reconstruction of post-traumatic high-energy maxillary defects: establishing the effectiveness of early reconstruction. *Plast Reconstr Surg* 2007;120:103s–117s.

Clark JR, Vesely M, Gilbert R. Scapula angle osteomyogenous flap in postmaxillectomy reconstruction: defect, reconstruction, shoulder function, and harvest technique. *Head Neck* 2008;30:10–20.

Brown JS, Shaw RJ. Reconstruction of the maxilla and midface: introducing a new classification. *Lancet Oncol* 2010;11:1001–1008.

23 THE HEMIMAXILLECTOMY DEFECT: THE SCAPULAR TIP FREE FLAP

Ralph W. Gilbert

INTRODUCTION

The scapula has been used for maxillary reconstruction and offers several advantages when compared to other reconstructive options. These advantages primarily relate to the chimeric nature of the subscapular vascular system allowing for harvest of multiple, independent skin paddles, serratus muscle with or without rib, latissimus dorsi muscle, and up to 14 cm of lateral scapular bone. This makes it an excellent option for the reconstruction of complex composite defects of the head and neck with large soft tissue requirements. In reconstructing a hemimaxillectomy defect, the advantage of the scapular tip free tissue transfer is the shape of the osseous component of the flap and how it mirrors the shape of the resected maxilla and palate. The primary disadvantage of the traditional scapular flap based on the circumflex scapular artery is the short vascular pedicle, which has led to increasing interest in the scapular tip supplied by the thoracodorsal system of vessels. The tip of the scapular flap is supplied by the angular branch of the thoracodorsal artery rather than the circumflex scapular artery. This design increases the available pedicle length (up to 12 to 14 cm) and allows for the use of the serratus anterior and teres major musculature along with the potential for integrating a latissimus dorsi myocutaneous flap or a thoracodorsal artery perforator flap.

HISTORY

Malignant lesions of the maxilla include adenocarcinoma arising from minor salivary glands, squamous cell carcinoma of the palate, or the maxillary sinus primary osseous malignancies such as osteosarcoma or odontogenic tumors. (Fig. 23.1). Patients may have a visible lesion of the oral cavity with pain, loose dentition, and bleeding. Occasionally, pain and paresthesias may indicate a cancer of the maxillary sinus that is not obvious in the oral cavity. It is important to elicit a history of prior surgery or trauma to the donor site.

PHYSICAL EXAMINATION

The physical examination of patients presenting with malignant tumors of the maxilla is relatively straightforward. The extent of the lesion should be evaluated intraorally to determine the size of the lesion and structures involved such as the maxillary alveolus, soft palate, buccal mucosa, and/or pharynx. Evaluation of the patient's dentition for resection and reconstructive planning is paramount. The donor site must be examined to evaluate for signs of trauma or prior surgery. Flexible fiberoptic examination should be performed to evaluate the involvement of the floor of the nose as well as the nasal cavity and middle meatus.

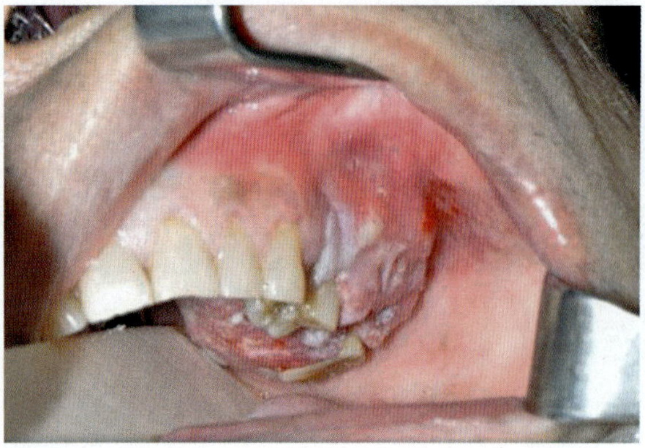

FIGURE 23.1
Squamous cell carcinoma of the maxilla requiring hemimaxillectomy and reconstruction.

INDICATIONS

Indications for maxillary reconstruction are listed below. The most common indications are malignant lesions of the maxilla, usually squamous cell carcinoma. Additional malignant or benign lesions are common indications for maxillectomy. Congenital anomalies requiring free tissue transfer are relatively rare.

- Malignant lesions of the maxilla (squamous cell carcinoma [SCCA], cancers of minor salivary gland origin, osteosarcoma)
- Benign lesions of the maxilla (ameloblastoma, giant cell tumors, meningioma)
- Traumatic avulsion/gunshot injuries
- Congenital anomalies

CONTRAINDICATIONS

There are no specific contraindications to maxillary reconstruction with the scapular osteomyogenous free tissue transfer. General medical conditions may prohibit complex reconstructive efforts, and a discussion with the patient regarding the use of an obturator should be undertaken in these cases. The selection of a reconstructive approach versus obturation requires a careful evaluation of the benefits of reconstruction versus the benefits of obturation. In general terms, the more extensive the defect, the more likely I am to recommend reconstruction given the low probability of satisfactory retention of a denture or an obturator. In smaller defects, reconstruction may be considered by patients who have the resources to consider osseointegrated implants for dental rehabilitation. In the rare event that the scapular donor site is contraindicated by previous trauma or surgery, other osseous reconstructive options may be entertained.

PREOPERATIVE PLANNING

The preoperative planning for maxillectomy and reconstruction is relatively standard. Nevertheless, several considerations merit mention.

Anatomy

The circumflex scapular arterial system provides the vascular supply to a number of reconstructive options related to the donor site (Fig. 23.2). The circumflex artery arises from the subscapular artery, which is a branch of the axillary artery in the upper thorax. The scapula and surrounding muscle are supplied by the distal muscular and periosteal branches of the circumflex scapular artery. The cutaneous territories overlying the scapula receive blood supply via the transverse and descending cutaneous branches. The blood supply of the latissimus dorsi muscle is derived from the thoracodorsal artery, which arises from the circumflex scapular artery. Distal angular branches of the thoracodorsal artery supply the tip of scapula, and these form the basis of the scapular tip free tissue transfer.

Imaging Studies

The imaging studies required for successful maxillary reconstruction will vary depending on the situation; however, in general, computed tomography with contrast enhancement is relatively standard. The preoperative imaging required is usually driven by the ablative surgical plan, as imaging of the scapular donor site vascular anatomy is unnecessary.

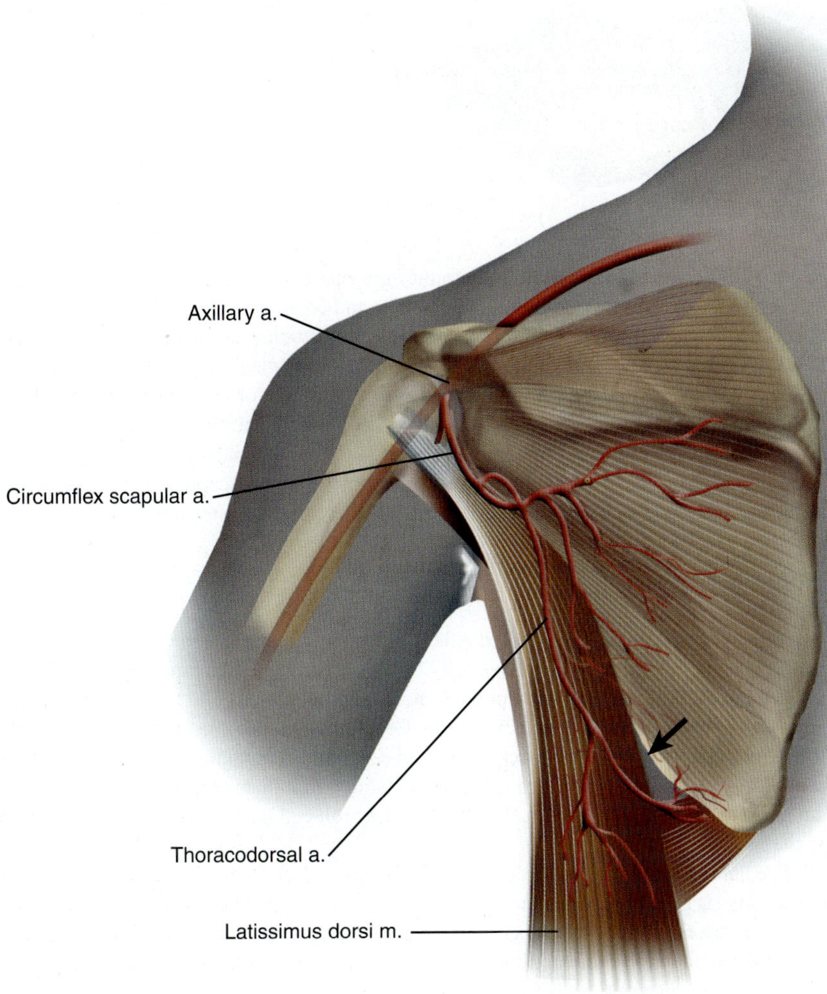

FIGURE 23.2 Anatomy of the subscapular arterial system. The *arrow* points to the angular branch.

SURGICAL TECHNIQUE

Flap Harvest

The patient is placed on a suction bean bag positioner prior to induction of anesthesia. After induction of anesthesia, the torso is turned approximately 45 degrees and the pelvis to 30 degrees. Access is sufficient when the tip of the scapula can be palpated easily, as shown in Figure 23.3. The contralateral arm is cradled without pressure on the shoulder, and all pressure points are padded. A pillow is placed between the knees and padding placed circumferentially around the feet and ankles. The patient is then secured with straps and wide tape to the operating table so that the table can be rotated without patient movement. Surgical technique starts with the incision design. If there is no plan for harvesting the skin, the incision is placed along the posterior axillary line. The anterior border of latissimus dorsi is identified, and the dorsal surface of the latissimus is mobilized to allow retraction if necessary (Fig. 23.4). Dissection of the pedicle will be anteromedial to latissimus (however, the osteotomies will be performed by retracting it anteriorly).

The vascular anatomy is then defined. The anterior border of the latissimus is mobilized and the teres major muscle identified. The branches of the thoracodorsal artery to the serratus muscle are identified and followed in an antegrade dissection identifying the branches to the latissimus dorsi muscle. The branching pattern of the circumflex scapular system is somewhat variable, and great care must be taken to avoid dividing individual branches until the entire anatomy and the position of the angular branch is identified. The angular branch usually arises from the thoracodorsal artery although it may also arise from the branch to the serratus muscle or form a trifurcation with these vessels. There is some variability in the distal course of the angular branch, and there may be multiple branches supplying the tip of the scapula as well as the serratus anterior muscle. If a separate branch supplying teres major is identified, it is preserved. If a combination scapula or parascapular cutaneous flap is planned, the proximal pedicle needs to be defined, as the thoracodorsal artery arises directly from the axillary artery in approximately 5% of cases.

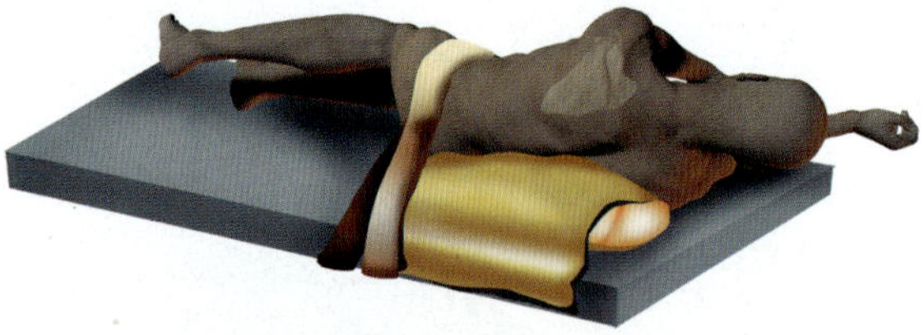

FIGURE 23.3
Positioning of patient for angular tip of scapular flap (note vacuum bag positioner and taping of patient to prevent movement with rotation).

The pedicle is fully mobilized before the osteotomies are made to avoid injury to the blood supply. The placement of the osteotomies depends on the desired quantity and contour. The length of bone supplied by the angular branch is approximately 6 cm based on cadaveric injection studies; however, based on our experience, larger amounts of bone may be harvested safely (up to 10 cm). I usually leave a small cuff of serratus anterior muscle anteroinferiorly to protect the angular branch and vary the volume of the teres major cuff dependent on the need for volume filling or revascularization in the maxillary defect. The final dissection of the pedicle of the flap is taken to the circumflex scapular vessels, with assessment of the viability of the flap before division. Serratus anterior, subscapularis, and teres major muscles are reattached to the scapular bone using drill holes and heavy absorbable suture. A large suction drain is used because of the extensive muscle dissection.

Maxillary Reconstruction

The osseous component of the flap can be oriented either horizontally to replace the palatoalveolar complex in infrastructure resections (Fig. 23.5A and B) or vertically to restore the zygomaticomaxillary and nasomaxillary buttress (Fig. 23.6A and B). The muscular component, including the serratus and teres major muscles, can be used as a vascularized covering for the bone (Fig. 23.7). Osteotomies are not generally recommended due to the periosteal blood supply, however "greenstick" fractured segments maintaining the periosteal blood supply, and improve contouring. Fixation is performed using rigid titanium miniplates from 1.5 to 2.0 mm, and the flap is secured to the residual maxilla and zygoma. The floor of the orbit can be reconstructed with additional bone from the donor site when necessary.

The vascular pedicle is then tunneled through the buccal space deep to the facial nerve and over the mandible. Vascular anastomosis is then performed using a single recipient artery and vein, most commonly the facial artery and vein. Other vessels such as the superficial temporal system or the superior thyroid vessels may be used depending on the length of the pedicle. With the angular modification, vein grafting is not usually required.

POSTOPERATIVE MANAGEMENT

Postoperative management of the patient is relatively straightforward with standard flap monitoring protocols using the Doppler pen, and the external skin paddle if present. For muscle flaps allowed to mucosalize the color of the intraoral component will often appear dark and/or purple, and this is not usually a sign of vascular compromise. The duration of NPO status varies depending on the patient and the reconstruction with longer periods indicated in the setting of preoperative radiotherapy. After 5 to 7 days, a soft diet is generally initiated. Chlorhexidine rinse may be used without detriment to the reconstruction. Nasal obstruction is common postoperatively, and intranasal saline spray may be used for comfort and to prevent crusting.

Regarding the donor site, shoulder movement commences on the first postoperative day, and a shoulder sling is unnecessary. Shoulder abduction exercises are performed daily after discharge. Formal physiotherapy is not required, but patients are advised that shoulder movement may take 6 months for full recovery.

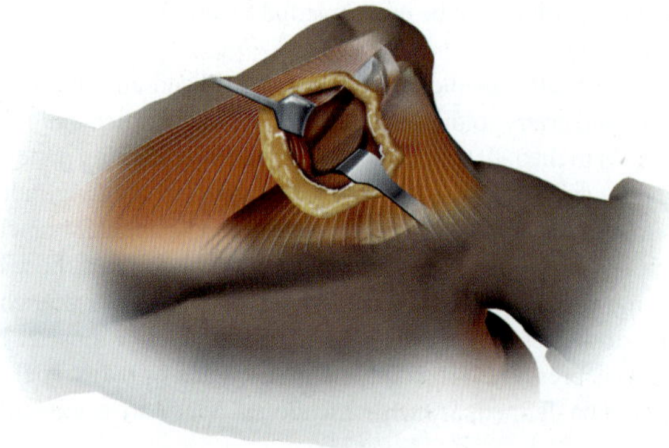

FIGURE 23.4
Surgical anatomy latissimus muscle is retracted anteriorly demonstrating the teres major muscle and lateral border of the scapula.

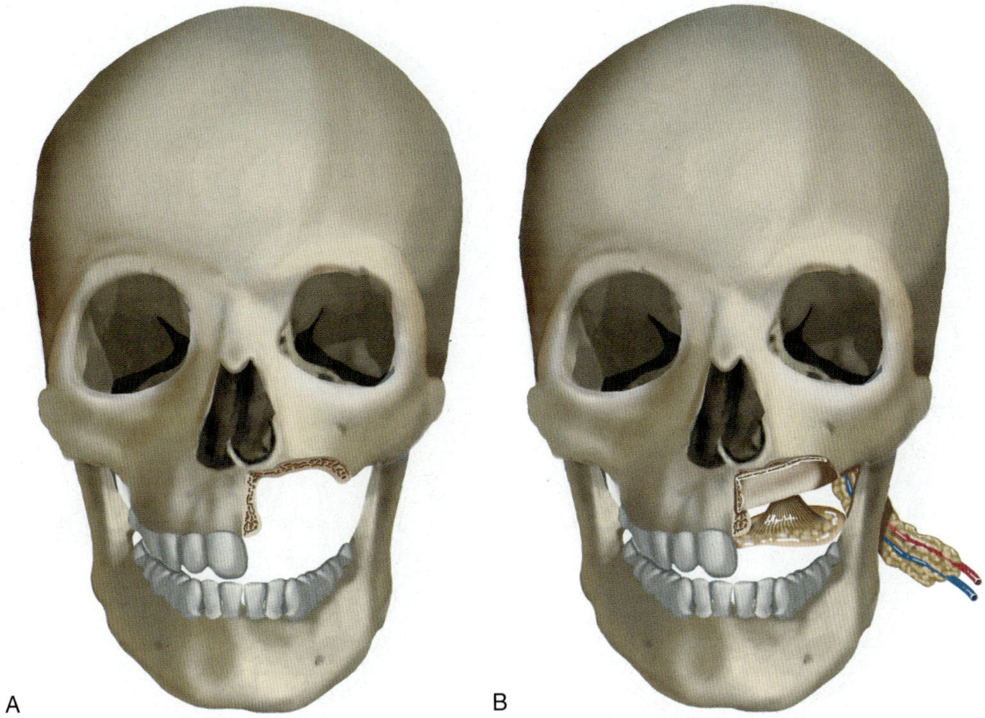

FIGURE 23.5 A. Demonstrates the infrastructure defect. **B.** Demonstrates the horizontal orientation of the scapula bone graft.

COMPLICATIONS

Complications from maxillary reconstruction with the scapular free tissue transfer include infection, hematoma, and seroma at the donor site. The scapular donor site commonly requires prolonged drainage due to the large muscle surface dissected during harvest. Long-term complications of maxillary reconstruction include malposition of the globe, ectropion, epiphora, palatal fistula, and aesthetic compromise due to inadequate bulk. Palatal fistula after reconstruction with muscle occurs in approximately 15% to 20% of patients; however, the majority close spontaneously, and additional surgical closure is rarely required. Exposure of the hardware occurs rarely and usually after radiation therapy. Preliminary data indicate that significant shoulder dysfunction is rare after scapular harvest; however, patients with previous neck surgery and radiation ipsilateral to the donor site may be at increased risk of shoulder dysfunction.

RESULTS

Patients undergoing reconstruction of the maxilla with the scapular free tissue transfer or other myoosseous flaps usually heal quickly with rehabilitation time dependent on the speed of remucosalization of the palate defect. A hemimaxillectomy may require 4 to 6 weeks to remucosalize; however, the final functional result is far superior to transferred intraoral cutaneous paddles. Most patients prefer oral competence with separation of the nasal cavity using an obturator, and normal diet is usually achieved. Involvement of significant portions of the soft palate commonly results in velopharyngeal insufficiency, which is a characteristic of the ablative procedure rather than the reconstructive technique selected.

The innate shape of the scapular tip offers an excellent option for maxillary reconstruction and allows the goals of maxillary reconstruction to be achieved with minimal donor site morbidity, relatively low complication rates, and excellent functional results.

PEARLS

- The branching pattern of the circumflex scapular system is somewhat variable, and this may alter dissection considerably. The dissection from distal to proximal starting with the serratus branch of the thoracodorsal system will allow the entire vascular territory to be identified prior to harvesting the flap.
- Use "greenstick" osteotomies to maintain the periosteal blood supply when contouring the osseous portion of the flap.

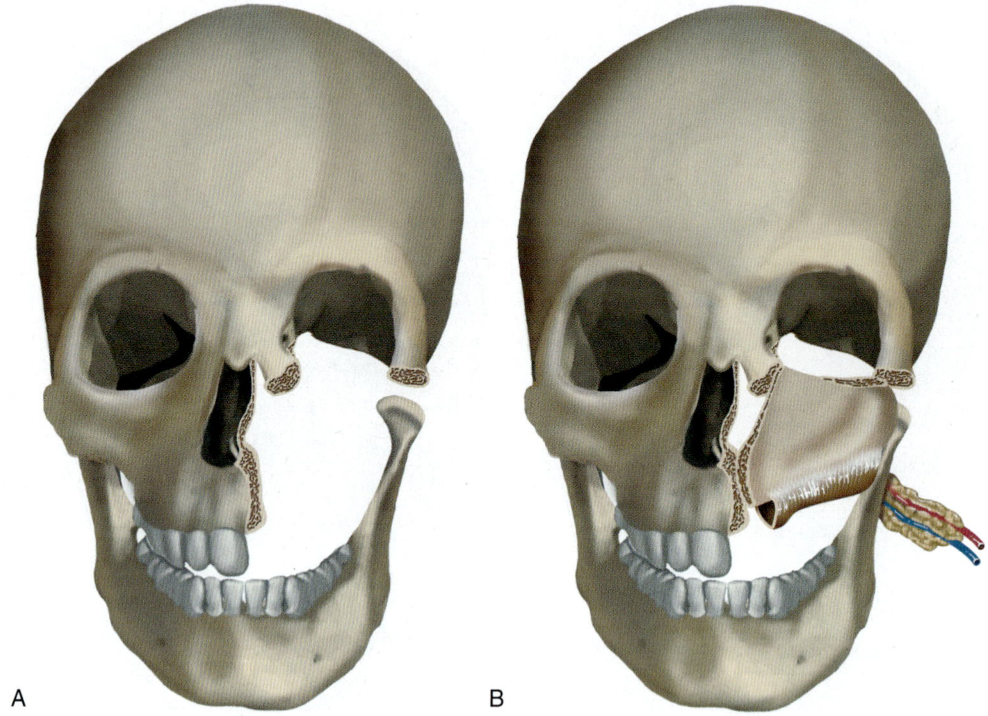

FIGURE 23.6
A. Demonstrates the vertical defect. **B.** Demonstrates the vertical orientation of the scapula.

- Vein grafting is not usually required with the angular modification.
- The scapular donor site commonly requires prolonged drainage due to the large surface area involved during harvest.
- Shoulder movement commences from postoperative day one.

PITFALLS

- Prone positioning lengthens the procedure and is unnecessary for scapular harvest.
- Careful attention to recipient vessel length in the neck will avoid unnecessary vein grafting.
- Identify the entire vascular system prior to performing osteotomies to avoid compromising the flap.
- Harvest adequate muscle bulk to cover the osseous transfer and provide closure of the oral cavity defect.

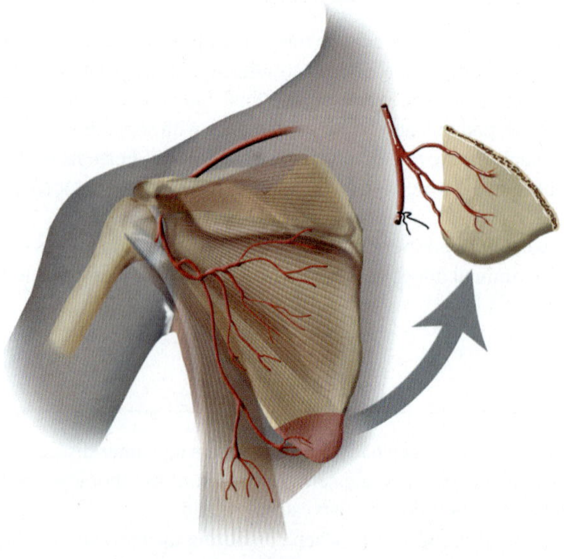

FIGURE 23.7
This illustration demonstrates the vascularization of the scapular tip and the teres muscle. The teres muscle can be harvested with the tip to provide soft tissue coverage of the palatal mucosal defect.

INSTRUMENTS TO HAVE AVAILABLE

- Standard head and neck surgical set
- Reciprocating bone saw
- Titanium plating system (1.5 mm)

SUGGESTED READING

Clark JR, Vesely M, Gilbert R. Scapular angle osteomyogenous flap in postmaxillectomy reconstruction: defect, reconstruction, shoulder function, and harvest technique. *Head Neck* 2008;30(1):10–20.

Brown J, Bekiroglu F, Shaw R. Indications for the scapular flap in reconstructions of the head and neck. *Br J Oral Maxillofac Surg* 2010;48(5):331–337.

Dolderer JH, Kelly JL, McCombe D, et al. Maxillofacial osseous reconstruction using the angular branch of the thoracodorsal vessels. *J Reconstr Microsurg* 2010;26(7):449–454.

Miles BA, Gilbert RW. Maxillary reconstruction with the scapular angle osteomyogenous free flap. *Arch Otolaryngol Head Neck Surg* 2011;137(11):1130–1135.

24 THE HEMIMAXILLECTOMY DEFECT: OSTEOCUTANEOUS RADIAL FOREARM FREE FLAP

Neal D. Futran

INTRODUCTION

The radial forearm free flap (RFFF) was first developed at the Shenyang Military General Hospital in China, and a large clinical series indicated that the flap was used very successfully to reconstruct defects of the head and neck. In 1983, Soutar et al. noted the benefits of this flap, with and without bone, for the reconstruction of intraoral defects. The radial forearm fasciocutaneous flap is ideally suited for intraoral reconstruction due to its pliability and thickness. The availability of vascularized bone for reconstruction of the mandible was later described, and the flap has been used by some for mandibular and maxillary reconstruction. While other donor sites have become popular for reconstruction of the mandible, the radial forearm flaps provides sufficient bone stock to reconstruct infrastructure and alveolar maxillary defects.

HISTORY

When evaluating a patient as a candidate for an RFFF reconstruction, I elicit any history of injury to the forearm, upper extremity vascular compromise, or osteopenia. Any history of osteopenia or osteoporosis should alert the surgeon that if the flap is going to be harvested with a segment of bone, there is an increased risk of fracture at the donor site.

PHYSICAL EXAMINATION

The physical examination should consist of a careful evaluation of the volar surface of the forearm to identify any prior injury, surgery, or congenital or acquired deformity. Additionally, an Allen test to evaluate the continuity of the deep and superficial palmer vascular arches is important to insure that the patient will tolerate harvest of the flap and the radial artery. The physical examination must also include a careful evaluation of the maxillary defect. Because the size of the bone graft is limited, the indications for this donor site are different from other vascular bone graft donor sites.

INDICATIONS

The radial forearm donor site provides a limited bone graft that is well suited for the reconstruction of alveolar and infrastructure defects but less than ideal for extensive maxillary defects involving a combination of the alveolus, infraorbital rim, and zygoma.

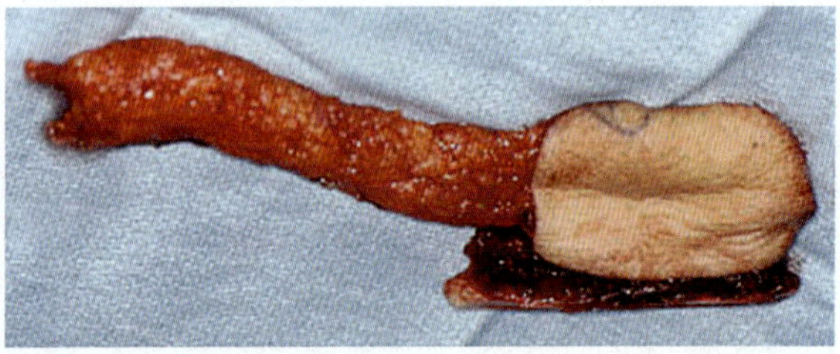

FIGURE 24.1 Osteocutaneous radial forearm free flap.

CONTRAINDICATIONS

The contraindications for this donor site for maxillary reconstruction are related to limitations of the donor site and the defects. The donor site limitations include any patient with a history of injury or vascular compromise of the forearm. Prior surgery, such as carpal tunnel surgery, and any history of radial fracture are contraindications to using this donor site. Other considerations are a history of osteopenia of the radial bone that may represent a high risk of postoperative fracture.

PREOPERATIVE PLANNING

The radius bone and skin paddle are both supplied through a relatively short intermuscular septum (5 to 6 cm long) that is 2 to 4 cm wide (Fig. 24.1). This allows for a degree of freedom when rotating the skin paddle relative to the bone segment, which is superior to other bone flaps such as the fibula and iliac crest. The length of the bone is limited to 10 to 12 cm by the insertions of the pronator teres and the brachioradialis muscles (Fig. 24.2). Also, to maintain the structural integrity of the radius bone, it is reported that only 40% of the circumference of the bone should be harvested. Thus, the quality of the bone stock is usually insufficient to support dental implants.

In an effort to reduce the morbidity at the donor site and therefore safely make use of the superior soft tissue characteristics of the volar forearm, biomechanical studies demonstrated greatly improved strength when a reconstruction plate is prophylactically applied to the donor radius after graft harvest. Studies from two institutions assessing over 100 patients, who underwent osteocutaneous radial forearm free flap (OCRFFF) harvest and prophylactic plating, reported only two instances of postoperative fracture of the radius. In both cases, the fracture occurred distal to the reconstruction plate after the patient fell. The OCRFFF has the advantage of tremendous soft tissue versatility. A long vascular pedicle, large amounts of thin pliable skin, and reliable sensory innervation make the soft tissue components of the RFFF ideal for the reconstruction of the tongue, floor of the mouth, alveolar ridge, pharyngeal wall, and soft palate. The available radius bone (9 to 12 cm) is of adequate length for reconstruction of many limited defects of the mandible and maxilla.

SURGICAL TECHNIQUE

Flap Harvest Technique

The RFFF is based on the radial artery, which branches from the brachial artery in the antecubital fossa. Its venous drainage is provided by the paired venae comitantes that run with the radial artery, and the superficial venous system, which contains the cephalic and basilic veins. The lateral intermuscular septum, which contains perforators from the radial artery supplying the periosteum of the radius, passes between the flexor carpi radialis and the brachioradialis muscles and must be preserved. Sensation of the flap is provided by the lateral and medial antebrachial cutaneous nerves.

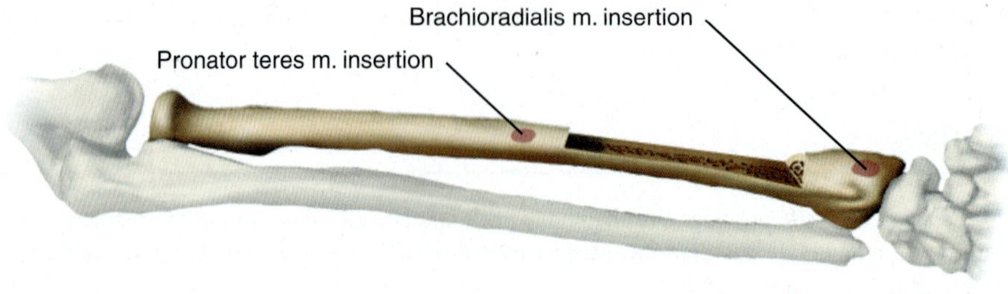

FIGURE 24.2 Diagram noting the extent of radial bone that can be harvested between the brachioradialis and pronator teres muscle insertions.

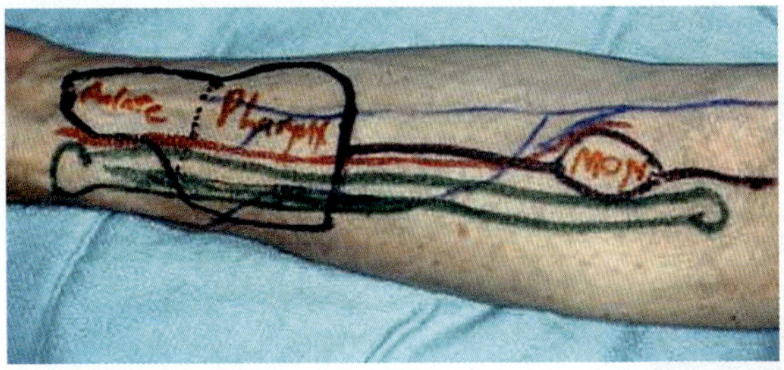

FIGURE 24.3
Outline of the osteocutaneous radial forearm free flap in anticipation of flap harvest.

Preoperatively, an Allen test is performed to confirm adequate circulation to the hand via the ulnar artery and to assist in the selection of the donor arm. At surgery, the radial artery and cephalic vein are marked, along with the proposed skin paddle. The soft tissue component is measured, and the flap outline is drawn on the volar aspect of the forearm (Fig. 24.3). The skin paddle is positioned at least 2 cm proximal to the wrist crease and with an ulnar bias. This ensures adequate skin coverage of the internal fixation plate. The soft tissue component of the flap is raised in the standard fashion, with care taken to preserve the lateral intermuscular septum. An incision is made in the skin proximal to the paddle up to the antecubital fossa, and the skin flaps are reflected. The skin paddle is the outlined and raised with the deep fascia to the level of the brachioradialis and flexor carpi radialis tendons. Careful dissection medial to the cephalic vein and radial artery to the vascular pedicle preserves the superficial branch of the radial nerve intact. The radial artery and the vena comitans are ligated, and the pedicle and the fascia are raised for approximately 1 to 2 cm. The available bone lies in between the insertion of the pronator teres muscle and the insertion of the tendon of the brachioradialis muscle. Lateral retraction of the brachioradialis tendon exposes the radial surface of the bone.

The bone is harvested between the pronator teres and brachioradialis tendon insertions. The flexor digitorum superficialis is released from the radius, allowing visualization of the flexor pollicis longus. The flexor pollicis longus muscle belly is divided over the midline of the volar surface of the radius with electrocautery or scalpel until the necessary length of radial bone is exposed. The required length of bone is marked. The distal osteotomy must be made at least 2.5 cm from the radial styloid to allow later fixation of the radius. Proximally, the osteotomy can be made even beyond the pronator teres insertion; however, the pronator teres tendon will require reinsertion. The sagittal saw with a fine blade is used to make a longitudinal osteotomy in the radius through its midportion. This osteotomy is placed to allow harvest of approximately 40% to 50% of the circumference of the radius with beveled osteotomies at the proximal and distal ends (Fig. 24.4). The periosteum is then incised dorsally, completing the harvest of the bone graft. The deep vascular pedicle and the cephalic vein are skeletonized up to the antecubital fossa. The lateral antebrachial cutaneous nerve can then be easily separated from the cephalic vein for approximately 8 to 10 cm. The flap is then left to perfuse on its pedicle, which is divided proximally and distally just before transfer of the flap to the recipient site.

Prophylactic fixation of the radius is begun by exposing the dorsal aspect of the radius proximally and distally. Distally, the radial wrist extensors are retracted. Proximally, the supinator is visualized. Great care is taken to protect the posterior interosseus nerve, which passes through the supinator but is not usually adjacent to the fixation area. An appropriately sized 2.4-mm locking reconstruction plate (Synthes, Davos, Switzerland) is positioned over the radius and bent to the contour of the bone with three holes on either side of the osteotomy site (Fig. 24.5). Bicortical screws are placed only in the three proximal and distal holes.

After standard closure of the forearm defect including split-thickness skin grafting, the arm is placed in the rigid ulnar gutter splint for approximately 7 days, at which time the splint is removed and the wound inspected. The patient is then encouraged to resume full activity of the wrist and fingers, including weight bearing and rotation, with the donor arm protected with a soft dressing until the wound has healed.

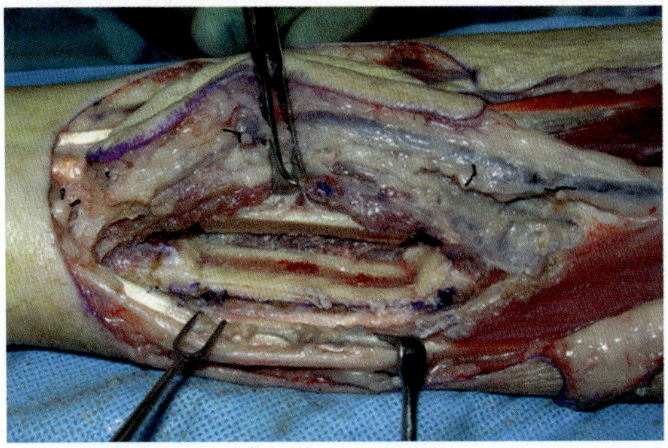

FIGURE 24.4
An osteotomy of the radial bone at approximately 40% of its thickness is carried out between the brachioradialis and pronator teres muscle insertions.

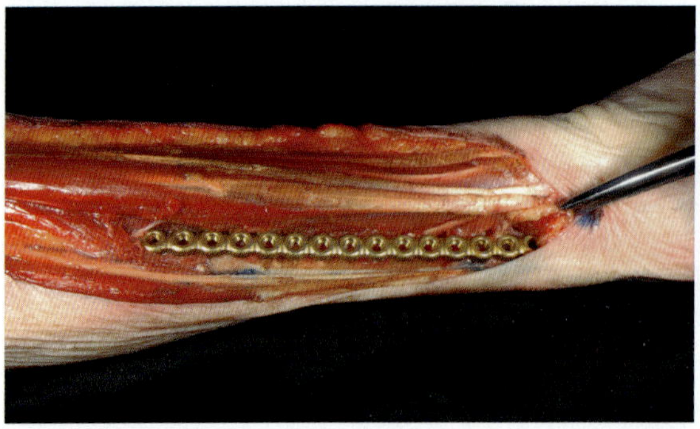

FIGURE 24.5
A 2.4-mm locking reconstruction plate (Synthes, Davos, Switzerland) is placed over the radial bone, so three holes are on either side of the osteotomy site in the radius. Appropriate-length bicortical screws are placed only in these holes.

Maxillary Inset Technique

A main indication for the use of this flap is in the reconstruction of limited maxillectomy defects. The thin radial bone that is harvested with this flap closely approximates the thin bone stock of the maxilla. The soft tissue from the forearm also conforms nicely to the palate and separates the oral and nasal cavities reliably. If implants are to be used for the upper denture, I have placed them in the native maxilla lateral to the radial bone. Usually, I do not place implants in the upper arch, because dentures can be formed to fit the slightly altered anatomy of the new anterior maxillary arch, with stabilization of the prosthesis coming from the normal lateral alveolar ridges. If a larger area than the premaxilla is involved, then I tend to choose either the fibula or iliac crest flaps, because dental implants become necessary to hold dentures in place.

The maxillary defect is prepared either by removal of tumor for neoplasm or by debridement of the wound in cases of traumatic injury (Figs. 24.6A–C). A limited neck dissection is done on the ipsilateral side for recipient vessel exposure. Any branch of the external carotid artery can be used, but typically, the facial artery or superior thyroid artery provides optimal vessel geometry and ease of anastomosis. The external jugular vein, internal jugular vein, or facial vein is readily available for venous anastomosis. A subcutaneous tunnel is made from the maxillary buccal area to the neck lateral to the mandible for passage of the flap vascular pedicle. This avoids trauma to the marginal mandibular nerve. The width of this tunnel should be two fingerbreadths to avoid compression of the flap pedicle. After the flap is passed under direct vision through this tunnel, the inset of the radius bone to the maxilla takes place. A single osteotomy can be made in the radius, if necessary, for optimal contour of the neomaxilla. This can be done prior to passage of the flap, and fixation is done with a 1.5-mm titanium miniplate (Fig. 24.6D). The bone is then trimmed to maximize bony contact with the remaining maxilla and fixated with 1.5-mm titanium miniplates. A minimum of two holes in the radius and maxilla is necessary for sufficient fixation (Fig. 24.6E). The soft tissue portion of the flap is then inset into the maxillary defect with 3-0 resorbable suture in an interrupted fashion (Fig. 24.6F). The vascular anastomoses are then performed in the conventional fashion, and the wounds are closed. Long-term results are noted in Figure 24.6G–J.

POSTOPERATIVE MANAGEMENT

Postoperatively, the patient is managed with a volar splint for 5 to 7 days. Physical therapy is initiated 2 to 3 weeks after surgery. The maxillary reconstruction requires 5 to 6 weeks for the bone union to occur, so patients are typically instructed to maintain a liquid diet for 5 to 6 weeks to alleviate pressure on the bone graft.

COMPLICATIONS

Complications are largely restricted to the risk of donor site morbidity. Postoperative radial fracture is considered the most serious complication. Plating the fracture site has been demonstrated to be effective in preventing this complication.

RESULTS

My results with this technique for maxillary reconstruction have demonstrated that this approach is reliable for small and moderately sized maxillary defects. The bone graft is substantial enough to accommodate osseointegrated dental implants.

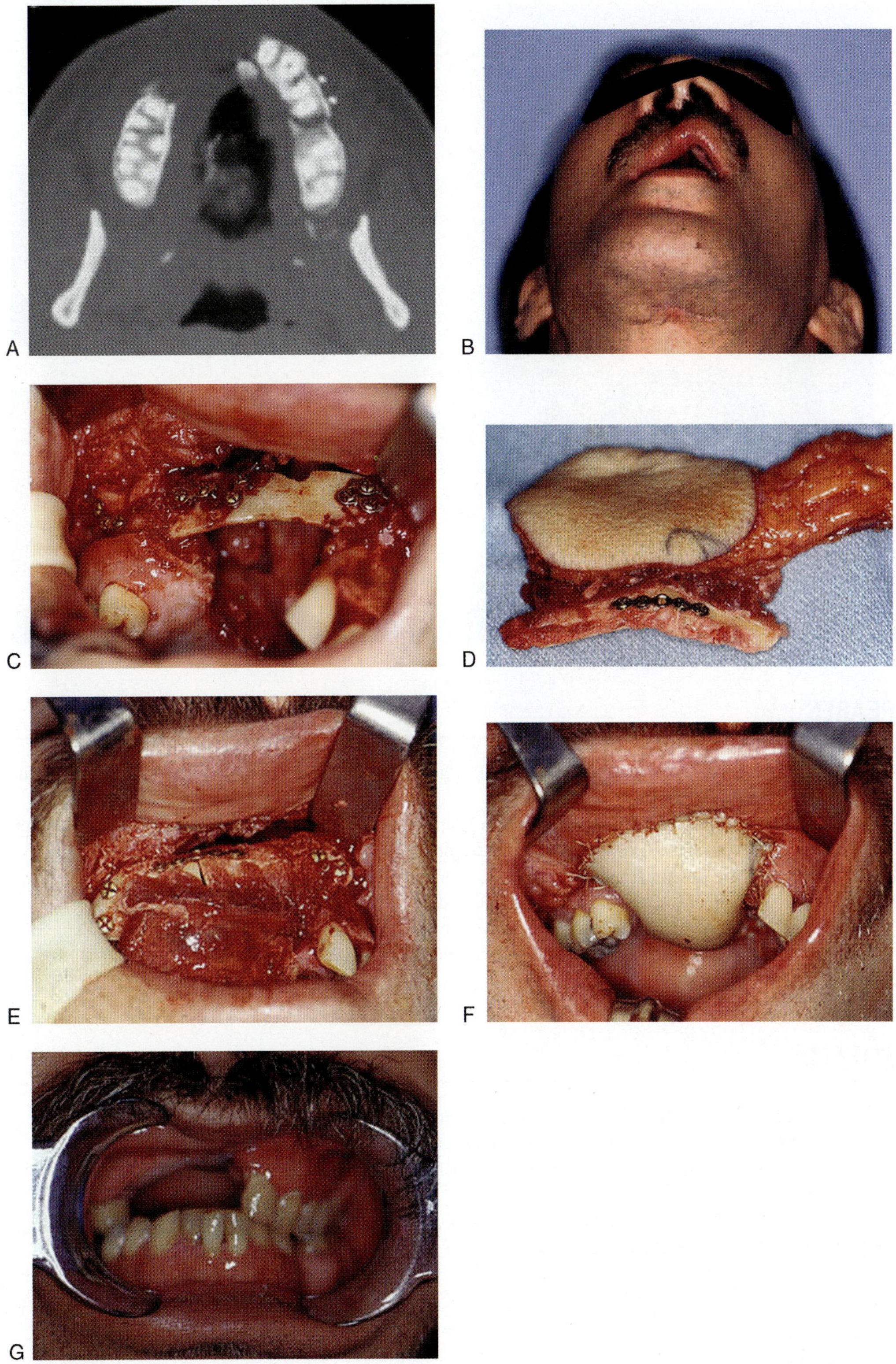

FIGURE 24.6 A. A axial CT scan of a 32-year-old man status post a gunshot wound to the anterior palate with a persistent oronasal and oroantral defect after Phase I treatment. **B.** Submental view of the collapsed premaxilla. **C.** The wound is exposed revealing non-viable bone grafts and necrotic tissue. **D.** A radial forearm osteocutaneous free flap. The bone is osteotomized to provide the proper contour for the premaxilla. **E.** The bone is fixated to the remaining maxillary bone with 1.5-mm titanium miniplates. **F.** The soft tissue component of the flap surrounds the bone and restores the palatal and nasal linings. **G.** At 1-year follow-up, the flap has conformed to the natural shape of the palate and provides a suitable base for a dental prosthesis.

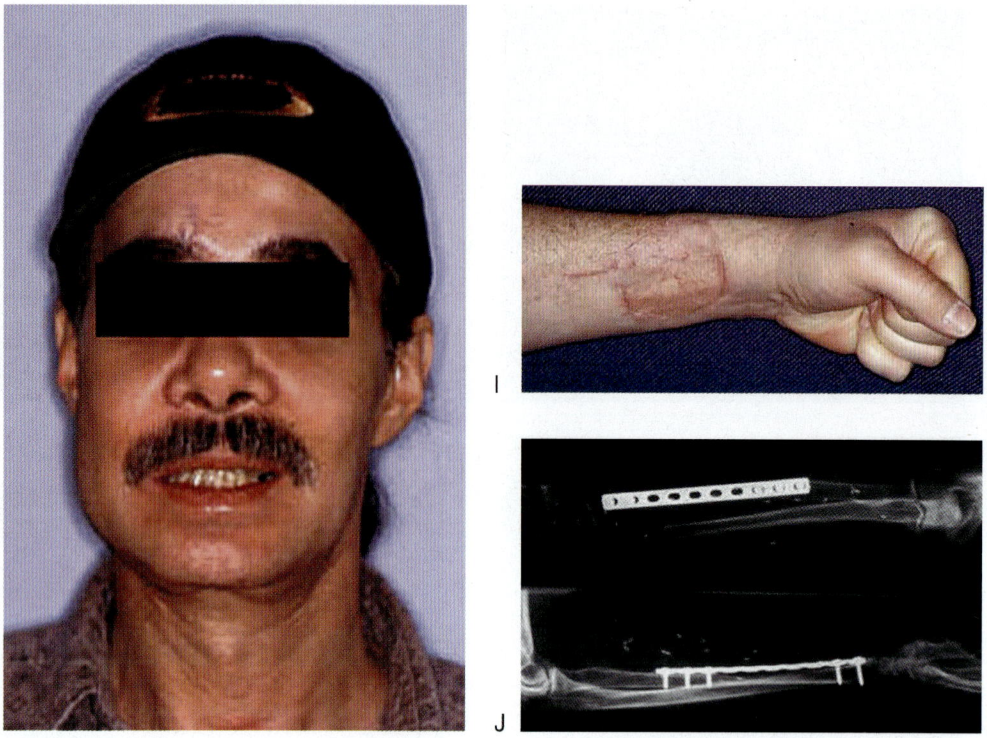

H I J

FIGURE 24.6
(*Continued*) **H.** Anterior view of the patient 1 year after free tissue transfer with restored form and function. **I.** Patient with intact donor site function at 1-year follow-up. **J.** Donor site radiograph at 1-year follow-up showing intact radius.

PEARLS

- Design the skin paddle with an ulnar bias such that there is more skin remaining on the radial aspect of the defect for advancement closure over the bone.
- Detach the flexor digitorum superficialis muscle from the radius bone during graft harvest. It can be repositioned over the top of the flexor carpi radialis tendon to improve closure over the defect and enhance skin graft takeover of the flexor carpi radialis tendon.
- Harvest 40% to 50% of the circumference of the radius.
- Place a locking reconstruction plate over the ostectomized radius.
- Remove the arm splint after 7 days to allow early mobilization of the wrist to avoid disuse, stiffness, and weakness in the donor arm.

PITFALLS

- Mobilize radial nerve adequately to allow retraction and prevent injury.
- Best use of this flap is for limited maxillectomy defects, not those involving both the orbit and alveolus.
- Radius will tolerate a maximum of one osteotomy and maintain adequate blood supply to the bone.

INSTRUMENTS TO HAVE AVAILABLE

- Reciprocating saw
- Mandibular plating system
- Mini plating system

SUGGESTED READING

Song R, Gao Y, Song Y, et al. The forearm flap. *Clin Plast Surg* 1982;9:21–26.

Soutar DS, Scheker NS, Tanner NS, et al. The radial forearm flap: a versatile method for intra-oral reconstruction. *Br J Plast Surg* 1983;36:1–8.

Swanson E, Boyd JB, Mulholland RS. The radial forearm flap: a biomechanical study of the osteotomized radius. *Plast Reconstr Surg* 1990;85:267–272.

Meland NB, Maki S, Chao EY, et al. The radial forearm flap: a biomechanical study of donor-site morbidity utilizing sheep tibia. *Plast Reconstr Surg* 1992;90:763–773.

Smith AA, Bowen CV, Rabeczak T, et al. Donor site deficit of the osteocutaneous radial forearm flap. *Ann Plast Surg* 1994;32:372–376.

Bowers KW, Edmonds JL, Girod DA, et al. Osteocutaneous radial forearm free flaps. *J Bone Joint Surg Am* 2000;82:694–704.

25 THE HEMIMAXILLECTOMY DEFECT: RECONSTRUCTION WITH THE FIBULA OSTEOCUTANEOUS FREE FLAP

Marita S. Teng

INTRODUCTION

The hemimaxillectomy defect arises most frequently from ablative surgery for malignant tumors, although severe facial trauma is another etiology. This type of defect is very complex, as a large oronasal and oromaxillary fistula is present, along with loss of bone support for the lip, orbit, and cheek. Midface projection and dentition are also sacrificed, resulting in significant impairments in speech and swallowing.

In general, reconstruction of the maxillectomy defect has multiple important goals, including the following:

- Separate the nasal and sinus cavities from the oral cavity to restore normal speech and swallowing
- Provide projection for the midface and palatal arch
- Reestablish functional occlusion
- Support the orbit or fill the defect in the case of orbital exenteration
- Maintain a patent nasal airway

Traditionally, these defects were lined with a split-thickness skin graft and a prosthetic obturator placed. Though this technique achieves separation of the nasal and oral cavities, maintenance of the prosthesis can be challenging, especially for older patients and particularly those who are edentulous. Furthermore, simple tasks such as swallowing and speaking are impossible without the obturator in place.

Free tissue transfer has become a very useful modality for single-stage reconstruction of these complex defects. Free flaps with bone include the fibula, iliac crest, and scapula osteocutaneous free flaps. The fibula free flap is an excellent choice for reconstruction of the hemimaxillectomy defect because of its ability to achieve all of the above reconstructive goals, while being relatively simple to harvest, and having minimal to no donor site morbidity. This flap has the additional advantages of having a long enough pedicle to reach the ipsilateral neck without requiring vein grafting, as well as suitable bone stock for osseointegrated implants.

HISTORY

As with any reconstructive surgery, midfacial reconstruction may be performed primarily (at the time of ablative surgery) or secondarily. History-taking will obviously differ depending on which situation is applicable, but in general, probably the most important aspect to assess is the patients' preoperative ability to eat and their postoperative expectations. For example, if a patient is restricted to a liquid diet preoperatively and has neither the desire nor the capability of eating a regular solid diet postoperatively, then one might reconsider the indications for reconstruction with bone. Other factors that should be assessed are the patient's age and medical comorbidities, as well as the importance that they place on the cosmetic result. For the fibula free flap, it is also critical to evaluate for a history of peripheral vascular disease or lower extremity trauma or gait disorders that could eliminate the fibula as a potential donor site.

PHYSICAL EXAMINATION

From a reconstructive standpoint, examination of the head and neck region should be focused on the anticipated defect. It is useful to think of the potential defect in terms of hard and soft tissue elements, as well as horizontal and vertical components. The most widely used classification for maxillectomy defects is Brown's classification, which divides the vertical component of the defect into classes 1 to 4 and the transverse extent of the defect into subtypes a-c (Fig. 25.1) (see Chapter 22). By assessing the anticipated defect in this manner, the surgeon can prioritize the most critical elements of the reconstruction and design the flap accordingly.

It is also important to assess the suitability of various free flap donor sites. Specifically for the fibula free flap, the legs should be examined for any evidence of arterial insufficiency, venous stasis, or previous scars from trauma or surgery. The AAI (ankle–arm index) can be used as a rough screen of lower extremity vascular perfusion, with an AAI of less than 1.0 being an indication of likely peripheral vascular occlusion.

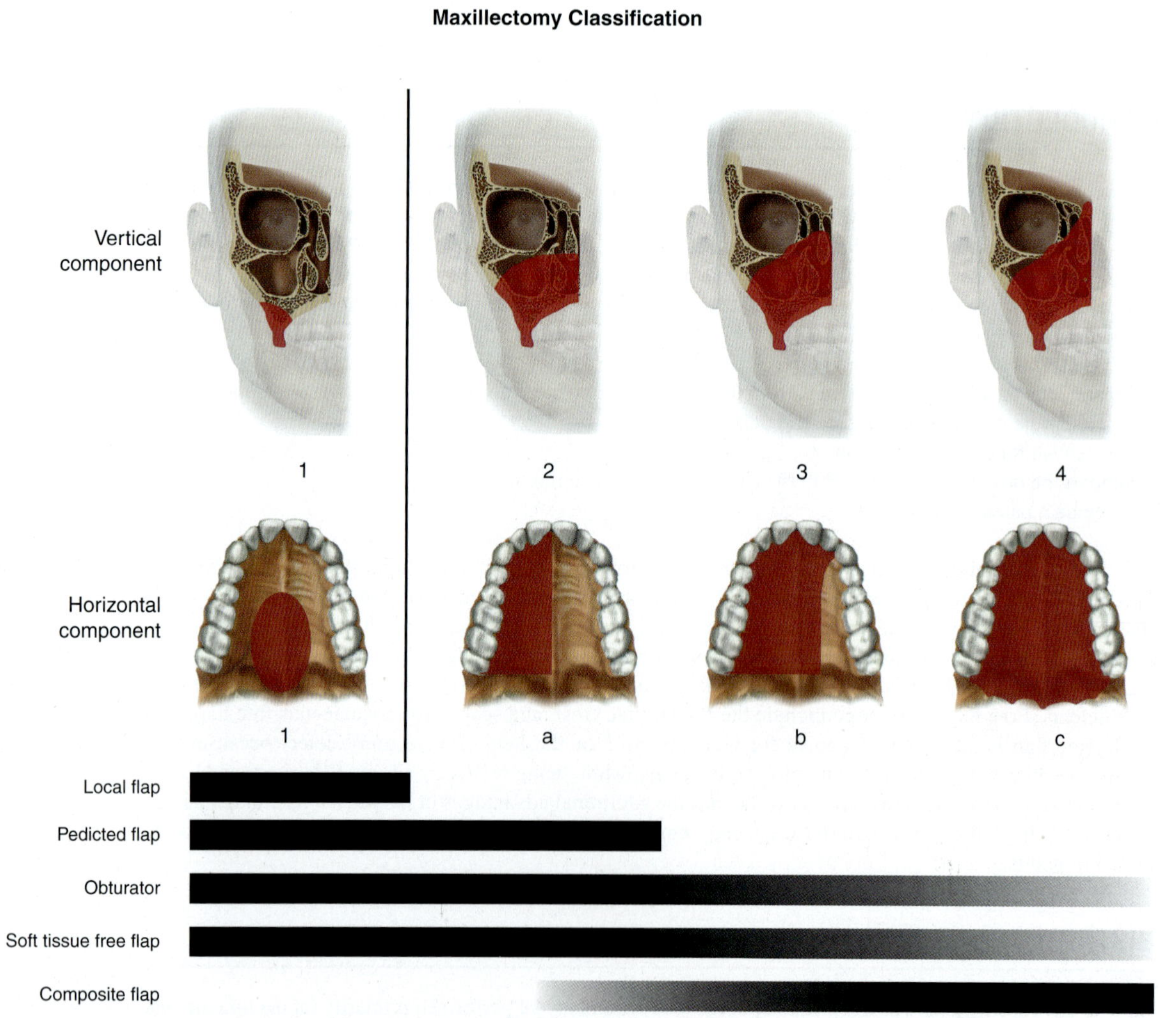

FIGURE 25.1 Brown's classification of maxillectomy defects, including vertical and horizontal components. This classification system provides a reconstructive algorithm to guide the reconstructive surgeon, which is useful in the decision-making process. (Redrawn from Brown JS, Shaw RJ. Reconstruction of the maxilla and midface: introducing a new classification. *Lancet Oncol* 2010;11(10):1001–1008. doi: 10.1016/S1470-2045(10)70113-3.)

INDICATIONS

The indications for fibular free flap reconstruction includes defects in the infrastructure or alveolus of the maxilla. The nature of the bone graft is such that it cannot be used to address vertical defect involving the orbital rim and/or lateral aspect of the zygoma. Vertical defects are best managed with a scapular or iliac graft. In contrast, the fibula free flap is ideally suited for the reconstruction of infrastructure defects. The bone stock is hearty and will accommodate osseointegrated implants.

CONTRAINDICATIONS

The most obvious and important contraindication to the use of the fibula free flap is vascular insufficiency, either to the flap (peroneal artery) or to the distal leg and foot after flap harvest (anterior and posterior tibial arteries). Rarely, the fibula bone may be absent or severely diminished in size, or even replaced by a fibrous band.

Relative contraindications include severe edema or venous stasis, as well as bulky overlying soft tissue in the lateral lower leg. Finally, though the fibula is a non–weight-bearing bone, careful consideration must be given to harvesting from a patient's only remaining leg or only remaining weight-bearing leg.

The fibula flap has limitations in terms of the arc of soft tissue rotation, as well as lack of bulk of soft tissue. Thus, when a large volume soft tissue defect exists, an alternative reconstructive method should be considered. In particular, defects that involve the orbital rim and/or lateral aspect of the zygoma require the vertical bone height that can only be achieved with an iliac or vertically oriented scapular bone flap (Fig. 25.2).

PREOPERATIVE PLANNING

As mentioned above, it is essential to plan out the structure and layout of the flap reconstruction based on the anticipated surgical defect. The fibula free flap contains ample length but limited caliber of bone; furthermore, the skin paddle is typically well vascularized but with limitations in terms of amount and arc of rotation. These characteristics make the fibula flap ideal for defects in the inferior maxilla, those which do not require extensive bone stock for reconstruction of the orbital floor or soft tissue (e.g., orbital exenteration) reconstruction.

Imaging Studies

Imaging studies of the head and neck must be obtained and are critical in planning ablative surgery. In addition, some form of imaging is imperative to evaluate the blood flow in the lower extremity and determine the

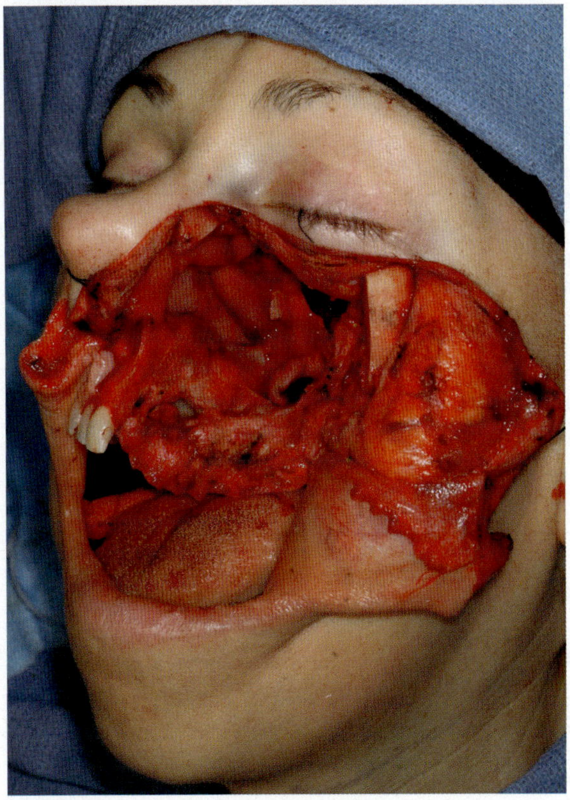

FIGURE 25.2
A maxillary defect with a vertical component that involves the orbital rim is difficult to manage with a fibular graft because there is no support for the orbital rim.

suitability of fibula free flap harvest. It is imperative to confirm that the tibioperoneal trunk gives adequate runoff to the foot via the anterior and posterior tibial arteries and the peroneal artery. Patency of the peroneal artery is also critical to the viability of the free flap. If three-vessel runoff is identified, fibula harvest can easily be performed with no risk to the vascularity of the foot. If only two-vessel runoff is identified, then harvest of the peroneal artery will leave only one artery to supply the foot, which is very tenuous, and use of the fibula flap should be carefully reconsidered.

Many surgeons advocate the use of magnetic resonance angiography to obtain detailed anatomic information about the tibioperoneal anatomy, as well as to possibly localize perforator vessels on the peroneal artery and their course in the posterolateral intermuscular septum. Others have traditionally advocated color flow Doppler as a less costly and invasive method of imaging the lower extremity. In an experienced ultrasonographer's hands, this technique can also identify septocutaneous perforators from the peroneal artery, thus aiding in the design of the skin paddle.

SURGICAL TECHNIQUE

In conceptualizing the fibula flap for reconstruction of a hemimaxillectomy defect, it is important to remember that the vascular pedicle should come off the posterior neomaxilla, creating a natural drape of the vessels into the ipsilateral neck for anastomosis. As such, the most distal end of the fibula will be inset into the anterior aspect of the defect, and the palatal soft tissue defect will best be reconstructed with a distally situated skin paddle. With these geometric considerations, it is preferable to use the ipsilateral leg as a donor site, as the skin paddle will naturally fall onto the intraoral/palatal surface when the pedicle is oriented posteriorly (Fig. 25.3A).

Landmarks for harvest of the fibula free flap are the fibular head proximally and the lateral epicondyle of the ankle distally. A line between these two points denotes the fibula bone itself. The posterior intermuscular septum, in which the septocutaneous perforators run, is located in a plane angled slightly posteriorly from the fibula bone (Fig. 25.3B). Furthermore, the dominant perforators are generally located more distally in the leg, so a skin paddle is centered over the middle and distal third of the bone. As mentioned above, consideration should be given to the desired location of the skin paddle relative to the bone once it is inset.

Six to seven centimeters of bone should be preserved at both the knee and ankle in order to maintain joint integrity. A thigh tourniquet is inflated to 350 mm Hg, and the anterior skin incision is performed first and carried subfascially. This incision exposes the peroneus longus and brevis muscles, which are retracted anteriorly to expose the fibula. The skin paddle is gently retracted posteriorly, and perforating vessels are identified in this manner. The bone is then skeletonized with cautery, taking care to avoid injury to the perforators by maintaining a small cuff of peroneus muscle around the visible perforators (Fig. 25.4). The dissection then proceeds anteriorly around the fibula, through the extensor muscles and to the interosseous septum. The interosseous septum is then incised along the length of the fibula, preserving several millimeters to protect periosteal vessels. It is sometimes necessary, especially in younger patients with less tissue laxity, to perform the osteotomies prior to incising the septum. Also, the posterior skin incision can be made, taking care to incorporate the perforators in the skin paddle (Fig. 25.5). Once the bone has been cut, it is distracted laterally to reveal the posterior compartment muscles. The peroneal vessels are then identified distally in the ankle, ligated, and divided. The tibialis posterior and flexor hallucis longus muscles are divided with cautery. A cuff of the flexor hallucis muscle, as well as of the soleus muscle, is preserved in order to maintain the integrity of any musculocutaneous perforators to the skin.

The bone is then shaped with closing osteotomies in order to create a shape that resembles a "mini-mandible" in order to restore the midface contour while recreating the palatal arch (Fig. 25.6). Miniplates are used to fixate the bone to the anterior palate as well as the remaining zygoma. The skin paddle is oriented to fill the palatal mucosal defect.

Closure of the donor site over a suction drain may be performed primarily or with a split-thickness skin graft. The decision about whether to use a skin graft is made not only based on the size of the harvested skin paddle but also by the laxity of the patient's skin and tissue.

POSTOPERATIVE MANAGEMENT

Immediately postoperatively, the patient should have neurovascular checks of the lower extremity at each flap check, which is performed every 4 to 6 hours. The donor leg should be elevated and immobilized in a neutral splint. On postoperative day (POD) 2, patients may begin ambulating with the aid of a walker and with the assistance of a nurse or a physical therapist. After POD 5, patients may weight-bear as tolerated, but throughout the first 2 to 3 weeks after surgery, the leg should be elevated while supine or seated. The splint is removed on POD 7 and the incision and/or skin graft examined, and the splint is replaced for protection of the leg for the second postoperative week before it is completely removed.

Postoperative care of the free flap itself is standard, with vigilant flap checks over the first 72 hours, in order to identify any microvascular issues early. Because the skin paddle may be quite edematous in the first

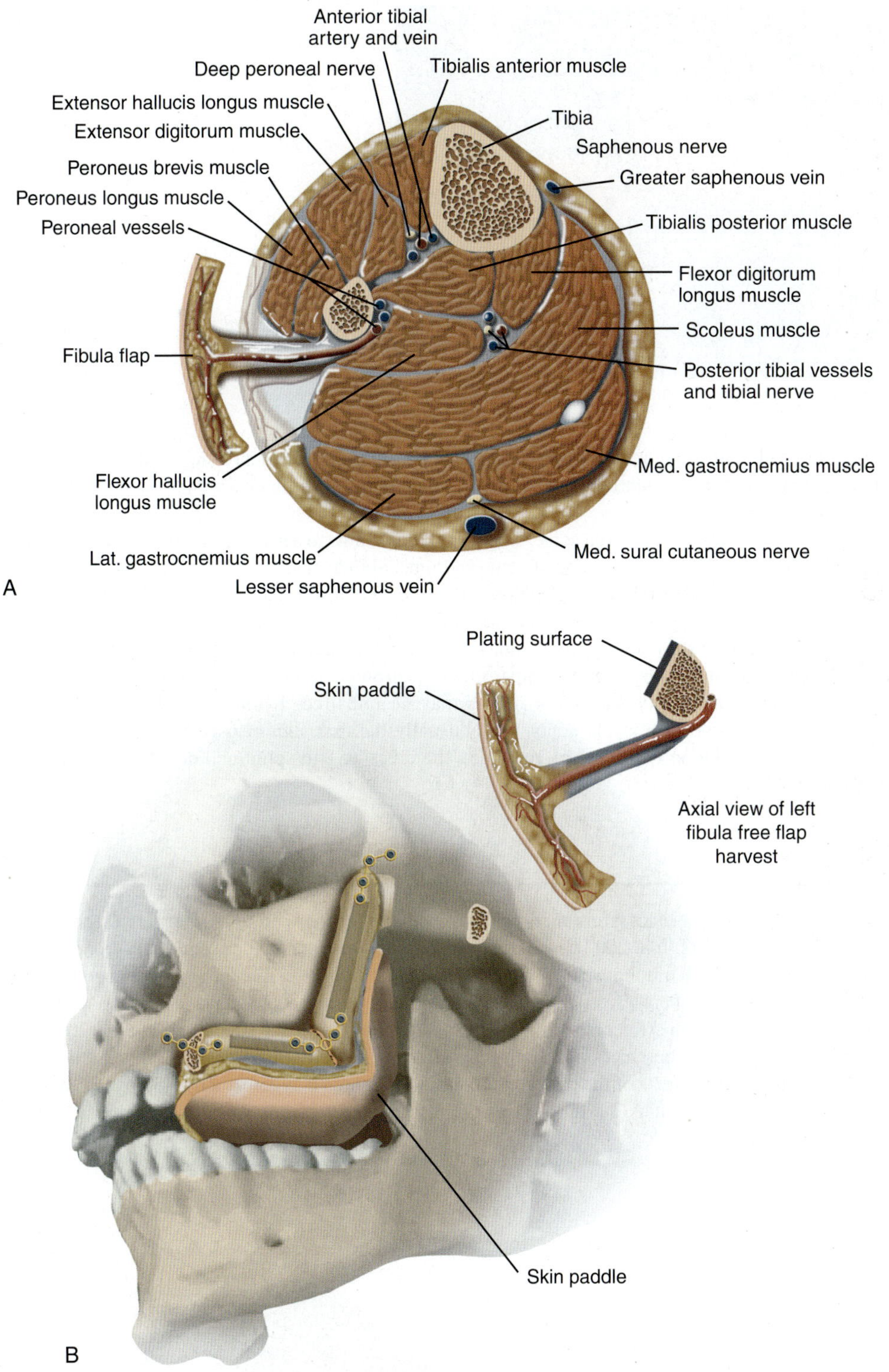

FIGURE 25.3 A. Axial view of the contents harvested with a left fibula free flap. **B.** Depiction of the plating surface of the fibula flap and how it is oriented into an ipsilateral maxillectomy defect. In this case, a left fibula flap is being inset into a left maxillectomy defect. The skin paddle naturally sits in an orientation to fill the palatal defect.

week, the paddle is at risk for excessive pressure or trauma from the mandibular teeth. Patients should be cautioned against biting on the skin paddle.

COMPLICATIONS

Minor complications to the donor extremity include cold intolerance or edema of the lower leg. When the muscles scar or branches of the peroneal nerve are injured, patients may experience weakness in dorsiflexion

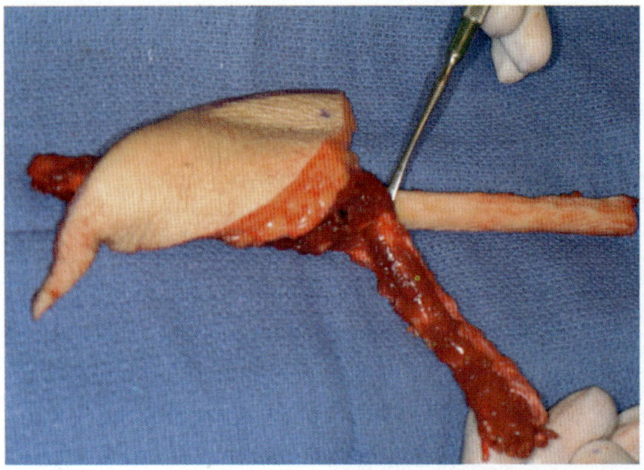

FIGURE 25.4
The bone can be skeletonized with cautery, taking care to avoid injury to the perforators by maintaining a small cuff of peroneus muscle around the visible perforators. This will lengthen the vascular pedicle.

of the big toe. Other uncommon complications include hematoma of the donor site or of course, flap failure. As usual, patients must be vigilantly followed for early recognition of problems with the donor site or with flap compromise.

Wound complications range from some simple skin breakdown to sensory or motor deficits resulting from tight closure that can cause a pseudocompartment syndrome. Shindo et al. determined that though multiple factors contribute to donor site wound complications after fibula harvest, if tension is present at the suture line, a skin graft should be strongly considered to minimize the risk of complications.

Extreme tension on the closure, which, due to tissue edema, can worsen after the closure is completed, may result in a very damaging pseudocompartment syndrome. In such a circumstance, the leg muscles can necrose, and both sensory and motor nerves may be impaired. If unrecognized, nerve damage can be permanent. Excessive pain at the donor site is usually the first sign of pseudocompartment syndrome and should immediately be examined by removing the dressing and splint and doing a full neurovascular examination.

RESULTS

Many series have reported successful functional and cosmetic results with fibula free flap reconstruction for hemimaxillectomy defects. In a 2002 case series by Futran, 27 patients underwent fibula reconstruction for this type of defect, with all of them achieving a regular or soft diet, 18 maintaining osseointegrated implants, and 22 being judged by themselves, their significant others, and the physician as having an "excellent" or "good" cosmetic outcome. Recently, Sun et al expanded the use of the fibula flap in their 2011 series of 20 patients undergoing reconstruction of high maxillectomy defects. Because of the increased complexity of reconstruction due to defects of the orbital floor, nasal wall, and/or zygoma, they employed titanium mesh to help support the anterior maxilla. In four cases, either a second flap or a zygomatic implant was used to

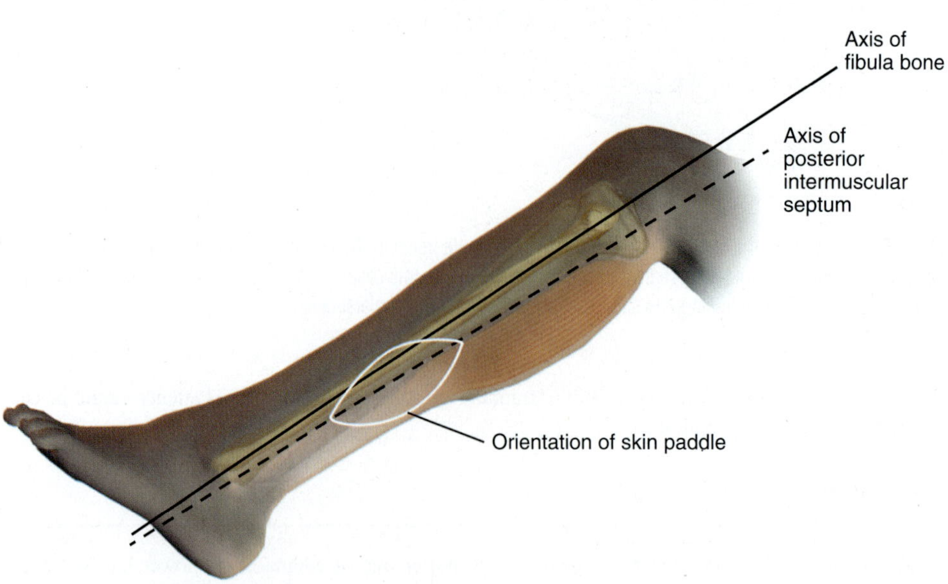

FIGURE 25.5
The axis of the posterior intermuscular septum is angled and posterior to the axis of the fibula bone. This fact is important to recognize when designing the skin paddle. The majority of skin perforators are generally located distally.

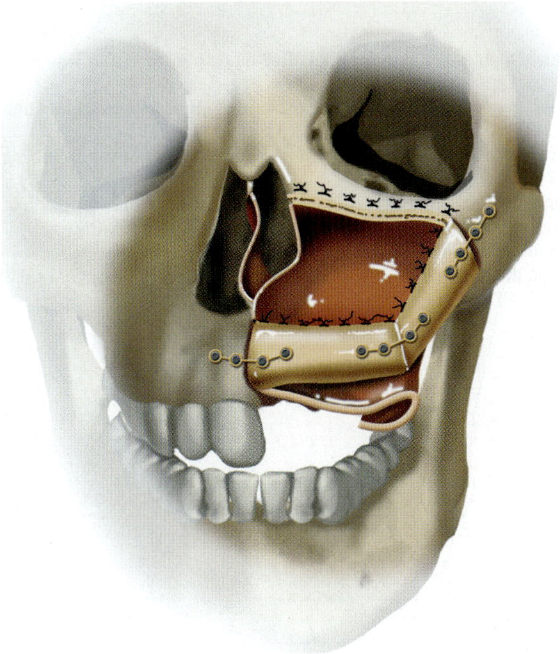

FIGURE 25.6
The fibula flap is fashioned into a "mini-mandible," secured to the remaining native palatal bone and root of the zygoma.

further augment the defect. Nineteen of these twenty patients achieved bony union and closure of the oronasal cavities, as well as intelligible speech. Both Futran and Sun admit that exposure or infection of titanium mesh is not uncommon, and its use should be employed cautiously in patients requiring or having a history of radiation therapy.

PEARLS

- The ipsilateral leg donor site orients the skin paddle in the most favorable position to restore the palatal defect.
- The posterior crural septum is often visible, especially in older patients with more tissue laxity. This plane is most noticeable when the soleus and gastrocnemius muscles are manipulated while the leg is relaxed, flexed at the knee. Marking out this septum facilitates design of the anterior skin incision to help incorporate the septocutaneous perforators.
- The skin paddle must be designed carefully, not only to incorporate the most likely dominant perforators but also to be placed in a favorable location relative to the bone in order to seal the palatal defect.
- When a long skin paddle is harvested, a portion may be used to reline the lateral nasal wall if necessary. The intervening skin between the neopalate and nasal wall can be deepithelialized to facilitate this.
- The vascular pedicle must be brought off the posterior (and superior) aspect of the maxillectomy defect, such that the vessels may be tunneled into the neck for anastomosis.
- Generally, the soft tissue tunnel into the neck is most easily created on the medial surface of the mandible. The technique creates the least angulation in the vessels and obviates the risk to branches of the facial nerve, which are at risk if a lateral tunnel is created.

PITFALLS

- Excessive traction on the common peroneal nerve during harvest can result in an equinovarus deformity, as well as numbness to the lateral leg and dorsum of the foot.
- Joint instability can occur if a proper (6 to 7 cm) length of fibular bone is not preserved at the knee and ankle joints.

INSTRUMENTS TO HAVE AVAILABLE

- Standard head and neck surgical set
- 2.0 locking plating set
- Reciprocating saw

SUGGESTED READING

Futran ND, Stack BC, Zaccardi MJ. Preoperative color flow Doppler imaging for fibula free tissue transfers. *Ann Vasc Surg* 1998;12(5):445–450.

Brown JS, Jones DC, Summerwill A, et al. Vascularized iliac crest with internal oblique muscle for immediate reconstruction after maxillectomy. *Br J Oral Maxillofac Surg* 2002;40:183–190.

Chang DW, Langstein HN. Use of the free fibula flap for restoration of orbital support and midfacial projection following maxillectomy. *J Reconstr Microsurg* 2003;19(3):147–152.

Genden EM, Okay D, Stepp MT, et al. Comparison of functional and quality-of-life outcomes in patients with and without palatomaxillary reconstruction: a preliminary report. *Arch Otolaryngol Head Neck Surg* 2003;129(7):775–780.

Futran ND, Mendez E. Developments in reconstruction of midface and maxilla. *Lancet Oncol* 2006;7:249–258.

Dalgorf D, Higgins K. Reconstruction of the midface and maxilla. *Curr Opin Otolaryngol Head Neck Surg* 2008;16:303–311.

26 TOTAL MAXILLECTOMY DEFECT: RECONSTRUCTION WITH THE FIBULAR FREE FLAP

Derrick T. Lin

INTRODUCTION

Reconstruction of the total maxillectomy defect is among the most challenging faced by the head and neck reconstructive surgeon. Defects in this area are most often due to resection for malignant tumors but also may occur with trauma, osteoradionecrosis, or infection/inflammation.

Anatomically, the two paired maxillae form the structural support of the midface. These paired structures provide separation of the oral, antral, and orbital cavities, forming the foundation necessary for facial contour and expression, mastication, speech, and deglutition.

The goals of palatomaxillary reconstruction are therefore to restore separation of the oral and antral cavities, correct hypernasal speech, and prevent regurgitation of foods and liquids into the nasal cavity. The simplest rehabilitation option is the use of an obturator. The advantages are short operative time, short post-operative stay, and complete visualization of the maxillectomy defect for oncologic surveillance. However, in larger defects where the anterior projecting element of the maxilla has been removed, reconstruction with bone is preferred.

The fibular osteocutaneous free flap was described by Taylor et al. in 1975. It is based on the peroneal artery and its two venae comitantes and was initially used for the reconstruction of an open fracture of the lower extremity. Hildalgo in 1989 was the first to adapt its uses for the head and neck in the reconstruction of a segmental mandibulectomy defect.

The fibula provides a large segment of bone for reconstruction where approximately 22 to 25 cm of bone can be harvested. The fibular flap can be transferred as either a free osseous or a free osteocutaneous flap. In the setting of the palatomaxillary defect, the cutaneous portion is necessary for reconstruction of the palatal surface. The width of the skin paddle is often defined by the ability to achieve primary closure of the donor site. If the donor site cannot be closed without excessive tension, a skin graft may be required.

Although the pedicle length may reach up to 12 cm, it is often limited by the bifurcation with the posterior tibial artery. The vascular supply to the skin paddle arises from either a septocutaneous perforator arising between the peroneus longus and the soleus muscles or a musculocutaneous perforator through the flexor hallucis longus and soleus muscle.

HISTORY

When considering the fibula as a donor site for reconstruction of the total maxillectomy defect, the history should include the patient's expectations. While some patients will be pleased with a soft tissue reconstruction, others will demand dental restoration. The fibula provides the opportunity to restore the dentition by providing a bony infrastructure for osseointegrated implants. This is not possible with other forms of soft tissue reconstruction.

PHYSICAL EXAMINATION

The physical examination should include a careful evaluation of the defect and the donor site. The fibula is ideal for infrastructure defects that do not require reconstruction of the orbital rim. High vertical defects require more bone that the fibula can provide. The donor site should be evaluated to assure that there is no evidence of trauma or prior surgery that may preclude using this donor site. The donor site must also be carefully inspected for venous stasis ulcers, lesions, or varicose veins. The overall thickness of the skin, subdermal component, and muscle must be carefully evaluated to ensure a good match for the defect.

INDICATIONS

The palatomaxillary defect involving the anterior projecting element is ideal for the use of an osteocutaneous flap. Radial forearm osteocutaneous, scapular, iliac crest, and fibular free flaps have been reported for reconstruction of this defect.

The fibular free flap should be considered in the setting of an intact orbital floor and rim and a total maxillectomy defect extending beyond the anterior projecting element. The bone provides the anterior projection, contouring, and support; the cutaneous component is used to recreate the palatal mucosal defect; and the muscle of the flap is used to fill in the midface volume defect. Additionally, the bone of the fibula can allow for future osteointegrated implants.

The fibular free flap, however, would not be the preferred reconstruction if a significant portion of the orbital floor and rim has been resected. Although many options have been reported in this setting, the scapular free flap using the tip for the orbital floor and rim would be my choice of reconstruction.

CONTRAINDICATIONS

There are some rare anatomic anomalies that would preclude the use of the fibular free flap. Three vessel runoff to the foot is a prerequisite for the use of the fibular flap, unless the peroneal artery is the nonrunoff vessel. Preoperative MRA is used to determine the patency of the arterial vasculature.

Mönckeberg calcinosis is a relative contraindication for fibular free flap reconstruction. This entity is characterized by calcium deposits in the medial layer of the artery and therefore cannot be diagnosed by MRA but only by plain radiography of the lower extremities. The arteries are firm and nonpliable making it difficult to accomplish a secure anastomosis in these patients.

The patients' donor site must be carefully inspected. Evaluation of the thickness of the lower extremity is critical in the reconstruction of the palatomaxillary defect. In patients with circumferentially large lower extremities, consideration of other donor sites may be necessary. The presence of venous stasis, varicose veins, and previous surgery or trauma to the lower extremity may be a relative contraindication for the use of the fibular flap.

PREOPERATIVE PLANNING

An MRA is performed for all patients being considered for a fibular free flap. Three-vessel runoff or anterior and posterior tibial artery runoff to the foot is required for successful harvest. I also recommend a preoperative radiograph of the lower extremity to exclude Mönckeberg calcinosis.

SURGICAL TECHNIQUE

The leg is positioned with a bump under the foot and the knee flexed at approximately 45 degrees. A tourniquet is placed on the upper thigh and the leg rotated slightly medially. The leg is then prepped and draped from the thigh to the foot.

The topographical anatomy is outlined on the lateral aspect of the leg. The bony landmarks of the posterior aspect of the fibular head superiorly and the lateral epicondyle of the ankle inferiorly are identified. A line is drawn from the posterior aspects of these bony landmarks. The intermuscular septum corresponds to this line with a slight 10-degree angle posteroinferiorly. The peroneal nerve runs approximately 1 to 2 cm below the fibular head.

A Doppler is used along the intermuscular septum to identify the skin perforator. Using a "pinch test," the skin is grasped using the skin perforator as the epicenter of the flap. The width of the proposed cutaneous portion is based on this maneuver to ensure primary closure of the donor site. A 6-cm strut of bone is left both superiorly and inferiorly to ensure stability of the ankle.

The tourniquet is then elevated up to 350 degrees of mercury. The anterior skin incision is made through the level of the muscular fascia. A subfascial plane overlying the peroneus longus and brevis muscles is dissected posteriorly allowing identification of the cutaneous perforators. These perforators are marked for future reference.

The peroneus longus and brevis muscles are then retracted anteriorly allowing access to the intermuscular septum medial to the fibular bone. The intermuscular septum is divided allowing access to the anterior compartment consisting of the extensor hallucis and extensor digitorum longus. This muscular complex is then elevated off the fibula exposing the interosseous septum. Sharp incision of the interosseus septum completes the anterior dissection revealing the posterior tibialis muscle.

The posterior skin incision is made to the level of soleus muscle. Similarly, dissection is performed into the subfascial plane. A cuff of soleus muscle is routinely taken at this point to protect the cutaneous perforators. Deep to the soleus lies the flexor hallucis longus muscle. The fascia of the flexor hallucis longus muscle is incised, allowing release of the posterior tibial vessels medially away from the flap harvest.

Using a right-angle clamp, the distal aspect of the fibular bone is isolated allowing 6 cm of bone to be left in both the distal and the proximal aspects of the fibular bone. The osteotomies are then made using the sagittal saw. A window of fibular bone is taken superiorly to allow for later pedicle dissection. The fibular bone is then distracted. The flexor tendon is identified and divided taking the entire flexor hallucis longus with the fibular free flap. The distal vascular pedicle is identified, clamped, divided, and ligated. The dissection continues with division of the posterior tibial muscle at the level of the chevron. This is done from a distal to proximal fashion until the pedicle is identified and dissected to its junction with the posterior tibial artery.

The peroneal artery is then identified and isolated in 360-degree fashion with its two venae comitantes. The tourniquet is released allowing reperfusion of the flap. The skin is examined carefully to ensure flap viability. A minimum of 15 minutes of reperfusion is necessary prior to harvest.

Once the defect is created (Fig. 26.1), the flap is then harvested from the leg. The flap is brought to the back table, and under microscopic guidance, the artery and veins are dissected from each other (Fig. 26.2).

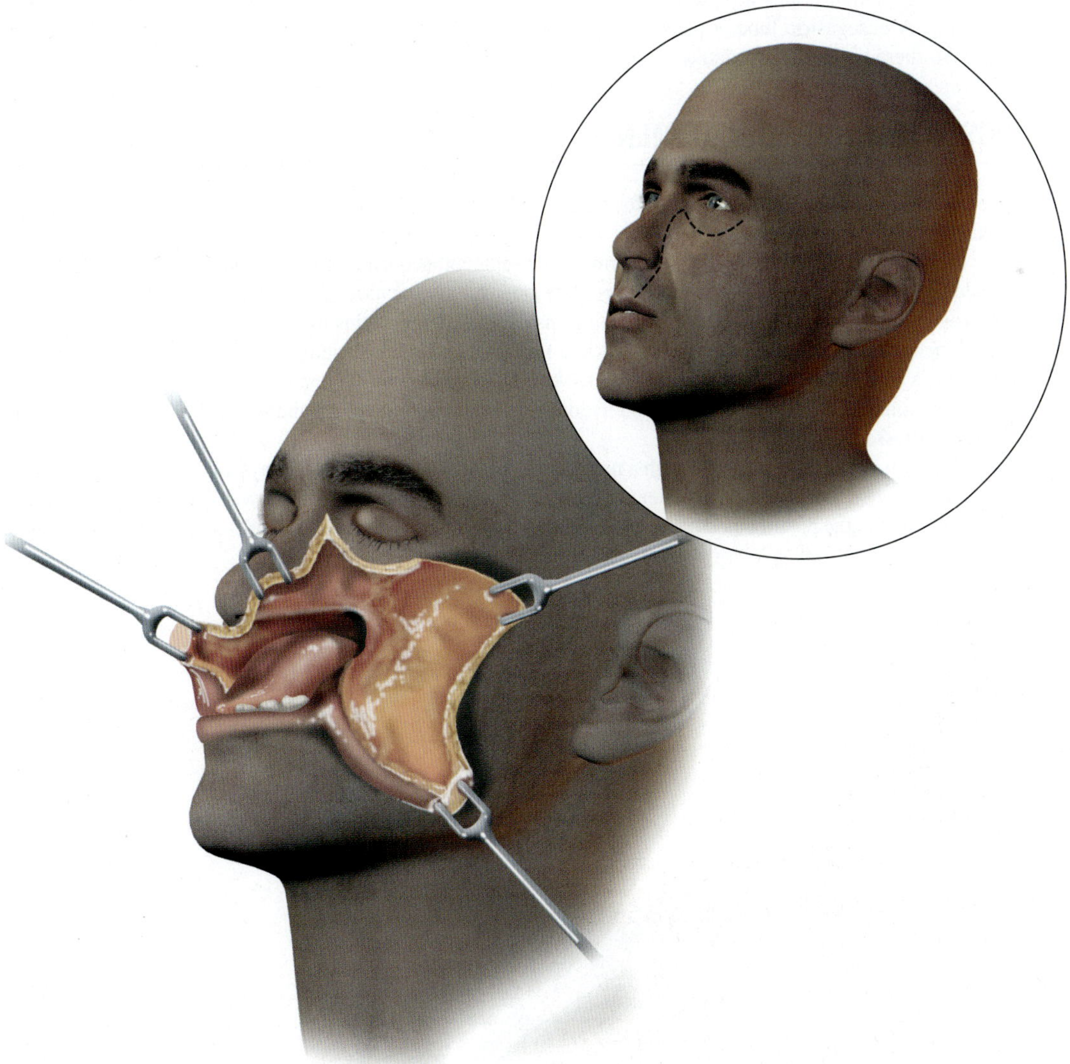

FIGURE 26.1 The total and near-total defect of the maxilla is typically approached through a Weber-Ferguson incision (**inset**). The maxillectomy defect can easily be accessed through this approach.

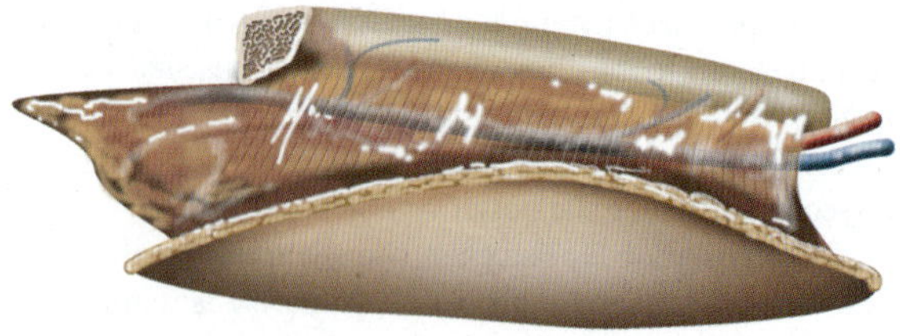

FIGURE 26.2
The fibular free flap provides a cylindrical bone graft. The peroneal artery and vein run parallel to the bone graft. The vessels can be dissected from the graft to gain length on the vascular pedicle.

The defect is then carefully analyzed. The contouring of the maxilla is created using a template fashioned to the resection specimen. The length of the fibular bone and appropriate closed osteotomies are determined based on this template.

To achieve appropriate length, the proximal periosteum is dissected to allow for the longest pedicle length possible. Using a sagittal saw, the bone is then contoured to the appropriate length (Fig. 26.3). The previously determined closed osteotomies are then performed to create the contour of the maxilla. Using 2.0 miniplates, the bone is then fashioned in place. Anteriorly, the bone is secured to the remnant maxilla. Laterally, the bone is secured to the remnant zygoma (Fig. 26.4).

The combination the flexor hallucis longus, soleus muscle are then brought into the midface to recreate fullness. The skin overlying the flap is then sewn into the mucosal defect. Prior to insetting the flap, a submucosal tunnel is made within the buccal fat into the subperiosteal plane lateral to the mandible and into the neck. The facial artery and vein are taken at the level of the mandible for microvascular anastomosis. The arterial anastomosis is done under microscopic guidance using a 9-0 nylon suture, and the venous anastomosis is usually completed using either a coupler or 8-0 nylon sutures.

Closed suction drains are placed both in the neck and in the donor site. A cast is placed on the lower extremity. A nasogastric tube is placed on the contralateral side. A temporary tracheostomy should be performed if there is significant edema.

POSTOPERATIVE MANAGEMENT

The cast is kept on the lower extremity for 5 days. Once the cast is removed, physical therapy is started with partial weight bearing.

Doppler monitoring of the flap is essential. The septocutaneous/musculocutaneous perforator to the skin should be identifiable with the Doppler. Pinprick testing can also be used as an adjunct to Doppler monitoring. Immediate exploration is indicated if there are signs of arterial/venous insufficiency.

A hematoma must also be carefully watched for either in the head and neck or the donor site. In the head and neck, a small blood collection could lead to venous congestion of the flap.

Hematoma in the donor site may lead to compartment syndrome or breakdown of the wound and should also be addressed immediately.

Nutrition is typically given through a nasogastric tube for a minimum of 7 days depending on the amount of tongue resected and whether the patient has received radiation therapy. I usually wait 2 weeks prior to initiating an oral diet in the postradiated patient. I recommend speech and swallow evaluations in all of these patients.

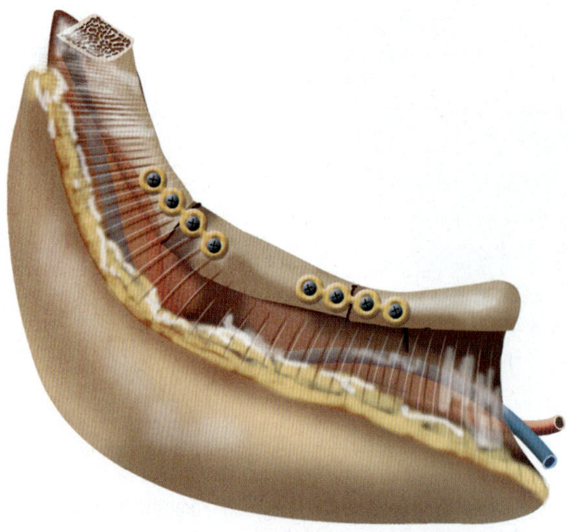

FIGURE 26.3
Multiple osteotomies can be made in the bone to provide the contour required for reconstruction of the maxilla.

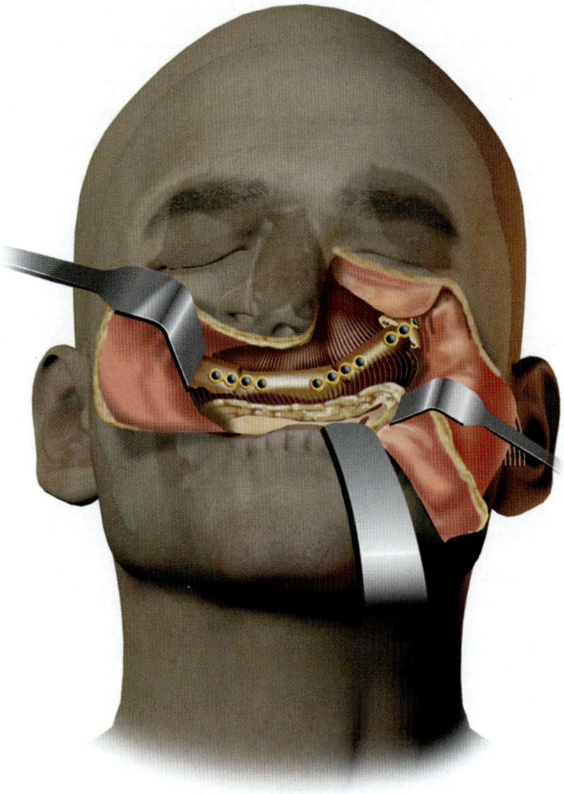

FIGURE 26.4
The bone graft is fixated to the native bone using miniplates. The soft tissue and skin paddle are used to line the palatal mucosal defect.

COMPLICATIONS

Hematomas were previously reported in up to 25% of patients with long bone reconstruction attributed to oozing from the exposed medullary surfaces of the fibular bone. My rate for hematoma in the head and neck is about 10%. As previously mentioned, immediate exploration is required once a hematoma is diagnosed.

Flap failure occurs at a rate of 2% at our institution, the majority of which are related to venous congestion. Emergent exploration is essential when there is presumed arterial or venous insufficiency. Leeches may be used when there is continual venous congestion where exploration reveals patency of the venous anastomosis or successful revision is performed. Donor site complications include a risk of footdrop secondary to injury to the common peroneal nerve. This complication may be avoided by meticulous dissection of the nerve early in the dissection. A 6-cm segment of bone should be left distally above the lateral malleolus to ensure ankle stability. Compartment syndrome may also rarely occur due to tight closure donor site. Judicious use of a skin graft should be considered in the setting of difficult donor site closure.

RESULTS

Reconstruction of the midface is one of the biggest challenges in head and neck reconstruction. Evaluation of the defect and possible reconstructive sites are essential for success. The fibular free flap is an excellent option in defects involving the anterior projection with an intact orbital floor and rim. Flap failure is rare in my experience. Patients undergoing successful repair should expect good cosmesis, speech, and swallowing function.

PEARLS

- Preoperative MRA and plain radiographs of the lower extremity are necessary.
- Patients with thin lower extremities are ideal for palatomaxillary reconstruction.
- Harvest with flexor hallucis longus allows for obliteration of the maxillary defect.
- Use of a premade template of the defect or the resection specimen is useful for accurate reconstruction.

PITFALLS

- Footdrop may occur if the peroneal nerve is not carefully preserved.
- Avoid using this flap in patients in whom the peroneal artery is the major blood supply to the foot.
- Avoid using this flap in patients with venous stasis ulcers, varicose veins, edema of the lower extremity, or a history of previous surgery or trauma to the drain site.
- Not an ideal flap for reconstruction in patients with defects of the orbital floor or orbital rim
- Ankle stability may be threatened unless 6 cm of distal bone above the lateral malleolus is preserved.

INSTRUMENTS TO HAVE AVAILABLE

- Standard head and neck surgical set
- A reciprocating saw
- Plating set

SUGGESTED READING

Hildalgo D. Fibula free flap: a new method of mandible reconstruction. *Plast Reconstr Surg* 1989;84:71.

Beppu M, Hanel D, Johnston G, et al. The osteocutaneous fibula flap: an anatomic study. *J Reconstr Microsurg* 1992;8: 215–233.

Futran ND, Wadsworth JT, Villaret D, et al. Midface reconstruction with the fibula free flap. *Arch Otolaryngol Head Neck Surg* 2002;128:161–166.

Kim DD, Dreher MA. The fibula free flap in maxillary reconstruction. *Atlas Oral Maxillofac Surg Clin North Am* 2007;15:13–22.

Dalgorf D, Higgins K. Reconstruction of the midface and maxilla. *Curr Opin Otololaryngol Head Neck Surg* 2008;16: 303–311.

27 PRIMARY RECONSTRUCTION OF THE TRACHEA

Eric M. Genden

INTRODUCTION

The history of tracheal reconstruction dates back more than 200 years. While many initially viewed the trachea as merely an airway conduit that could be replaced by an alloplastic tube, investigators and surgeons have gained a greater respect for the complex biology of the airway. The tracheal airway plays a critical role in mucociliary transport, airway hygiene, and antigen processing. Ideally, reconstructive techniques should strive to maintain these important functions.

Tracheal airway defects can be classified into three categories: Defects less than 4 cm, defects between 4 and 6 cm, and defects greater than 6 cm in length. Defects less than 4 cm are usually amenable to primary end-to-end anastomosis. Defects between 4 and 6 cm may require a multistaged reconstruction, and defects greater than 6 cm continue to represent a reconstructive dilemma; although a variety of techniques have been used to manage the latter group including allograft reconstruction, alloplastic reconstitution, and tracheal transplantation, none has proven effective.

HISTORY

A careful preoperative history and physical examination are essential. I feel that a detailed history is important in trying to understand the nature of the tracheal problem particularly a history of prior surgery, infection, and compromised wound healing. The underlying cause of the tracheal problem is important because it will help to determine the best approach to the reconstruction and often estimate the risk of restenosis. Tracheal defects may be the result of trauma, tumor resection, congenital stenosis, inhalational injury, or acquired idiopathic disease. While defects from trauma and tumor resection are often focal in nature, congenital and inhalational tracheal disease may result in more diffuse injury and therefore more extensive defects. In contrast, idiopathic disease often involves the cricoid cartilage and therefore presents a separate set of challenges. A thorough history can help to elucidate the underlying cause of the tracheal disease as well as to predict the nature of the defect and the best approach for reconstruction.

Factors of a general nature in the patient's history include infection or adverse wound healing. Both issues can compromise the outcome and, in some cases, may result in a catastrophic complication. Patients with brittle diabetes, collagen vascular disease, or prior surgery represent the greatest challenge.

PHYSICAL EXAMINATION

The physical examination includes both preoperative and intraoperative evaluations. Preoperatively, pulmonary function studies, computed tomography (CT), and endoscopy represent the three pillars of the evaluation. The pulmonary function studies are not essential for every patient but may provide information

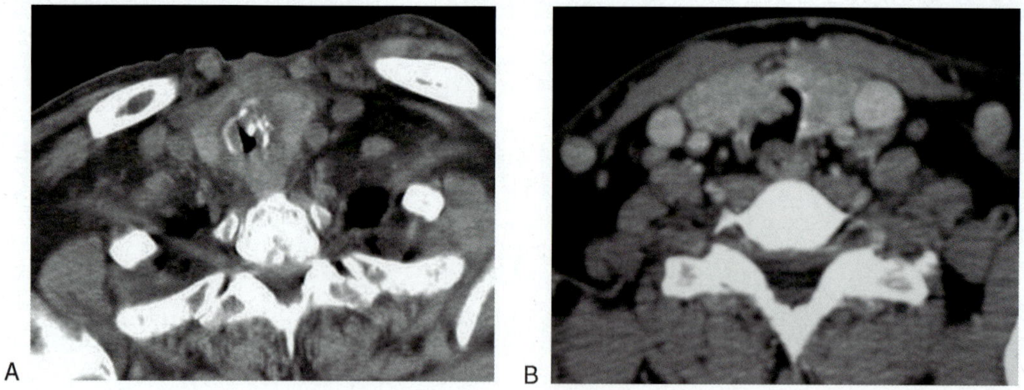

FIGURE 27.1
A,B. The high-resolution CT scan (1-mm cuts) provides a sensitive method to evaluate the infraglottic airway. These images demonstrate invasion of the trachea that may not be appreciated on office endoscopy.

about whether the airway obstruction is fixed or dynamic. Dynamic obstruction, such as tracheomalacia and vascular compression syndrome, is often more challenging to manage than is focal fixed obstruction. The CT scan and the endoscopic evaluations often provide information related to the length and site of the stenosis. Flexible tracheoscopy can be performed in the office to evaluate the airway and determine if an obstruction is dynamic or fixed. Unfortunately, not all patients will tolerate such an examination. The high-resolution CT scan (1-mm cuts) is a highly sensitive method used in the evaluation of the infraglottic airway, and I find that the axial, coronal, and sagittal views each offer important information (Fig. 27.1A and B). Three-dimensional reconstruction can also provide important information related to the site of the stenosis (Fig. 27.2).

The intraoperative endoscopy typically provides the best examination. A rigid fiberoptic endoscope provides a high-resolution evaluation of the airway that can be exceptionally helpful in determining the nature of the disease and predict the best approach to reconstruction (Fig. 27.3).

INDICATIONS

The indications for primary (end-to-end) tracheal reconstruction are defects that are less than 4 cm in length. In select patients, defects that are less than 6 cm can be managed with primary end-to-end reconstruction but may require infrahyoid muscle release and/or a suprahyoid muscle release. However, these techniques impede elevation of the larynx during swallowing and may result in aspiration.

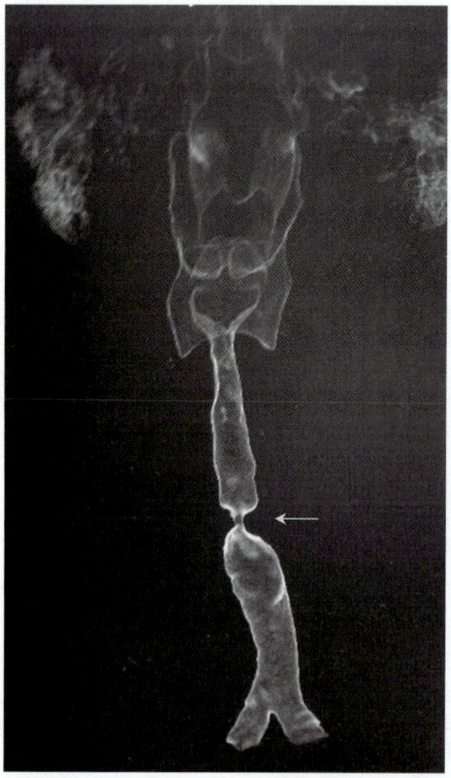

FIGURE 27.2
Three-dimensional reconstruction can provide important information related to the site of the stenosis.

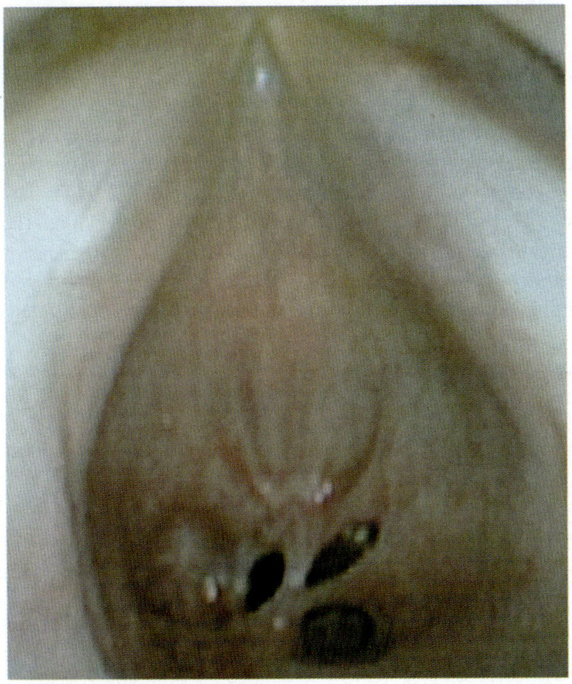

FIGURE 27.3
High-resolution endoscopy of a tracheal lesion.

CONTRAINDICATIONS

The contraindications to primary tracheal reconstruction are patients with defects greater than 6 cm in length and patients with defects greater than 4 cm in length if there is a history of a previously failed reconstruction, external beam radiation therapy, or compromised healing. It is critical to understand that every patient is an individual and therefore each patient should be evaluated as such. Most contraindications are "relative" contraindications. The patient's anatomy, body habitus, and personal disposition all play a role in the decision-making process concerning reconstruction.

PREOPERATIVE PLANNING

Prior to surgery, I evaluate airway resistance in all subjects. A flow-volume loop is generated by having the patient inhale deeply to total lung capacity (TLC), forcefully exhale until the lungs have been emptied to residual volume, and rapidly inhale to reach TLC. A maximal expiratory flow 50%: Maximal inspiratory flow 50% ratio is, therefore, usually less than 1. In variable extrathoracic lesions, the ratio is increased (usually >1), while in variable intrathoracic lesions, the ratio is diminished (0.2 or less). In fixed obstructions, the ratio is expected to be close to 1. This study provides an excellent method to determine diagnosis and eligibility for surgery.

SURGICAL TECHNIQUE

Primary reconstruction of the trachea can be achieved through a straight end-to-end technique or a sliding technique depending on the defect and the needs of the patient. Independent of the approach, the basic technique is similar. Prior to oral–tracheal intubation, I perform a rigid endoscopy using an apneic technique or with a ventilating bronchoscope. This provides an opportunity to reevaluate the nature of the tracheal disease and it thoroughly acquaint me with the location of the pathology. After the endoscopy, the patient is intubated orally, and the standard sterile preparation is performed. The neck is exposed through a standard collar incision. The trachea is exposed through a midline strap-splitting approach.

The trachea is isolated by dissecting along it with Metzenbaum scissors and bipolar cautery to achieve a bloodless field. Careful attention is dedicated to the recurrent laryngeal nerves, and as the dissection progresses peripherally, the soft tissue enveloping the recurrent laryngeal nerves is gently dissected off of the trachea.

Once the trachea is isolated, the cuff of the endotracheal tube is deflated and a transverse incision is made into the airway above and below the stenosis. The resection of the tracheal disease should include both the cartilaginous trachea and the membranous posterior segment.

Once the tracheal resection is complete, the distal trachea can be dissected from the esophagus and surrounding soft tissue to release and advance the airway cephalad. The mediastinal release can be achieved through careful blunt finger dissection. In short defects of the trachea, a mediastinal release may be appropriate; however, in more extensive defects, an infrahyoid and/or suprahyoid release may be required. In either case, the hyoid attachments can be cut with electrocautery at a low setting in an effort to prevent injury to the superior laryngeal nerves.

Once the tracheal release has been achieved, the anastomosis can be performed. I begin the procedure by deflating the cuff of the endotracheal tube to expose the defect in the posterior wall (Fig. 27.4A). The posterior wall of the trachea is reconstructed using 3-0 glycolide suture (Monocryl, Ethicon, Somerville, NJ). The sutures are placed interrupted with the knots directed outside of the lumen (Fig. 27.4B). Once the posterior membranous wall has been reconstructed, the remainder of the cartilage tracheal anastomosis can be completed using 2-0 polypropylene suture (Prolene suture, Ethicon, Somerville, NJ). The sutures are placed interrupted, and the knots are directed outside the lumen (Fig. 27.4C).

I like to place a "tension-releasing suture" across the tracheal anastomosis to alleviate tension on the tracheal anastomosis. The strap muscles are closed over the trachea, and a suction drain is placed.

POSTOPERATIVE MANAGEMENT

Postoperatively, the patient is extubated in the operating room. The patient is then transferred to a monitored bed for 24 hours. I consider discharge from the hospital on postoperative day 4 or 5. Patients are instructed on open-mouth sneezing and minimal coughing.

COMPLICATIONS

Complications of airway reconstruction can range from minor infections to catastrophic anastomotic breakdown. Careful routine evaluation of the patient is important to identify complications and institute early management. Minor complications such as subcutaneous air can result in wound infection and tracheal anastomotic breakdown without early intervention. More significant complications such as wound breakdown require aggressive management that should not be delayed.

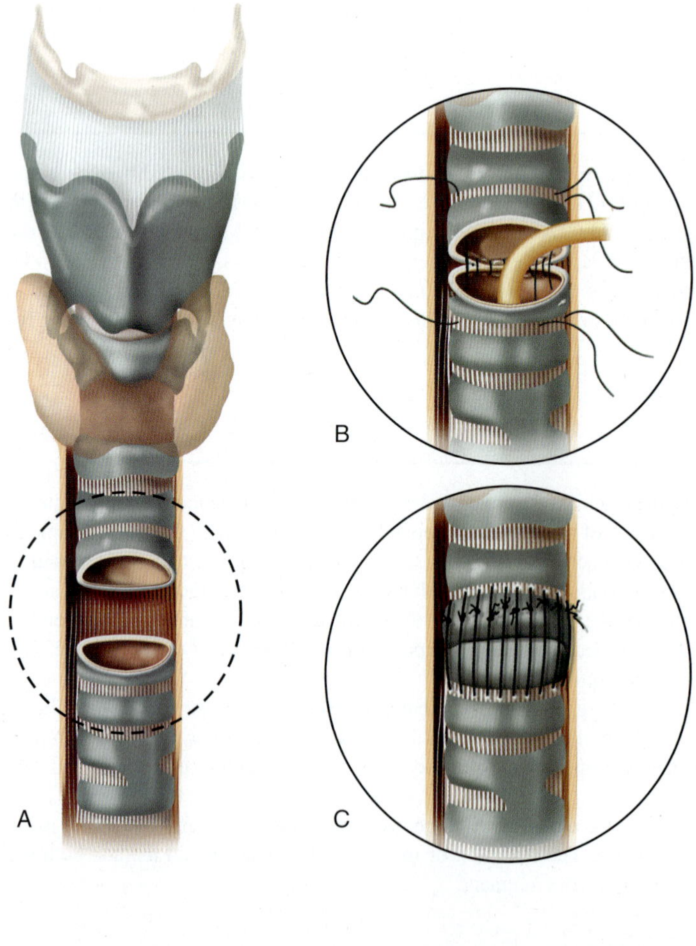

FIGURE 27.4
A. The tracheal defect resulting from resection of the airway. **B.** Reconstruction of the membranous posterior tracheal wall with absorbable sutures. **C.** Interrupted nonabsorbable sutures used to reconstruct the anterior tracheal wall.

RESULTS

I have found that this technique is reliable and safe in my personal series of more than 150 such cases. Meticulous surgical technique tends to limit the risk of minor complications such as intraluminal granulation tissue and restenosis. Extubation in the operating room is helpful in identifying problems early so that the patient can be managed in a safe and monitored setting. My complication rate is less than 1%, and my restenosis rate is less than 3%.

PEARLS

- Endoscopy and CT scan are essential aspects of the preoperative evaluation.
- Endoscopy performed in the operating room prior to surgery is helpful in evaluating the pathology and predicting the defect.
- Meticulous surgical technique will help to prevent granulation tissue in the tracheal lumen.
- When the tracheal ends are brought together, it is important to oppose the ends and not prolapse them.

PITFALLS

- Early recognition of an anastomotic leak can be made at the time of extubation. It can also be managed immediately before subcutaneous air and infection ensue.
- If the suture knots are placed intraluminal, granulation and restenosis are more common.

INSTRUMENTS TO HAVE AVAILABLE

- Standard head and neck surgery set
- Rigid fiberoptic endoscopy

SUGGESTED READING

de Alarcon A, Rutter MJ. Cervical slide tracheoplasty. *Arch Otolaryngol Head Neck Surg* 2012;138:812–816.
Delaere PR. Tracheal transplantation (Review). *Curr Opin Pulm Med* 2012;18:313–320.
Rich JT, Gullane PJ. Current concepts in tracheal reconstruction. *Curr Opin Otolaryngol Head Neck Surg* 2012;20:246–253.

28 STAGED RECONSTRUCTION OF THE CERVICAL TRACHEA

Peak Woo

INTRODUCTION

The laryngotracheal system is a challenge for all reconstructive surgeons. Physiologic restoration requires that the reconstruction performed after ablation satisfies the specific physiologic requirements for breathing, speaking, and swallow. Any permanent loss of any of the above functions results in severe quality of life deficiencies that can cause great emotional distress for the patient. The unique nature of the composite tissue required for adequate reconstruction of the trachea has challenged reconstructive surgeons over many decades. Consistent results for replacement of longer trachea loss after tumor surgery, trauma, and intubation have eluded excellent surgeons despite reports of grafts, prosthesis, and free flaps. This situation continues today.

Multiple very sophisticated techniques have been proposed since the use of local flaps was initially proposed for laryngotracheal reconstruction. These include mucosal flaps, muscle flaps, pedicled flap, perichondrium flaps, and free tissue transfer flaps. Despite this, great challenges remain in the reconstruction of tracheal and laryngeal defects after ablation for cancer and defects caused by trauma and infection. Any use of metallic or foreign materials has a tendency for extrusion due to pressure necrosis. In the trachea, repetitive motion from respiration and infection are the main factors contributing to long-term failure. Despite these challenges, the staged cervical tracheal reconstruction approach is worthy of consideration in selected patients with long-segment tracheal defects.

HISTORY

Resection of the cervical trachea, sometimes in conjunction with resection of the skin of the neck with the larynx still being intact, requires reconstructive techniques that will bring tissue together as a hollow tube. The hollow tube is necessary in order to permit continued respiration, phonation, and swallowing through an intact larynx and pharynx. While the trachea may be thought of as a static tube for airway maintenance, the cervical trachea is subject to great movement during flexion, extension, and swallowing. Small regional flaps in the neck may routinely be used for rehabilitation of limited defects if the surgical defect is less than 50% of the circumference of the larynx and trachea. Larger defects in this area may require resection and anastomosis, use of free tissue transfer, or staged reconstruction. For example, a small primary cancer of the subglottis or localized tracheal invasion by a low-grade cancer of the thyroid may result in a small defect that can be immediately repaired by rotation of composite tissue or a small muscle flap with free graft of cartilage into the area to maintain stability of the segment. With endolaryngeal or tracheal stenting, such small defects can be reliably reconstructed immediately. The reconstructive procedure of choice for small to medium circumferential defects of the trachea is by primary resection and anastomosis as popularized by Grillo, however, some patients are not suitable candidates. If this stenosis or tumor involvement involves less than four tracheal rings and the patient's neck anatomy is favorable, primary resection and anastomosis of up to 4 cm may be accompanied easily by primary resection, tracheal release, and direct approximation of the two ends of the trachea. In the patient with a short neck, in patients who have had previous radiation therapy, and in the patient with previous surgery involving the mediastinum, the ability to transpose the trachea superiorly in order to perform primary anastomosis is much more limited. This is especially so in the patients who have previously failed attempted laryngotracheoplasty. When the defect goes beyond the limits of primary anastomosis or the surgery is limited by an ability to mobilize and transpose the trachea without tension, a staged augmentation approach should be considered.

Complications that result in tracheal stenosis should be separated on the basis of whether it is due to tumor resection, to mechanical external trauma, or to trauma from prolonged intubation or tracheostomy. Defects due to resection of primary cancer in the cervical trachea are rare and more likely are due to tracheal invasion by thyroid cancer. In this group of patients, primary tracheal reconstruction usually has a favorable outcome due to the uninvolved nature of the trachea from scarring and intubation. In patients with complications of the trachea due to motor vehicle trauma or industrial accident, early diagnosis and treatment and primary treatment may be able to be performed by primary repair and stenting around an indwelling T tube or Montgomery laryngeal stent. Early diagnosis and treatment in most instances can prevent the progression to late cicatricial stenosis.

Management of acute tracheal trauma is dictated by the need for establishment of an adequate airway, to control bleeding, and by the urgency of medical attention needed for other systems injury treatment. If possible, the laryngeal and tracheal area suspected of injury should be inspected early. Hematoma, fracture, and laceration and dislocations may be sutured and reconstituted by internal stenting. Endotracheal stent using a soft Silastic tube or endotracheal tube is usually left for 2 to 3 weeks. Small fragments and lacerations may be repaired with sutures, and stabilization of the indwelling stent using wires or external fixation with Silastic buttons. If there has been extensive mucosal loss from trauma, the airway lumen should be stabilized by indwelling stent for 3 weeks to 2 months depending on the extent of mucosal injury. By use of early stenting, there is less likelihood of need for late staged reconstruction.

In patients who develop laryngeal or tracheal stenosis as a complication of intubation, the defect is usually recognized late. This occurs as failure of decannulation from tracheotomy, or the patient may present with progressive stridor after decannulation. This group of patients with iatrogenic intubation-related injury should be considered separately from tumor or trauma cases. They can be considered to be at higher risk for development of laryngeal and tracheal stenosis. Poor wound healing and scar formation risk factors for laryngeal tracheal stenosis include diabetes mellitus, asthma and chronic obstructive pulmonary disease, acid reflux and nonacid reflux of abdominal contents into the trachea, autoimmune disease, and systemic illness that require chronic corticosteroid use. In these patients, preoperative evaluation of the position and size of the stenosis before surgery should be accompanied by medical evaluation to optimize systemic factors such as diabetes, pulmonary disease, and acid reflux. The use of 24-hour pH hour probe study should be entertained if there is persistent granulation or chronic inflammation at the stenosis site. The patient should be weaned off all systemic steroids before surgery. The ideal state of the patient before undergoing tracheal reconstruction should be a mature white scar at the site of the tracheal stenosis. Granulation tissue and chronic inflammation should be reversed or limited only to the area that is to be resected.

PHYSICAL EXAMINATION

Accurate assessment of the laryngotracheal stenosis is accomplished by radiography as well as by endoscopy. Endoscopic examination with biopsy will be able to check the area of stenosis as well as to differentiate the area of stenosis as to whether it is circumferential or local. Examination under anesthesia with bronchoscopy will also identify areas of malacia that may need resection. A biopsy of the area of concern will usually be able to tell if the stenosis is a mature scar or whether this is actively inflamed with chronic and acute inflammatory changes. If there is chronic inflammation on the preoperative tissue biopsy, surgical resection should go beyond the area of chronic inflammation into more healthy tissue in order to avoid repeat stenosis. Radiographic imaging is accomplished by CT scan with 1-mm cuts through the trachea. This scan can be reconstructed as a virtual bronchoscopy with three-dimensional reconstruction. In addition, a CT scan can differentiate easily between circumferential wine bottle–type stenosis versus isolated tracheal stenosis. In the patient who has already failed previous laryngotracheal reconstruction, evaluation using CT scan can be especially helpful to decide whether the restenosis can be treated by endoscopic means or whether open surgical intervention may be needed.

Some patients with tracheostomy dependence and laryngotracheal stenosis are not good candidates for reconstruction. Poorly controlled diabetes mellitus, renal failure with cortical steroid dependence, chronic bacterial tracheitis, and chronic bronchitis are some of the reasons for deferment of patients for tracheal reconstruction. One example of such is the patient with poor mucosal hygiene and tracheotomy care. Chronic infection of the tracheotomy site in patients with chronic indwelling tracheostomy tubes results in copious granulation tissue, tracheitis, and mucopurulent discharge. Despite the best efforts of the health care team, sometimes it is not possible to restore the tracheostomy stenosis site to a healthy enough state to consider reconstruction. In these patients, premature surgical intervention can result in worse outcome with stricture formation, granulation tissue, and complete stenosis. In these patients, it may be preferable to delay reconstruction as long as possible until the traumatized area has undergone complete cicatricial formation. Attention in the meantime should be directed to allow all the necrotic tissue to be absorbed, the granulation to become healthy epithelium, and the tracheostomy site to be odorless and clean. This may take as long as 18 months after the initial injury.

If the stenosis is less than 2 cm in length, a direct resection and approximation of the proximal and distal ends may be done without tension. This can be performed as a single-stage procedure. If the two ends of the tracheal cartilage of the anastomosis are solid, internal stenting is not necessary. In patients who have favorable anatomy to permit a tension-free closure and when the site can be directly approximated, this is the most expedient technique with the least complications.

INDICATIONS

The indications for staged tracheal reconstruction are defects greater than 4-cm circumferential tracheal stenosis, long-segment tracheal stenosis where pull-up primary anastomosis is not possible, combined laryngeal and tracheal stenosis, tracheal stenosis after ablative surgery without donor vessels for free tissue transfer, and tracheal stenosis in patients with prior resection.

CONTRAINDICATIONS

When surgery involves multiple sites such as cricoid cartilage and tracheal resection, direct closure may not be feasible. After primary resection of the scar tissue, the lumen can be established. For short segments of raw tissue devoid of mucosa, resurfacing by allowing the surrounding epithelium to grow in may need to be followed by prolonged internal stenting. Stabilization of the lumen with the use of an internal stent is usually done with a soft Silastic T tube or a conforming internal laryngeal stent made of soft Silastic. Local mucosal flaps have a limited role in the trachea. The trachea does not lend itself easily to mucosal flaps from other tracheal tissue due to damage to the donor site. Small rotation flaps from the posterior wall of the trachea are limited to a small triangle of tissue that is at most 5 mm in length. In selected situations, a small mucosal flap may be transposed to cover defects. An alternative technique is to transfer the mucosal by a mucosal grafting technique. This requires stenting and is sometimes unreliable due to excessive movement of the stent against the trachea.

PREOPERATIVE PLANNING

Evaluation: The patient will have already undergone the appropriate radiographic study and endoscopy to determine the necessity of a staged procedure. Consent is obtained for excision of tracheal stenosis with cervical advancement flap and placement of endoluminal stent.

The use of a staged rehabilitation by flap transposition technique has a long and colorful history that first challenged reconstructive surgeons after the First World War. Rehabilitation by flap transposition may be accomplished using local or regional flaps, flaps in combination with skin or mucosal grafting, or distant flaps migrated into position. More recently, the development of free tissue transfer has made a significant contribution to the need for staged reconstruction. However, staged reconstruction continues to have a role in tracheal reconstruction since free tissue transfer is often limited by soft tissue bulk. The development of tracheal staged reconstruction follows the staged reconstruction techniques for the esophagus.

Many surgical procedures have been devised to manage laryngotracheal stenosis resulting from trauma. Laryngotracheal atresia is the most severe form and the most difficult to repair. To correct larger defects without primary repair, epithelial grafting may be considered. Free partial-thickness skin grafts can be used around a stent. This is hard to stabilize, and infection and slough of the graft are common. The contraction of the split-thickness graft after placement is another concern that prevents its use in the trachea.

Since the trachea is a composite tissue of thin soft and hard tissue, the geometry of reconstruction of the composite tissue is critical. Single-stage autologous tissue transfer is difficult to simulate the architectural requirements of the defects after trauma, intubation, or disease processes. Composite tissue can be transferred after creation in a distant donor site and transferred into place, or there may be staged procedures whereby soft and hard tissue is fabricated in the recipient site. For small defects of the anterior trachea, the use of solid tissue support may not be necessary, and Eliacher has advocated the use of the rotatory trap door flap as a single-stage procedure. This has the advantage of a single-stage procedure and does not need rigid expansion or support, but it is limited by the small anterior defects. For small defects of the anterior trachea, muscle flaps with titanium plates have also been proposed.

Some regenerative capacity of the trachea from the resection margin can be expected over time. This mucosa can be expected to resurface the muscle or perichondrium placed over the defect so that it could more closely simulate normal tracheal mucosa. This technique requires placement of a long-term endoluminal stent of 6 to 12 months until secondary contraction and scar healing is complete. Long-term stenting is used to avoid the need for treatment of secondary stenosis. This approach is best used when the posterior trachea is still intact so that there is sufficient healthy mucosa to grow into the defect.

For long-segment stenosis, a staged reconstruction is necessary. Reconstruction of the cervical trachea using cervical skin was described by Montgomery in 1964. This is one of the first descriptions of staged reconstruction. He reported the use of a staged procedure with rib grafting to maintain patency in a single patient. Conley described a similar approach in 1970. The tracheal trough is first lined by thin non–hair-bearing skin. The trough is then matured by inserting a semisolid mold or a T tube that traverses the defect. After a suitable period of maturation that is variable from 3 to 6 months, a secondary procedure is done by placing a roof over the trough. Since the initial reports in the 60s, other reconstructive surgeons have reported successful use of this approach for longer segments of the trachea where primary anastomosis is not feasible.

Extraluminal integrity to maintain the semisolid state of the trachea can be maintained by internal stenting with secondary reconstruction with Silastic, rib cartilage, or titanium mesh. For very long segments, it is best to maintain long-term stenting using a long indwelling T tube with a permanent tracheotomy without attempt at complete decannulation. In this way, the problem of longer-term tracheal collapse over time and plugging can be overcome by easy removal and cleansing of a long-term internal stent by having a permanent tracheal stoma. For long-segment stenosis that requires long-term stenting, one then has to be satisfied with having a phonatory system using lung-powered speech with plugging of the internal stent. The patient has to be satisfied with long-term internal stenting without decannulation.

The Meyer procedure is a three-stage operation that provides structural support that is covered with mucosa. A laryngotracheal trough is created, and a carved trough-shaped cartilage graft is placed above and lateral to it in the first stage. The skin over the graft is replaced by buccal mucosa in the second stage. In the last stage, the cartilage graft with overlying mucosa is swung onto the trough as a composite flap replacing the anterior and lateral laryngeal and tracheal walls.

The creation of a new tracheal conduit using cervical flaps first came out of creation of laryngotracheal stoma after cancer extirpation. Especially, for peristomal recurrent cancer, regional flaps were used to cover great vessels and avoid wound breakdown after radiation therapy. When tracheal resection was performed as part of oncologic surgery, it became necessary to split the sternum in order to gain access to the mediastinum. Placement of the inferior stump of the trachea required chest flaps or regional flaps in order to secure a tracheal stoma. Myocutaneous flaps were used to obliterate large dead space and protect the great vessels. It is from the experience of oncologic surgery that experience was gained for reconstruction of the trachea for air passage using cervical skin flaps.

Surgeons using regional flaps must take into consideration factors of wound healing. Patients who have received external beam radiation therapy in the past will have progressive fibrosis with telangiectasia. Postradiated skin rarely can be used as a regional skin flap. Similarly, skin grafts placed into a radiated bed have a high incidence of infection and failure. Patients who are on corticosteroids or on immunosuppression similarly risk failure of the reconstruction from wound breakdown while patients with chronic inflammation and autoimmune disease suffer the risk of repeat stenosis from progressive wound contracture.

Local cervical flaps use the inverted cervical skin for internal lining of closure of a stoma. Large non–hair-bearing cervical flaps from the inferior aspect of the neck are obtainable from the female but may be a problem in the male. In tracheal reconstruction, the approach is similar to that of reconstruction of the cervical esophagus with the exception of need for a semirigid tube that does not collapse with inspiration. After excision of the stenosis, the tube and the end of the tracheal stoma are sutured onto the cervical flap. Subsequently, the stoma and the skin from the cervical flap are then tubed with various degrees or types of hard tissue to permit the reconstruction of a rigid tube. Regional tissue from the cervical flap is then used to construct a roof over the rigid trough. The local skin defect after construction of the skin-lined tube is closed by a second flap to accomplish external skin surface closure. The closure of the skin donor defect may be accomplished by a local rotation cervical flap or by the use of a deltopectoral flap. Although the deltopectoral flap is a highly versatile flap that has been used for esophageal reconstruction, its use in reconstruction of the lining of the trachea has been limited.

SURGICAL TECHNIQUE

The staged procedure is classically described as a three staged procedure. The first and second stage may be combined in some patients. The first stage is the resection of the stenosis and bridging of the tracheal defect by the cervical skin flap to create a trough. The second stage is performed to create a rigid wall for the conduit for air by the insertion of titanium mesh or cartilage into the wall of the skin flap. The third stage is the closure of the trough by using the local reinforced tissue to close the "roof" of the trough and close the skin donor defect. In large defects, there may even be a fourth stage where the third stage is closed but still leaving a small tracheostomy in place for later decannulation after it is certain that the patient can tolerate removal of the tracheostomy. Clearly, some patients with extensive defects or those with major medical morbidities may complete only some stages of the reconstruction. In those cases, the patient has the benefit of speech and can be plugged with long-term indwelling internal stent. The patient is taught the care for indwelling long-term T tube and the rest of the reconstruction is delayed, sometimes indefinitely.

Stage I

Resection of the Stenosis Followed by Skin-Lined Trough Creation

The patient is placed in a supine position with the indwelling endotracheal tube sutured downward. The anesthesiology team is on the patients left side. The tracheostomy tube is removed and replaced with an anode tube. The anode tube is sutured in the midline on the sternum with two 2-0 silk sutures with a 2- to 3-cm distance of endotracheal tube to the stoma. The cuff is prepped into the wound. The above maneuver is to allow the surgical team to remove and replace the endotracheal tube at will during the operation. The surgical team is at the head and each side of the neck. The prep incorporates the head, neck, and any local flaps that may be anticipated to do the resection and the first stage of the reconstruction. If the plan is to insert rib cartilage at the time of the first stage, the right chest over the lower costal cartilage is also prepared. One goes from the clean to the dirty operative site. So before the resection and insertion of the costal cartilage graft, the costal cartilage graft would be harvested and set aside for later use.

Planning of the Incision

Most of the patients with tracheostomy dependence and tracheal stenosis will already have a hypertrophic scar in the midline. When the segment of stenosis is long, a vertical incision is preferred to perform the resection. In some selected cases, two parallel horizontal incisions can be used if the skin in the midline is healthy. This requires an exact knowledge as to the size of the defect to be lined. It also makes it a bit more difficult to do the resection. For this reason, the majority of tracheal resections are done with a vertical incision. After the tracheal resection is complete and the size of the defect is known, the cervical advancement flap is designed and completed. At the end of the resection of the stenosis, a double cervical advancement flap from each side is used to suture together on top of the cervical esophagus. This is usually not a problem by simple advancement since the trachea has been resected. To achieve a tension-free closure, a Burroughs triangle may be resected as part of the flap design (Fig. 28.1).

Resection of Stenosis

Resection of stenosis is done by resection of the abnormal skin and the scarred trachea. It is critical to resect the abnormal skin and reach healthy tissue both at the skin level and the trachea. In the trachea, it is usually necessary to resect the entire tracheal stoma in order to reach healthy tissue. This may need dissection behind the sternum, and the cervical trachea must be mobilized adequately as in a tracheal resection and anastomosis. Healthy, granulation-free tissue must be reached both proximally and distally in order to become the two ends of the new tracheal conduit (Fig. 28.2.)

Creation of the Flap

The distal tracheal stump is secured by sutures to the skin of the neck at the inferior end of the incision. The skin of the neck that is sutured to the inferior wall of the trachea may need to have the adipose tissue removed so that full-thickness skin is advanced without tether. The angulations of the trachea should not be disturbed by the suture and kinking of the trachea should be avoided. 4-0 Vicryl suture is used for this purpose.

Bilateral cervical advancement skin flaps are now created and advanced to the midline. The size of the skin flap should be just enough to fill the tracheal defect without tension. The skin advanced to create the new lining

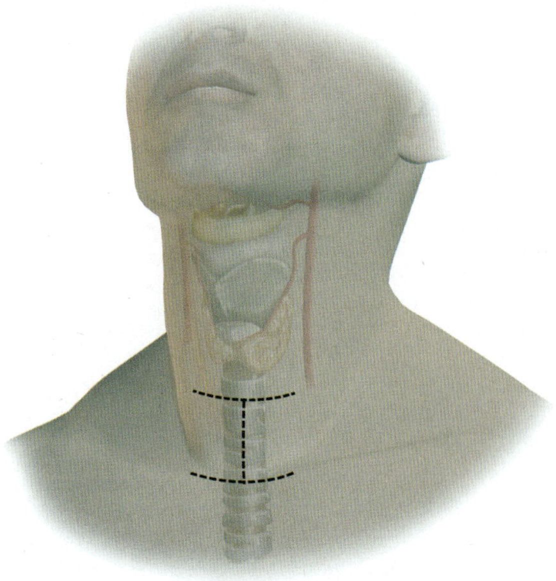

FIGURE 28.1
Incision for the advancement flap and resection of the poor quality skin and the tracheal stenosis. The final design of the cervical advancement flap should be created after the resection is complete.

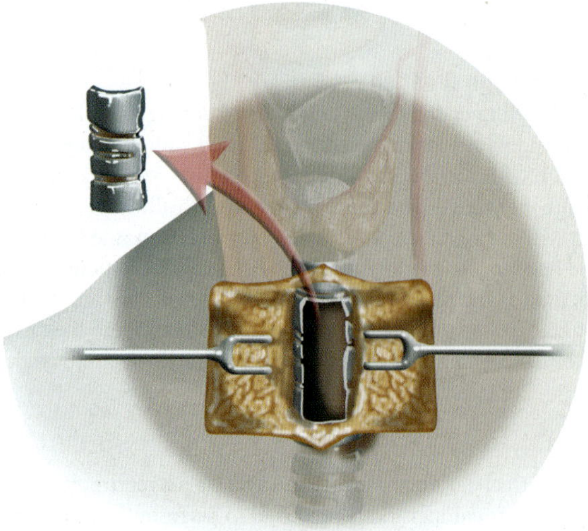

FIGURE 28.2
Resection of the stenosis from the cervical tracheal stenosis.

of the trachea should be full thickness and should not include platysma muscle. Therefore, the distal 2 cm of each flap is thinned out until only the skin is present. The distal end of the flap is trimmed of excessive adipose tissue such that the skin flap that is laid down is skin on muscle (Fig. 28.3).

If the posterior tracheal wall is intact, the skin is advanced as a bilateral cervical advancement flap. The skin is sutured to the membranous portion of the trachea using 4-0 Monocryl. If there is complete stenosis and a complete relining of the trachea is necessary, the skin flaps are approximated in the midline using a 4-0 Vicryl. Sutures are buried, so there are no knots in the lumen side.

Several tacking sutures are placed on to the cervical advancement flap against the sternomastoid muscle. This reduces the tension on the cervical skin flaps and allows the new tracheal skin trough to be formed around a stent. The proximal and the distal ends of the trachea are sutured to the horizontal portion of the cervical flap. It is important that the skin flap lies flat and the skin and tracheal tissue make a smooth transition without redundancy of the skin.

Insertion of the T-tube stent for maintenance of the trough packing is done last (Fig. 28.4). Penrose drain is placed under the flap for drainage. Soft Silastic T-tube or finger cot packing is used. The finger cot pack is made by using iodoform gauze packed into a no. 8 finger cot glove and coated with antibiotic ointment. The finger cot is then sutured into the skin flap so as to create the trough by using a Prolene suture through the top and bottom of the skin flap and pulling the flaps to each other. The Prolene is placed through the top of the finger cot so as to keep the finger cot to prevent displacement. Two sutures secure the packing in place and keep the stent in place while maintaining the trough. The tracheostomy is used to replace the endotracheal tube at the end of the case.

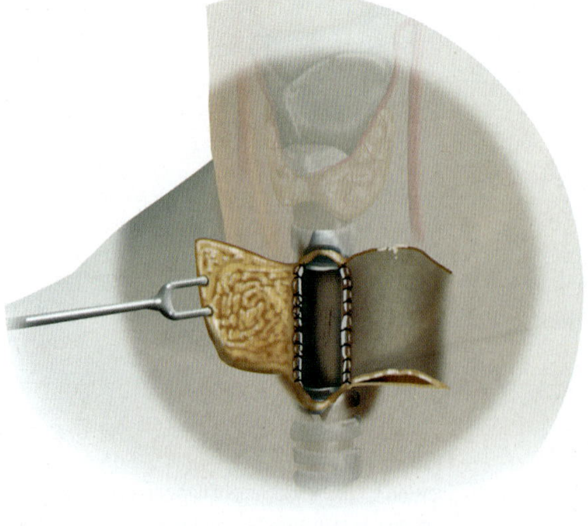

FIGURE 28.3
Bilateral cervical skin advancement flaps are created and advanced into the tracheal defect. Thinning of the cervical flap at the most medial 1 cm of the flap to a full-thickness flap to line the trough is necessary to create the trough.

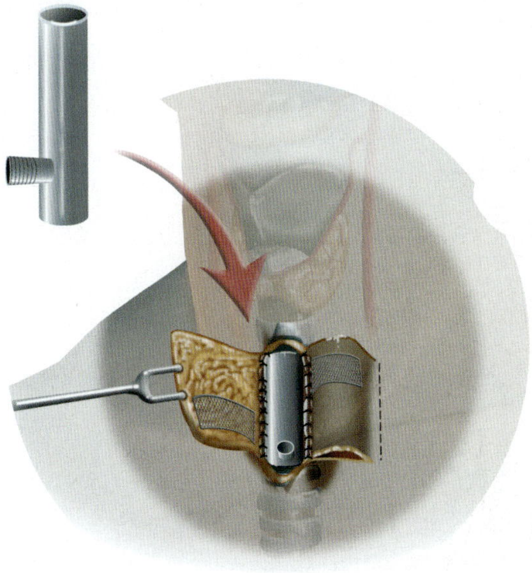

FIGURE 28.4
A T tube or a Montgomery laryngeal stent is placed into the defect and secured in order to create and allow the trough to mature.

Stage II

Stage II is done by inserting the cartilage or titanium mesh for hard tissue reconstruction.

Once the flap has matured, the patient is brought into the operating room for the second stage. At least 6 weeks should elapse after the first stage for the trough to mature and the flap to revascularize. This procedure can be done under local anesthesia and uses titanium mesh inserted below the skin to make the lateral wall of the new trachea. Alternatively, cartilage from the ear or costal cartilage can be used. This depends on the surgeon's preference.

The skin over the skin flap is infiltrated with lidocaine. The strips of titanium (1.3-mm mesh screen, Synthesis, West Chester, PA) are cut into 8 mm × 4-mm strips. Several 5- to 7-mm incisions are made over the top of the trough and the skin is elevated as several tunnels for the placement of the mesh. Each mesh is separated from the others by 4 to 5 mm of soft tissue. It is important to create a pocket bigger than the mesh to be implanted so that during the insertion of the mesh there is no kinking of the mesh. The pocket must be created just under the skin so that there is no excessive bulk. Once the strips of titanium mesh are placed, the skin incisions are closed with 4-0 Monocryl.

Stage III

Closure of the Tracheal Defect

Central to the concept of bringing cervical skin to reline the air conduit is the building of an epithelial-lined tube that will stand up to the rigors of respiration, cough, and phonation. The final stage of the reconstruction is performed when the skin flap has returned to good perfusion along the site of the mesh. If the local skin is used for the roof of the tracheal trough, it must be thin and viable. It must also be closed with enough room for swelling to accommodate the edema of the skin flap that invariably accompanies the tubing of the flap for the final stage. Therefore, the decision as to when it is appropriate to perform the final stage is based on the evaluation of the skin and the donor site. If the skin has good perfusion and it is not edematous, it should stand up to the rigors of the final stage.

Most of the time, the surgeon will want to know if closing the tracheal stoma will cause any airway distress. One can test for this by removing the T tube and inserting a tracheostomy tube below. The stoma above the tracheostomy tube can be taped closed in order to see if there is any collapse of the newly constructed tube. One can even put in a fenestrated no. 5 Jackson tracheostomy tube ahead of time and tape the whole area closed. In this way, one can be sure if there is any other narrowing of the airway such as laryngomalacia, sleep apnea, paradoxical airway closure, or psychological barrier to decannulation. One would obviously like to be quite secure that the last stage will not result in unwanted return to the operating room for replacement of the tracheostomy tube. The final closure of the tracheostomy should therefore be done only if the first two stages have been completed successfully and all the factors that can be optimized for success have been done. Figure 28.5 shows a schematic of the closure of the skin-lined tube. Closure of the roof of the tracheal trough is done under anesthesia and is done with an endotracheal tube in place.

Closure with slight tracheal skin tube redundancy is the key to success. The skin flap is incised lateral to the end of the titanium mesh. Usually, a 1-cm flap is all that is necessary. The full-thickness skin flap is raised

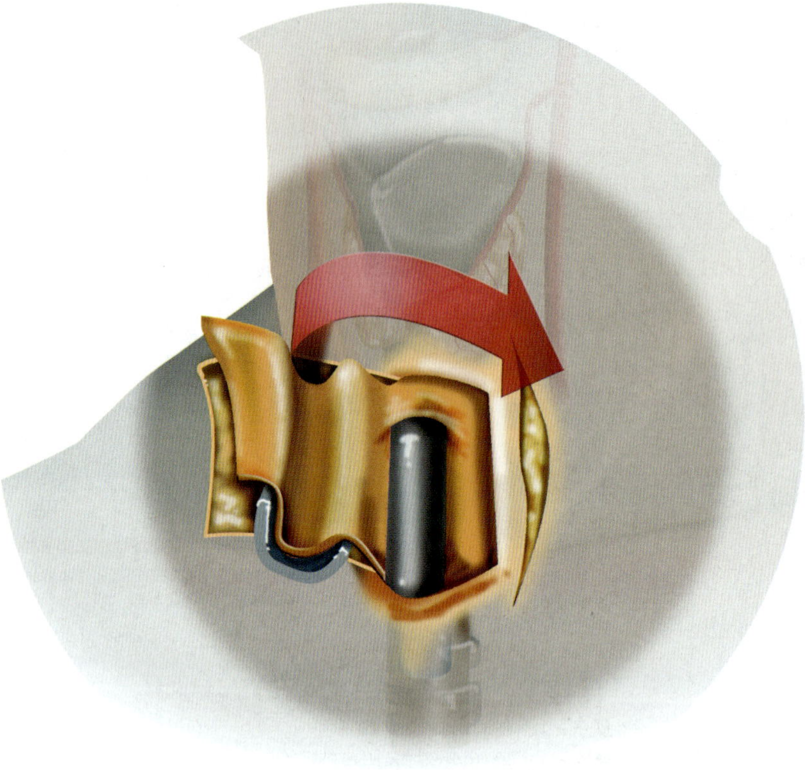

FIGURE 28.5
A schematic of the closure of the skin-lined tube at the last and final stage. This shows the design of the skin-lined flap used to cover the tracheal defect.

to the edge of the titanium mesh. If the titanium mesh is splayed outward too much, dissection is done sharply to go deep to the mesh. The skin flap and the titanium mesh are then raised as a composite flap. It is important not to go too deep on the dissection and to free up the entire mesh and skin as the scarring laterally gives some integrity and provides the blood supply to the flap.

On the opposite side, only the skin is incised right at the old incision for the insertion of the titanium mesh and it is elevated only enough to achieve closure with the skin flap from the other side. The skin flap is sutured over to edge of the opposite side. Closure is done with interrupted sutures with no tension. Figure 28.6 shows the design of the skin flap at the third stage prior to closure for reconstruction of the cervical trachea. Figure 28.7 shows the defect without the T tube or the Montgomery laryngeal stent in place.

A single cervical rotation flap or a double rotation flap is done. Design of the skin flap should be done without pinching the tubed new trachea below. A drain is placed. The key to tubing the flaps for internal lining is to maintain a rectangular airway with the rigid structural support laterally. By keeping the flaps approximated with some redundancy, postoperative edema of the flap will not compromise the airway (Fig. 28.8). Figure 28.9 shows the final coverage of the reconstruction with the cervical advancement flap to cover the skin defect after tracheal reconstruction.

POSTOPERATIVE MANAGEMENT

Decannulation is either carried out at the final stage of reconstruction or by leaving a small tracheostomy in place for later decannulation. If the patient has a well-established trough that has been occluded without a T tube in place, the third and final stage of closure is done with the tracheostomy removed. The patient is then admitted to the hospital afterward for observation of air leak and airway management. The patient is given humidified air and antitussives. Discharge is done if the patient is infection free after 1 day. In large defects of greater than 4 cm, the T tube is removed at the time of the final reconstruction and a small metal Jackson tracheostomy tube is left in place. The patient is discharged the next day with a small indwelling tracheostomy tube. Once the edema from the surgery has subsided, the tracheostomy can be capped and removed as an outpatient. The remaining small fistula can be closed under local anesthesia in the office or in the operating room once the reconstruction is complete and the absence of a need for tracheostomy is verified by capping the tube for 2 weeks. Beside more security for decannulation, the residual tracheostomy diverts the airway away from the reconstruction, prevents air leak into the cervical flap, and allows the reconstruction of a safety valve from the dynamics changes that may be experienced from coughing, swallowing, and respiration during the immediate postoperative period.

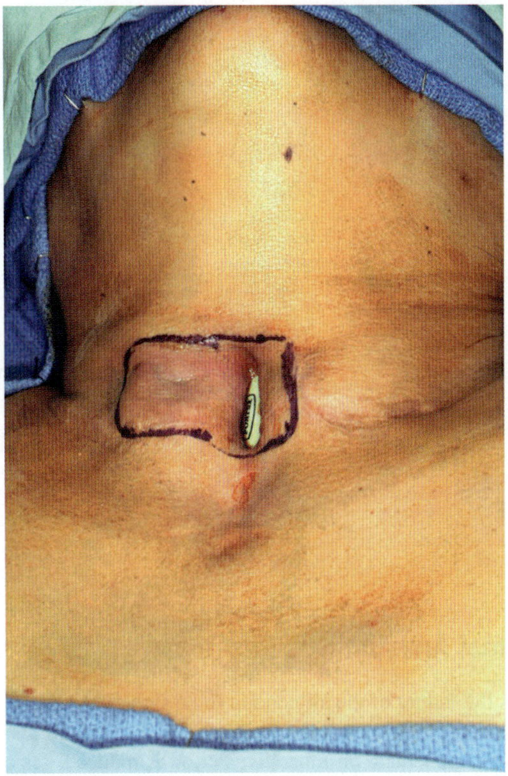

FIGURE 28.6
This clinical photograph shows the design of the skin flap incision at the third stage prior to closure for reconstruction of the cervical trachea. Note that the patient has been intubated from above.

COMPLICATIONS

Complications after staged reconstruction can be divided into short-term complications and long-term complications. Short-term complications include edema, granulation, and infection with compromise of the airway. Long-term complications include positional stridor, skin and hair in the transposed tube, malacia of the reconstructed segment, and restenosis.

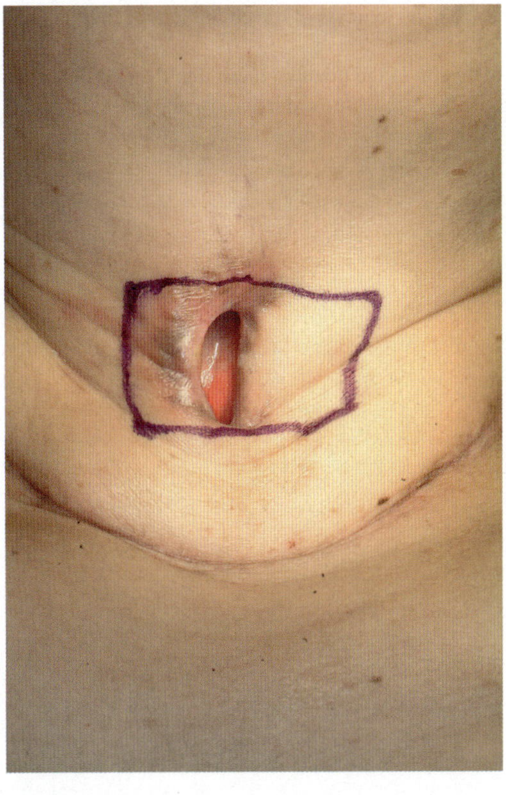

FIGURE 28.7
This clinical photograph shows the defect without the T tube or the Montgomery laryngeal stent in place.

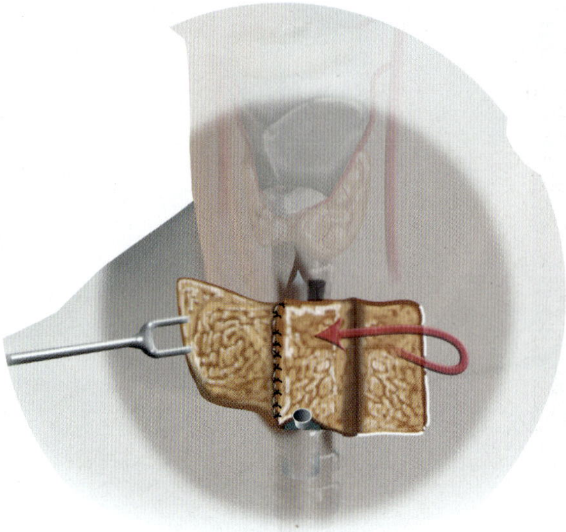

FIGURE 28.8
Closure of the tracheal trough is done by rotating the skin flap and the titanium mesh to close the tracheal defect using skin supported by the titanium mesh.

Management of Local Stenosis at the Stomal Anastomosis Site

The worst complication that occurs with this approach is the failure of the air conduit to be stable through all the requirements for the patient. Stomal stenosis and malacia is the most common problem. By keeping the reconstruction of the roof high, the chance of edema in the immediate postoperative period is reduced. This, however, increases the size of the keratin-bearing skin that is in the neck over the long term. This can result in infection and foul odor.

If the patient has severe chronic obstructive lung disease, malacia of the tissue may occur over time. This may need dynamic evaluation to assess the presence of malacia. This can be done by fiberoptic laryngoscopy with bronchoscopy or a dynamic CT scan. Management of late tracheal malacia is difficult and the use of long-term T tube should be considered.

The CO_2 laser can be used to trim local stenosis and granulation tissue. This can be accompanied by the use of Mitomycin and steroid injection. Radial dilation of the stenosis may be helpful but should be reserved for thin areas of restenosis.

In some male patients, the hair-bearing skin causes infection and disturbance due to obstruction. CO_2 laser debulking of flap may be done. In severe cases, open resection and removal of the epithelium of the flap may be necessary.

In some patients with titanium mesh, there may be extrusion of the titanium mesh into the skin. This can occur many years after the completion of the reconstruction. This can cause local irritation, and the patient must return for removal of the mesh.

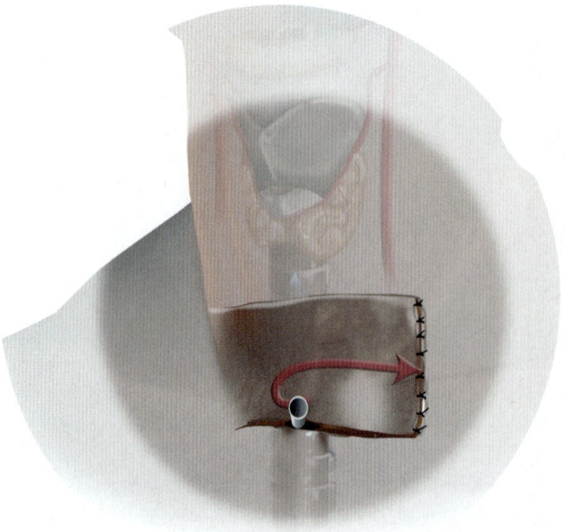

FIGURE 28.9
The overlying donor skin defect is then closed by a cervical advancement flap from the contralateral side.

RESULTS

Staged reconstruction of the trachea using local skin flaps should be considered when immediate end-to-end anastomosis cannot be performed. The different stages can be halted without completion to complete decannulation to allow creation of a skin-lined tube that is clean and permit lung-powered speech by internal stenting. Its utility is good in allowing the patient to go on to a clean conduit with lung-powered speech and regain quality of life without an open tracheotomy tube. With care in long-segment tube creation, thin full-thickness skin reinforced by titanium mesh or cartilage can be created to allow for a stoma-free existence.

PEARLS

- When creating skin flaps for the stage I, make sure the flaps are well perfused and designed on a broad pedicle.
- Meticulous stage I reconstruction will result in less granulation tissue and a better long-term result.

PITFALLS

- If the skin flaps are not carefully sutured to the mucosa of the trachea, granulation tissue will form.
- Patients who have been previously exposed to radiotherapy may not heal well.

INSTRUMENTS TO HAVE AVAILABLE

- Standard head and neck surgical set

SUGGESTED READING

Grillo HC. Surgical treatment of postintubation tracheal injuries. *J Thorac Cardiovasc Surg* 1979;78(6):860–875.

Grillo HC. Primary reconstruction of airway after resection of subglottic laryngeal and upper tracheal stenosis. *Ann Thorac Surg* 1982;33(1):3–18.

Eliachar I, et al. Combined rotary door flap and epiglottic laryngoplasty for reconstruction of large laryngotracheal defects in dogs. *Laryngoscope* 1986;96(10):1154–1158.

Maddaus MA, et al. Subglottic tracheal resection and synchronous laryngeal reconstruction. *J Thorac Cardiovasc Surg* 1992;104(5):1443–1450.

Wang Z, et al. Endoscopic diode laser welding of mucosal grafts on the larynx: a new technique. *Laryngoscope* 1995;105(1):49–52.

29 MANAGEMENT OF THE LARYNGECTOMY/PARTIAL PHARYNGECTOMY DEFECT

Daniel G. Deschler

INTRODUCTION

The reconstruction of the laryngectomy–partial pharyngectomy (LPP) defect has presented one of the greatest challenges in the history of head and neck reconstruction. This considerable defect is the result of the extension of the standard laryngectomy defect to include a significant portion of the pharynx, which precludes the primary closure done after standard laryngectomy. At least 2 cm of remaining viable mucosa is acceptable for primary closure, and anything less than this requires some form of reconstruction in order to avoid the inevitable stenosis that follows primary closure with insufficient mucosa. The more considerable defect is that of the total laryngopharyngectomy in which the entire larynx and pharynx is resected.

A review of the reconstructive efforts that have been introduced to address this challenging defect demonstrates the great creativity and perseverance exemplified by reconstructive surgeons over many decades. The first technique with proven success was introduced by Wookey and modified by Montgomery. This involved a staged sequence of cervical rotation flaps to achieve eventual reconstruction of a neopharyngeal conduit. Later introduction of reconstruction using regional flaps including the deltopectoral flap and the pectoralis major flap were considerable advances in the field. These were the first flaps to be used in the immediate reconstruction of major wounds in the head and neck since they brought their own robust circulation. They also had the major advantage of being outside the radiated field and therefore more reliable.

The current state of the art for reconstruction of the partial and total laryngopharyngectomy defect is the use of free tissue transfer techniques. The major options include the use of enteric flaps such as the jejunal or gastroomental flaps, as well as fasciocutaneous free flaps such as the radial forearm and anterolateral thigh flaps. These techniques have met with great success, yet clinical situations may arise in which free tissue transfer is not achievable. Therefore, familiarity with alternative methods is mandatory.

Soon after the introduction of the pectoralis major myocutaneous (PMM) flap in the late 1970s by Ariyan and Biller in separate publications, the use of the PMM flap for reconstruction following laryngopharyngectomy was described. In the early 1980s, numerous small series were reported by Schuller and Fabian demonstrating the successful use of the PMM flap in the management of the LPP defect. These publications demonstrated an acceptably low failure rate of the flap of less than 5% with a similarly low fistula rate in the 10% to 20% range. Likewise, the stenosis rates were demonstrated to be acceptable in the 20% range. This marked a significant improvement over previously described techniques. Based upon their success, free tissue transfer reconstructive methods have largely supplanted the use of the PMM flap for this defect. However, clinical situations may still arise in which the PMM flap becomes the favored option for pharyngoesophageal reconstruction.

HISTORY

Taking a detailed history is essential when considering a reconstruction using a PMM flap. The history should emphasize prior chest wall surgery and restrictive lung disease since prior chest wall surgery may interrupt the blood supply to the flap. Similarly, a patient with restrictive lung disease may not tolerate the tight chest wall closure that is often necessary after harvesting a PMM with a large skin paddle. It is also important to consider whether the patient has had a prior vascular port for administration of chemotherapy. This can cause scarring and disruption of the pectoralis tissue planes.

PHYSICAL EXAMINATION

The physical examination should include a general medical examination to assess for cardiac, pulmonary, and renal disease. Additionally, the examination should include an evaluation of the donor site to evaluate for prior chest wall surgery that might rule out the use of the pectoralis donor site. The donor site may require reconstruction with a split thickness skin graft if the defect is too extensive for primary closure. In general, the PMM flap can be used for extensive defects but defects that extend into the nasopharynx may represent a challenge for the pedicled pectoralis flap. A free flap is the best option to reach the nasopharynx.

INDICATIONS

The decision to use the PMM flap for pharyngoesophageal reconstruction is usually because of the inability to use free tissue transfer techniques. Factors precluding the use of a free flap include the failure of a previous reconstruction using free tissue transfer, a reoperation in a significantly vessel-depleted neck, no available donor sites for reconstruction due to previous surgery, or significant medical comorbidities precluding a potentially long-duration surgery, which is characteristic of certain reconstructions using free tissue transfer.

CONTRAINDICATIONS

The only absolute contraindication to PMM flap reconstruction for the pharyngoesophageal defect is previous surgery involving the pectoralis major donor site. Any skin elevations in previous procedures, which have separated the myocutaneous perforators, as well as any interventions in the subclavicular area affecting the vascular pedicle eliminate the use of this flap. Previous median sternotomy is not a contraindication as such since it does not affect the viability of the flap. Likewise, the previous use of the internal mammary artery system has no effect on flap survival. A relative contraindication is significant tissue bulk overlying the PMM, which may preclude the placement of such tissue in the neck. This can be notable in obese patients as well as women with large breasts.

PREOPERATIVE PLANNING

Surgical Technique

There are three options for pharyngoesophageal reconstruction using the PMM flap. The first is the PMM flap used as a cutaneous "patch" to complete circumferential closure of the neopharynx following a partial pharyngectomy with a small segment of pharynx remaining. A second option is reconstruction of a total laryngopharyngectomy defect in which the PMM flap is tubed to create an entirely skin-lined neopharynx. The third option is the use of the flap in a 270-degree fold over fashion with attachment of the skin island to the prevertebral fascia as described by Fabian. Although myofascial flap reconstruction of the partial and total laryngopharyngectomy defect has been reported, the technical details of this will not be discussed.

My technique for harvesting the PMM flap for laryngopharyngeal reconstruction is a subtle modification of the standard technique. Specific subtleties for this defect are highlighted. The flap is usually elevated in a fashion such that the skin territory of the deltopectoral flap is preserved for use in a later reconstruction should this be required. A curvilinear line is drawn extending from the axilla down toward the xiphoid process. A long ellipse is then planned around this line extending from the medial edge of the nipple to the skin overlying the pectoralis muscle's medial attachments to the sternum. The ellipse will measure approximately 15 × 7 to 8 cm in width. This will make adequate tissue available to roll into a neopharyngeal conduit without significant tension. The elongated ellipse is used so that sequential closure of the chest can be done in a simplified fashion without the need for skin grafting. The large ellipse of skin can then be easily modified to the specific laryngopharyngectomy defect once it is delivered into the cervical region.

The procedure begins with the incision of the lateral skin ellipse and extending toward the axilla (Fig. 29.1). The incision is taken through the underlying dermis and then sloped slightly to harvest a greater amount of subcutaneous adipose tissue over the muscle. This allows a greater potential capture of perforating vessels to the skin island. The lateral chest flap is now elevated down to the level of the pectoralis major muscle and then elevated laterally until the lateral border of the PMM is identified (Fig. 29.2). At this point, the surgeon

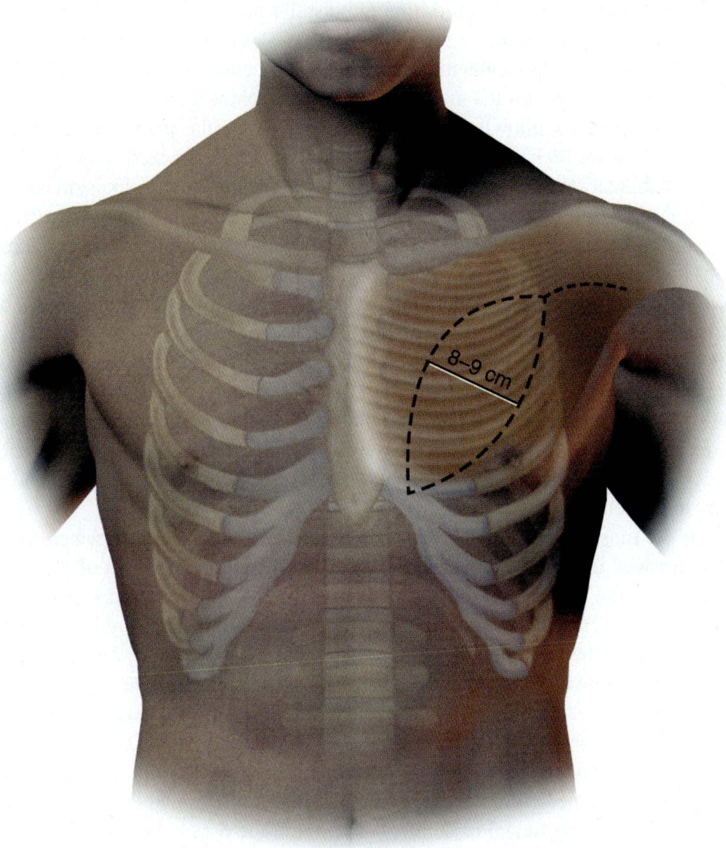

FIGURE 29.1
The incision design for the harvest of the PMM flap. The incision for the skin paddle is designed as an ellipse centered over the pectoralis major muscle. This allows a greater potential capture of perforating vessels to the skin island. The ellipse also facilitates closure of the donor site.

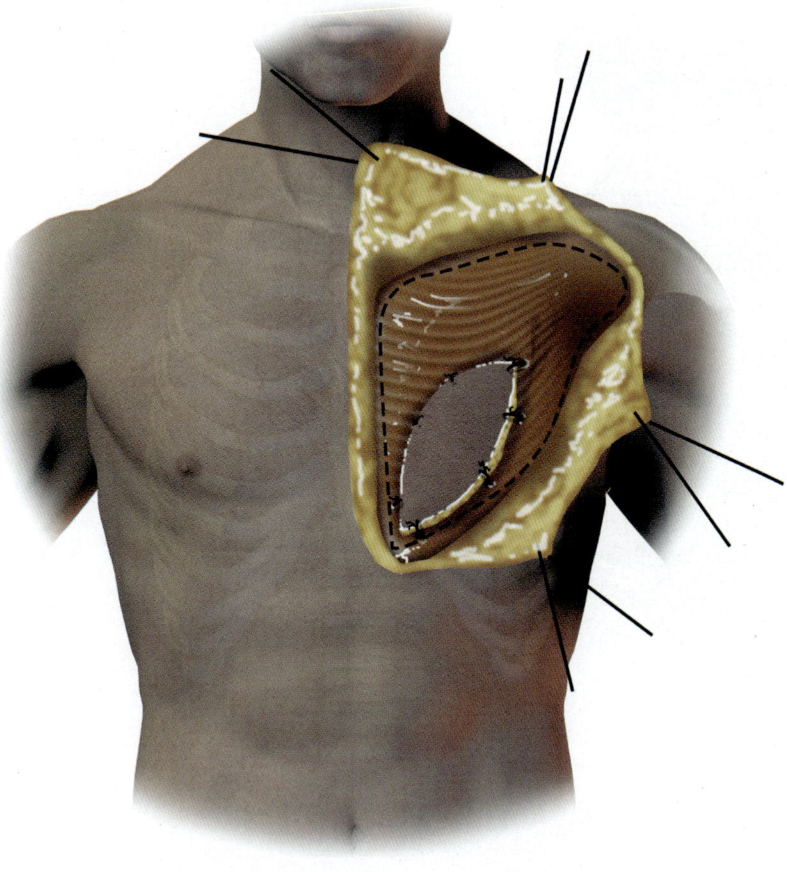

FIGURE 29.2
The incision is taken through the underlying dermis and then sloped slightly to harvest a greater amount of subcutaneous adipose tissue over the muscle. This allows a greater potential capture of perforating vessels to the skin island.

can assess whether the skin island is optimally placed. Should it be too distally placed and have a significant random component, the skin island can be readjusted more proximally to have a greater capture of perforating vessels. With the lateral border identified, the pectoralis muscle is then gently elevated with its underlying fascia in the plane superficial to the fascia of the pectoralis minor muscle. Gentle blunt dissection is done with the fingertips in this plane up toward the clavicle, allowing identification of the vascular pedicle early in the procedure. Three to four absorbable sutures are then placed in the skin subdermally and tacked loosely to the fascia of the muscle laterally to allow stabilization of the skin island (Fig. 29.2). The medial skin incision is now created through the underlying dermis and adipose tissue to the pectoralis major muscle attachments medially. The superior skin flap is elevated in the plane just deep to the fascia of the pectoralis major muscle elevating this with the corresponding skin flap of the deltopectoral flap. The superior flap elevation is done over the clavicle until the neck incision from the laryngopharyngectomy is encountered. A tunnel admitting the entire width of the hand should be created to allow the muscle to be passed easily into the cervical region.

At this point, similar tacking sutures are placed in the medial portion of the skin island securing it to the muscle. The tacking sutures are removed once the flap is delivered into the neck, and the skin island inset contouring is begun. There will usually be a distal segment of the large ellipse that will overlie the rectus fascia. A small square of rectus fascia overlying the lower ribcage is harvested with this distal segment of flap. This fascia will have adhesions to the pectoralis major muscle and will maintain its connection with it upon elevation. The potential use of the fascia later in the reconstruction is described.

With the skin island secured to the muscle and the vascular pedicle identified, the flap is elevated from inferiorly to superiorly off of the chest wall using electrocautery (Fig. 29.3). At the inferior level of the sternum, the muscle can be taken directly off the ribcage as it is elevated superiorly. As the first and second ribs are approached, it is important to leave a 2-cm cuff of muscle medially to preserve the perforating vessels toward the deltopectoral flap. The skin flap is then completely elevated superiorly to the clavicle. Dissection of the muscle as it approaches the clavicle is done carefully with visualization of the main pedicle of the flap to preserve its integrity. The humeral head of the pectoralis muscle must be severed to allow adequate rotation of the flap into the cervical defect, and this is done with direct visualization of the pedicle. Full mobilization of the flap will often require sacrifice of the lateral vascular pedicle, which can be done with minimal risk to the viability of the flap if there is a prominent main pedicle. The flap is then folded superiorly, and the distal rectus fascia is held with a clamp and pulled through the tunnel to deliver the flap into the cervical region. The skin island should now be facing toward the spine.

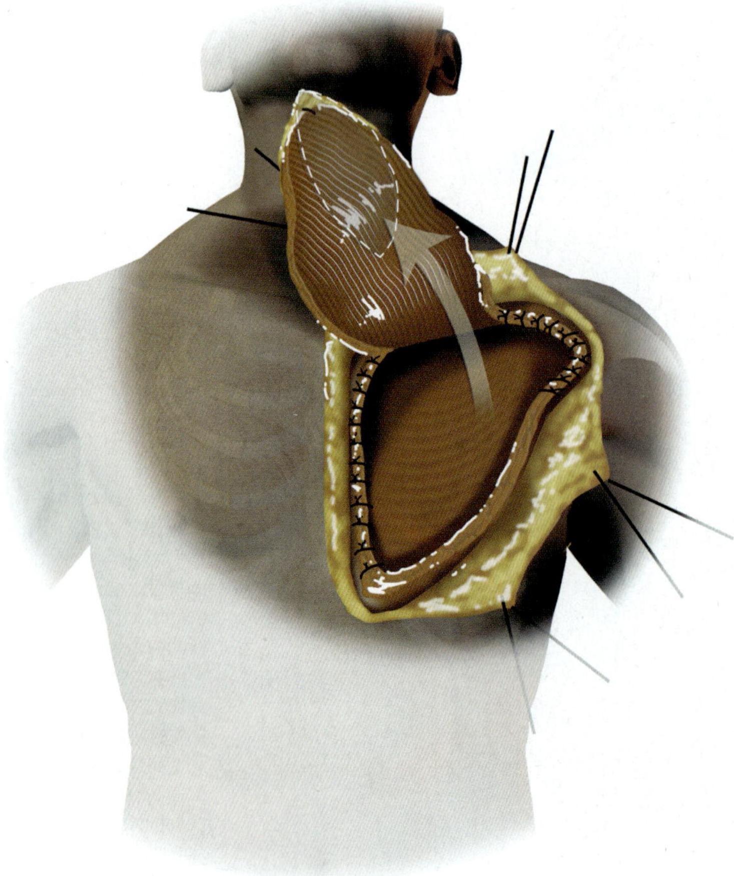

FIGURE 29.3
The pectoralis muscle is then gently elevated with its underlying fascia in the plane superficial to the fascia of the pectoralis minor muscle.

Complete hemostasis is obtained at the donor site. Specific care is then taken to insure that all of the perforating vessels from the thorax to the muscle have been adequately addressed. Specific care is taken during elevation not to burn or injure the perichondrium and periosteum of the ribcage as this can lead to poor wound healing. The stump of the pectoralis muscle at the humeral head is now oversewn using a large suture in a running locking fashion. Two large-bore drains are placed exiting inferiorly. The skin flaps are mobilized laterally and medially to allow primary closure with the least amount of tension.

Prior to closing the donor site, the positioning of the vascular pedicle is examined as is the skin color and integrity of the skin island to confirm that there are no venous or arterial problems after transfer into the cervical region. Perforating motor nerves are severed during the elevation off the pectoralis minor muscle. There still can be significant neural elements closely approximated to the vascular pedicle, which may upon inspection have a constricting effect on the pedicle. If this is the case, these nerves can be severed using a nerve stimulator for guidance. Unlike reconstructive efforts that require rotation of the skin island to lie externally, in which these pedicle-associated nerves should always be severed, these nerves may not require direct attention during pharyngoesophageal reconstruction.

Partial Laryngopharyngectomy Defect

Using the PMM flap for partial laryngopharyngectomy defects is a straightforward endeavor. The flap is now placed into the midline cervical region overlying the proposed defect. The proximal part of the skin island, which will correspond to the lower portion of the neopharyngeal closure, is trimmed in appropriate fashion to have an adequate tension-free position. In a similar manner, the decision is made as to the appropriate length of the flap and width of the distal segment of the pectoralis skin island to fit into the defect of the base of the tongue (Fig. 29.4). Care is taken to leave the underlying rectus fascia as this will be used to reinforce closure at the base of the tongue.

Attention is first turned to completing the closure at the lower esophageal segment taking care to contour the lower flap and allow the 270-degree closure around the esophagus. Usually, 3 cm of skin is required for this. Now 3-0 Vicryl sutures are used in an interrupted fashion to closely approximate the skin to the mucosa and submucosa of the esophagus and remaining posterior pharyngeal mucosa (Fig. 29.5). This is usually done by placing the knots on the inside with close attention to having a subdermal to submucosal approximation creating a watertight closure with good epithelial abutment. Closure of the lateral aspect of the pharyngeal remnant is now completed on the side of the pectoralis major elevation. This is done with 3-0 Vicryl or the larger 2-0 Vicryl suture in a horizontal mattress fashion to further ensure watertight closure with good mucosal and cutaneous abutment. The flap is closed up to the base of the tongue, and the distal aspect of the previously contoured ellipse of skin is now rolled medially to achieve closure at the base of the tongue. Again, it is critical that the width of the distal flap be sufficient to cover the entire base of the tongue. This usually involves the broadest width of the harvested flap. The flap is now closed to the midline tongue base using 2-0 sutures in a horizontal mattress fashion. Attention is now turned to the contralateral lateral closure, which is done as previously described. Again, all suturing is done internally under direct visualization to ensure good mucosal and skin abutment. As the contralateral side is brought up to the base of the tongue, it will now cross toward the

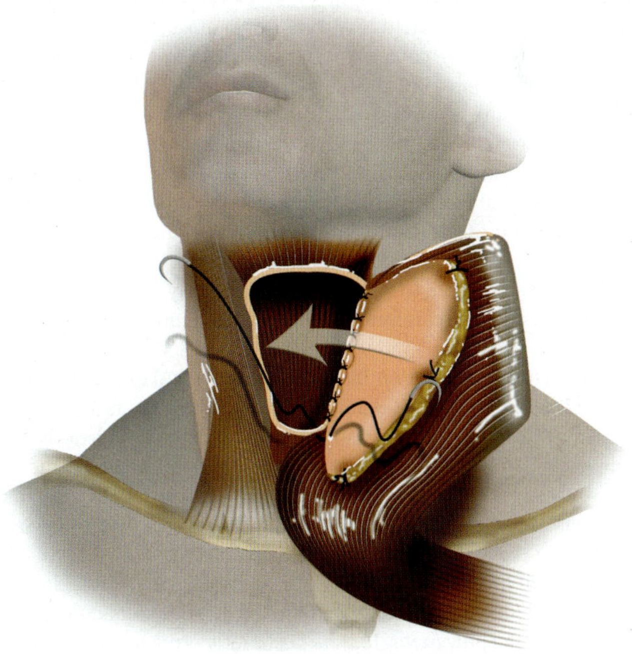

FIGURE 29.4
The pectoralis muscle and skin paddle are rotated into the pharyngeal defect for the final reconstruction.

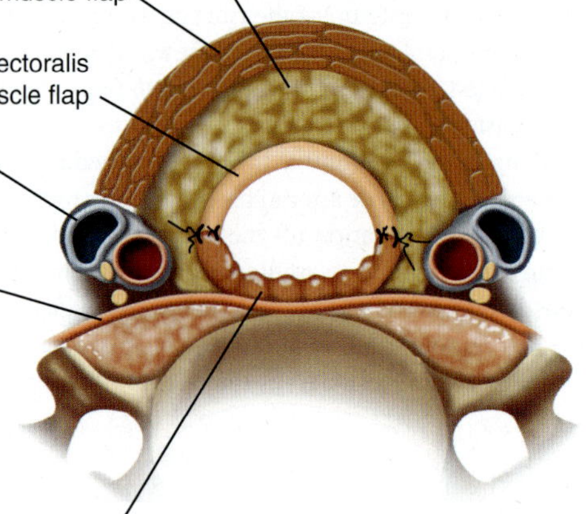

FIGURE 29.5
The technique of wrapping the flap 270 degrees around the anterior and lateral aspects of the defect and securing it to the remaining posterior pharyngeal mucosa posteriorly.

midline. At this point, the sutures can no longer be tied intraluminally and are therefore placed in the subdermal and submucosal fashion with a large bite to achieve closure at the base of the tongue. With this completed, the large remnant of pectoralis muscle that was elevated during the initial flap harvest is now draped over the closure. Using 3-0 Vicryl sutures in horizontal mattress fashion, the muscle is secured on the contralateral side to either the prevertebral fascia or the remnant of the pharyngeal musculature (Fig. 29.5). Superiorly, muscle as well as the rectus fascia is draped over the base of the tongue supporting the closure in this fashion. The muscle is then draped and secured around the neopharyngeal closure on the side ipsilateral to the harvest.

The previously elevated apron flap is now draped over the wound, and in most cases, primary closure can be achieved. If there is not sufficient skin for primary closure of the neck or if such closure would have a constricting effect on the flap pedicle, a skin graft can be placed on the pectoralis major muscle. Suction drains are applied bilaterally, placed under and superior to the flap on the side of the harvest. A soft laryngectomy tube may be necessary because of the initial bulk of the flap, but this will usually not be required long term as the muscle atrophies. The laryngectomy tube should be sewn in place, and potentially constricting tracheostomy ties should not be used.

Total Laryngopharyngectomy

Two options for closure of the total laryngopharyngectomy defect using the PMM flap are available. In patients who do not have significant bulk to their PMM flap, a complete tubulation of the flap can be undertaken for the reconstruction of the neopharynx. Care must be taken in the initial elevation to have sufficient tissue to allow complete rotation of the flap upon itself. Complete tubing is usually not achievable when the flap is large and bulky. Similar to the partial pharyngectomy defect, the flap is delivered into the cervical region and then the previously harvested ellipse is contoured to fill the specific defect. The superior skin component must be wide enough to allow complete closure at the base of the tongue. The lower skin edge can be shorter at the esophageal anastomosis that is narrower. The skin island of the flap is laid over the midline with the skin edge at the perisagittal plane just lateral to the midline on the contralateral side. The muscle and rectus fascia are secured superiorly to the prevertebral fascia to limit the amount of pull inferiorly related to time and gravity. The superior contoured component of the flap is now sewn directly to the cut edge of the pharyngeal mucosa using a horizontal mattress technique taking care to take good deep bites of tissue to support this closure. The distal aspect of the flap is then secured to the esophagus inferiorly in a similar manner usually using a 3-0 suture at this level. The flap is now circumferentially rotated and inset superiorly and inferiorly (Fig. 29.6).

The longitudinal closure of the newly formed tube is closed on the side opposite the flap harvest. This closure is done by abutting the skin island to itself with 2-0 Vicryl sutures in horizontal mattress fashion. This is done from superior to inferior for approximately 40% of the defect and then from inferior to superiorly for approximately 40% of the defect. The last component is closed with subdermal sutures to complete the closure. A size 8 to 10 Montgomery salivary bypass tube is placed in the neopharynx prior to complete closure. In a fashion similar to the partial pharyngectomy defect, the muscle harvested with the flap is now draped over the closure and reinforced to the prevertebral fascia and to the base of the tongue. Drains are similarly placed.

In the majority of cases, a complete tubulation of the pectoralis major flap to reconstruct the total laryngopharyngectomy defect is not achievable. The technique of wrapping the flap 270 degrees around the anterior and lateral aspects of the defect and securing it to the prevertebral fascia posteriorly provides an excellent

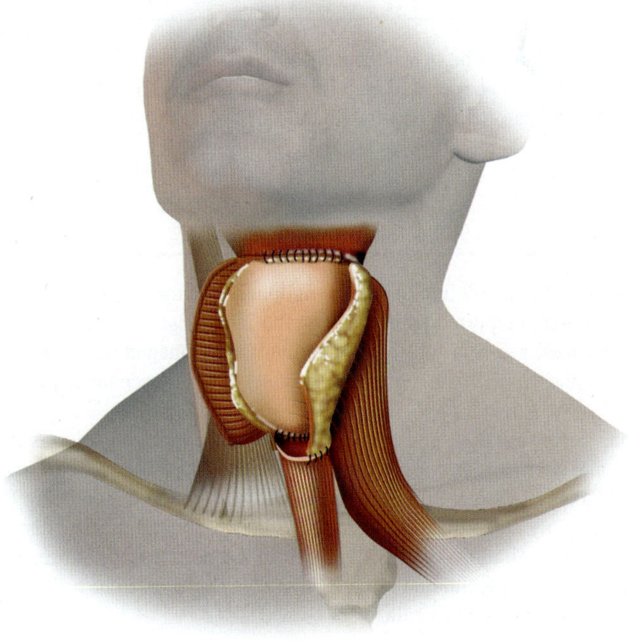

FIGURE 29.6
Technique for complete tubulation of the PMM for the TLP defect after securing to the posterior pharynx superiorly and the esophagus inferiorly.

alternative (Fig. 29.7). In this technique, the flap again is contoured to the specific defect from the previously elevated ellipse. The posterior pharyngeal mucosa is now sutured to the prevertebral fascia superiorly. Inferiorly, the posterior esophageal mucosa is likewise secured to the prevertebral fascia. The pectoralis skin island is contoured to fit in this defect with attention being placed on leaving enough skin superiorly to complete the closure at the base of the tongue. Although the early descriptions of this technique discuss placing of a skin graft over the prevertebral fascia, subsequent experience has shown this to be unnecessary. The skin island on the side ipsilateral to the flap elevation is now secured to the prevertebral fascia using 2-0 Vicryl in an interrupted or horizontal mattress fashion. Large bites of the subdermis are secured to the prevertebral fascia and tied externally. This places close abutment of the dermis to the underlying prevertebral fascia and muscle. The prevertebral fascia may be scored along the line of the proposed closure to expose the more vascular muscle. The ipsilateral closure is completed in a linear fashion. Closure of the skin to the esophageal component is now done rolling it toward the contralateral aspect side. This is likewise done at the base of the tongue. The subdermis of the flap is now secured to the prevertebral fascia on the contralateral side providing complete closure of the defect. The use of a salivary bypass is recommended. The muscle again is draped over the closure and then secured contralaterally to the prevertebral fascia. Drains are placed as described previously.

As with the partial laryngopharyngectomy, the apron flap is closed over the neopharyngeal reconstruction. If there is insufficient tissue or pedicle constriction, then a skin graft is applied. Drains are left in place until criteria are met for removal.

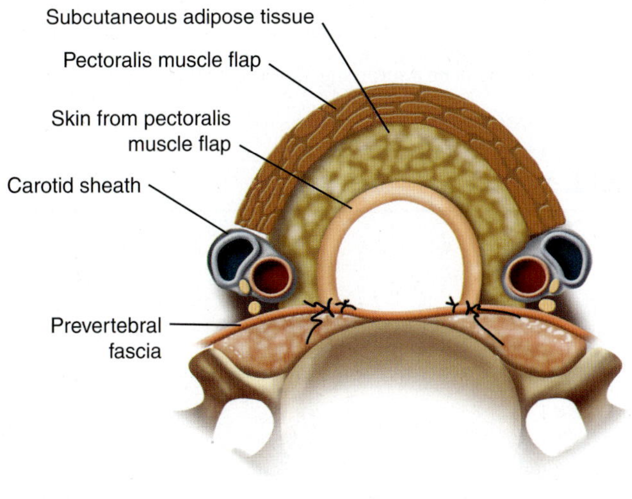

FIGURE 29.7
The technique of wrapping the flap 270 degrees around the anterior and lateral aspects of the defect and securing it to the prevertebral fascia posteriorly provides an excellent alternative when tubing is not possible.

POSTOPERATIVE MANAGEMENT

Tube feeds are given through a preexisting gastrostomy tube or via a nasogastric tube placed through the salivary bypass tube. Patients are kept NPO for at least 2 weeks. This may be extended if significant preexisting conditions favoring fistula formation exist. A pharyngogram is done, with the salivary bypass tube in place. If no leak is noted, then the salivary bypass is removed in the office and oral diet is begun.

COMPLICATIONS

The most common complication after PMM flap reconstruction of the laryngopharyngectomy defect is fistula formation. The series prior to the chemoradiation era reported fistula rates in the 20% range, which are higher now for salvage surgery. In the majority of cases, a fistula will be self-limited and managed with standard wound care. The salivary bypass tube is left in place to aid with management of secretions. Once the fistula has closed, an oral diet is begun.

Flap failure is rare with pectoralis flap reconstruction, and to avoid this complication, meticulous flap elevation and inspection of pedicle integrity and geometry during closure are critical. If flap failure occurs, then the contralateral PMM flap can be used. Stenosis is another common complication with the fistula being the primary risk factor. Stenosis occurs most commonly at the distal anastomosis and is best diagnosed by history and pharyngogram. Management is with judicious dilation. Excess flap bulk in the neck and its subsequent effects on stomal geometry is a common sequel of this technique rather than a complication. Time will allow muscle atrophy and relief of the functional problems related to bulk.

Donor site complications are likewise rare. Hematoma is the most common and should be addressed with expeditious drainage. After standard donor site closure, a significant depression should be present below the clavicle. If this concavity flattens, then hematoma formation is highly unlikely. Formal ligature of the humeral head of the pectoralis muscle as well as attention to the perforators from the ribcage should help to prevent hematoma. Wound dehiscence can be avoided with appropriate mobilization of the PMM flap and positioning at the time of closure. If the closure was felt to be tight, then the skin staples can be left in place for 2 weeks.

Tumor implantation at the chest donor site has been reported, but fortunately, it is an exceedingly rare occurrence.

RESULTS

The results with this technique are reliable and, in general, excellent. The donor tissue is ideal for patients who have been radiated and are at risk for fistula formation.

PEARLS

- The harvesting of a large ellipse of skin usually allows for primary closure of the donor site as well as providing sufficient tissue for the reconstruction of the pharyngectomy defect.
- Dependable and effective tracheoesophageal voice restoration is achievable after PMM flap reconstruction of the pharyngoesophageal defect.

PITFALLS

- Fistula formation is common enough in the current era to not be a surprising development for the experienced reconstructive surgeon.

INSTRUMENTS TO HAVE AVAILABLE

- Standard head and neck surgical set

SUGGESTED READING

Wookey H. The surgical treatment of carcinoma of the pharynx and upper esophagus. *Surg Gynecol Obstet* 1942;75:499–506.

Montgomery WW. Reconstruction of the cervical esophagus. *Arch Otolaryngol* 1963;77:609–620.

Bakamjian VY. A two stage method for pharyngoesophageal reconstruction with a primary pectoral skin flap. *Plast Reconstr Surg* 1965;36:173–184.

Fabian RL. Reconstruction of the laryngopharynx and cervical esophagus. *Laryngoscope* 1984;94:1334–1350.

Schuller DE. Reconstructive options for pharyngoesophageal and/or cervical esophageal defects. *Arch Otolaryngol* 1985;111:193–197.

30 MANAGEMENT OF THE PHARYNGEAL DEFECT: THE ANTEROLATERAL THIGH FLAP

Donald T. Weed

INTRODUCTION

The surgical management of cancer of the hypopharynx is a challenge for both the ablative and the reconstructive head and neck surgeon. Cancers arising from this subsite in the upper aerodigestive tract are characterized by a propensity for early metastases to the cervical lymph nodes. Local growth is equally problematic, as compromise of the critical junction between the pharynx and esophageal inlet presents not only a reconstructive challenge but also the potential for underestimation of the full extent of the local disease. Preoperative imaging accurately predicts the extent of bulky disease, but submucosal spread may not be well defined by either imaging or staging endoscopy. The successful reconstructive strategy must, therefore, anticipate a range of surgical defects in order to achieve consistently good oncologic and functional outcomes.

Reconstruction of the neopharynx following laryngopharyngectomy is critical to the oncologic success of treatment, a point sometimes underestimated by the reconstructive surgeon. Successful oncologic treatment of hypopharyngeal cancer depends first and foremost on the adequacy of the surgical resection. The extent of resection, or the decision whether or not to proceed with surgical resection, should not be compromised by limitations in reconstructive options. Similarly, the reconstruction must be accomplished safely, with a goal of timely healing and recovery with limited risk for complications. Primary closure of a previously radiated pharynx may be adequate from the perspective of the anticipated luminal diameter of the reconstructed neopharynx but may place the patient at undue risk for fistula formation and the potential for additional complications, major or minor, that may accompany that fistula. Failure of a particular reconstructive technique, because of flap loss, significant fistula formation, or other related complications, may also introduce a critical delay in beginning adjuvant therapy necessary to the oncologic success of treatment.

The importance of the surgical reconstruction of hypopharyngeal defects is more obvious with regard to its impact on the functional outcomes of treatment. A successful swallowing outcome following laryngopharyngectomy depends on an adequate luminal diameter of the neopharynx. This, in turn, depends on two factors. The first is the selection of a reconstructive technique that provides for an adequate-sized neopharynx. The second is the avoidance of a fistula and its attendant risk of stricture formation when healing occurs by second intention. Successful speech rehabilitation following laryngopharyngectomy also depends on an adequate luminal diameter of the neopharynx and esophageal inlet when tracheoesophageal or esophageal speech is anticipated in the postoperative period. While a patent alimentary tract is necessary for tracheoesophageal speech, the quality of speech achieved may also be affected by the choice of cutaneous versus gastrointestinal flaps. These factors must all be considered in the planning and surgical reconstruction of the hypopharyngeal defect.

The surgical treatment of hypopharyngeal cancer depends, therefore, on a sophisticated analysis of the extent of surgical resection, the appropriate execution of this resection with clear surgical margins, and the selection of a reconstructive option that is tailored to the defect size and extent. The choice among reconstructive options is critically dependent on patient factors, such as comorbidities, and history of previous treatment, both surgical and nonsurgical, as these relate to the likelihood of achieving an uncomplicated postoperative course. The goal of the reconstructive surgeon is to insure the patient's safe and timely return to optimal functional status. Successfully achieving this goal will not limit further cancer treatment and will maximize quality of life in patients whose overall prognosis may be poor.

HISTORY

Dysphagia, odynophagia, and aspiration are the most common presenting symptoms of cancer in the hypopharynx or esophageal inlet. Other symptoms include otalgia, dysphonia, dyspnea, or a mass in the neck. A history of weight loss is important as this often correlates with the local extent of disease and suggests compromised nutritional status. A thorough assessment of patient comorbidities and their impact on treatment options is critical to the development of the multidisciplinary treatment plan.

PHYSICAL EXAMINATION

Physical examination, aided by flexible fiberoptic laryngoscopy, is generally adequate to establish a presumptive diagnosis in patients with cancer of the hypopharynx, as most lesions will be visible on fiberoptic examination. The functional status of the larynx is important to the initial treatment plan. The patient who presents in respiratory distress with bilateral vocal cord paralysis and a mass in the postcricoid hypopharynx will require a tracheostomy to establish a safe airway and is more likely to benefit from initial surgical treatment rather than a strategy focusing on organ preservation. The patient who has been previously treated for hypopharyngeal cancer with radiation or chemoradiation therapy may present with many of the same symptoms mentioned above, but the diagnostic challenge is usually greater in these patients. These symptoms may occur as a consequence of prior therapy rather than as a sign of recurrent cancer. Recurrence may be more difficult to detect on physical examination in the patient whose laryngeal and pharyngeal mucosa may be chronically edematous after previous therapy. The extent of disease recurrence is also more difficult to assess under these circumstances.

An important aspect of the examination relates to examination of the donor site. Although rare, occasionally an injury or prior surgery can preclude use of the anterolateral thigh (ALT) donor site. Similarly, a patient with gait disturbance should be carefully evaluated to determine if this donor site could further impair ambulation.

INDICATIONS

Three important factors must be considered when deciding among reconstructive options for defects of the hypopharynx and cervical esophagus. These are the extent of involvement of the posterior pharyngeal wall, the distal extent of disease and the anticipated distal extent of resection, and the involvement of cervical skin. The options for patch reconstruction of the neopharynx when an adequate amount of posterior pharyngeal mucosa remains are more varied as compared with reconstructive options for a total laryngopharyngeal defect. The distal extent of the resection is the critical determining factor when choosing a gastric pull-up rather than a regional pedicle flap or free flap alternative. Some reconstructive options are suitable for combined simultaneous use for neopharyngeal and cervical skin reconstruction, while other reconstructive options for neopharyngeal reconstruction would require an additional flap or technique for cervical skin coverage. Once these three factors have been considered with regard to the optimal choice of flap for the extent of the surgical defect, this choice must then be made in the context of other patient factors such as body habitus, donor site morbidity, and patient comorbidities.

CONTRAINDICATIONS

With the exception of prior injury to the donor site, there are no contraindications to this procedure.

PREOPERATIVE PLANNING

Imaging Studies

After history and physical examination have established a high suspicion of new or recurrent cancer in the hypopharynx, the extent of disease can accurately be assessed by high-resolution contrast-enhanced computed tomography (CT) scan. This will allow for accurate assessment of cartilage invasion, and generally reliable assessment of invasion of prevertebral musculature or encasement of the carotid artery and other factors that may establish the resectability of the cancer. Positron emission tomography combined with CT (PET–CT) is

particularly useful in evaluating the local extent of disease in patients who have undergone previous radiation or chemoradiation therapy more than 3 months prior and whose physical examination is limited by diffuse posttreatment mucosal edema. PET–CT also provides for assessment of distant metastatic disease, which is important to identify in this patient population. MRI with contrast is generally reserved for those patients whose resectability is in doubt, particularly as this relates to involvement of the prevertebral fascia or involvement of the deep cervical musculature by clinically fixed lymph nodes where CT imaging does not reveal obvious muscle invasion. MRI without contrast typically can provide more diagnostic information than CT scan without contrast in patients with severe contrast allergy or poor renal function and should also be considered in these cases. Preoperative modified barium swallow (MBS) is useful in establishing baseline swallowing status in order to guide decisions regarding percutaneous gastrostomy (PEG) placement preoperatively and to assess preoperative history of aspiration as this may relate to equivocal findings on chest imaging or risk of postoperative pulmonary complications. It is also the most reliable study in evaluating invasion of the prevertebral fascia as it studies the mobility of the pharynx over the prevertebral fascia during swallowing. The MBS is not as useful as a tool to assess the extent of the disease.

Surgical Evaluation and Biopsy

Tissue biopsy to establish the presence of cancer is mandatory. Fine needle aspiration biopsy is useful to quickly and easily establish the presumptive diagnosis of cancer in patients with palpable neck disease; but false positives can occur with inflammatory neck masses. While some patients do undergo laryngopharyngectomy for complete esophageal inlet stricture or a nonfunctional larynx, or both, following chemoradiation therapy in the absence of recurrent cancer, it is critical that the difficult decision to proceed with ablative surgery in this context is made only after a thorough attempt to rule out recurrent cancer has been made. This attempt should include biopsy of the primary site.

Proceeding with ablative surgery without a positive biopsy is reasonable in some instances as long as the patient is fully apprised of the potential for no viable cancer to be found in the surgical specimen, as microscopic or multifocal disease may at times only be identified at surgical ablation rather than directed biopsy. In either case, a rigid upper endoscopy is important to accurately assess the extent of mucosal abnormality whether or not a tissue diagnosis has been established. This is especially important in assessing the extent of involvement of the posterior pharyngeal wall and the likelihood of tubed versus patch pharyngeal reconstruction. Similarly, the distal extent of cancer in the cervical esophagus must be established to determine the potential need for a gastric pull-up. When complete or near complete obstruction of the esophageal inlet precludes visualization of the distal extent of disease, the small diameter transnasal esophagoscope may sometimes traverse a tight stricture or obstruction by tumor.

When endoscopy from above cannot establish the extent of the distal disease, preoperative imaging should give a reasonably accurate assessment of whether or not tumor extends distally enough to warrant consideration of the gastric pull-up. If the concern is high but imaging is equivocal, then another option to consider is retrograde esophagoscopy via a gastrostomy tube. Placement of a gastrostomy tube will be necessary in these patients preoperatively as their dysphagia will be severe and their nutritional status compromised. A PEG in place does not preclude the ability to subsequently perform a gastric pull-up if necessary.

Patient Assessment for Reconstruction

Once the defect has been assessed as described above and is limited to a mucosal defect above the thoracic inlet with or without associated cutaneous involvement, patient factors must be evaluated to determine their suitability for ALT flap reconstruction. These include an assessment of the recipient site, the donor site, and the patient's comorbidities. The status of the surrounding tissues in the neck beyond that of the surgical defect is critical in determining the patient's suitability for free flap reconstruction. This includes the overall condition of the tissues and the local impact of previous therapies such as previous surgery and radiation therapy. This is generally evident by physical examination with regard to the suppleness of the soft tissues to manipulation, but the status of suitable donor vessels will be less evident and may require careful review of previous operative reports. Ultimately, this determination is definitively made at the time of the ablative procedure, so backup reconstructive plans need to be in place should a microvascular reconstruction be considered inadvisable based on operative findings.

Evaluation of the donor site is critically important when assessing the role of the ALT flap in hypopharyngeal reconstruction. While contraindications to ALT harvest exist, such as extensive prior trauma to the local site, these are uncommon. The patient's body habitus and anticipated thickness of the flap is a crucial point to consider as this relates to the expected surgical defect. Preference should be given to the radial forearm free flap (RFFF) in patients with excess subcutaneous adipose tissue in the thigh and in whom a circumferential defect is anticipated. The jejunal free flap would be an alternative consideration in this case. A modestly thick ALT flap will still work well for a patch flap reconstruction. Finally, a careful assessment of comorbidities is important as this relates to safe perioperative medical management, and the patient's suitability for the anticipated greater length of anesthesia required for most patients undergoing free flap reconstruction.

SURGICAL TECHNIQUE

General Considerations

When possible, reconstruction of the hypopharynx and cervical esophagus with the ALT flap is performed as a two-team procedure with the tumor ablation performed by a surgical team separate from the reconstructive surgeon. This provides many advantages, most important of which is the overall shorter operative time facilitated by flap harvest performed simultaneously with the surgical resection. Equally important is the elimination of the ablative surgeon's concern for compromising the surgical margins based on limitations of reconstructive options. This is not to say that the ablative surgeon should resect posterior pharynx or cervical esophagus with abandon, and a familiar working relationship between ablative and reconstructive surgeon is immensely helpful with regard to establishing consistent outcomes. The preoperative assessment of the extent of the anticipated defect is as important from an oncologic perspective as it is from a reconstructive perspective, and the patient will benefit from a careful assessment of this important point by both surgeons who are in direct communication with each other about their findings and surgical plans.

The primary goal of the preoperative planning period is to define the best operation for the patient while minimizing the chances of intraoperative surprises. When this coordinated evaluation is done properly with the ablative and reconstructive teams, then the harvest of the appropriate flap of appropriate size and design can be accomplished simultaneously with the tumor ablation to minimize operative time. Unexpected findings occasionally do occur intraoperatively despite the most careful preoperative planning, however, and unless sequential flap harvest following ablation is planned, then the flap should be harvested with some contingencies in mind. This generally means harvesting a skin paddle somewhat larger than required to allow for modification as necessary.

Flap Harvest

The patient is placed on the operative table in the supine position. Following induction of general endotracheal anesthesia, the bed is rotated 180 degrees with the feet facing the anesthesiologist. Tracheostomy is performed initially or at the time of laryngectomy depending upon the status of the airway preoperatively. Paralysis is not required for flap harvest and is generally not used with dissection simultaneously occurring in the neck. Flap harvest is performed according the technique described by Prof. Fu-Chan Wei of Taiwan. The selection of which leg to use is generally guided by patient preference, as the harvest site is sufficiently distant from the resection site such that either leg can be used for simultaneous flap harvest. A bump is sometimes placed under the ipsilateral hip but is usually not necessary. The skin paddle is centered on a line drawn from the anterior superior iliac spine to the lateral aspect of the patella. This line approximates the location of the intermuscular septum between the rectus femoris and vastus lateralis muscles. The center point between the anterior superior iliac spine and the superior aspect of the lateral patella is marked as a means of localizing the majority of skin perforators. As described by Mardini et al., a circle with a 3-cm diameter is drawn from this center point, localizing the majority of cutaneous perforators in the distal posterior quadrant of this circle (Fig. 30.1). The skin paddle is drawn to incorporate this entire circle, erring on centering the skin paddle more on this distal posterior quadrant of the circle rather than the

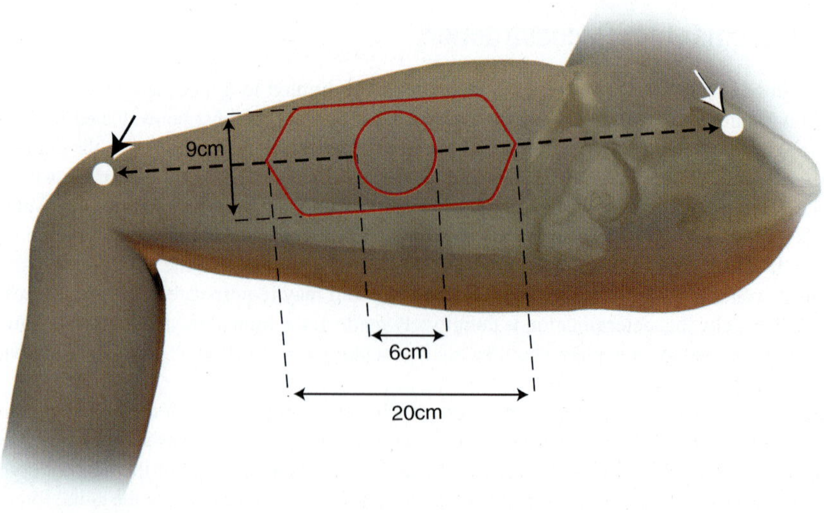

FIGURE 30.1 A line is drawn from the anterior superior iliac spine to the lateral aspect of the superior border of the patella. This line is bisected, and at this central point, a circle is drawn with 6-cm circumference. The skin paddle is designed to incorporate this circle, with the posterior–inferior quadrant most reliably harboring the cutaneous perforators. The skin paddle is then drawn to include sufficient skin for reconstruction of the defect while tapering the ends to facilitate closure of the donor site.

line approximating the intermuscular septum per se. A Doppler probe can be used to localize skin perforators both within or near this circle, or cephalad or caudad to it, with the skin paddle modified to incorporate at least two perforators if possible. Due to the occasional difficulty encountered in localizing skin perforators with the Doppler probe, this circle as described is always incorporated in the skin paddle near its center point.

Determination of the appropriate size skin paddle is based on standard factors consistent with every pharyngoesophageal defect, as well as factors specific to the individual defect as assessed by the preoperative surgical plan. One of the main advantages of the ALT flap is that it provides the reconstructive surgeon with the ability to reconstruct total pharyngeal defects in tubed fashion as well as on-lay patch reconstruction of partial pharyngeal defects. Even if the preoperative assessment suggests that a significant (>2 cm) strip of posterior pharyngeal mucosa can be preserved, it is prudent to harvest a skin paddle of at least 9 cm in diameter. This is done in the event that assessment of the margins dictates sacrifice of the remaining posterior pharyngeal strip thought initially to be clear of tumor or if the remaining posterior pharyngeal strip appears to have insufficient vascularity to maintain a dual vertical suture line. Mucosal strips narrower than 2 cm will ultimately have two mucocutaneous suture lines running parallel to each other 1 cm or less apart, and the benefit of preserving this narrow strip in comparison to a single suture line in an appropriately vascularized cutaneous skin paddle is controversial. The mucosal strip is more frequently discarded in the previously irradiated patient as compared with nonirradiated mucosa. Even a narrow strip of mucosa is not discarded until the flap is determined to be well vascularized in the unlikely necessity of using an alternative reconstructive technique at the same operative setting.

If a pectoralis major myocutaneous (PMM) flap is chosen, then depending upon its thickness the preservation of this mucosal strip may have greater benefit. The 9-cm width is selected to ensure a neopharyngeal tube diameter of nearly 3 cm. A 9.4-cm wide skin paddle will create a 3-cm diameter tube when folded on itself, and this approximate width is also standardized between all patients. If a posterior strip of pharyngeal mucosa is successfully preserved, then the flap can be narrowed after harvest to avoid redundancy. The length of the skin paddle harvested is dependent on the location of perforators identified outside of the central circle and the need for additional skin for cervical skin reconstruction. A longer flap will allow for creation of an external skin paddle based either on a localizable skin perforator or by virtue of deepithelializing a portion of the skin paddle to enable the distal skin paddle to be folded and oriented externally. This may require horizontal rather than vertical flap inset (see *Flap Inset*). A horizontally inset flap will likely require a greater width to accommodate the vertical length of the defect and may not be suitable for defects including significant amounts of cervical esophagus.

Once the skin paddle is marked, the leg is circumferentially prepped and draped. The flap is harvested with loupe magnification (3.5×) in the subfascial plane. Incision is first made the length of the medial aspect of the skin paddle, subsequently incising the rectus femoris fascia on a line paralleling the skin incision (Fig. 30.2). A subfascial plane is elevated laterally to expose the intermuscular septum between rectus femoris and vastus lateralis. Regardless of the preincision localization of cutaneous perforators by Doppler probe, the elevation of the skin paddle off of the rectus femoris muscle is performed carefully to localize the cutaneous perforator(s) either within the intermuscular septum or traversing the vastus lateralis muscle. In either case, the rectus femoris muscle is widely exposed and then retracted medially to expose the primary vascular pedicle of the flap, the descending branch of the lateral circumflex femoral artery (LCFA). In this fashion, the cutaneous perforators will be localized along with the LCFA. The lateral aspect of the skin paddle is incised and elevated in a subfascial plane off of the vastus lateralis muscle and then dissection of the cutaneous perforators is performed. If these traverse the muscle, the muscle fibers anterior or medial to these perforators are elevated with a fine clamp and divided. An irrigating bipolar cautery allows for control of hemostasis with limited heat transfer to the delicate perforators. Larger muscular perforators are divided between small Ligaclips. This technique allows for elevation of the skin paddle with minimal additional bulk, a circumstance generally preferable for hypopharyngeal defect reconstruction, particularly if a tubed skin paddle is anticipated. Alternatively, a segment of vastus lateralis muscle may be harvested that incorporates a significant component of the muscle between the perforators or beyond if greater bulk is required or if vascular muscle for cervical vessel coverage is desired. This vascularized muscle may also be skin grafted for external coverage in carefully selected cases.

Microvascular Anastomoses

Donor vessels are selected in the neck based on availability. The ALT flap vascular pedicle is of sufficient length to support anastomoses either low or high in the neck and from the contralateral side for partial pharyngeal defects if necessary. The facial artery is used in the majority of cases mobilized to its takeoff from the external carotid artery. Transverse cervical vessels are usually available in the previously dissected neck when branches of the external carotid artery may be unavailable and represent an excellent alternative to the facial vessels. Most common venous anastomoses are to the facial vein, external jugular vein, internal jugular vein, and transverse cervical vein. Two venous anastomoses are often performed with both venae comitantes of the LCFA, although these two venae comitantes often join if dissected thoroughly, allowing for a single venous anastamosis in such cases.

Flap Inset

Flap inset is relatively straightforward where a significant posterior pharyngeal strip of mucosa has been preserved. If the vascular anastomoses have been performed with the facial vessels, the proximal aspect of the skin paddle is inset in the base of the tongue and tonsil region while the distal skin is inset at the esophageal inlet.

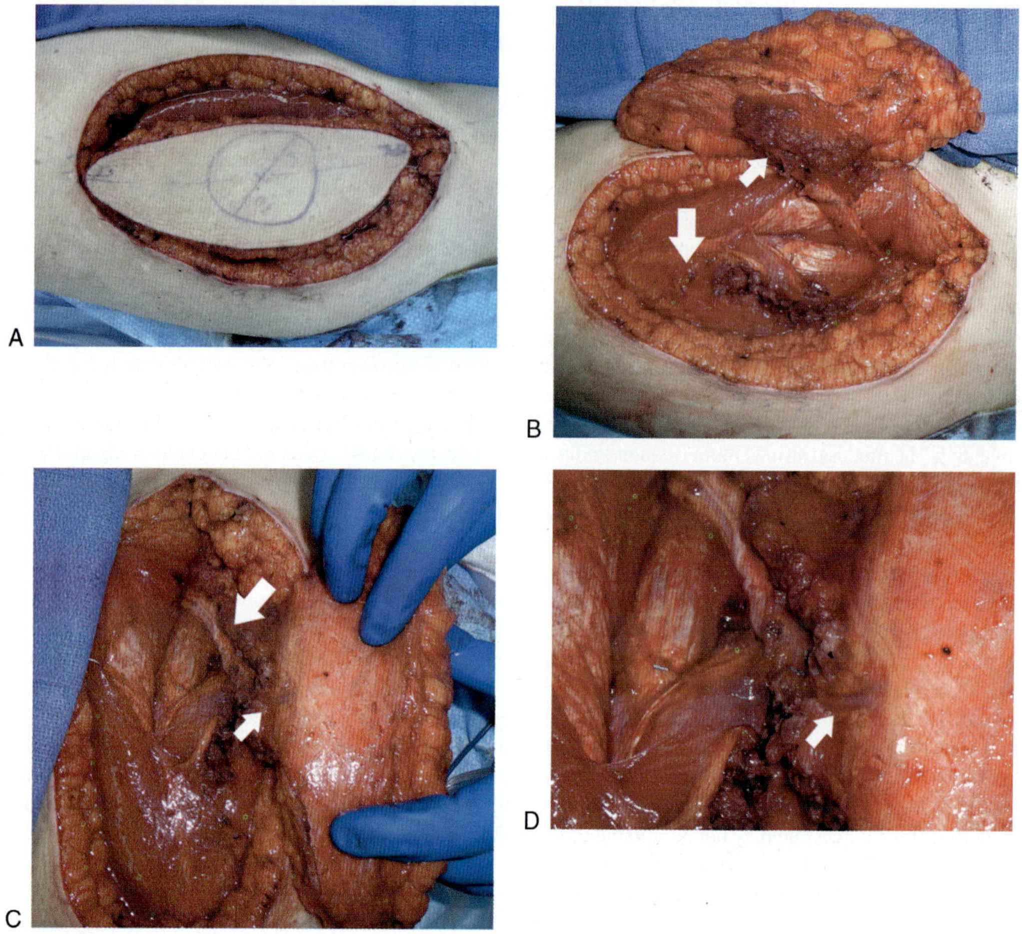

FIGURE 30.2 **A.** A 9 × 20–cm skin paddle has been elevated and replaced in its normal position on the leg. Note the thickness of the subcutaneous fat in this mildly obese patient. This represents the upper limit of ideal thickness for a tubed skin paddle. **B.** The undersurface of the flap is shown with a small cuff of vastus lateralis muscle elevated with the cutaneous perforator (*small arrow*), leaving the majority of the vastus lateralis undisturbed (*large arrow*). Minimizing the amount of muscle harvested with the flap is especially important in a more obese individual with a thick layer of subcutaneous fat. **C.** *Large arrow* shows the vascular pedicle with the *small arrow* showing a dominant single cutaneous perforator. **D.** The cutaneous perforator is shown at higher magnification (*arrow*).

The size and shape of the skin paddle is tailored to the specific defect size after flap revascularization both to avoid redundancy of the skin paddle and to ensure that all areas of the skin paddle utilized in the mucosal reconstruction bleed appropriately. Redundancy of the skin paddle is avoided to prevent a patulous neopharynx with outpouchings of nonmucous secreting surface area that in turn will contribute to decrease bolus transit time with swallowing or possibly trap and retain portions of the bolus. The unused cutaneous portions of the skin paddle are discarded or can alternatively be harvested for split-thickness skin graft if necessary for reconstruction of the external defect. Rather than discard the full thickness of any unused portion of the skin paddle, however, the excess skin paddle is deepithelialized to preserve the well-vascularized subcutaneous adipose tissue. This can then be used as a second layer to cover the adjacent suture lines. An alternative technique described by Yu et al. is to harvest an extra width of fascia with the skin paddle such that this can be used to bolster the suture line.

Inset for a circumferential pharyngeal defect requires the creation of the alimentary tract tube by suture of the flap to itself. In most cases, this is done with the flap oriented vertically to provide sufficient length to reconstruct the pharyngeal defect without undue tension on either proximal or distal pharyngeal anastomoses. Care must be taken to approximate the circumferential size of the defect as closely as possible at the larger proximal or oropharyngeal end where an additional length of skin paddle may be preserved as an extension that both lengthens the anastomotic circumference, while also providing for inset of the flap more superiorly into the oropharynx as needed (Fig. 30.3). The opposite problem typically exists at the esophageal inlet where the normal size of the lumen is smaller, and this can be further narrowed by inset of a skin paddle with a circumferential suture line. This is offset by vertically incising the esophagus for a length of at least 1.5 cm and spatulating this mucosal edge to the 3-cm-wide cutaneous tube (Fig. 30.4). The skin paddle is closed over a Dobhoff nasogastric feeding tube if a PEG tube is not already in place, but otherwise no tube is left in the neopharyngeal lumen. Murray et al. described a small series in which no fistulae occurred and a stricture rate of 14% in 14 patients reconstructed with an ALT flap tubed over a salivary bypass tube as an alternative to consider. Any excess portions of skin paddle proximally and distally are deepithelialized, and the retained vascularized adipose tissue is used to bolster proximal and distal suture lines.

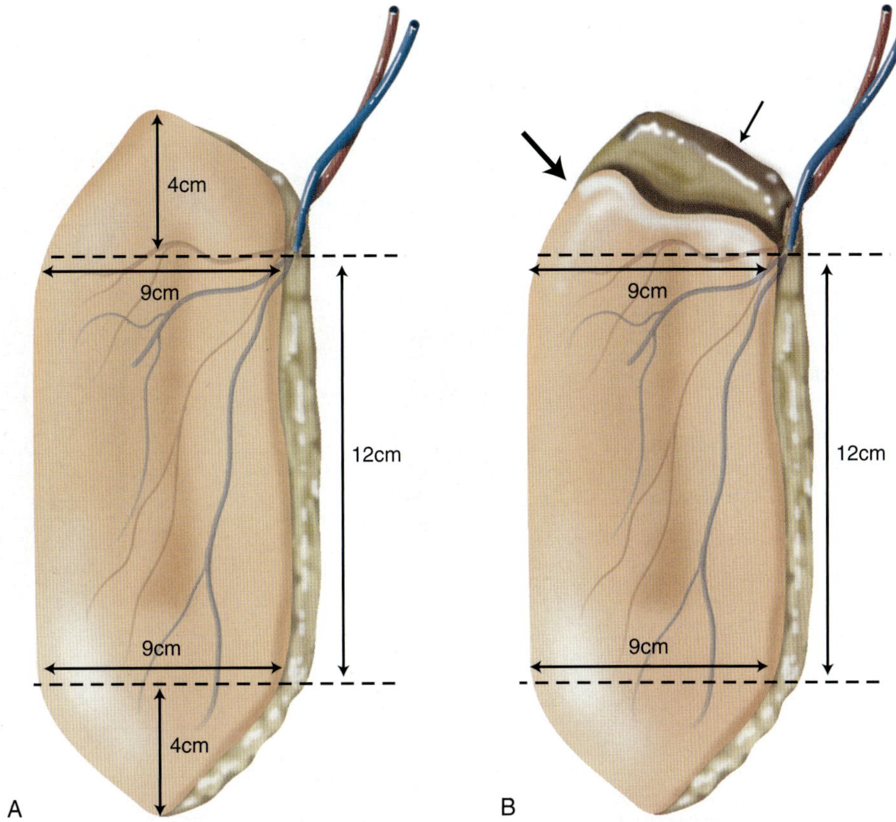

FIGURE 30.3 **A.** A 9-cm-wide skin paddle has been harvested. The skin paddle is designed for a defect length of approximately 12 cm. The central portion of the flap approximates this 9 × 12–cm defect (to accommodate a neopharyngeal tube with nearly 3 cm diameter). Approximately 4 cm of additional skin are harvested proximal and distal to this central 12-cm-long segment, tapering each end of the skin paddle to facilitate closure of the donor site defect. These proximal and distal tapered ends of the skin paddle can then be tailored for the specific defect. **B.** In this example, the superior extent of the defect extends unilaterally into the oropharynx. This results in a defect length longer than 12 cm on one side and a superior defect circumference longer than that of the more uniform midportion or typically smaller inferior portions of the defect. This is addressed by extending the proximal skin paddle in a rounded fashion on one side to extend into the oropharynx (*long arrow*) while drawing a curvilinear line to the opposite side of the flap. This curvilinear line effectively lengthens the suture line (*circumference*) of the superior aspect of the neopharyngeal and oropharyngeal anastomosis without harvesting a wider flap with its greater donor site morbidity. The skin proximal to this curvilinear line is deepithelialized (*short arrow*), preserving the subcutaneous fat to reinforce the suture line.

Relatively short vertical segment defects can be closed with the flap inset horizontally. This may provide better orientation of the vascular pedicle in the neck and therefore reduce the risk of vessel kinking. Alternatively, this may also provide for better orientation of an external skin paddle harvested as the distal aspect of the skin paddle based either on a separate cutaneous perforator or as a distal segment of skin separated from its proximal aspect by a deepithelized strip of subcutaneous adipose tissue. An externally oriented skin paddle provides for an excellent means of monitoring the flap but is not universally used if not required for skin reconstruction.

Closure of the Donor Site

Closure of the donor site usually requires split-thickness skin grafting for defect widths of greater than 9 cm. Wide undermining of the adjacent skin edges can allow for sufficient laxity to permit primary closure in many cases where the defect width is limited to 9 cm or less. Cut edges of the vastus lateralis muscle are reapproximated with 3-0 Vicryl sutures. Closed suction drain is placed between the muscle bellies of vastus lateralis and rectus femoris to prevent seroma formation and is usually well separated from the skin graft if necessary to permit suction to be retained in the postoperative period. Early mobilization and physical therapy is encouraged in the postoperative period, although this is delayed if a bolstered skin graft is in place until the bolster is removed on postoperative day 5.

POSTOPERATIVE MANAGEMENT

Patients are observed with surgical drains in the neck typically for 3 to 5 days. The volume and character of the drainage is closely monitored for signs of salivary leakage. If none is seen, then drains are removed when

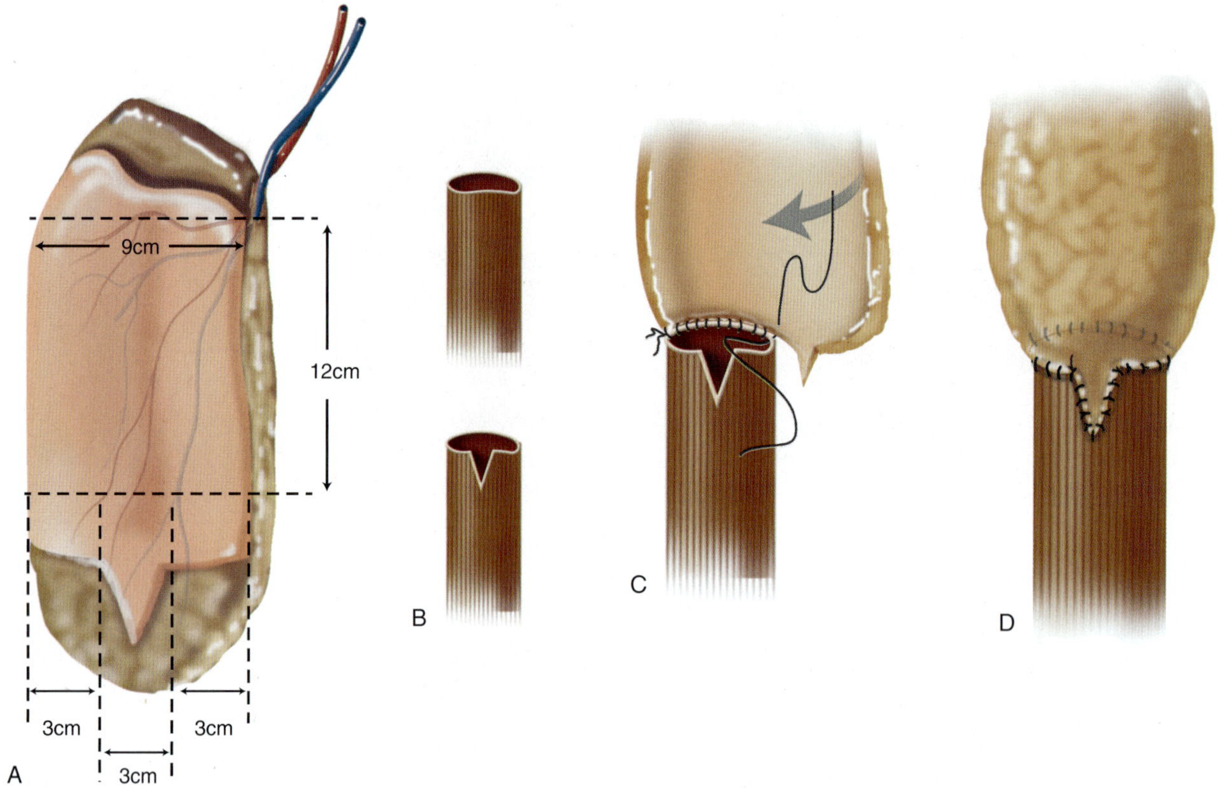

FIGURE 30.4 **A.** A triangular extension of the skin paddle is drawn to extend into the distal tapered end of the flap. The remainder of the distal tapered end skin is deepithelialized. **B.** A vertical incision is made in the anterior wall of the cervical esophagus. This incision is made approximately 2.5 to 3 cm in length and corresponds to the length of the legs of the triangle drawn in (A). **C.** The posterior wall of the esophagus is approximated to the skin paddle. **D.** The skin paddle triangle is inset into the anterior cervical esophagus as the distal neopharyngeal—esophageal anastomosis is completed. This spatulates the distal anastomosis, lengthening its suture line (*circumference*), thereby reducing likelihood of stricture.

output is less than 30 mL/d. Tube feeding is initiated on postoperative day 1 but started only at a low continuous rate and advanced slowly to minimize risk of reflux. Routine stoma care is performed. Monitoring of the flap is performed with Doppler checks of the localized vascular pedicle every 1 hour while in the intensive care unit and confirmed by bedside portable color flow Doppler on postoperative day 1 to more accurately define the course and patency of the arterial and venous vascular pedicles if a monitoring skin paddle is not used.

Discharge planning begins when tube feeding has been advanced to a bolus regimen and is able to be administered by the patient and his or her family, when the patient is able to demonstrate adequate care of the tracheostomy, and if there are no clinical signs of fistula formation by postoperative day 6. Discharge typically occurs between postoperative days 6 and 9 if no postoperative complications have occurred. Follow-up is scheduled as an outpatient on postoperative days 13 to 14. Assuming no clinical signs of fistula are evident, then liquids are started by mouth under direct observation. Adequate swallowing function demonstrated at that time may allow for removal of the nasogastric feeding tube if in place. Any concern for the presence of a fistula or demonstration of difficulty with swallowing of liquids will prompt a formal MBS study to be obtained to assess overall swallowing function. Once liquids are initiated, the diet will be restricted to full liquids for 1 week, soft diet for the following week, and then a regular diet as tolerated will be initiated. For patients undergoing postoperative radiotherapy, it is essential that daily swallowing of liquids at least be maintained throughout treatment. This will help maintain patency of the neopharynx and pharyngoesophageal anastomoses through the course of therapy. Maintaining a PEG tube in these patients is still advisable to be sure they do not become dehydrated and suffer prolonged breaks in treatment as a result, but their daily swallowing must be strongly encouraged and supported by adequate pain management as needed.

Speech rehabilitation begins with the early use of an electrolarynx. Preoperative teaching by the speech therapist is important to hasten early and effective use of the device in the postoperative period. Tracheoesophageal puncture (TEP) for placement of a TEP is considered by 3 months postoperative if minimal to no dysphagia is evident. If significant dysphagia is noted, then an MBS to assess for stricture formation is performed, and consideration of dilation is entertained. If minimal dilation is necessary, then TEP can be performed at the same operative setting. Significant stricture formation may require serial dilation prior to creation of the speech fistula. These time schedules are modified as needed by the presence or absence of concomitant adjuvant therapy.

COMPLICATIONS

The ALT flap itself is associated with few complications; however, the reconstruction of the pharynx can be fraught with complications including fistula and wound breakdown. This occurs more commonly in the malnourished and radiated patients.

RESULTS

Richmon and Brumond provide a thorough summary of the various reconstructive options for hypopharyngeal defects in a recent review. The PMM flap is well suited to patch reconstruction of the neopharynx in many patients. Its advantages are its reliability, its technical ease of harvest without need for reanastomosis of its vascular supply in the neck and its versatility. The optimal patient for PMM flap reconstruction of the hypopharynx is one with a relatively thin chest wall whose neck has not received previous treatment that would impact the availability of donor vessels for microvascular reconstruction and whose preoperative risk of fistula is determined to be high based on the overall condition of the tissues in the neck after previous radiation. The published rates of stricture (0% to 16%) and fistula formation (0% to 47%) with PMM flap reconstruction are likely influenced heavily by patient selection; however, the well-vascularized pectoralis muscle that accompanies its skin paddle usually provides excellent protection of critical vascular structures in the neck should a fistula occur and is itself resistant to flap loss or vessel thrombosis in the context of a fistula. The pectoralis muscle may be skin grafted for external skin coverage if necessary. The PMM flap also provides a reliable alternative to microvascular reconstruction should free flap failure occur or in the properly selected patient with significant comorbidities as a first treatment option. The PMM flap is not well suited for the reconstruction of circumferential hypopharyngeal defects unless the chest wall is quite thin, as does occur in some patients who present with a prolonged history of dysphagia and weight loss.

The RFFF avoids many of the disadvantages of the PMM flap for hypopharyngeal reconstruction by virtue of its thin, pliable skin paddle. In the majority of cases, the RFFF can be harvested of sufficient width to reconstruct a circumferential defect provided that the distal pharyngoesophageal anastomosis remains accessible in the neck. Reported stricture (10% to 36%) and fistula (17% to 28%) rates are still significant, and the donor site morbidity of the RFFF is an important consideration. While rates of tendon exposure and limitation of hand function are low, these issues are important considerations in certain individuals whose occupation depends on precise control of hand and finger function. The donor site scar is also quite noticeable with the RFFF. Restoration of tracheoesophageal speech is reliable with the RFFF, but reconstruction of associated cervical skin defects requires an adjunctive procedure such as simultaneous PMM flap.

Gastrointestinal flaps play a significant role in reconstruction of hypopharyngeal defects. The gastric pull-up remains the procedure of choice for defects whose distal extent is beyond the thoracic inlet by providing for simultaneous complete resection of the entire esophagus as wide distal margin and a single pharyngeal anastomosis at the level of the base of the tongue. Its disadvantages are its donor site morbidity, with mortality rates reported as high as 10%. In a more recent series, Shuangba et al. reported a perioperative mortality of 2% and anastomotic leak of 9.1% in a series of 208 patients over a 20-year period. Adjunctive flaps must be considered when external coverage is required or when a significant oropharyngeal defect accompanies the hypopharyngeal defect. Free intestinal flaps are suitable for reconstruction of defects whose distal extent is above the thoracic inlet. The reported rates of stricture formation vary from 15% to 22% with the jejunal free flap, although a recent report by Sharp et al. describes 18 of 19 patients tolerating an oral diet with mean follow-up time of 4 years. Fistula rates for jejunal free flaps are similar or slightly lower than reported for RFFF. Tracheoesophageal speech has been more difficult to achieve with jejunal free flap reconstruction of the hypopharynx. Sharp et al. reports 15 of 19 patients successfully using tracheoesophageal speech, with 11 of 19 having no or mild dysphonia. Yu et al., however, reported of only 22% of 31 patients achieving fluent tracheoesophageal speech following jejunal free flap reconstruction. Other disadvantages of the free jejunal flap are its associated abdominal harvest site morbidity and the need for three intestinal anastomoses, as well as its relative size mismatch at the level of the oropharynx.

The ALT flap has gained great popularity in the reconstruction of head and neck defects by virtue of its versatility and its low donor site morbidity. A typically large skin paddle can be harvested whose thickness varies based on body habitus. This large skin paddle can be subdivided into separate skin paddles for cases in which reconstruction of a mucosal defect and external skin coverage is required based either on individual skin perforators from the vascular pedicle or by deepithelializing portions of the skin paddle whether or not separate skin perforators are identified. Vascularized muscle can also be transferred with the ALT skin paddle if additional bulk or vascular protection is required. Yu et al. have reported results of 114 patients with pharyngoesophageal defects reconstructed with the ALT following total laryngopharyngectomy. Pharyngocutaneous fistula occurred in 9% while strictures developed in 6%. Ninety-one percent of patients tolerated an oral diet without need for feeding tube supplementation. TEP for speech rehabilitation was performed in 51 of 114 patients, with 81% of patients achieving fluent speech with secondary TEP, while 41% of patients achieving fluent speech following primary TEP. A disadvantage of the ALT flap for pharyngoesophageal reconstruction is its increased bulk in some patients. This is less disadvantageous where posterior pharyngeal wall mucosa has been preserved but may be unsuitable for circumferential defect reconstruction.

In the properly selected patient, the ALT flap provides the surgeon with the flexibility to reconstruct a variety of potential defects. These include hypopharyngeal defects where sufficient posterior pharyngeal mucosa is preserved to create an on-lay patch, total pharyngeal defects where a tubed skin paddle is required provided that sufficient cervical esophagus remains for the esophageal anastomosis to be performed in the neck, and combined mucosal and external skin defects where a single flap is preferable to two flaps. This flexibility is critical to consistently achieving acceptable short-term and long-term functional outcomes in this challenging patient population whose true extent of the disease may not be evident until the resection has been completed. While all of the reconstructive options mentioned above may provide the best alternative for any given patient, the ALT will provide the best option for the majority of patients whose hypopharyngeal and esophageal mucosal defects are above the thoracic inlet.

PEARLS

- Preoperative assessment of the extent of the anticipated surgical defect is critical in the reconstruction of the hypopharynx.
- Accurate assessment of the size of the defect depends on anatomic imaging such as CT and MRI, although PET–CT may be very helpful in localizing the extent of tumor in previously irradiated patients whose examination or conventional imaging may be limited by posttreatment changes.
- Staging endoscopy is an important adjunct to imaging for localization of disease at or beyond the esophageal inlet.
- The ALT provides for effective reconstruction of the defect for both partial and total pharyngeal defects and may also allow for simultaneous reconstruction of an external cervical skin defect. This versatility provides important leeway in the reconstructive plan should the ablative defect prove larger than anticipated.
- The skin paddle should be designed for a minimum width of 9 cm to create a nearly 3-cm-diameter neopharynx.
- Redundancy of the skin paddle should be avoided at flap inset in order to avoid a patulous neopharynx likely to be associated with increase transit times of the food bolus.
- Inset of the skin paddle at the esophageal inlet should include inset within a vertically oriented incision in the esophagus to broaden the esophageal inlet at the location of the distal anastomosis.

PITFALLS

- Consider an alternate flap reconstruction if the ALT is significantly thick. This will be adequate for an on-lay patch reconstruction but inadequate for a tubed reconstruction of the total pharyngeal defect. Consider a tubed RFFF in this case.
- An accurate assessment of the distal extent of disease is imperative to avoid a circumstance where the distal defect is beyond the limit of what can be safely reconstructed with a fasciocutaneous flap. If there is significant doubt about this point, then flap harvest can be delayed until a distal mucosal incision has been made and margin cleared, with the gastric pull-up to be used instead if the resection extends beyond the cervical esophagus. This reconstructive eventuality must be prepared for with an appropriate surgical service on standby if sufficient concern for this exists.

INSTRUMENTS TO HAVE AVAILABLE

- Standard head and neck surgical set

SUGGESTED READING

Murray DJ, Gilbert RW, Vesely MJJ, et al. Functional outcomes and donor site morbidity following circumferential pharyngoesophageal reconstruction using an anterolateral thigh flap and salivary bypass tube. *Head Neck* 2007;29:147–154.

Richmon JD, Brumund KT. Reconstruction of the hypopharynx: current trends. *Curr Opin Otolaryngol Head Neck Surg* 2007;15:208–212.

Chan YW, Ng RW, Lun Liu LH, et al. Reconstruction of circumferential pharyngeal defects after tumour resection: reference or preference. *J Plast Reconstr Aesthet Surg* 2011;64(8):1022–1028.

Joo YH, Sun DI, Cho KJ, et al. Fasciocutaneous free flap reconstruction for squamous cell carcinoma of the hypopharynx. *Eur Arch Otorhinolaryngol* 2011;268:289–294.

Takes RP, Strojan P, Silver CE, et al. Current trends in initial management of hypopharyngeal cancer: the declining use of open surgery. *Head Neck* 2012;34(2):270–281

31 THE GASTRIC PULL-UP

D. Gregory Farwell

INTRODUCTION

Cancer involving the cervical esophagus, pyriform sinuses, and larynx may require removal of the cervical esophagus creating a major continuity defect of the upper digestive tract. Reestablishing a conduit for swallowing is essential to rehabilitate patients and give them an optimal quality of life after extensive extirpative surgery. Other rare diagnostic entities that may leave patients in need of esophageal reconstruction include atresia and other congenital anomalies such as tracheoesophageal fistula, caustic ingestions, and trauma. Several techniques have been used to reconstruct the cervical esophageal defect including the creation of local skin flaps (Wookey flap), tubed locoregional flaps, or tubed cutaneous flaps and microvascular enteric flaps. In certain patients, either the defect may be too large or the particular needs of the patient require the technique of pedicled enteric flaps from the abdomen such as the gastric pull-up or a colonic interposition graft. These techniques provide vascularized enteric tissue, which reestablishes a communication between the oropharynx and the rest of the gastrointestinal tract.

The gastric pull-up is the most frequently performed pedicled enteric flap used to reconstruct the esophagus. Most patients with advanced cancer involving the larynx and pyriform sinus require a laryngectomy. However, for thoracic esophageal pathology, the patient may be able to retain the larynx. These patients, with their larynx intact, have additional potential postoperative problems including aspiration and vocal fold immobility that may complicate their recovery. All patients undergoing gastric pull-up are at risk for significant morbidity and potential mortality due to the extensive nature of the surgery.

HISTORY

The majority of patients in need of cervical esophageal replacement have been diagnosed with cancer of the larynx, hypopharynx, or cervical esophagus. As such, they may present with dysphonia, dyspnea, dysphagia, weight loss, or pain. Often, these cancers present at a late stage due to the extensive submucosal lymphatics of the hypopharynx and cervical esophagus. As such, a careful diagnostic evaluation including a staging endoscopy is critical before embarking on aggressive surgical therapy. Any suggestion of cervical lymphadenopathy should be carefully noted and further evaluated. These cancers usually interfere with optimal alimentation so that these patients are often malnourished. An assessment of the degree of weight loss should be included in the pretreatment history. One of the major decision points in these surgical procedures is whether the larynx can be preserved. A history of hoarseness or aspiration implies laryngeal involvement with the cancer and should be carefully elicited.

A systematic evaluation should include a careful assessment of pulmonary status, a history of gastrointestinal disorders, prior abdominal surgery, and overall conditioning. Special attention should be paid to the degree of pulmonary dysfunction including prior home oxygen use and limited exercise tolerance. If the patient has had prior pulmonary function testing, these records should be obtained and reviewed. Prior gastrointestinal conditions such as peptic ulcer disease, prior percutaneous gastrostomy tube placement, and prior laparotomy may make the procedure more complex or prevent the use of a gastric conduit for esophageal replacement. The patient's intake of tobacco and alcohol should be elicited to take steps to avoid withdrawal effects that are physically dangerous and add tremendously to hospital costs.

PHYSICAL EXAMINATION

Examination will often require the use of in-office flexible and operative rigid endoscopy to map out the extent of the tumor and to determine resectability and extent of the surgical procedure. Special attention should be paid to the function of the larynx and the proximity of the cancer to the postcricoid and pyriform sinus regions of the hypopharynx. These findings will help to determine whether the larynx can be saved or if it will have to be resected with the esophagus. Lymph nodes should be palpated looking for any evidence of metastasis. The larynx, pharynx, and esophagus should be palpated to make sure that these structures are mobile off of the prevertebral fascia indicating lack of invasion.

INDICATIONS

The indications for a gastric pull-up reconstruction include the presence of any complete defect of the cervical and upper thoracic esophagus.

CONTRAINDICATIONS

Contraindications to gastric pull-up include tumor-specific and patient-specific factors. Obviously, it is contraindicated to perform this surgery for cancers that have distant metastasis or are unresectable due to local extension into the prevertebral fascia. Many surgeons also consider involvement of the carotid artery as a relative contraindication to surgical resection.

Patient-specific contraindications include medical comorbidities such as advanced pulmonary disease that would preclude them from tolerating the procedure. Additional patient-specific contraindications would include prior abdominal or gastric surgery that might eliminate the use of the stomach as a conduit.

PREOPERATIVE PLANNING

Imaging Studies

Historically, the esophagus was evaluated with a barium swallow esophagram. While this study can still be used to look for a mass within the esophagus, it has been largely supplanted by rigid and more recently flexible esophagoscopy. As such, barium swallow evaluations are rarely used in modern practice. Detailed anatomical imaging studies with computed tomography (CT) and/or magnetic resonance imaging are helpful in determining the extent of the lesion and the presence of metastatic lymphadenopathy. These studies can be used to evaluate for extraesophageal extension of the cancer especially in the region of the prevertebral area and the carotid artery as these may negatively impact the resectability of the cancer. Transesophageal ultrasound is commonly used to evaluate distal esophageal cancers to determine the thickness and extraesophageal extension of the cancer.

Staging of the chest and abdomen is very important in the evaluation of these cancers, and historically, chest and abdominal CT was used. Currently, PET–CT is increasingly used to stage cancers of the head and neck. This modality is especially useful for lesions involving the esophagus and hypopharynx due to their aggressive nature and tendency for metastasis to the neck, mediastinum, and lungs. Due to the morbidity and mortality of surgical treatment of these cancers, adequate staging is essential before embarking upon surgery.

Staging Endoscopy

Preoperative endoscopy should be undertaken to determine the extent of the cancer and its resectability. The proximal extent of the cancer is important as the gastric pull-up will reliably reach the inferior tonsil fossa in most patients but becomes increasingly unreliable with defects further superior. Careful evaluation of the distal esophagus is essential in determining the inferior extent of the cancer and whether the entire esophagus must be resected. Some surgeons recommend mapping biopsies of the distal esophagus despite normal-appearing mucosa due to the tendency for skip lesions and submucosal spread of the tumor. At the time of the endoscopy, evaluation of the stomach is helpful to look for any pathology that might preclude the use of the gastric conduit.

Preoperative Testing

In addition to the endoscopy and staging workup, preoperative testing should include evaluation of pulmonary function. The gastric pull-up procedure is associated with pulmonary complications that are predicted by poor presurgical pulmonary function. Additional consultation with the patient's primary care physician or preoperative anesthesia consultation is advisable to estimate the patient's perioperative risk and to evaluate for modifiable risk factors.

SURGICAL TECHNIQUE

The gastric pull-up technique was first described by Ong and Lee in 1960. Since that time, minor modifications have been made to optimize the reliability of the tissue transfer. The procedure is initiated with the cervical esophagectomy and often neck dissections for oncologic cases. The creation of the gastric tube and abdominal procedure is frequently performed by a colleague in surgical oncology or thoracic surgery who is skilled in working in the abdomen and mediastinum. Since cancers of the hypopharynx and cervical esophagus require resection of the larynx for complete extirpation, most patients will have had a laryngectomy as part of their procedure, and the airway is controlled through a tracheostomy for the remainder of the procedure.

A laparotomy is made, often through a bilateral subcostal chevron incision or a midline incision. The blood supply of the stomach is multifaceted and includes contributions from the right and left gastric artery, the right gastroepiploic artery, the short gastrics, and the pancreaticogastric arteries (Fig. 31.1). For mobilization into the neck, the stomach is pedicled on its right gastroepiploic and right gastric arteries, and the remainder of the blood vessels are ligated allowing the stretch necessary to reach the pharynx (Fig. 31.2). The proximal portion of the stomach is at high risk due to vascular compromise as its blood supply is dependent upon the submucosal blood supply off of the gastroepiploics.

Several techniques have been described to optimize the chance of a successful gastric transfer. These include careful preservation of the gastroepiploic arcade during the dissection and meticulous dissection in the region of the gastrocolic ligament, capturing the arcade that is often present in this ligament to supply the proximal stomach. Blunt transhiatal dissection is then carried out from below to mobilize the thoracic esophagus (Fig. 31.3). This can often be done under direct vision to approximately the carina. Similarly, blunt dissection is performed from superiorly to carefully mobilize the superior thoracic esophagus. With blunt dissection, the recurrent laryngeal nerves are preserved laterally as the esophagus is completely mobilized from the gossamer fascia within the mediastinum and chest. A pyloromyotomy or pyloroplasty is often performed to achieve adequate drainage.

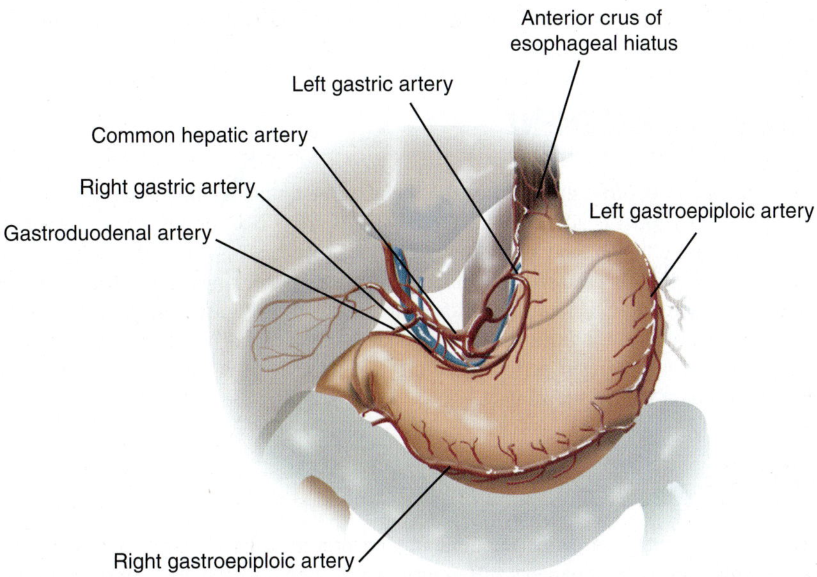

FIGURE 31.1 The stomach is shown in its relation to the diaphragm and abdominal viscera. The stomach will be mobilized, fashioned into a tube primarily vascularized by the right gastroepiploic artery and right gastric artery.

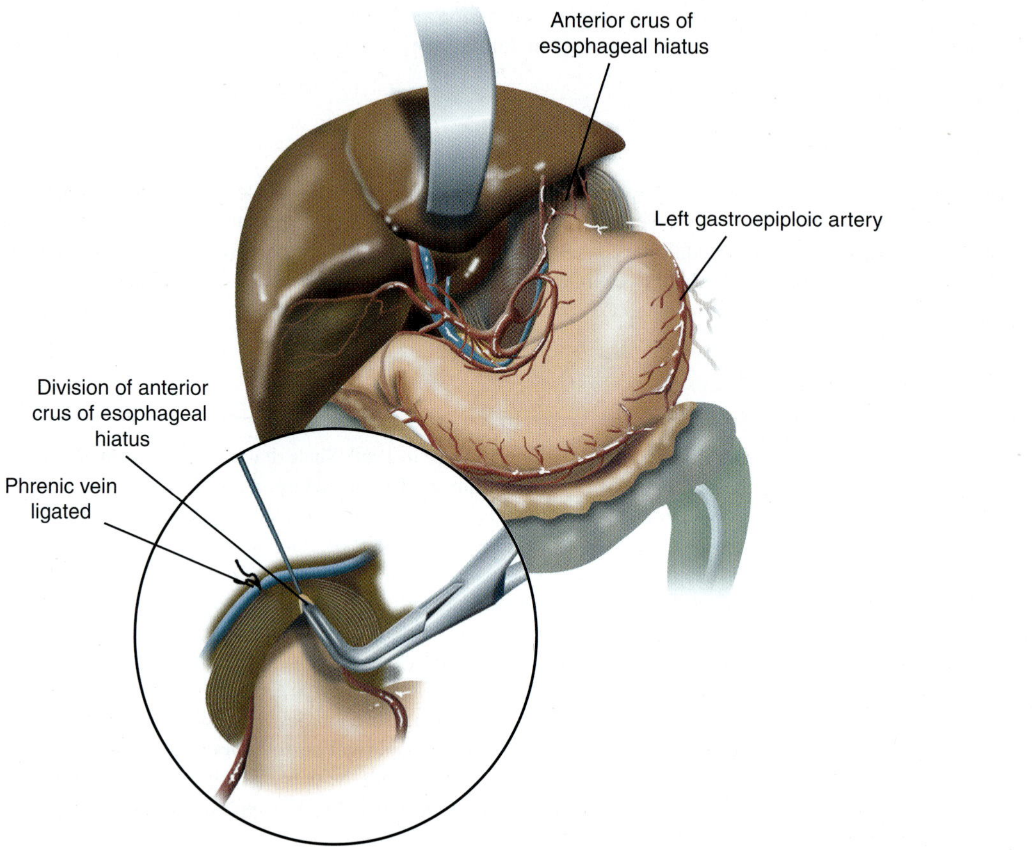

FIGURE 31.2
For mobilization into the neck, the stomach is pedicled on its right gastroepiploic and right gastric arteries, and the remainder of the blood vessels are ligated allowing the stretch necessary to reach the pharynx.

The stomach is transformed into a tube by using surgical staples to transect the extra stomach opposite the gastroepiploic artery. An approximately 4-cm-diameter tube is created to allow it to be passed retrocardiac into the neck (Fig. 31.4). Sutures are utilized to augment the staple line and minimize the chance of a leak into the thorax. The gastric tube is then passed under the heart and up into the neck for anastomosis (Fig. 31.5). Care is taken in the transfer of this tube to minimize traction on the stomach to preserve the blood supply. The diaphragm is then closed to minimize the risk of a diaphragmatic hernia.

The gastric tube is then secured to the hypopharyngeal mucosal margin in two layers with a deep layer involving the constrictor muscles of the pharynx and the serosa of the stomach. A second layer is performed from the mucosa of the pharynx to the mucosa of the stomach. A salivary bypass tube may be used to stent and divert secretions away from the suture line. After assuring a watertight closure, the abdomen and neck are closed over appropriate drains.

POSTOPERATIVE MANAGEMENT

Postoperatively, the patient is often managed in the intensive care unit for initial surveillance and monitoring. Aggressive pulmonary toilet is advocated as these patients are at risk for pulmonary morbidity including pulmonary edema, pleural effusion, and aspiration pneumonia (especially with laryngeal preservation). Deep venous thrombosis prophylaxis is used with pneumatic compression stockings and subcutaneous heparin. The drains are removed as appropriate. Patients are allowed to eat 7 to 14 days after the procedure as long as there is no evidence of anastomotic leak. The diet of patients undergoing a gastric pull-up is altered, and most require frequent small meals and a prolonged period of sitting upright at least 30 inches postprandial to minimize regurgitation or aspiration if the larynx is intact.

COMPLICATIONS

Unfortunately, a large percentage of patients undergoing this procedure have complications. In a recent review of over 200 gastric pull-ups, 42% of patients suffered a complication. The range of complications is from 22% to 89%. The most common acute complications are respiratory in nature including pneumonitis, pleural effusion, and hemothorax (Table 31.1). Pulmonary complications are often the cause of perioperative mortality. Delayed complications are listed in Table 31.2. Mortality is a well-known possibility due to the extensive

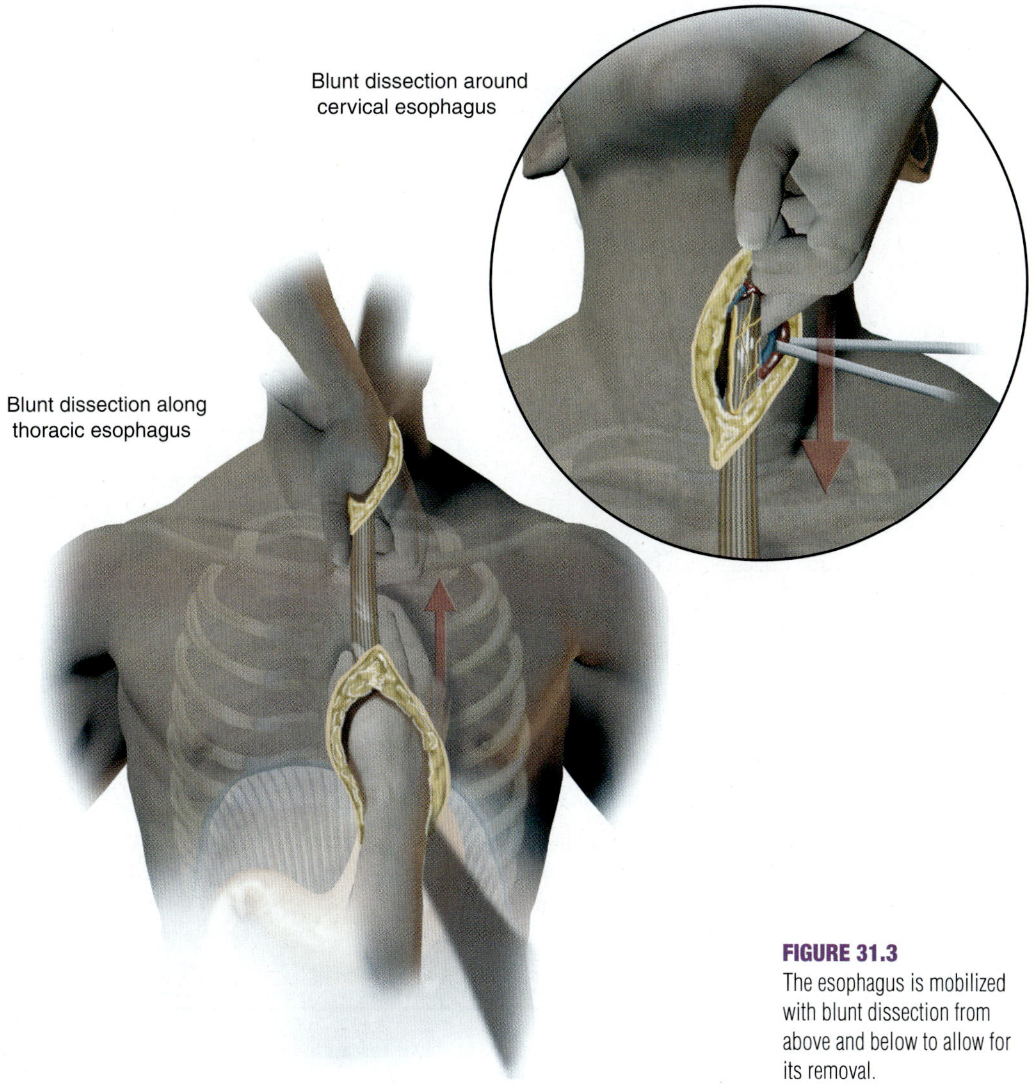

FIGURE 31.3
The esophagus is mobilized with blunt dissection from above and below to allow for its removal.

surgery and coexisting conditions in many of these patients. The rate of mortality may be as much as 15%, but most recent studies range between 2% and 11%.

RESULTS

Surgical reconstruction of a cervical esophagectomy defect with a gastric pull-up is a relatively reliable technique. A percentage of these patients will demonstrate postoperative stenosis at the neopharynx and require dilation. However, most patients achieve an oral diet and can be rehabilitated with a tracheoesophageal puncture for speech. Despite an overall survival ranging from 11% to 47%, the quality of life afforded by this procedure is acceptable with excellent global and functional results but expected low results in areas of smell, taste, speech, and sexuality.

PEARLS

- Prior to surgical management, an exhaustive staging workup should be performed to evaluate the local resectability of the cancer and the presence of regional or distant metastasis due to the advanced stage of these cancers at presentation.
- Patients need to be aware of the gravity of their situation but understand that survivors can expect an acceptable quality of life.
- Preoperative pulmonary function testing may predict which patients are at higher risk for postoperative complications.

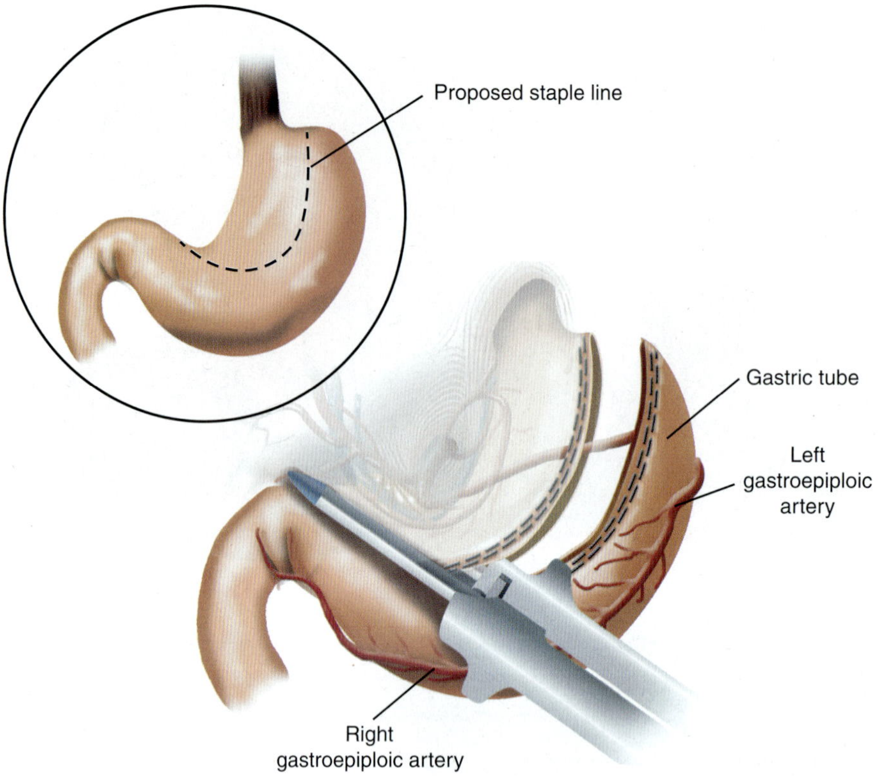

FIGURE 31.4
The lesser curvature of the stomach is then excised with a surgical stapler to create a conduit tube for transfer through the mediastinum and into the neck.

- The gastric tube must be harvested with great care to preserve the right short gastric and gastroepiploic arteries to insure adequate perfusion of the proximal stomach. This can reliably reach the postcricoid region and as high as the inferior tonsillar fossa in most patients.

PITFALLS

- Cancers that require resection of the base of the tongue or tonsil fossa are associated with higher complication rates as the proximal stomach is more prone to ischemia and anastomotic leak with more superior anastomoses.

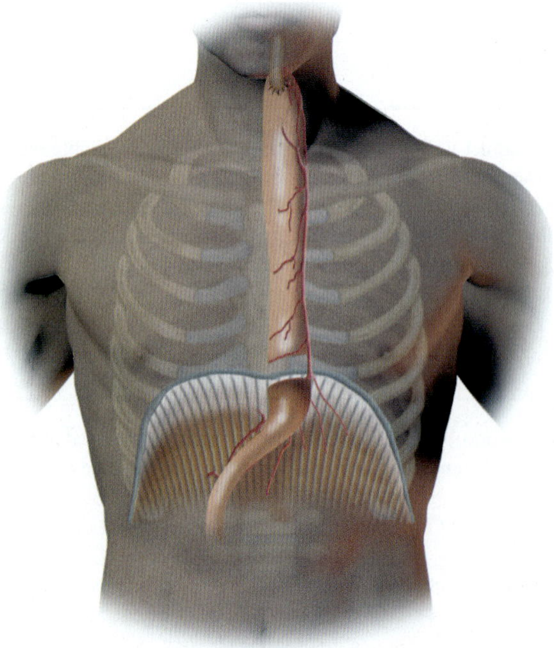

FIGURE 31.5
The gastric tube is then "pulled up" into the neck to allow for anastomosis with the pharyngeal remnant.

TABLE 31.1 Acute Complications After Gastric Pull-up Reported in the Literature
Anastomotic leakage
Chylous fistula
Heart failure
Hemoperitoneum
Hemothorax
Ischemia and necrosis of the stomach
Peritonitis
Pleural effusion
Pneumonitis
Recurrent laryngeal nerve paralysis (larynx preserving surgeries)
Wound infection

TABLE 31.2 Delayed Complications from Gastric Pull-up Reported in the Literature
Dumping syndrome
Stricture at the neopharynx anastomosis
Tracheostoma stricture

- Postoperative care is necessary to prevent and manage the complications associated with this procedure, which most frequently are pulmonary and wound.

Instruments to Have Available

- Standard head and neck surgical set

SUGGESTED READING

Wookey H. The surgical treatment of the pharynx and upper esophagus. *Surg Gynecol Obstet* 1942;75:499–506.

Ong GB, Lee TC. Pharyngogastric anastomosis after esophageal pharyngectomy for carcinoma of the hypopharynx and cervical esophagus. *Br J Surg* 1960;45:193–200.

Dumont P, Wihlm JM, Hentz JG, et al. Respiratory complications after surgical treatment of esophageal cancer. A study of 309 patients according to the type of resection. *Eur J Cardiothorac Surg* 1995;99(10);539–543.

Wei WI, Sham JST. Extent of resection of hypopharyngeal cancer. In: Wei WI, Sham JST, eds. *Cancer of the larynx and hypopharynx*. Oxford, UK: Isis Media Medical Ltd, 2000:95–104.

Ferguson MK, Durkin AE. Preoperative prediction of the risk of pulmonary complications after esophagectomy for cancer. *J Thorac Cardiovasc Surg* 2002;123(4):661–669.

32 RADIAL FOREARM FREE TISSUE TRANSFER

Brett A. Miles

INTRODUCTION

Surgical management of cancer of the hypopharynx, cervical esophagus, and larynx often results in defects in the cervical esophagus requiring reconstruction with free tissue transfer. Esophageal strictures requiring free tissue reconstruction are often a result of surgical and nonsurgical therapies for these malignancies. Patients with traumatic injuries and ingestion of caustic substances may rarely require esophageal reconstruction.

Perhaps the most challenging pharyngeal/cervical reconstruction is the free tissue transfer reconstruction of the cervical esophagus while maintaining an intact larynx. Previous surgery and radiation therapy often result in significant motor and sensory dysfunction of the cervical esophagus and larynx that is further complicated when reconstructive efforts are entertained.

Chronic aspiration, dysphagia, chondroradionecrosis, and pain may result in a nonfunctional larynx as a result of nonsurgical organ preservation strategies. In many such cases, total laryngectomy may be indicated despite a successful oncologic outcome of the initial treatment. Perhaps the least appreciated aspect regarding this patient population is the fact that resection of the cervical esophagus and successful free tissue reconstruction establishing a patent conduit does not always lead to successful swallowing outcomes. This is especially relevant in the context of adjuvant radiotherapy.

A variety of esophageal reconstructive options exist in the management of total laryngectomy, including gastric transposition, pectoralis major myocutaneous flap, jejunal flap, colonic interposition, anterolateral thigh flap, and the radial forearm flap. When the larynx is intact, a thin and well-vascularized flap is essential for reconstructing an isolated defect in the cervical esophagus in order to maximize functional outcome and provide reliable healing for the esophageal conduit. The radial forearm free tissue transfer offers several advantages in this situation including thin, well-vascularized tissue that conforms to the defect and has an extremely reliable vascular pedicle. The technique of esophageal reconstruction with the radial forearm free tissue transfer is reviewed.

HISTORY

In general, the presenting history of a patient requiring esophageal reconstruction is relatively straightforward. Dysphagia, regurgitation, aspiration, odynophagia, or complete inability to tolerate oral intake are common complaints in patients with malignancy and/or stenosis/stricture from a variety of etiologies as noted above. Any historical insult to the cervical esophagus may be relevant in these patients including surgery, radiation, caustic ingestion, and trauma and should be considered by the surgeon prior to selecting the best reconstructive technique.

PHYSICAL EXAMINATION

While the physical examination of patients requiring cervical esophageal reconstruction may be normal, findings such as masses in the neck, cervical fistula, pain, and soft tissue fibrosis/scarring may be present and should be evaluated by the surgeon. Mobility of the tongue and soft palate should be documented in order to identify factors contributing to the dysphagia. Flexible fiberoptic examination should be performed to evaluate the postcricoid space, laryngeal structures, epiglottis, and the base of the tongue. The sensation of the larynx should be tested and documented. The patient should be asked to swallow, and observation of the mobility of the tongue and pharynx, mucosal surface hydration, laryngeal elevation, and aspiration/coughing should be noted. More formal swallowing evaluation should be used in the majority of cases as noted below.

INDICATIONS

Indications for esophageal reconstruction vary and are listed below. The most common indications are cancers of the upper aerodigestive tract and thyroid. Sequelae from the treatment of these lesions such as surgery and radiation resulting in stricture or fistulae are common indications. Congenital anomalies requiring free tissue transfer are relatively rare. Functional abnormalities such as perforated Zenker diverticula, achalasia, or other esophageal abnormalities occasionally require more advanced reconstruction after failure of previous therapy.

- Cancer of the esophagus
- Cancer of the larynx or thyroid with invasion of the esophagus
- Caustic ingestion/chemical injury
- Esophageal stricture
- Cervicoesophageal fistulae
- Traumatic injuries
- Congenital abnormalities
- Functional abnormalities

CONTRAINDICATIONS

There are no specific contraindications to cervical esophageal reconstruction. General medical conditions may prohibit reconstructive efforts; however, in most patients, reconstruction of the cervical esophagus can be performed. In the event that thoracic or abdominal access is required for reconstruction, the risk profile as well as the associated contraindications change. Candidates with complicated prior abdominal/thoracic surgery may not be candidates for gastric pull-up or thoracic access for esophageal reconstruction. An obvious contraindication for radial forearm free tissue transfer is inadequate ulnar arterial flow as evaluated by a preoperative Allen test or ultrasonographic vascular studies of the upper extremity. In these situations, another reconstructive option such as the jejunum or anterolateral thigh flap is used.

PREOPERATIVE PLANNING

The underlying etiology resulting in esophageal compromise often drives the preoperative evaluation in patients undergoing radial forearm free tissue transfer for esophageal reconstruction. Nevertheless, several considerations merit mention.

Anatomy

While the anatomy pertinent to esophageal reconstruction is beyond the scope of this chapter, several anatomical considerations are pertinent to reconstruction in this area. Perhaps the most important factor is body habitus in terms of technical difficulty. Overweight/obese patients are significantly more challenging and may require additional incisions and early thoracic access when compared to thinner patients. The surgeon should assess the distance between the mandible and the clavicle preoperatively to determine the relative working area and plan for surgical access accordingly. Patients with a previous history of cervical surgery, or injury, or range-of-motion limitations from kyphosis or secondary to radiotherapy are significant challenges. In these patients, mobilization of the distal esophagus may be problematic, and preemptive thoracic consultation is warranted in the event that reconstruction is not feasible without a combined approach.

In terms of the radial forearm donor site, the most important anatomical consideration is the preoperative Allen test, which is used to evaluate the vascular integrity of the palmar arch to ensure adequate blood supply to the hand after radial arterial harvest. In the event that the Allen test is questionable, an ultrasound flow

Doppler Allen should be performed. Previous injury or surgery to the upper extremity may preclude the use of the radial forearm harvest.

Imaging Studies

The imaging studies required for successful esophageal reconstruction vary depending on the situation; however, in general, computed tomography (CT) with contrast enhancement is relatively standard. In addition, traditional esophagram will provide information regarding the anatomy of the lumen, which is not readily appreciable on CT scans. The esophagram will provide an accurate assessment of the length of the esophagus involved with the pathologic process to allow for reconstructive planning. This is especially true for patients with an esophageal stricture. Additionally, information regarding preoperative aspiration in patients who have undergone previous adjuvant therapies or surgery will be assessed, which is critical when preservation of the larynx is entertained. Modified barium esophagram is critical if preoperative swallowing dysfunction or aspiration is present, which is often the case, in order to determine the presurgical dysfunction and better determine the likely postoperative outcome. Somewhat less frequently MRI may be employed in cases where prevertebral soft tissue involvement with malignancy is suspected or other information related to the soft tissue is required.

Laryngoscopy/Endoscopy

It is difficult to overstate the importance of preoperative endoscopy in the evaluation of the cervical esophagus prior to embarking on resection and reconstruction. Functional evaluation of the motor and sensory components of the larynx is critical, if the larynx is to be preserved. Severe sensory or motor deficits and/or anatomical deficits due to previous surgery are contraindications to laryngeal preservation in conjunction with esophageal reconstruction due to functional disturbances and aspiration. In these situations, laryngectomy is often indicated. In addition, the length and magnitude of the stricture or pathologic process must be adequately evaluated prior to surgery.

Rigid and flexible esophagoscopy offer vital information for surgical planning and allow the surgeon to anticipate problems prior to surgery. Occasionally, retrograde esophagoscopy is required via a gastrotomy tube to adequately determine the existing anatomy. Problems such as thoracic involvement limiting access for esophageal anastomosis or extremely long strictures requiring gastric mobilization must be identified prior to surgery for appropriate planning.

SURGICAL TECHNIQUE

The transcervical approach to the cervical esophagus is relatively well described and similar to preparation for laryngectomy. Subplatysmal flaps are raised to the level of the hyoid bone superiorly and inferiorly to the level of the sternum and clavicles. The sternocleidomastoid muscles are exposed. The structures of the carotid sheath must be identified and protected prior to reconstruction of the cervical esophagus. The extent of the dissection varies depending on the location of the proposed reconstruction; however, it is advisable to widely prepare the site as the bulk of the radial forearm flap and its associated vascular pedicle require adequate access for esophageal/pharyngeal anastomosis. In patients in whom laryngeal preservation is warranted, the larynx must be rolled laterally to expose the esophagus. Placement of a nasogastric tube early in the operation (when possible) will allow for identification of the esophagus and avoid inadvertent injury. Removal of the thyroid lobe on the ipsilateral side may be required to create room for the reconstruction and also allows for preparation of the superior thyroid vessels for microvascular anastomosis. The parathyroid glands are preserved if possible. Identification and preservation of the recurrent laryngeal nerve on the side of the reconstruction are necessary to preserve the swallowing function for the patient and prevent postoperative aspiration. Similarly, the superior laryngeal nerves should be preserved if possible. When the esophagus has been separated from the trachea, and the carotid structures are lateralized, the stenotic segment may be resected. Careful attention to the dissection inferiorly is required to avoid compromising the vascular supply of the distal cervical esophagus, which will be used for the neoesophageal anastomosis. In oncologic cases, the resection of the cancer with negative margins dictates the approach and extent of the resection. The defect can then be evaluated, and the reconstruction can be planned.

The harvest of the radial forearm free tissue transfer has been well described and is currently a very popular method of reconstruction of structures in the head and neck. Briefly, the flap is designed over the radial surface of the flexor surface of the forearm with the appropriate size measured from the defect. The distal portion of the incision should be approximately 1 cm proximal to the wrist crease, and the flap should include the cephalic vein if possible. Under tourniquet, the skin and dermis is incised and the cephalic vein, lateral antebrachial cutaneous nerve, and brachioradialis tendon are identified on the radial side of the flap. The ulnar artery lies medial to the flexor carpi ulnaris and lateral to the palmaris tendon, and preservation of the overlying fascia is mandatory to avoid inadvertent injury of the ulnar artery. The dissection in either a subfascial or suprafascial plane from lateral to medial to isolate the radial artery pedicle and the fasciocutaneous flap. At this point, the radial artery can be ligated distally after division of the extensor retinaculum and identification of the artery and its associated venae comitantes. Dissection of the vascular pedicle is then performed from a distal to proximal

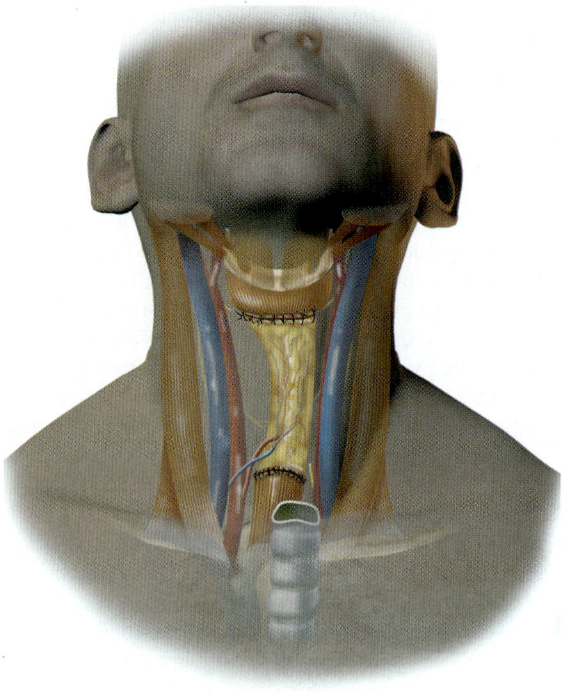

FIGURE 32.1 After laryngectomy. Note anastomosis suture lines may be oriented anteriorly or posteriorly, as long as potential leak areas are away from the vascular pedicle.

direction with the radial artery located between the brachioradialis muscle and flexor carpi radialis muscle. The proximal limit of the dissection is the antecubital fossa where the radial artery joins the brachial artery and the superficial cephalic/median cubital vein joins the deep venous system. At this point, the tourniquet can be released and flap perfusion verified. Perfusion of the distal extremity must be verified at this point in the event that vascular compromise is present requiring repair of the radial artery and aborting the flap procedure.

At the conclusion of the harvest, the radial forearm flap is inset into the esophageal defect (Figs. 32.1 and 32.2). In partial defects it is best to close the distal and proximal portions of the reconstruction and leave the

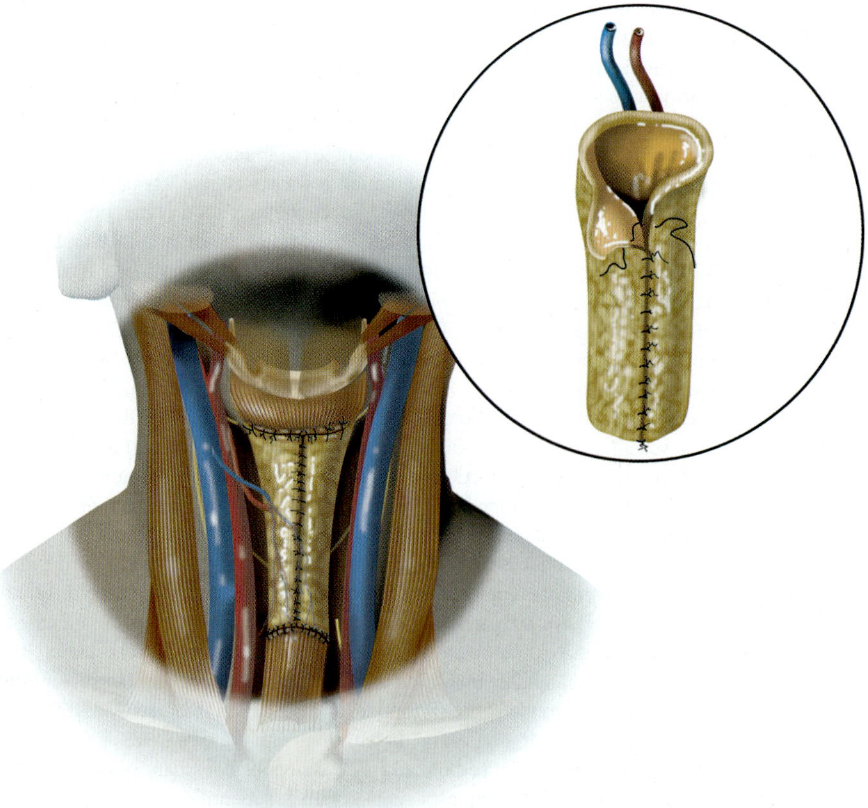

FIGURE 32.2 Radial forearm flap sutured in tubed technique (salivary bypass tube may be used, unless larynx remains intact).

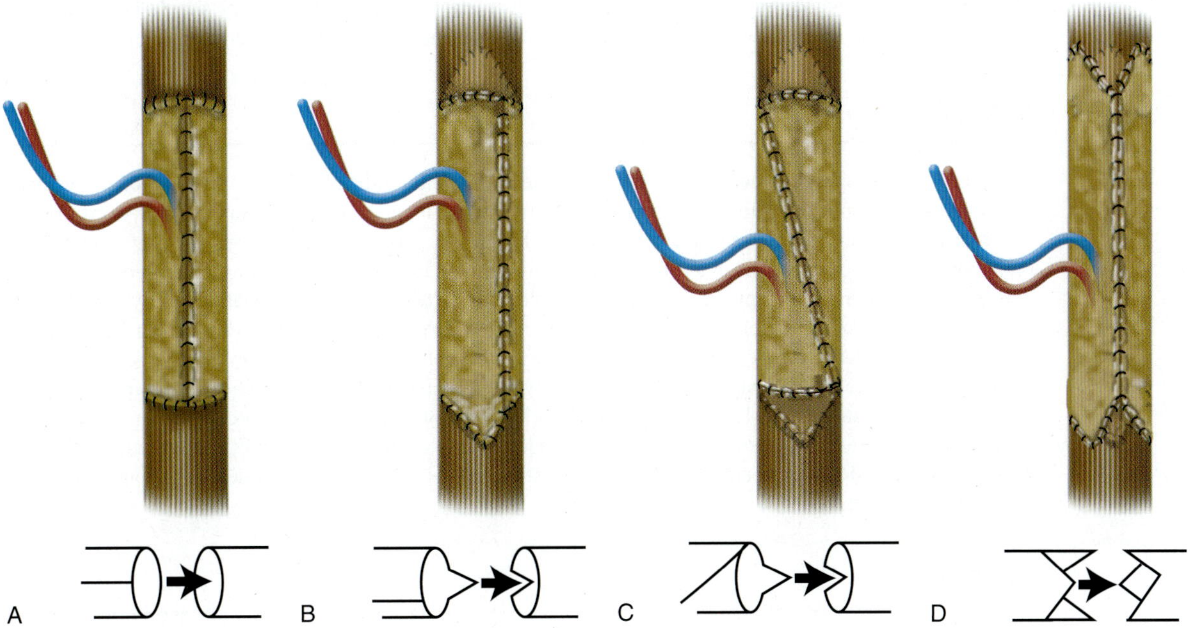

FIGURE 32.3 **A.** Standard circumferential inset may result in contraction and stricture proximally and distally. **B.** Dart modification for stricture prevention. **C.** Oblique/twisted flap orientation, with dart modification. **D.** Running Z-plasty/triple dart type modification.

central portion to close last for greatest access during closure. Additionally, insetting with a small triangle of flap into the distal esophagus may prevent stricture formation (see Fig. 32.3, Complications).

POSTOPERATIVE MANAGEMENT

Postoperative care of the patient is relatively straightforward with standard flap monitoring protocols using the Doppler pen, and an external skin paddle if used. The duration of NPO status varies depending on the patient and reconstruction with longer periods indicated on a patient with a history of preoperative radiotherapy. Approximately 7 to 10 days is generally appropriate prior to obtaining a postoperative esophagram to verify that there is no anastomotic leak. If negative, a clear liquid diet may be instituted and advanced as tolerated to a soft diet. The nasogastric tube may now be removed.

COMPLICATIONS

The most devastating complications of esophageal reconstruction with the radial forearm free tissue transfer include complete flap loss secondary to vascular thrombosis, salivary fistula, hematoma, and infection, all of which may lead to a prolonged postoperative course. The risk of salivary fistula with radial forearm reconstruction is approximately 15% to 20%. Risk factors vary; however, previous radiotherapy is statistically correlated with fistula formation and increases the risk in pharyngeal/esophageal reconstructions. Preventative measures such as fibrin glue have been described with positive results but remain unproven as a reliable way to prevent salivary leakage. Positioning the longitudinal suture line posteriorly in contact with the prevertebral fascia has also been advocated. Conservative local management including packing/diversion and antibiotics are effective in approximately 60% to 65% of cases with the remaining requiring surgical revision and additional reconstruction. Regarding the location of the fistula, it appears that fistula occurring in the longitudinal portion of the anastomosis (partial reconstructions) is less common than distal/proximal fistula formation, which occurs at a rate of approximately 50%, respectively. Use of a salivary bypass tube may reduce the incidence of salivary fistula. Early exteriorization and local wound care are warranted to prevent additional complications.

Another potential complication, which is often challenging to manage, is postoperative stricture formation. The presence of a stricture is usually related to the occurrence of a salivary fistula. Some authors have advocated the use of alternative flaps for cervical reconstruction to avoid additional suture lines and stricture formation, while others prefer the radial forearm flap for its previously noted advantages. Technical recommendations include a small dart or angled interdigitation techniques, which may decrease the stricture rate when compared to circumferential anastomotic techniques (Fig. 32.3). Early recognition and management of postsurgical strictures may prevent failure of the reconstruction. Esophageal dilations should be initiated as soon as possible after initial healing (approximately 3 to 4 weeks), and serial dilations may be required.

RESULTS

The results after esophageal reconstruction often relate to the initial indication for the reconstruction. Primary resection of the esophagus with reconstruction will often result in an adequate salivary conduit; however, the flap is insensate and without muscular contraction. Therefore, partial reconstructions may fare better than total esophageal reconstructions in terms of swallowing as some muscular contractions are preserved. In cases where surgery and radiotherapy are indicated, the rates of stricture, fistula, and swallowing dysfunction are increased. The risk of aspiration must be evaluated in cases which the reconstruction involves an intact larynx, especially if laryngeal dysfunction is present (i.e., cervical esophageal reconstruction for thyroid malignancy with associated vocal cord paralysis). This is especially relevant in patients with significant pulmonary disease. In general, most patients will be able to resume oral intake; however, in cases where significant swallowing dysfunction is present, long-term gastrostomy dependence may occur. This possibility should always be discussed with the patients preoperatively. Caustic ingestion results vary significantly depending on the severity and length of the injury.

PEARLS

- Preoperative education of the patient regarding realistic postoperative swallowing results is critical to success.
- Suprafascial or subfascial dissection of the radial forearm flap is feasible.
- A nasogastric tube should be used to help identify the esophagus in difficult situations such as prior surgery and/or radiotherapy
- Do an elective tracheostomy.
- Interdigitation of the esophageal anastomosis may prevent stricture formation.
- Meticulous anastomotic closure is required to prevent salivary leakage.
- Early recognition with exteriorization of a salivary fistula is critical to minimize complications.
- The radial flap has a superior ischemia time and decreased donor site morbidity when compared to enteric flap options.
- The radial flap has a long, reliable vascular pedicle of excellent diameter for microvascular anastomosis.
- Dissection of the radial artery performed superficial to the flexor retinaculum improves visualization of the distal vascular pedicle.
- Avoid violation of flexor retinaculum overlying the ulnar artery.
- Meticulous attention to vascular perforators to prevent postoperative hematoma.
- Verify distal extremity perfusion after tourniquet release prior to completing flap harvest.
- External skin paddle may be used for monitoring if desired.

PITFALLS

- Improper preoperative evaluation of the esophageal segment requiring reconstruction is inadequate surgical planning and may result in a complication.
- Preservation of the larynx may not be possible in cases with multiple previous insults such as surgery and radiotherapy.

INSTRUMENTS TO HAVE AVAILABLE

- Head and neck surgical tray
- Steven tenotomy scissors, curved 6 inch (15 cm) Baby Metzenbaum 5 1/4 inch (14 cm)
- DeBakey Straight 1.5 mm tip Petit-Point mosquito 7 1/8 inch curved Jarit Flat Tip Scissors 5 inch
- Jamison Scissors Curved 7 inch Jamison-Metz Scissors Curved 6 inch
- Semken Needle Forceps, carbide, delicate 6 inch
- Gerald Forceps 1 × 2 teeth
- Adson Forceps, toothed Delicate Allis Clamps 7 1/2 inch
- Petit-Point Mixter 7 1/4 inch Polar/Army Navy retractors Medium Clip Appliers
- Small Clip Appliers
- Bipolar Insulated 4 inch 0.5 mm tip Monopolar Cautery, insulated tip Kittner dissector sponges Microvascular instrumentation

SUGGESTED READING

Varvares MA, Cheney ML, Gliklich RE, et al. Use of the radial forearm fasciocutaneous free flap and Montgomery salivary bypass tube for pharyngoesophageal reconstruction. *Head Neck* 2000;22(5):463–468.

Marin VP, Yu P, Weber RS. Isolated cervical esophageal reconstruction for rare esophageal tumors. *Head Neck* 2006;28(9):856–860.

Stile FL, Sud V, Zhang F, et al. Reconstruction of long cervical esophageal defects with the radial forearm flap. *J Craniofac Surg* 2006;17(2):382–387.

Andrade P, Pehler SF, Baranano CF, et al. Fistula analysis after radial forearm free flap reconstruction of hypopharyngeal defects. *Laryngoscope* 2008;118(7):1157–1163.

Murray DJ, Novak CB, Neligan PC. Fasciocutaneous free flaps in pharyngolaryngo-oesophageal reconstruction: a critical review of the literature. *J Plast Reconstr Aesthet Surg* 2008;61(10):1148–1156.

33 FREE SEGMENTAL AND PEDICLED SUPERCHARGED JEJUNAL TRANSFER

Jesse C. Selber

INTRODUCTION

Esophageal reconstruction is a demanding and highly coordinated multidisciplinary effort. It requires meticulous planning, exacting intraoperative execution, and vigilant postoperative management. Complications are common but often avoidable. Speech and swallowing function, which are the goals of esophageal reconstruction, can be restored in most, but not all, cases.

In this chapter, I first examine indications, focusing on what types of reconstruction are appropriate based on defect characteristics. I then describe the operative technique in detail for both the free jejunal segment and the pedicled supercharged jejunum. There is a certain amount of overlap in the abdominal approach, recipient vessel identification, and bowel and microvascular anastomoses, but there are also critical differences. I conclude with a discussion of postoperative management, results, and complications.

HISTORY

The most important aspect of the history when considering a jejunal reconstruction is a careful history of previous abdominal surgery. When there has been extensive abdominal surgery, the jejunum may be compromised. Injury to the vascular mesentery or excessive adhesions can preclude the use of the jejunal flap.

PHYSICAL EXAMINATION

The physical examination should include a careful evaluation of the recipient site within the neck and the abdomen. The examination of the recipient site should include an evaluation of the distal defect. If the distal esophageal defect is too inferior in the neck or in the chest, a gastric pull-up or colonic interposition may be more appropriate. An examination of the abdomen may reveal surgical scarring which may impact the choice of the donor site.

INDICATIONS

The most important factor in selecting the appropriate reconstructive method is the length and location of the esophageal defect. If the defect is limited to the cervical esophagus, the two choices are to reconstruct using a jejunal free flap or a tubed fasciocutaneous flap, either a radial forearm or anterolateral thigh flap. If just a patch rather than a circumferential conduit is required, a radial forearm flap is more than adequate to provide reconstruction. For circumferential defects of the cervical esophagus, I prefer to use an anterolateral thigh flap. The reasons for this are multiple. The radial forearm flap is well known to have a significantly

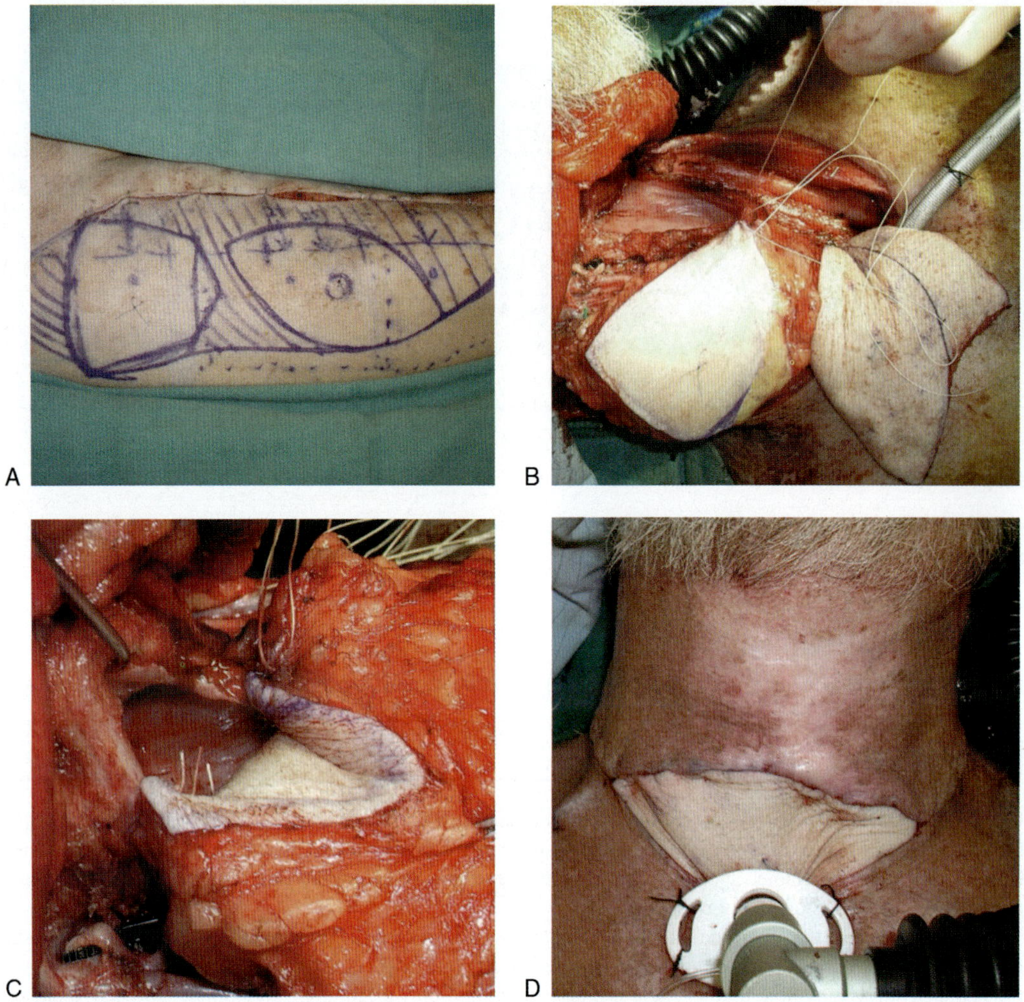

FIGURE 33.1 Pharyngoesophageal deconstruction using the anterolateral thigh flap. **A.** The design of a two-skin island flap permits a trapezoidal design for the conduit and an elliptical design for the skin resurfacing. **B.** The proximal skin island based on the proximal perforator is tubed or used as a patch to form the conduit. **C.** This is sutured into the base of the tongue and posterior pharynx proximally and distally into the esophageal inlet. **D.** The external skin island is used for monitoring and resurfacing the defect in the neck.

higher fistula rate (approximately 17%) than either the anterolateral thigh flap or the free jejunal flap (both approximately 9%). Patients who have cancer of the head and neck often have multiple medical comorbidities. The thigh donor site is less taxing on the patient than is the intra-abdominal donor site, which may result in significant fluid shifts and increased cardiopulmonary complications, not to mention the associated risks of a bowel anastomosis. The anterolateral thigh flap can be harvested in a trapezoidal shape to form a wider opening to accommodate the pharyngeal anastomosis if a laryngopharyngectomy is performed, and in these cases, speech outcomes following tracheoesophageal puncture (TE) puncture are better than with a free jejunal segment. Finally, a second skin paddle can be designed, perforator anatomy permitting, to resurface the neck in cases of injury secondary to radiation therapy (Fig. 33.1).

Occasionally, circumferential defects of the cervical esophagus occur in patients in whom the anterolateral thigh donor site is unavailable. Reasons include previously harvested flaps, previous hemicorpectomies, obese thighs, critical atherosclerotic damage to the profunda femoris, or critical atherosclerotic disease of the superficial femoral artery, which is being effectively bypassed via the descending branch of the lateral femoral circumflex artery. In these cases, a jejunal free flap is the best option. Jejunal free flaps, which are often used in cases of cancer of the hypopharynx and cervical esophagus, are limited to short esophageal defects due to the segmental blood supply. The flap is based on a single branch of the superior mesenteric artery and vein. Generally speaking, one mesenteric branch supplies 15 to 20 cm of bowel. Therefore, in defects of 15 cm or less, for which the distal portion of the esophagus is accessible through the neck, the jejunal free flap is an excellent option.

For defects greater than 15 cm and for which the distal esophagus is inaccessible due to its intrathoracic location, a gastric conduit is the first choice for reconstruction due to its robust blood supply and requiring only one bowel anastomosis to reestablish continuity; however, in certain situations, the stomach is unusable. Colon interposition has been employed for several decades as an alternative to the gastric conduit; however, patients with atherosclerosis, inappropriate vascular anatomy, previous colon resection, or intrinsic colon disease, such as inflammatory bowel disease, cancer, or diverticulosis, are not candidates.

The pedicled supercharged jejunum is the preferable alternative because it closely approximates the size of the native esophagus, possesses peristaltic activity, and is typically free of intrinsic diseases. The addition of microsurgical techniques has allowed for the replacement of the entire esophagus using longer conduits through "supercharging." Longmire described the first supercharged jejunal flap for reconstruction of the esophagus in 1947. Since then, the field of microsurgery has advanced significantly and the use of these techniques has become more widespread, making the supercharged jejunal flap the best option for total esophageal reconstruction when the stomach is unavailable.

CONTRAINDICATIONS

Total esophageal reconstruction using a free, segmental, or pedicled, supercharged jejunal flap is technically challenging and requires a multidisciplinary approach. Relative contraindications include a surgeon who is not working with a team to manage the patient and patients with prior extensive abdominal or specifically jejunal surgery.

PREOPERATIVE PLANNING

These procedures can be successfully performed as an alternative reconstruction when the stomach is unavailable with good long-term function and acceptable morbidity. Thorough surgical planning is critical to the success of this operation. When using the jejunum, preoperative planning requires that a careful operative history is taken to assess the potential for abdominal adhesions that may hinder the harvest of a jejunal segment.

SURGICAL TECHNIQUE

The initial approach to the abdomen is the same for both the free segmental and pedicled supercharged jejunum. Once resection is complete, the ligament of Treitz is identified and the small bowel with its mesentery is explored to ensure that no intrinsic abnormalities or iatrogenic injuries exist. The length of the esophageal defect is measured to estimate the length of the conduit needed (Fig. 33.2). The mesentery of the proximal and mid jejunum are closely examined using a fiberoptic light to transilluminate the tissues and elucidate the vascular anatomy (Fig. 33.3).

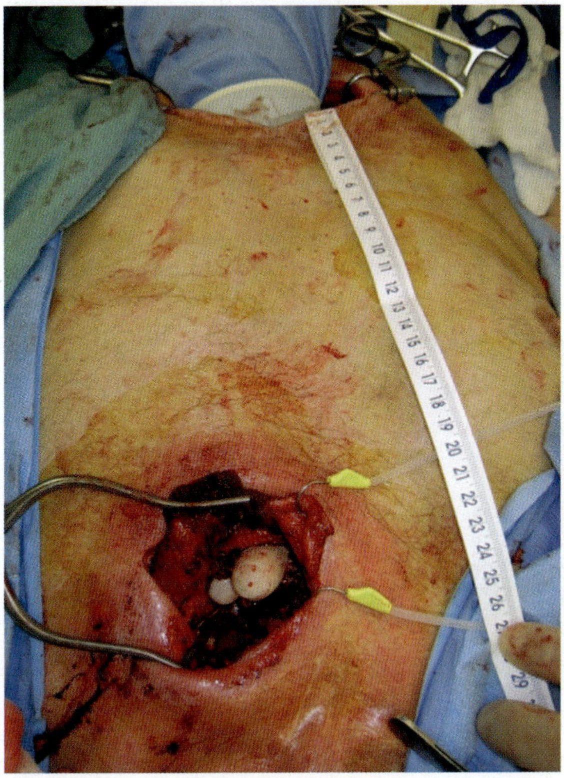

FIGURE 33.2
In esophageal reconstruction, the length of the conduit is measured by the distance from the proximal portion to the distal portion, often through the thoracic inlet and outlet.

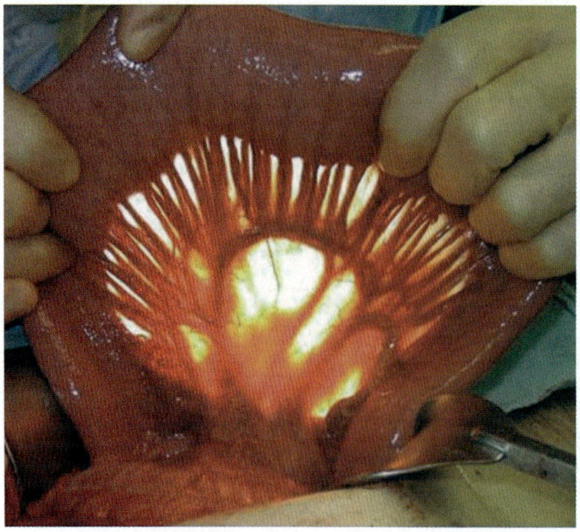

FIGURE 33.3
Transillumination of the small bowel is used to demonstrate the vascular anatomy of the inferior mesenteric artery and vein and identify the most appropriate vessels to divide and transfer.

Free Jejunal Segment

If a free jejunal segment is the reconstructive option of choice, a single mesenteric vessel is selected around 40 cm from the ligament of Treitz, which usually corresponds to the second or third mesenteric branch. The choice of these vessels yields the largest arc of mesentery and thus the longest vascular pedicle. Once the appropriate vessel is identified, it is dissected free from the mesentery. The secondary arcade emerging from this single mesenteric vessel must be kept intact to ensure vascularity of the entire segment. This is done by harvesting the wedge of mesentery between the pedicle and the jejunal segment (Fig. 33.4). Dissection through the mesentery can be assisted by transillumination. The mesenteric vessels are extremely friable, and great care should be taken to avoid rough dissection, which will result in a hematoma of the mesentery and obfuscate the dissection. This dissection is taken up to the serosal border distally, and the superior mesenteric artery and vein proximally, insuring maximum pedicle length and caliber.

Prior to dividing the bowel, the proximal or isoperistaltic portion of the jejunum is marked. This insures appropriate orientation in the neck. The bowel is divided with a standard endostapler. The pedicle is then ligated, and the flap is transferred to the head and neck. A stapled, side-to-side anastomosis of the remaining jejunum in the abdomen is performed, or a two-layer, hand-sewn end-to-end anastomosis, depending on surgeon preference, and the midline incision is closed in standard fashion.

Once in the neck, heparinized saline is run through the flap as is customary for all free flaps. The bowel is oriented appropriately, usually in an isoperistaltic fashion. Generally, I like to perform at least the distal esophageal anastomosis prior to the microvascular anastomosis since this will set the tension on the bowel. The proximal 3 to 5 cm of jejunum, based on one or two terminal arcade vessels, is exteriorized as a postoperative monitoring segment. The esophagojejunal anastomoses are then performed in the neck using a single layer of 3-0 Vicryl or polydioxanone suture (PDS) in an end-to-end fashion. In patients with a total laryngopharyngectomy, the proximal pharynx or the base of the tongue is larger than the jejunal diameter, so an end-to-side anastomosis is performed to accommodate the size discrepancy.

Recipient vessels are prepared prior to dividing the vascular pedicle and passing the jejunal conduit. The transverse cervical vessels (if the neck has been significantly damaged due to prior surgery and/or radiation),

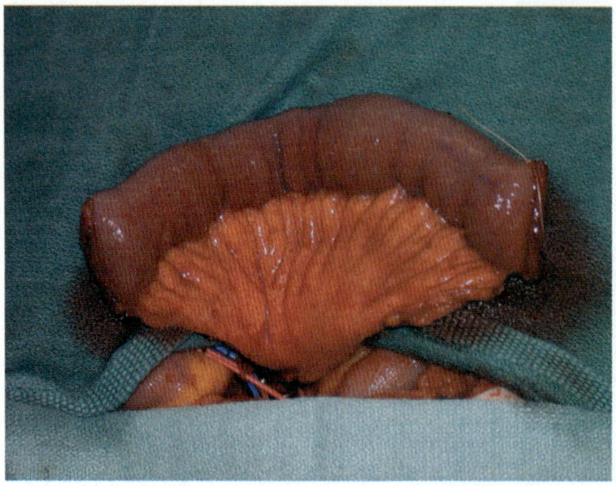

FIGURE 33.4
For a free jejunal segment, the mesenteric vessel that will yield the longest arc of mesentery is selected and dissected free from the mesentery. The secondary arcade emerging from this single mesenteric vessel must be kept intact to ensure vascularity of the entire segment. This is done by harvesting the wedge of mesentery between the pedicle and the jejunal segment.

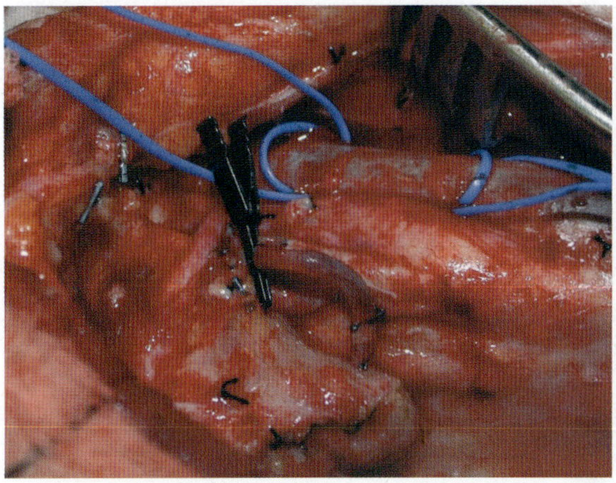

FIGURE 33.5
Recipient vessels are prepared prior to dividing the vascular pedicle and passing the jejunal conduit. The transverse cervical vessels (if the neck has been significantly damaged due to prior surgery and/or radiation), the external carotid system (the facial, lingual, or superior thyroid arteries), and jugular veins are common recipient vessels depending on the clinical scenario. In this case, the vessel loop is around the jugular vein, and the Ackland clamp is on the facial artery.

the external carotid system (the facial, lingual, or superior thyroid arteries), and jugular veins are common recipient vessels depending on the clinical scenario (Fig. 33.5). Arterial anastomoses are performed under the operating microscope using 9-0 Nylon sutures. Venous anastomoses are commonly completed using a venous coupling device (Synovis Surgical Innovations, St. Paul, MN).

Pedicled Supercharged Jejunum

For total or near total esophageal replacement, the supercharged jejunum is the best option. The esophagectomy and gastrectomy, when necessary, are performed by the thoracic and/or general surgeons. The surgical approach is through either two incisions (abdominal and cervical) as in a transhiatal esophagectomy or three incisions with the addition of a right thoracotomy. The initial abdominal approach mirrors that for the jejunal segment: the ligament of Treitz is identified, and the small bowel with its mesentery is explored to ensure that no intrinsic abnormalities or iatrogenic injuries exist. The length of the esophageal defect is measured to estimate the length of the conduit needed. The mesentery of the proximal and mid jejunum is closely examined using a fiberoptic light to transilluminate the tissues and identify the vascular anatomy.

The next steps are unique to the pedicled flap and are the most technically sensitive part of the procedure. The first mesenteric branch beyond the ligament of Treitz is identified and preserved to maintain blood supply to the distal duodenum and most proximal portion of jejunum, which is used to reestablish enteric continuity.

Typically, the second mesenteric branch is dissected down to the level of the superior mesenteric artery and vein, and ultimately divided to serve as the vascular pedicle for supercharging the proximal flap (Fig. 33.6). In the simplest cases, the mesentery between the second and third branches is divided up to the serosal border, allowing the jejunal segment to unfurl (Fig. 33.7). This step helps straighten the natural sinusoidal properties of the small bowel and reduce redundancy. If more length is required, the third mesenteric branch is ligated and divided (Fig. 33.8). Secondary arcade vessels between the third and fourth mesenteric branches are preserved so that the segment of bowel normally supplied by the third branch is now supplied by the pedicled fourth branch through intact arcade vessels. This approach is the most commonly used technique.

If still greater length is required, such as in patients with a very long torso or a concomitant total laryngopharyngectomy, the fourth mesenteric branch can also be ligated. In these cases, only the mesentery between the third and fourth branches is divided to the serosal border while the arcade connections are preserved between the second and third, and between the fourth and fifth branches (Fig. 33.9). The third segment receives perfusion from the supercharged second segment, and the fourth segment receives perfusion from the pedicled

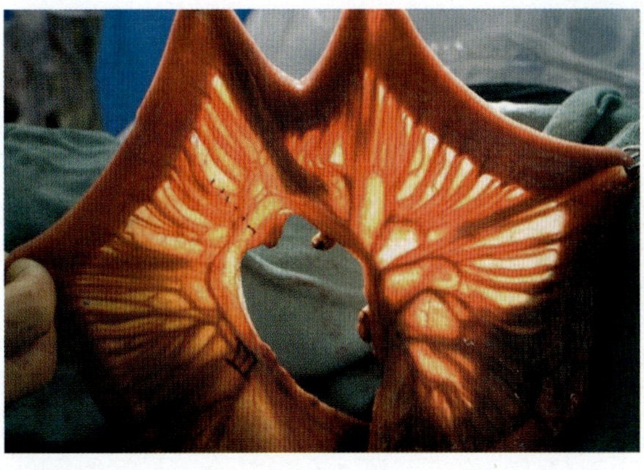

FIGURE 33.6
In planning the supercharged jejunum, typically, the second mesenteric branch is dissected down to the level of the superior mesenteric artery and vein and ultimately divided to serve as the vascular pedicle for supercharging the proximal flap.

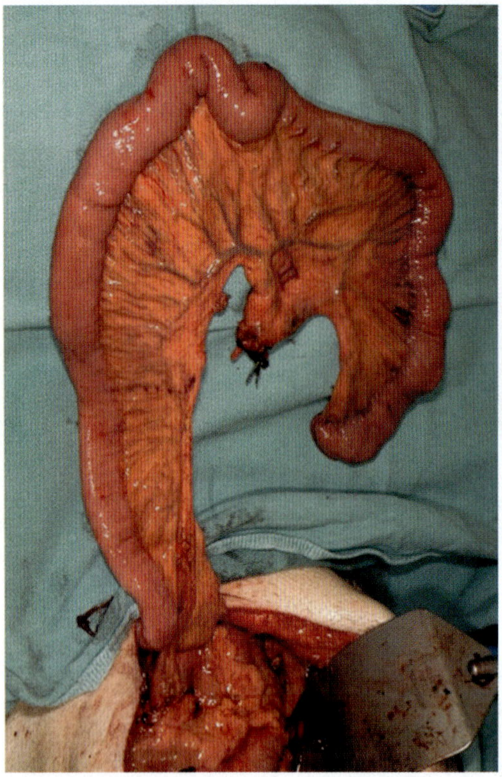

FIGURE 33.7 In the simplest cases of supercharged jejunums, the mesentery between the second and third branches is divided up to the serosal border, allowing the jejunal segment to unfurl. This step helps straighten the natural sinusoidal properties of the small bowel and reduce redundancy.

fifth branch. Once adequate length is achieved, the jejunum is divided proximally with a linear cutting stapler, typically 30 to 40 cm distal to the ligament of Treitz.

There are two potential routes for transferring the jejunal flap to the neck: retrocardiac, which is the orthotopic route, or substernal, which is the heterotopic route (Fig. 33.10). The former is used in patients undergoing immediate reconstruction. The latter is usually reserved for patients undergoing a delayed reconstruction after previous failed esophageal reconstruction. In these cases, a portion of the manubrium, clavicular head, and first rib are removed to enlarge the thoracic inlet and avoid constriction on the jejunal conduit. Whether the retrocardiac or substernal route is selected, transfer is accomplished using a sterile laparoscopic camera bag to protect the conduit and prevent traction and shearing forces on the delicate arcade vessels.

Recipient vessels are again prepared prior to dividing the vascular pedicle and passing the jejunal conduit. As in the free jejunal segment, the transverse cervical vessels, the external carotid system, and jugular veins are common recipient vessels depending on the clinical plan. The internal mammary vessels are used much more frequently in the supercharged flap because a manubriumectomy created for ease of conduit passage often leaves these vessels exposed. Once the jejunal flap is passed, arterial anastomoses are performed under the operating microscope using 9-0 Nylon sutures. Venous anastomoses are commonly completed using a venous

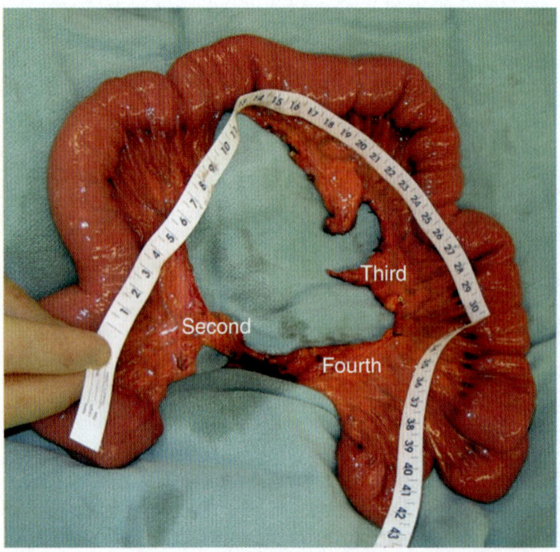

FIGURE 33.8 If more length is required on the jejunum, the third mesenteric branch is ligated and divided. Secondary arcade vessels between the third and fourth mesenteric branches are preserved so that the segment of bowel normally supplied by the third branch is now supplied by the pedicled fourth branch through intact arcade vessels.

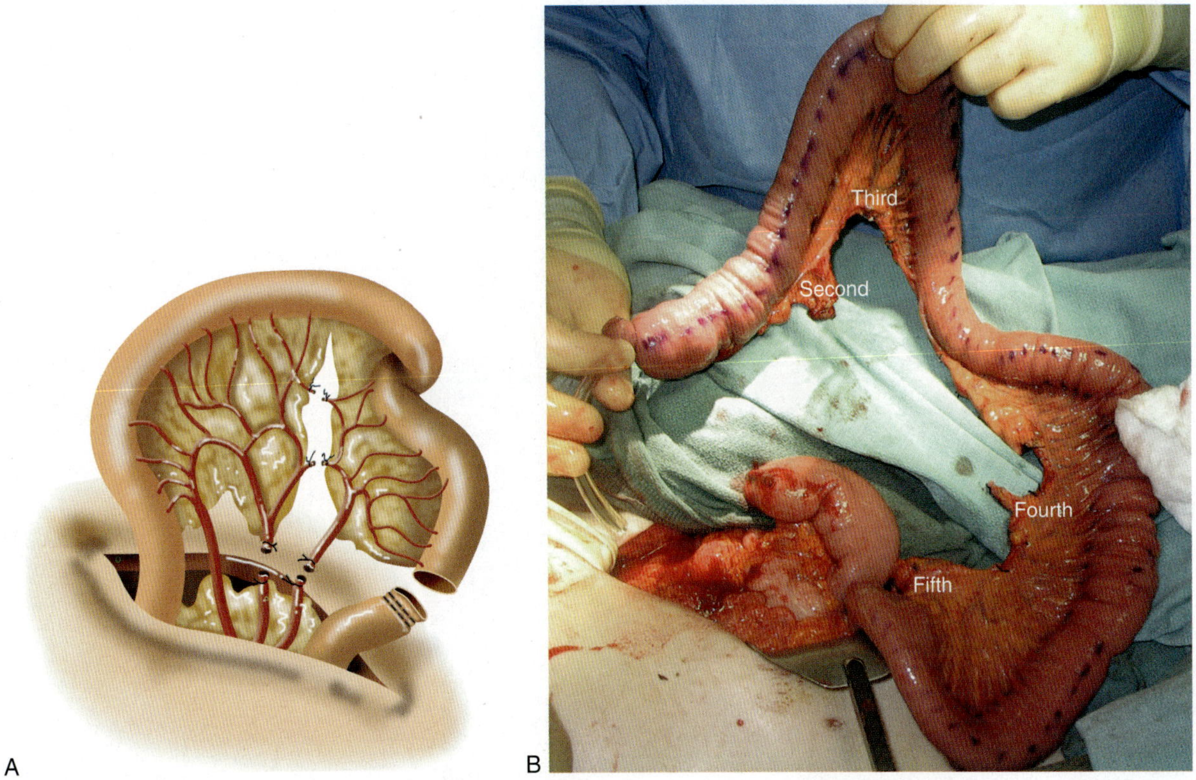

FIGURE 33.9 A. If still greater length is required, such as in patients with a very long torso or a concomitant total laryngopharyngectomy, the fourth mesenteric branch can also be ligated. **B.** In these cases, only the mesentery between the third and fourth branches is divided to the serosal border while the arcade connections are preserved between the second and third, and between the fourth and fifth branches.

coupling device (Synovis Surgical Innovations, St. Paul, MN). A vein graft is used in some cases to bridge the gap between the jejunal vascular pedicle and the recipient vessels.

Once the proximal jejunum is revascularized, any excess length of jejunal conduit is removed in order to minimize redundancy in the neck. As in the free segmental jejunum, the proximal 3 to 5 cm of bowel is exteriorized based on secondary arcade vessels as a postoperative monitoring segment (Fig. 33.11). The esophagojejunal anastomosis is then as described above. Intestinal continuity is reestablished in the abdomen by the thoracic or general surgical team through a gastrojejunal anastomosis using the posterior wall of the stomach or through a Roux-en-Y jejunojejunal anastomosis if a gastrectomy was performed. A feeding jejunostomy tube is routinely placed.

Advanced Techniques and Tips for Supercharging

After passing the bowel through the chest and into the neck, tension on the mesentery may compromise the perfusion of the middle jejunal segment. This segment should be carefully inspected before closing the abdomen. If the perfusion is questionable, it can be revascularized by anastomosing its mesenteric branch to the gastroepiploic, right gastric, or mesocolonic vessels or even the stump of the superior mesenteric vessels with or without a vein graft. Revascularization of the middle segment was successfully performed in four patients in my series.

Typically, three surgical services are involved in this type of cases: thoracic surgery, general surgery, and plastic surgery. To minimize the operating time, it is important to establish a coordinated flow between the various teams. If a thoracotomy is required, the patient is first placed in lateral decubitus position and then switched to supine. While the ablative surgical team is operating in the abdomen, the reconstructive surgeons can start to prepare recipient vessels in the neck. The teams then change positions. The reconstructive surgeons now prepare the jejunal flap while the ablative surgeons expose the proximal esophagus through the neck incision and remove the manubrium and clavicular head if a substernal approach is desired. The jejunal conduit is then passed through the chest and into the neck, and the teams switch positions again. The reconstructive surgeons revascularize the proximal jejunum, complete the esophagojejunal anastomosis, and fashion the monitoring segment while the other surgical team restores gastrointestinal continuity in the abdomen. When properly organized, no time is wasted for any of the teams involved. Clear communication between surgical teams and anesthesia regarding fluid resuscitation and avoidance of vasopressor medications is imperative as different disciplines may manage these issues differently.

Technically, three key steps are required in such a complex reconstruction: selecting the appropriate jejunal segment, choosing the optimal recipient vessels for microsurgical anastomosis, and creating a suitable conduit passageway.

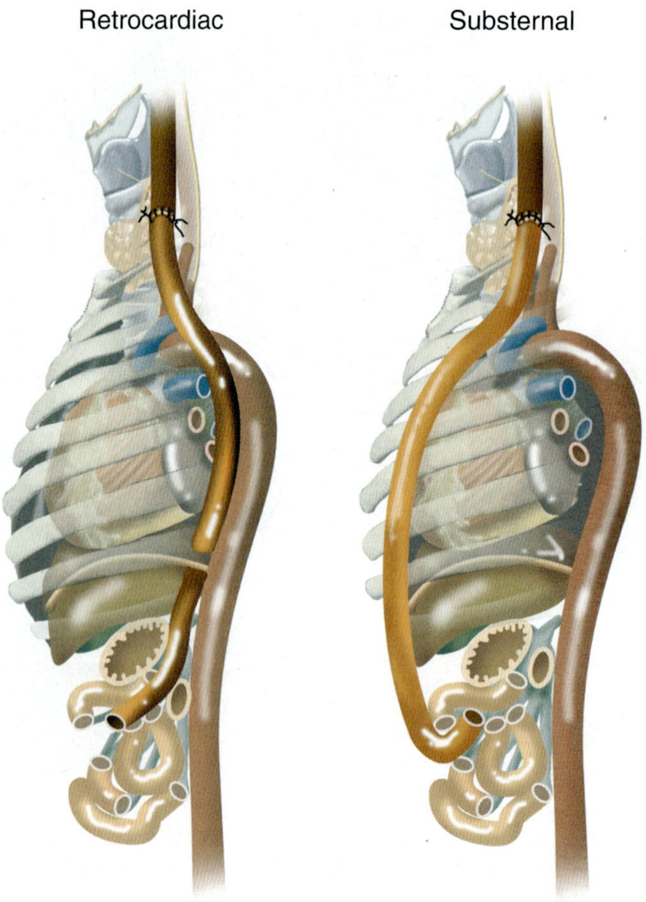

FIGURE 33.10
There are two potential routes for transferring the jejunal flap to the neck: retrocardiac, which is the orthotopic route, or substernal, which is the heterotopic route. The former is used in patients undergoing immediate reconstruction. The latter is usually reserved for patients undergoing a delayed reconstruction after previous failed esophageal reconstruction.

Careful consideration of the mesenteric anatomy is the most critical component in surgical planning. If possible, the most proximal jejunum beyond the first mesenteric branch should be included to avoid wasting of the proximal bowel. Thus, the second mesenteric branch is often selected for supercharging. However, this selection also depends on the anatomy of the mesentery since it is the arc length of the mesentery between branches, not the bowel itself, that determines the reach of the flap. Therefore, the segment of bowel with longer mesenteric vessels and wider mesenteric intervals between the vessels should be selected so the conduit can be adequately unfurled and lengthened. Transillumination of the mesentery can help to determine the vascular anatomy.

Choice of recipient vessels is another critical factor in the decision-making algorithm. In general, recipient vessels in the inferior part of the neck (transverse cervical vessels) or in the chest (internal mammary vessels) are preferred to facilitate reach of the mesenteric pedicle. The choice of recipient vessels also depends on conduit pathway, which is dictated by the clinical scenario of each individual patient (e.g., immediate vs. delayed reconstruction). A reconstructive algorithm is created to assist with surgical planning (Fig. 33.12).

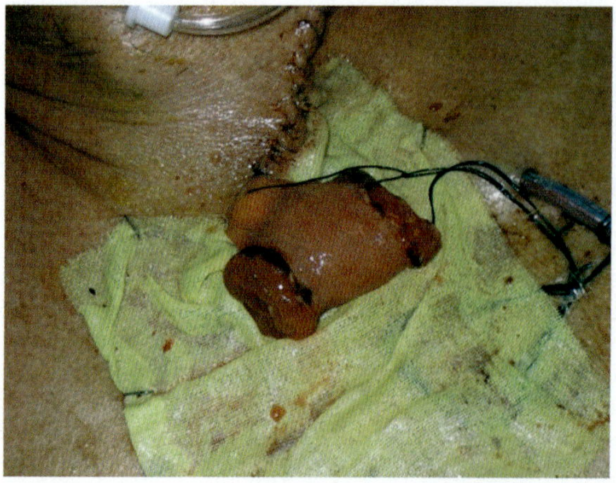

FIGURE 33.11
As in the free segmental jejunum, the proximal 3 to 5 cm of bowel in the supercharged jejunum is exteriorized based on secondary arcade vessels as a postoperative monitoring segment.

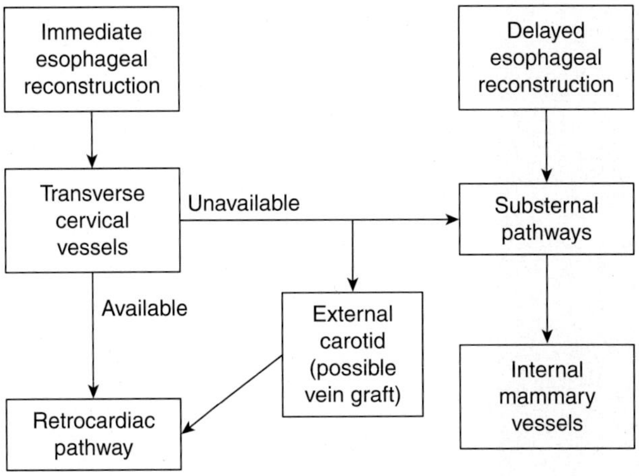

FIGURE 33.12
In general, recipient vessels in the inferior part of the neck (transverse cervical vessels) or in the chest (internal mammary vessels) are preferred to facilitate reach of the mesenteric pedicle. The choice of recipient vessels also depends on conduit pathway, which is dictated by the clinical scenario of each individual patient (e.g., immediate vs. delayed reconstruction). A reconstructive algorithm is created to assist with surgical planning.

For delayed reconstruction, the substernal pathway is chosen because the retrocardiac route is scarred from previous surgery or infection. The left manubrium and clavicular head are resected and the internal mammary vessels are easily exposed, making them the recipient vessel of choice. The vascular anastomosis is then completed in the upper chest in the space where the manubrium and clavicular head were removed. The left transverse cervical vessels are an alternate option.

For immediate reconstruction, the native retrocardiac pathway is available and preferred to avoid unnecessary resection of the manubrium and clavicular head. This pathway is also slightly shorter than the substernal pathway. The internal mammary vessels, which are located anteriorly, are not a good option with this pathway. The transverse cervical vessels lower in the neck are preferred to avoid vein grafting to the external carotid system. The substernal pathway, however, should be considered during an immediate reconstruction in the following clinical circumstances: (1) the transverse cervical vessels are unavailable, which may occur in 23% of the unilateral necks and (2) the patient suffers from severe kyphosis. One contraindication for choosing the substernal pathway is in patients with previous coronary artery bypass surgery where the internal mammary artery was used as the bypass graft. Therefore, for immediate reconstruction, I now prefer exploring the left transverse cervical vessels first. If they are adequate, the retrocardiac pathway is chosen. If not, then I opt for the substernal pathway and the use of the internal mammary vessels. The second option is to proceed with the retrocardiac pathway and use the external carotid system, such as the superior thyroid artery and internal jugular vein as recipient vessels. This option is less desirable because a vein graft is often necessary, making an already complex reconstruction even more so.

POSTOPERATIVE MANAGEMENT

Patients are recovered first in the intensive care unit and then transferred to the ward. The externalized monitoring segment of the jejunum is observed for 7 to 10 days postoperatively at which time its mesentery is ligated and the segment removed. If the patient's postoperative course is uneventful, a modified barium swallow (MBS) is performed 7 to 14 days postprocedure (Fig. 33.13). If no leak is detected, the patient is started on a liquid diet and slowly advanced to a postgastrectomy diet, as tolerated.

COMPLICATIONS

Major postoperative respiratory complications are particularly common and difficult to manage due to the involvement of multiple organs and body cavities, major fluid shifts, frequent need for fluid resuscitation, and the relative contraindications to using vasopressors in the setting of microvascular reconstruction.

Our conduit-related complications are comparable to those reported in the literature and the majority of those occurred in our early experience. All subclinical radiographic leaks healed spontaneously within 2 weeks. Once a leak is identified on the initial MBS, the patients are kept NPO for additional 2 weeks and then an MBS is repeated. Most clinical fistulas also heal with conservative management. Major leaks or anastomotic breakdowns should be surgical explored and possibly reconstructed to prevent catastrophic complications. Anastomotic strictures are typically managed with endoscopic dilatation, and repeated dilatations may be required. Two patients in my series developed a stricture in the watershed jejunal segment in the middle of the conduit requiring surgical intervention, which highlights the importance of selecting the appropriate jejunal segment based on the mesenteric anatomy and understanding the extent to which arcade vessels can be divided.

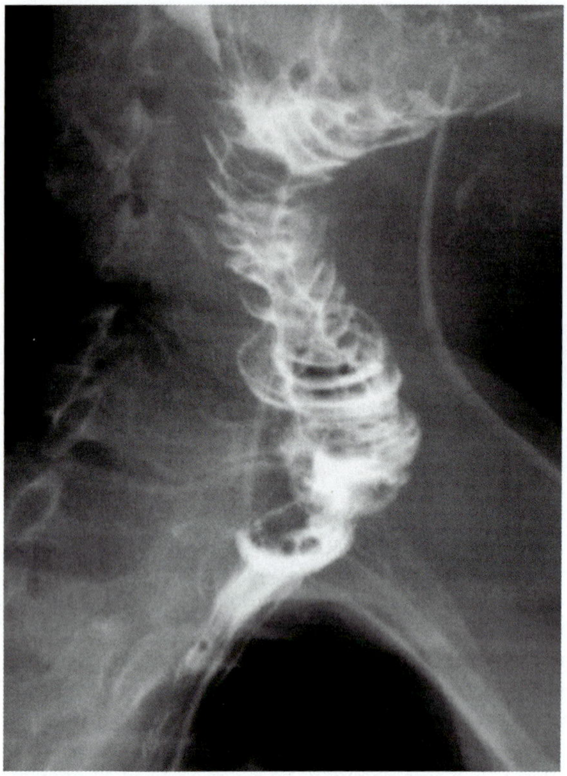

FIGURE 33.13
If the patient's postoperative course is uneventful, an MBS is performed 7 to 14 days postprocedure. If no leak is detected, the patient is started on a liquid diet and slowly advanced to a postgastrectomy diet, as tolerated.

RESULTS

Supercharged jejunal transfer is a technically demanding surgery, yet reasonable functional outcomes can be achieved. I published the largest series of supercharged jejunal flaps for total esophageal reconstruction to date. The majority of his patients were able to achieve a regular diet (90%) and discontinue their tube feeds (80%), which has a tremendous psychological and physical benefit to the patient. Reflux was infrequent and mild.

My overall success rate using an super-charged jejunal flap (SCJF) for total esophageal reconstruction was 94%, with three flap failures in my early experience. Two patients died during their hospitalization and medical and surgical complications occurred in 65% of patients, reflecting the fact that the SCJF is a challenging and complex procedure. Patients often have significant comorbid diseases and therefore need be nutritionally and medically optimized prior to surgery.

PEARLS

- For defects greater than 15 cm and for which the distal esophagus is inaccessible due to its intrathoracic location, a gastric conduit is the first choice for reconstruction.
- Free jejunal segments, which are often used in cases of hypopharyngeal and cervical esophageal carcinoma, are limited to short esophageal defects due to the segmental blood supply.

PITFALLS

- When using the jejunum, preoperative planning requires that a careful operative history is taken to assess the potential for abdominal adhesions that may hinder the harvest of a jejunal segment.
- If a leak is identified on the initial MBS, the patients are kept NPO for additional 2 weeks and then an MBS is repeated.
- Anastomotic strictures are typically managed with endoscopic dilatation, and repeated dilatations may be required.

INSTRUMENTS TO HAVE AVAILABLE:

- Abdominal surgical instruments
- Standard head and neck surgical set

ACKNOWLEDGMENTS

I gratefully acknowledge the contributions of Melissa M. Poh and Peirong Yu.

SUGGESTED READING

Anthony JP, Singer MI, Mathes SJ. Pharyngoesophageal reconstruction using the tubed free radial forearm flap. *Clin Plast Surg* 1994;21:137–147.

Reece GP, Schusterman MA, Miller MJ, et al. Morbidity and functional outcome of free jejunal transfer reconstruction for circumferential defects of the pharynx and cervical esophagus. *Plast Reconstr Surg* 1995;96:1307–1316.

Cho BC, Kim M, Lee JH, et al. Pharyngoesophageal reconstruction with a tubed free radial forearm flap. *J Reconstrt Microsurg* 1998;14:535–540.

Scharpf J, Esclamado RM. Reconstruction with radial forearm flaps after ablative surgery for hypopharyngeal cancer. *Head Neck* 2002;25:261–266.

Disa JJ, Pusic AL, Mehrara BJ. Reconstruction of the hypopharynx with the free jejunum transfer. *J Surg Oncol* 2006;94:466–470.

Yu P, Hanasono M, Skoracki R, et al. Pharyngoesophageal reconstruction with the anterolateral thigh flap after total laryngopharyngectomy. *Cancer* 2010;116(7):1718–1724.

34 THE RADIAL FOREARM FLAP

Francisco J. Civantos

INTRODUCTION

Cancer of the hypopharynx represents a unique challenge to the surgeon, both oncologically and in terms of reconstruction. These cancers are more aggressive than are lesions that occur nearby in the endolarynx, and there is a lack of anatomic barriers to contain them. While laryngeal cancers are contained by the surrounding cartilage, pharyngeal cancers rapidly invade through the constrictor muscles to involve the parapharyngeal and retropharyngeal spaces, as well as the soft tissues of the neck. There is a propensity to develop lymphatic metastases to the lateral neck and paratracheal regions. Furthermore, cancer of the hypopharynx generally occurs in patients who have a significant history of smoking tobacco and/or drinking alcohol, and because of this, significant cardiac and pulmonary comorbidities need to be managed. The cancers themselves interfere with deglutition, and patients are often in poor nutritional condition at the time of surgery, which can lead to difficulty in healing and other complications.

While early-stage cancers of the hypopharynx may be treated with radiation, chemotherapy combined with radiation, or partial laryngectomy; advanced-stage cancer will require a total laryngectomy, along with partial or total pharyngectomy, even if the larynx is not directly invaded, in order to reconstruct the patient in a manner that protects the airway from aspiration and provides for oral nutrition through successful deglutition. Primary treatment of advanced cancer will also involve postoperative radiation when possible, and in some circumstances, postoperative chemoradiation.

Resection of the cancer must be adequate, with wide margins, and in many cases, this mandates circumferential pharyngectomy. Cancer resection should not be compromised to facilitate reconstruction, and this tends to work best when a separate microvascular reconstructive team is available to enter the procedure fresh at the end of the cancer resection.

Reconstruction of the hypopharynx has passed through several phases. Early techniques involved local flaps of cervical skin, and several stages of surgery, with open fistulas during the intervening periods. These were fraught with complications and poor results in swallowing. The deltopectoral flap represented an important advance, but still usually required at least two stages and a controlled fistula, and hypopharyngeal strictures were common. Single-stage reconstruction became possible with the development of the pectoralis major myocutaneous flap, and this remains an important option in very thin patients or for subtotal pharyngeal reconstruction. It may be a preferred option in the medically infirm.

The type of reconstruction selected should not compromise the resection—for either the primary site or the lymphatic basins—a principle that has limited the use of platysma flaps and other local flaps. The reconstructive procedure should be reliable and should minimize the postoperative deformity, morbidity, and mortality. Failure of the reconstruction in the neck can lead to fistula and even death from vascular rupture. A variety of options now exist for reconstruction of the hypopharynx, including gastric pull-up, enteric microvascular flaps, regional flaps, and cutaneous microvascular flaps. Thinner, more pliable and reliable free flaps have now largely supplanted musculocutaneous pedicle flaps, particularly when a circumferential defect is a realistic possibility.

The gastric pull-up, while avoiding the need for a microvascular anastomosis, has several disadvantages. It has measurable mortality related to pulmonary complications and mediastinitis, neither of which are as significant when reconstructing with cutaneous flaps. Furthermore, primary site complications in the abdomen can occur, which are not an issue with cutaneous flaps. There can be situations where the stomach cannot be mobilized sufficiently to reach the upper portion of a pharyngeal defect or where the distal portion of the flap is lost, leading to a fistula and complications with healing.

Enteric microvascular flaps, such as those obtained from the jejunum or gastro-omental flap, solve some of these problems and have gained some popularity. However, they require not only a laparotomy but also an intestinal anastomosis, which entails additional risks. While laparoscopic techniques can reduce some of these risks, these remain a relatively invasive way to obtain donor tissue. Enteric flaps in general are less well suited for tracheoesophageal prosthetic speech rehabilitation due to the tendency toward excess secretions and a "wet" sounding voice. For all of these reasons, the majority of centers have returned to cutaneous flaps as a means of reconstructing the hypopharynx. The gastro-omental flap has been supported by some in the revision setting, for patients who can tolerate laparotomy because the omentum coats the pharyngeal repair and cervical blood vessels and may be protective in terms of fistula and vascular rupture.

For very thin patients with significant comorbidities, regional flaps, especially the pectoralis major flap, sometimes are the best option because of their relative simplicity. However, for most patients, the pectoralis major flap is very thick, and the lumen of the neopharynx can be obliterated in an attempt to tube thicker skin. It can also be difficult to close the cervical skin over the bulk of the pectoral muscle pedicle. Formation of an adequate stoma, contour of the neck, and ability to close the wound can all be compromised by this bulky muscular pedicle. The most anatomically favorable flaps for reconstruction of the hypopharynx are cutaneous free flaps, including anterolateral thigh, lateral arm, and radial forearm. While the anterolateral thigh flap has been gaining popularity, the reliable radial forearm flap currently continues to serve as the most popular flap for hypopharyngeal reconstruction at many centers.

The radial forearm free flap was originally described in cadaveric studies in 1978 and in a large clinical series in 1981, in the Chinese literature, as a free tissue transfer, by Yang Guofan et al. Its first use for reconstruction of the hypopharynx was described in 1987 by Takato et al. Since then, several large series have reported on the use of this flap for hypopharyngeal reconstruction, and it has become a popular mode of hypopharyngeal reconstruction and is favored over enteric flaps in most centers.

The radial forearm flap provides a sufficiently wide expanse of thin skin (Fig. 34.1) that can be easily tubed while maintaining both an inner lumen and minimizing bulk in order to allow closure of overlying skin and creation of a patent tracheostoma.

This chapter focuses on the technical details of reconstruction of the hypopharynx with a radial forearm free flap.

HISTORY

Unfortunately, the early symptoms of cancer of the hypopharynx are often nonspecific and include a foreign body sensation in the throat, mild discomfort with swallowing, or mild otalgia. These are generally persistent and continuous, rather than intermittent, and gradually become worse over time. It is common for patients to be misdiagnosed by primary physicians as suffering from pharyngitis or reflux and to be treated with multiple courses of antibiotics and antireflux therapies, prior to making the correct diagnosis, particularly since the presence of superinfection, combined with a placebo effect may lead patients to report improvement after initial antibiotic therapy.

Patients are usually diagnosed with advanced stages of cancer, by which time the patient has developed severe odynophagia, dysphagia, and/or otalgia, which can be unilateral or bilateral depending on the location of the cancer. Some patients will present with cervical adenopathy as the primary complaint, and 65% to 75% of patients will have clinically obvious metastasis to cervical lymph nodes at the time of presentation. Severe dysphagia and inability to eat solids can be a sign of involvement of the cervical esophagus. Exophytic hypopharyngeal cancer can cause the classic "hot potato" voice due to a change in the hypopharyngeal resonance, and direct invasion of the larynx can lead to fixation of the vocal cords, with hoarseness and breathiness of the voice, as well as chronic aspiration. Halitosis, inability to manage secretions, bloody secretions, hemoptysis, and hematemesis are all hallmarks of advanced cancer of the hypopharynx.

The vast majority of patients with cancer of the hypopharynx will have a significant history of tobacco and alcohol abuse. Unlike the nearby oropharyngeal subsite, cancers in this area are rarely related to HPV exposure. Due in part to delays related to alcohol abuse or poor access to medical care, in combination with dysphagia and anorexia related to the cancer itself, some patients who have hypopharyngeal cancer will suffer severe weight loss and present in a state of marked malnutrition, which can greatly compromise healing and the ability to withstand cytotoxic therapies.

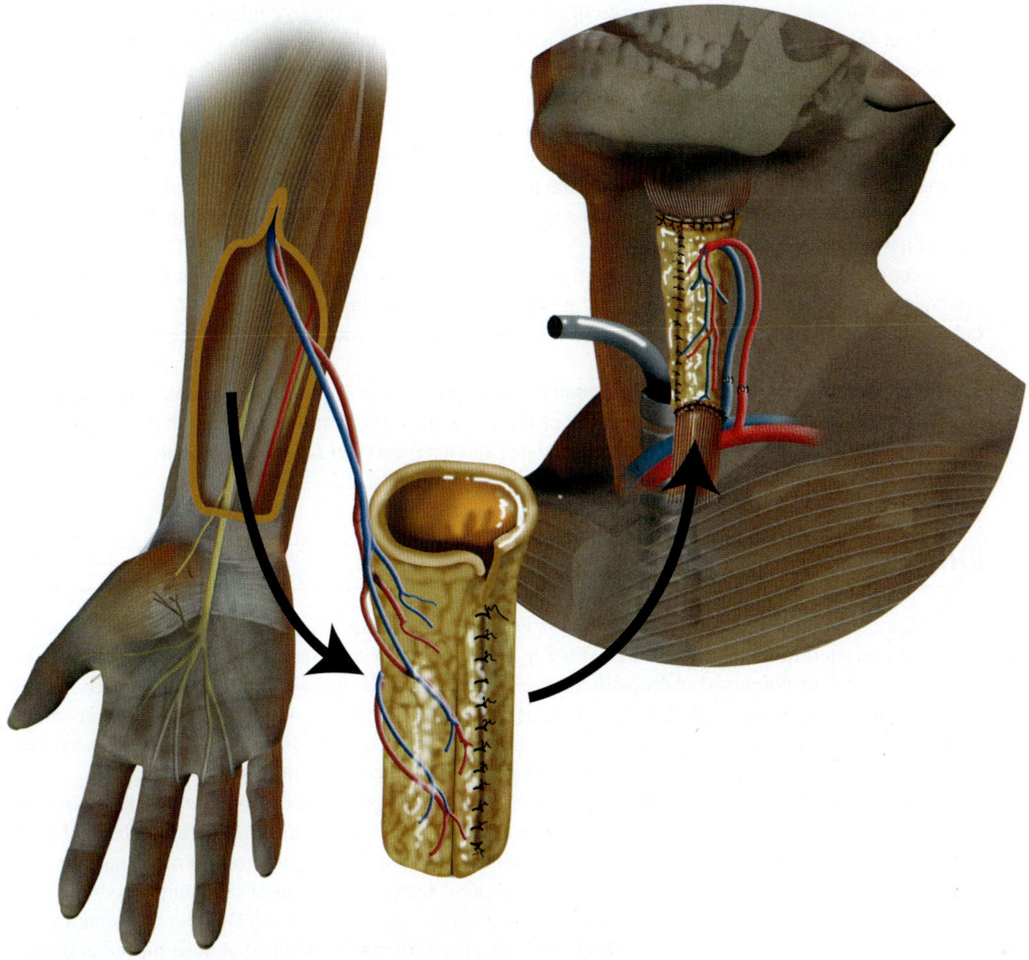

A

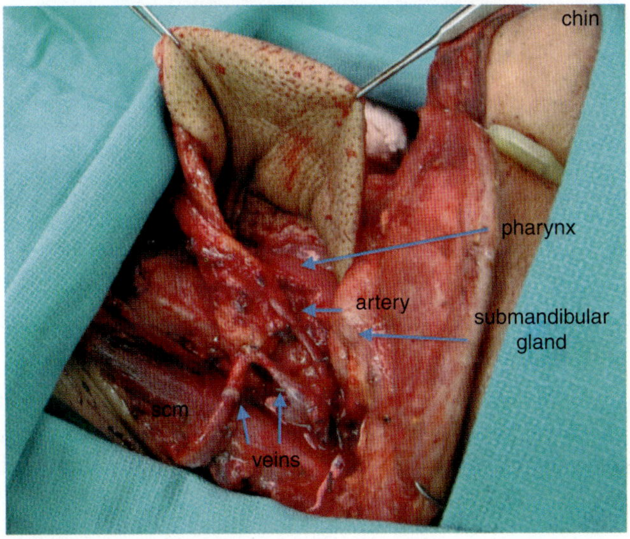

B

FIGURE 34.1
A. Diagram of forearm flap tubed to recreate the hypopharynx. The pharyngeal closure and microvascular anastomosis can be seen on the right. **B.** Surgical photograph similar to the diagram on the right side of (A). Two venous and one arterial anastomoses are seen. SCM indicates sternocleidomastoid muscle. Other anatomic landmarks are as designated. The pliable forearm flap is being held up to demonstrate the initial suture line on the right pharyngeal wall. In the photograph, there is a strip of mucosa posteriorly, while the prior diagram shows a circumferential reconstruction.

PHYSICAL EXAMINATION

When the patient presents to the otolaryngologist with a history of symptoms referable to the hypopharynx, the first step is a complete examination of the head and neck, including palpation of the neck, mirror examination of the larynx and hypopharynx, and in most cases, an office fiberoptic laryngopharyngoscopy is a part of the physical examination. In many cases, an irregularity in the mucosa will be seen that can be exophytic or infiltrative. Raised areas, with a combination of erythroplasia and blanched necrotic tissue, may be identified. More infiltrative cancers can be more difficult to detect visually but can be characterized by ulceration and edema of the overlying mucosa. Lesions may be present on the posterior wall of the hypopharynx above the level of the arytenoids or on the medial, anterior, or lateral walls of the piriform sinuses. Cancers of the postcricoid area or the apex of the piriform sinus cannot be seen directly on routine fiberoptic nasopharyngoscopy and laryngoscopy, but edema and pooling of secretions are usually present. A Valsalva maneuver may open the piriform sinus and assist in the visualization of a tumor. The diffusion of office transnasal esophagoscopes, with the ability to insufflate and suction without requiring specific scheduling and sedation, allows the surgeon to better visualize the more distal lesions at the time of the initial office evaluation. Fiberoptic esophagoscopy, however, can miss a lesion in the piriform sinus or postcricoid area due to loss of visualization at the constricted area of the cricopharyngeus muscle.

Cancer of the medial wall of the piriform sinus commonly extends submucosally at the deep margin into the paraglottic space, and fiberoptic laryngoscopy may reveal thickening or edema of the aryepiglottic folds and vocal fold paralysis. Cancers of the postcricoid area will typically produce edema of the arytenoids and may also lead to fixation of the vocal folds.

Palpation of the neck will allow the surgeon to assess the number of pathologic lymph nodes present, their size, unilaterality versus bilaterality, and whether there is reduced mobility or fixation that portends involvement of vascular structures, cranial and spinal nerves, and deep cervical muscles. The retropharyngeal lymph nodes may also be involved.

INDICATIONS

Laryngopharyngectomy, with cervical lymphadenectomy and reconstruction of the pharynx with a radial forearm flap, is indicated for advanced cancer of the hypopharynx. For early stage I and II cancer, partial laryngectomy, radiation, or combined chemoradiation are often excellent options. For stage III cancer, combined chemoradiation is commonly considered, and for certain tumor anatomies, stage III (T3N0) lesions might be considered for extended partial laryngectomy. However, for advanced T4 cancer of the hypopharynx, and for recurrent cancer after previous treatment, laryngopharyngectomy is usually indicated.

Radial forearm flaps are contraindicated in patients with inadequate circulation to the hand, as sacrifice of the radial artery in such a case would lead to vascular insufficiency and even gangrene of the hand. The Allen test is used to assess this on physical examination, with concurrent compression of the radial and ulnar arteries, followed by release of the ulnar artery and evaluation of revascularization of the hand by assessing color. When the Allen test is equivocal, the test can be repeated with the assistance of the Doppler ultrasound to assess blood flow and pressure in the fingers (digital Doppler-assisted Allen test). If a patient fails his or her Allen test, other reconstructive options must be considered. Generally, the pectoralis major flap, anterolateral thigh flap, or lateral arm flap provide reasonable alternatives.

CONTRAINDICATIONS

This procedure represents a major intervention and can take 10 or more hours to accomplish. Patients with severe comorbidities, such as severe cardiovascular disease, marked malnutrition and debilitation, end-stage renal or pulmonary disease, or dementia, may not tolerate such prolonged surgery.

PREOPERATIVE PLANNING

Fine Needle Aspiration

When patients present with palpable cervical lymph adenopathy and the primary cancer is not well visualized, fine needle aspiration and cytologic analysis can be used to establish the diagnosis of cancer and justify imaging and endoscopy. It is not mandatory if biopsy of the primary cancer is planned.

Endoscopy

The way to most accurately diagnose cancer of the hypopharynx is direct laryngoscopy with biopsy under general anesthesia. Failure to visualize a lesion on office examination should not dissuade the surgeon from proceeding with direct laryngoscopy in the presence of unexplained, persistent foreign body sensation in the throat, discomfort with swallowing, or otalgia. Typically rigid or flexible esophagoscopy is also performed to rule out direct extension or second primary cancers involving the esophagus. Screening bronchoscopy may also be performed. The risk of second primary cancers of the upper aerodigestive tract, esophagus, or lungs is estimated at 10% to 20% and is a particularly significant issue for hypopharyngeal cancers relative to other anatomic subsites in the head and neck. Early second primary cancers are not always seen on imaging and may occasionally be detected on careful endoscopy.

A biopsy is mandatory in order to establish a diagnosis and potentially recommend treatments that are radical or toxic. The biopsy is usually obtained with a cup forceps, and infrequently, other microsurgical instruments, such as sickle blades, microscissors, or lasers, are needed to perform incisions and obtain biopsies of submucosal or cartilaginous tumors, or indurated cancers that are difficult to enter with a cup forceps. Generous biopsies, including some performed at the interface between the cancer and normal adjacent tissue, should be performed, in order to ensure that sufficient viable tissue is obtained to make an appropriate pathologic diagnosis.

Head and neck oncologic surgeons will commonly receive patients who have already undergone direct laryngoscopy and carry a biopsy-proven diagnosis of cancer, most commonly squamous cell carcinoma. In this situation, the surgeon may develop a relatively complete understanding of the anatomy of the lesion, based on office nasopharyngoscopy or transnasal esophagoscopy, and imaging studies, and may elect to repeat the direct laryngoscopy immediately prior to ablative surgery, during the same intervention. In other cases, a repeat direct laryngoscopy and esophagoscopy at an earlier date may be indicated in order to ascertain whether circumferential involvement or esophageal involvement is present, and better plan the reconstruction, as well as to ensure adequate staging and make proper decisions regarding the use of chemotherapy and radiation as alternative approaches in the management of these cancers.

Imaging Studies

A barium swallow may be useful in a patient with symptoms of dysphagia in whom a visible lesion is not present, although in a setting of high suspicion, the surgeon will often elect to bypass this study and proceed to direct laryngoscopy and esophagoscopy. A negative barium swallow does not exclude cancer in the hypopharynx, and results of such a contrast study should be interpreted with caution.

When the diagnosis of cancer of the hypopharynx is strongly suspected or confirmed, an anatomic imaging study, most commonly a contrasted computerized tomography (CT) of the neck, is indicated in order to delineate the anatomy of the cancer, including its superficial and deep extension. The presence of cartilage destruction in the larynx is best identified on CT. The extent of invasion of larger metastatic nodes and the number of suspicious nodes can also be determined. Magnetic resonance imaging with or without gadolinium contrast can be used when the patient is allergic to iodine, or as a complementary study to assist in answering specific questions, such as the presence of invasion of the retropharyngeal fascia or vascular structures and the presence of gross perineural invasion, findings that may predict an inability to completely clear the resection margins of cancer.

Positron emission tomography–computerized tomography (PET–CT) can be useful in determining whether equivocal lymph nodes palpated or seen on imaging actually harbor malignancy. It can also identify mediastinal lymph node metastases, pulmonary nodules, and other distant metastases. However, false positives related to inflammatory processes are common, and the surgeon must be skeptical in the interpretation of PET and utilize anatomic imaging and clinical knowledge to make appropriate decisions regarding treatment. Alternatively, a CT of the thorax with contrast will image the highest risk sites, the mediastinum and lungs, for the presence of distant metastases.

Histopathology

More than 95% of malignant hypopharyngeal tumors are squamous cell carcinomas. In addition to the classic variant, subtypes of squamous cell carcinoma occasionally are described, such as adenosquamous, acantholytic, basaloid, spindle cell, papillary, and nasopharyngeal type (lymphoepithelial). Most of these behave similarly to classic squamous cell carcinoma. Verrucous carcinoma is well differentiated and indolent and most commonly is treated surgically in order to avoid purported risk of transformation to more aggressive histologies when treated with radiation therapy. It grows with pushing borders and rarely metastasizes. Verrucous carcinoma is infrequent in the hypopharynx and occurs most commonly in the oral cavity and occasionally in the larynx. Acantholytic and papillary squamous cell carcinomas can be less infiltrative than the classic variant. Nasopharyngeal-type carcinoma occurs rarely in the hypopharynx, and while high in grade, these cancers are characterized by exquisite sensitivity to chemotherapy and radiation.

Nonsquamous carcinomas, such as mucoepidermoid carcinoma and neuroendocrine carcinomas, can occur. Their behavior is often predicated by their grade, which can be high, intermediate, or low. Low-grade neuroendocrine carcinomas are referred to as carcinoid tumors and are much more common in the lower gastrointestinal tract. Sarcomas and lymphomas can also occur in the hypopharynx but are exceedingly rare.

SURGICAL TECHNIQUE

The patient is brought to the operating room and placed under general endotracheal anesthesia. If the presence of exophytic cancer makes standard intubation difficult, awake fiberoptic intubation is an option, but more commonly awake tracheostomy is performed to allow for induction of anesthesia, since a tracheostomy is planned as part of the procedure. After induction of anesthesia, the eyes are protected with tape and hard goggles, pressure points are padded, and the head of the bed is rotated 180 degrees away from the anesthesia station. Dynamic compression stockings are placed for the prevention of pulmonary embolus. Direct laryngoscopy is then performed to confirm the anatomy of the cancer. Rigid esophagoscopy and bronchoscopy are also performed. The presence of esophageal involvement below the cervical inlet, or involvement of the inferior aspect of the trachea, may make the planned procedure impossible; alternatives, including gastric pull-up, sternectomy, mediastinal tracheostomy, or nonsurgical options, may need to be considered. Appropriate preparation is performed with antiseptic solution and draping of the head and neck, forearm, and pectoral area (for a possible backup flap). I begin the open procedure by prepping and draping the patient to the neck as well as to the forearm.

The resection, tracheostomy, and neck dissections are open surgical procedures, and there are a wide variety of styles that surgeons have in accomplishing these procedures. I favor a meticulous dissection with the use of scalpel, bipolar cautery, DeBakey forceps, Gerald forceps with teeth, and fine Jamison scissors. I use electrocautery for the less delicate portions of the dissection, and ties or clips for control of vessels.

Elevation of the flap involves clipping multiple vascular branches that come off of the pedicle, and automatically reloading clips will expedite this procedure. A tourniquet is usually used during flap elevation to temporarily maintain hemostasis at the donor site. For the microvascular anastomosis, I have a tray of shorter microvascular instruments and a tray of longer microvascular instruments, including jeweler's forceps, microvascular needle holders, single and frame sizes 3 and 4 arterial and venous clamps, larger vascular bulldog clamps, and 9-0 nylon on a V100-3 needle. The Synovis GEM microvascular anastomosis coupler can be used for the venous anastomosis if adequate-sized matching vessels are found, and this can reduce operative time significantly.

The pectoralis major donor site is also prepared as a backup flap. It is preferable to use two teams, and one begins working on the forearm, while another works on the neck. Apron style incisions or horizontal incisions can be used, and subplatysmal flaps are raised up from the sternal notch to the submental area. Laterally, the flaps expose the sternocleidomastoid muscles and angle of the mandible. Neck dissections are performed that are most commonly bilateral. If palpable adenopathy is present, the surgeon may elect to dissect level 5 (posterior triangle), but most commonly, levels 2 through 4, the jugular chain, are dissected. If there are clearly indications for postoperative radiation, level 5 can be left undissected even in the presence of palpable jugular adenopathy, as level 5 will be included in the radiation field.

The neck dissections are performed in the following manner: The sternocleidomastoid muscle is sharply delineated with a no. 15 blade. Hemostasis is obtained with bipolar cautery. The spinal accessory nerve is identified as it exits the superior portion of the muscle and preserved. I follow the nerve with a McCabe nerve dissector and divides overlying tissue with a harmonic scalpel or bipolar cautery. I take the IIB nodes above the nerve either in continuity or as a separate specimen. The lymphatics are then reflected off of the deep cervical fascia, cervical plexus, and the sheath of the jugular and carotid artery using a no. 15 blade and bipolar cautery. If bulky adenopathy is present unilaterally, the jugular vein should be taken, but at least one jugular vein should be preserved to avoid complications, including cerebral edema. I elevate the tissues in a plane just above the superior thyroid vessels and come off the strap muscles. Anterosuperiorly the digastric muscle serves as the limit of dissection, and removal of level 1 is rarely indicated for hypopharyngeal lesions. An identical procedure is performed on the contralateral side. At this point, removal of levels 2 through 4 has been completed. Paratracheal and upper mediastinal lymph nodes will commonly also be resected in the context of the laryngectomy, particularly for hypopharyngeal lesions extending into the apex of the piriform sinus or esophagus.

During the neck dissections, specific care must be taken to dissect out arteries and veins that may serve as potential donor vessels, with sufficient length to provide for flexibility in designing blood vessel geometry at the time of the microvascular anastomosis. The facial artery is preserved, taking it at the angle of the mandible and clipping it distally, as well as the facial vein, and external jugular vein, again taken distally and clipped. Other potential donor blood vessels, such as the external carotid artery, internal jugular vein, superior thyroid veins, and transverse cervical veins, are often left intact during the neck dissection as their ligation is not necessary to facilitate the lymphadenectomy. These can be divided later if necessary for microvascular anastomosis. Microvascular clamps should not be placed on the vessels during the neck dissection, in advance of the microvascular anastomosis, as prolonged vascular compression can lead to ischemia of the endothelium at the clamp site and create a sluffed area that will lead to thrombosis. Instead, ligaclips are used, and the vascular clamps are placed when vessels are trimmed immediately before beginning the microvascular anastomosis.

Laterally, the retropharyngeal space is dissected, separating the carotid and jugular sheaths from the hypopharynx. If a circumferential pharyngectomy is planned, I do not divide the inferior pharyngeal constrictor muscle, but for partial pharyngectomy, the constrictor is divided at its attachment to the thyroid cartilage on the less involved side. The superior laryngeal vascular pedicle is ligated on the side where the thyroid is preserved, and the superior thyroid vessels are ligated on the side where the thyroid is resected. The suprahyoid muscles are then released from the hyoid bone, cutting directly onto the hyoid bone. A sensation of release is noted, and greater laryngeal mobility is achieved, when the suprahyoid muscles are completely transected and the submucosal space is entered.

If there is involvement of superior portions of the hypopharynx, adjacent or superior to the hyoid bone, the surgeon must dissect out the branches of the external carotid artery and the hypoglossal nerves and elevate these

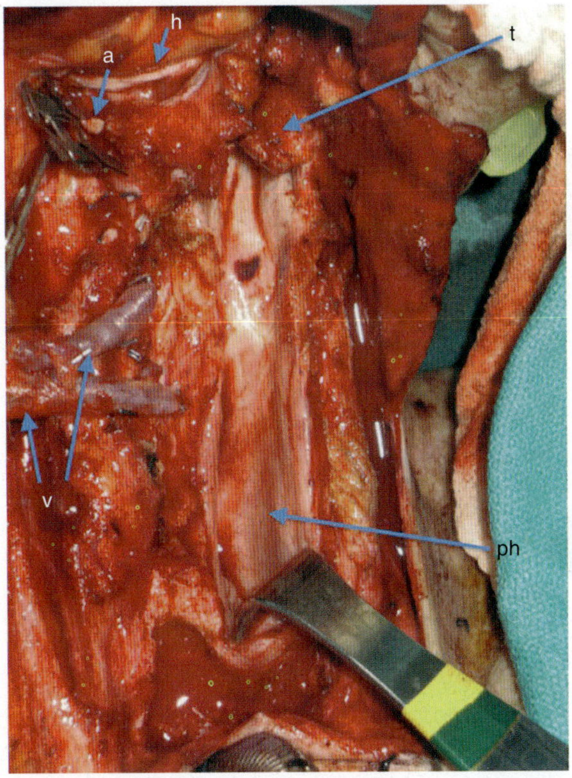

FIGURE 34.2
Pharyngolaryngectomy defect with posterior pharyngeal wall preserved. v, veins; a, artery; ph, pharyngeal remnant; t, base of the tongue; h, hypoglossal nerve. The endotracheal tube can be seen at the inferior aspect of the field.

off of the pharynx and the base of the tongue prior to making an incision into the pharynx. Some branches of the external carotid artery and even the hypoglossal nerve may need to be sacrificed due to deep extension of the cancer. At least one lingual artery and one hypoglossal nerve must be preserved in order to maintain viability and function of the oral tongue.

Once the hypopharynx has been skeletonized and the mentioned blood vessels and nerves protected, incisions are made into the mucosa, either saving a strip of hypopharynx posteriorly or circumferentially resecting the hypopharynx (Figs. 34.2 to 34.4).

The paratracheal nodes are dissected while awaiting the results of the frozen sections. The tissues from the medial aspect of the inferior portion of the common carotid artery and jugular vein, across the retroesophageal fascia, and off of the esophagus and trachea, including midline pretracheal tissue, are included in this dissection. When justifiable, a unilateral midline compartment dissection is performed in order to leave the parathyroids on the contralateral side undissected. The parathyroids are identified and preserved on the dissected side. The superior parathyroid can generally be left undisturbed superior to the dissection. Whenever possible, the

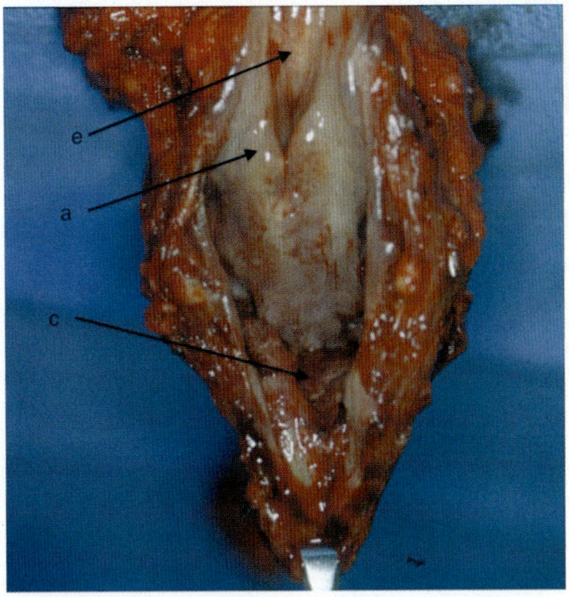

FIGURE 34.3
Total laryngopharyngectomy specimen. e, laryngeal surface of epiglottis; a, left arytenoid; c, cancer involving apex of piriform sinus, posterior wall of the hypopharynx, and cervical esophagus.

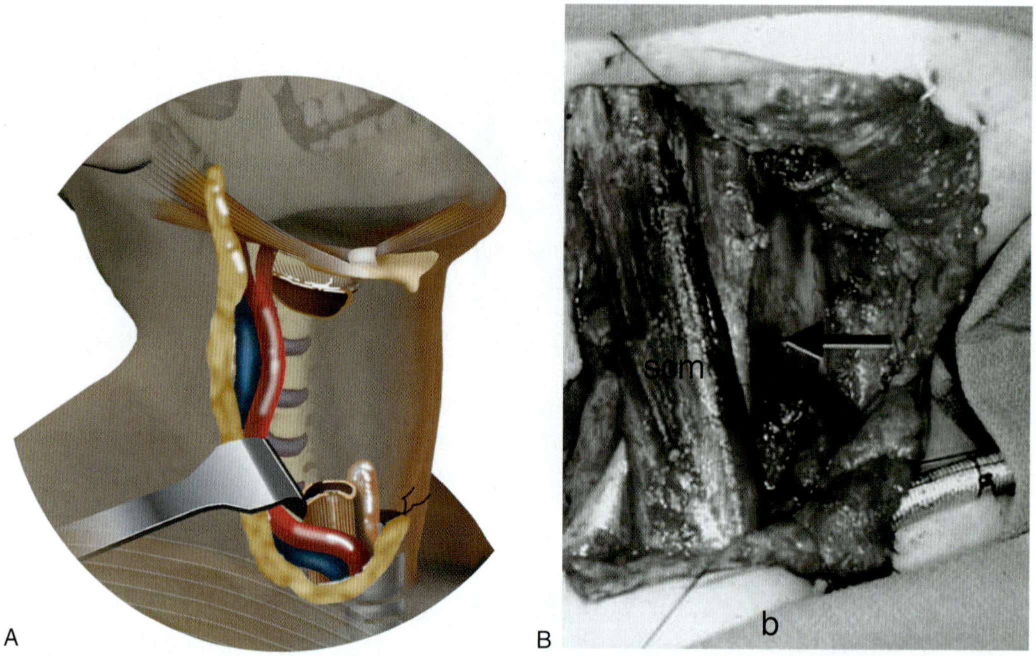

FIGURE 34.4 A,B. Circumferential pharyngectomy in (A) diagrammatic and (B) photographic image. The *black arrow* on the right designates the retropharyngeal fascia. SCM, sternocleidomastoid muscle. The sternocleidomastoid muscle is absent from the diagram on the left.

inferior parathyroid is visualized and reflected laterally on its vascular pedicle. Compromised parathyroids are minced and reimplanted in the sternocleidomastoid muscle.

While the tumor resection is proceeding in the neck, a second surgeon will begin elevating the forearm flap. The anatomy of the forearm is shown in Figure 34.5. Approximately a 13- by 10-cm flap will be sufficient

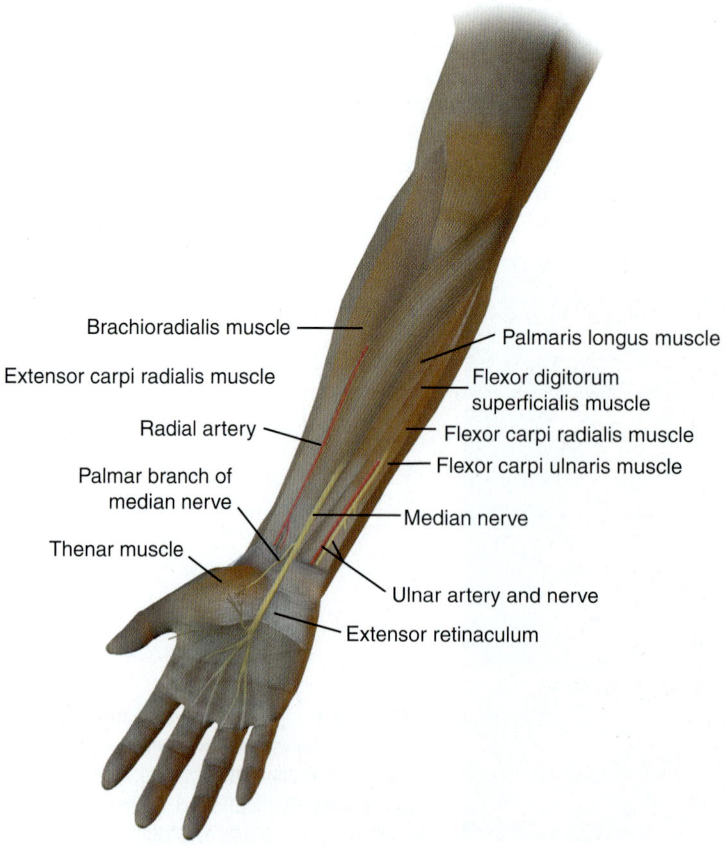

FIGURE 34.5
Anatomy of the forearm. Full-thickness flap of subcutaneous tissue is elevated off of the brachioradialis and the extensor carpi radialis medial to the radial artery pedicle (which runs with venae comitantes, not shown). The flap is also elevated from the flexor carpi radialis, palmaris longus, flexor digitorum superficialis, and flexor carpi ulnaris. Care is taken to leave the ulnar vessels, shown, under deep fascia. The paratenon is left on all tendons in order to facilitate take of the skin graft. The typical location of the skin flap is indicated by the blue rectangle.

for a complete circumferential pharyngeal reconstruction from the postcricoid area to the superior oropharynx. Generally, the nondominant arm is preferred. The Allen test is repeated in the holding area in order to confirm adequate circulation to the hand with sacrifice of the radial artery.

Once the primary site resection and lymphadenectomies are completed, the surgeon who will perform the reconstruction will begin preparing the blood vessels in the neck, using standard microvascular technique, including placement of arterial and venous bulldog microvascular clamps and recutting the blood vessels with a pair of sharp scissors or blade in order to achieve a straight, clean cut, and trimming excess adventitia from the ends of the vessels. The site of the vessel cut and position of the donor vessels are planned based on the anatomy of the already elevated flap pedicle. The vessels, and particularly the artery, are bled, in order to assess for adequate blood flow. In general, the forearm flap is not harvested until frozen sections are known to be clear, as additional ablative work could prove necessary, and it is preferable that this not be performed while the flap is ischemic.

The skin paddle is marked, and a proximal incision with a radial curve going all the way up to the antecubital fossa is drawn. The patient is prepped and draped to the arm up to the axilla with a tourniquet on the upper arm. The visible superficial forearm veins are marked. The upper extremity is then partially exsanguinated with an Esmarch elastic bandage wrapped around the arm in a raised position, in order to push the intravascular fluid back into the rest of the body, and the tourniquet is inflated to 300 mm Hg in order to minimize blood loss during flap elevation. The anatomy of the forearm is shown in Figure 34.5.

The order of steps in flap elevation can be flexible and varies between surgeons. I make a curvilinear incision above the flap first and elevate skin flaps in a subdermal plane over the proximal forearm and then dissect out the superficial forearm venous system, leaving a variable pannus of adipose tissue around the vessels depending on the reconstructive needs. The incision is then continued around the superior and medial aspects of the flap skin paddle. The skin is divided and subcutaneous adipose tissue transected with a 15-blade. Bipolar electrocoagulation is used for hemostasis, and small subcutaneous veins are clipped and transected as needed. The flap is commonly elevated from the ulnar side laterally going in a suprafascial plane until the tendon of the flexor carpi radialis muscle is reached. Care is taken to leave sufficient paratenon on the tendons, and the plane just deep to the subcutaneous adipose tissue can be followed in order to leave a thicker covering. All proximal and distal subcutaneous veins are elevated, clipped or ligated, and transected. Next, the radial aspect of the dissection is performed in a similar manner. The skin and subcutaneous adipose tissue are divided. Dorsal branches of the cephalic vein to the forearm are elevated and transected between clamps and tied using 3-0 Vicryl ties. The flap is elevated again in a suprafascial layer preserving the sensory branch of the radial nerve to the anatomic snuffbox with all its small ramifications. Dissection is continued until the medial aspect of the tendon of the brachioradialis muscle is reached. Next, the proximal incision is divided all the way up to the antecubital fossa. Fascial incisions are made on the bellies of the flexor carpi radialis muscle and brachioradialis muscle, and the muscles are rolled away from the septum. The radial vascular pedicle is identified, and numerous perforating vascular branches to the surrounding muscles were elevated, clipped, and transected. Dissection can be performed from distal to proximal or from proximal to distal, separating the tendons, and protecting the septum between the pedicle and the skin paddle. The deep aspect of the pedicle is freed, and perforating vessels to the surrounding muscles are clipped and transected. The distal aspect of the pedicle is identified as it exits the skin island distally. Multiple venae comitantes are clipped and transected, while the distal aspect of the radial artery is elevated and transected between clamps and ligated using 2-0 silk suture ligatures. The upper portion of the flap pedicle is completely freed distal to proximal and dissected until the recurrent radial artery is identified. At this level, numerous venous branches to the brachial comitantes system and the ulnar comitantes system, as well as proximal perforators to the surrounding muscles, are identified, clipped, and transected. A large connecting branch between the venae comitantes and the cephalic vein can commonly be found and protected and incorporated with the flap, and the cephalic vein dissected proximally until it is found to divide into significant branches, both of which were used for microvascular anastomosis. If a communicating branch between the venae comitantes and the superficial venous system is not present, the flap will survive quite well with venous anastomoses from either the superficial or deep systems. The superficial veins are much larger, and when available, incorporation of the superficial venous plexus is preferred. Occasionally in a patient who has had many intravenous lines, perhaps because of prior chemotherapy, only the venae comitantes are available. Once raised, the flap is set to rest in situ, placing tacking sutures in a favorable position in order to avoid kinking of the pedicle, while the resection is being completed. The tourniquet is deflated and completely removed in order to ensure that no arm compression persists.

Flap monitoring for a hypopharyngeal reconstruction can be challenging, as the flap is buried and cannot be visualized directly at the bedside during the postoperative period. For this reason, it can be beneficial when possible to exteriorize a marker skin paddle into one of the skin incisions in order to monitor the flap. This can be performed if a separate proximal perforator can be identified, in order to design a small additional skin paddle around it. De-epithelialization of a portion of the flap in order to exteriorize an area is not advisable, as the de-epithelialized dermis can compromise the pharyngeal repair and serve as a conduit for fistulization. If a separate skin paddle can be designed on a perforator, it can be brought out to the skin incision for monitoring. This may not be possible if all of the skin of the forearm is needed for a large pharyngeal reconstruction.

Once the cancer resection is completed, the reconstructive surgeon must turn his attention to the anatomy of the defect and the donor vessels in the neck. Limited areas may benefit from initial primary approximation of mucosa. This is common at the glossopharyngeal folds, and these sutures can be placed prior to inducing flap ischemia. The dimensions of the flap relative to the defect are assessed, and the geometry of the vascular pedicle is planned. Donor vessels are selected, vascular clamps are placed, and vessels are cut cleanly, dilated when necessary, and trimmed of excess adventitia. Aggressive excessive trimming of adventitia should be avoided as it can weaken and thin the walls of donor arteries and veins. Clamps are released to assess arterial flow. As clamps are placed and microvascular work is initiated, the surgeon should be careful to identify important neurovascular structures, such as the hypoglossal nerve, preserved lingual nerve, carotid artery, and vagus nerve, and ensure that the clamps and instruments are not placing pressure on these structures.

Once the frozen section results are returned as negative the flap can be harvested. The vessels are clamped proximally and transected. The radial artery is ligated using 2-0 silk suture ligatures, while the branches of the cephalic vein are ligated using 3-0 Vicryl suture ligatures. The sensory nerve is transected under the cephalic vein. In the setting of a hypopharyngeal reconstruction, there is no need to anastomose the sensory nerve. The flap is passed up into the neck, and the artery is irrigated with heparinized saline until clear fluid can be seen exiting the veins. Each vein is also irrigated with heparinized saline. In the meantime, a 0.018-inch split-thickness skin graft is harvested from the left thigh. It is trimmed to match the size of the defect in the forearm. The forearm is irrigated and checked for hemostasis. While the anastomosis proceeds in the neck, another team can begin closing the forearm donor site. The proximal aspect is closed in two layers using interrupted 3-0 Vicryl sutures, and skin staples over a 19-French suction drain. The distal aspect of the defect is covered with a skin graft, and 4-0 chromic sutures are circumferentially used. The skin graft is pie-crusted and tacked down to the muscles. It is secured with a Xeroform bolster tied to the distal forearm with 2-0 silk sutures. The wound is dressed, and the forearm is wrapped with Kerlix bandage. At the end of the procedure, a splint is used to stabilize the upper extremity with the wrist slightly extended and the fingers in neutral position.

In the meantime, the cut edges of the recipient vessels of the flap are freshened and cleaned. The vessels are dilated as needed to create a favorable size match with the donor vessels. The flap is partially inset in order to plan vessel geometry. However, the flap itself can overhang the vascular anastomosis, and once the geometry has been planned, the surgeon may elect to release tacking sutures and reposition the bulk of the flap farther away from the blood vessels in order to temporarily facilitate microvascular anastomosis.

Although some surgeons prefer to close the pharynx prior to microvascular anastomosis, I feel that this increases ischemia time excessively and I prefer to place a small number of sutures in order to plan vessel geometry and then proceed with microvascular anastomosis. Sufficient distance from the donor vessels to the flap is needed in order to allow for looping of the vascular pedicle without kinking. End-to-end arterial anastomosis is generally performed using interrupted 9-0 nylon sutures.

End-to-end venous anastomosis can be done either with sutures or using a coupling device. Some surgeons prefer to have at least one end-to-side venous anastomosis directly to the jugular vein. Plain 2% lidocaine or papaverine is used to irrigate the anastomosis and vascular pedicle in order to prevent vascular spasm. Clamps are removed, and the flap should revascularize. It is important to delay detailed assessment of color, warmth, and turgor of the skin paddle for at least 10 minutes in order to ensure adequate time to recover from the period of ischemia. Blood flow through the flap pedicle is assessed using the Doppler probe.

The pharyngoesophageal repair begins with cricopharyngeal myotomy to prevent stenosis and facilitate tracheoesophageal speech (see Fig. 34.1B). Extramucosal myotomy is done with a no. 15 blade or scissors, with a finger inside the digestive tract lumen protecting the mucosa. The circumferential muscular fibers are transected until the circular muscle band was completely released. The mucosa is completely preserved. A beveled cut at the level of the esophagus, if possible at the time of the resection, will serve to reduce the risk of stenosis. If this is not possible, a "fish-mouth" cut can be made in the esophagus, and the tip of the flap can be inset into it, in order to reduce the chances of stricture at a narrow, circumferential esophageal anastomosis. While suturing, I am careful to maintain the esophagus stretched to its maximal dimension during closure. A tracheal dilator placed into the esophagus can be helpful to determine the stretched diameter of the esophagus and not constrict it as the flap is sutured to it.

For the pharyngoesophageal repair, the flap can be positioned with the vascular pedicle oriented horizontally or vertically. The vessels are positioned with the pedicle resting on the prevertebral planes wherever possible, and the pedicle can exit the flap more superiorly or more inferiorly, based on the planned vascular geometry, and looped gently toward the donor vessels in a manner that will minimize the risk of kinking when the head is flexed or turned. Inverted vertical mattress (interrupted Connell) sutures with 3-0 Vicryl are used circumferentially to suture the skin of the flap to the mucosa of the esophagus and pharynx. In the early stages of the closure, when the lumen is open, standard vertical mattress sutures can also be used, as one might use on skin. The flap is anastomosed to the pharyngoesophageal stump inferiorly, and the upper corners are attached to the superior pharyngeal mucosal remnants. Superior circumferential closure is performed marching along the posterior pharyngeal wall, to the level of the contralateral superior pharynx or tonsillar fossa, and back to the base of the tongue. The flap is turned on itself and finally anastomosed to itself in a vertical plane (see Fig. 34.1A). A feeding tube is passed transnasally through the flap-lined lumen and esophagus, to the stomach, and sutured to the columella. The last sutures on the flap are placed while leaving several untied, to facilitate visualization, and then all are tied at the end of the closure.

Once the pharyngeal repair is complete, vessel geometry is checked. Occasionally, tacking sutures are used to maintain favorable pedicle anatomy. Wounds are irrigated and checked for hemostasis. A tracheostoma is fashioned after resecting skin from either the inferior or superior skin flaps as needed to ensure that the stoma does not collapse and maintains adequate dimensions. The tracheostoma is sutured using interrupted extramucosal Prolene or 3-0 Vicryl sutures, and ultimately running 4-0 chromic sutures between the mucosa and the skin. This can be facilitated by brief apneic episodes where the tube is briefly removed from the trachea to place a suture, and then replaced, resuming ventilation. Care should be taken during this maneuver to not allow the patients' oxygen saturation to drop below 90% and to ventilate sufficiently to maintain low CO_2 levels. Suction drains are placed in the neck. Wounds were closed in two layers using interrupted 3-0 Vicryl sutures and skin staples. If a marker skin paddle has been designed, it is incorporated into the skin closure, often just above the stoma. Prolene sutures are placed at various points on the neck to mark sites for postoperative Doppler checks. The procedure is completed at this point, and the patient is turned over to the care of the anesthesiology team to reverse general anesthesia.

POSTOPERATIVE MANAGEMENT

The patient is initially placed in an intensive care setting. Many surgeons use either aspirin, dextran, or other medications designed to prevent thrombus formation during the postoperative period. My own preference is to use aspirin only, administered rectally, immediately postoperatively, and to give a single dose of intravenous heparin, 5,000 units, in cases that have become problematic, either due to poor condition of the blood vessels or witnessed episodes of thrombosis.

Continuous cardiac monitoring and monitoring of oxygen saturation are performed. Dynamic compression stockings and subcutaneous heparin or fragmin are used to prevent deep venous thrombosis. Nursing care is focused on care of the tracheal stoma, with removal of crusts, and saline irrigation and suctioning of the trachea. Suction drains must also be cleansed, monitored, and emptied. Patients are weaned from mechanical ventilation rapidly when possible and required to get into a chair on the first day postoperatively and on subsequent days are ambulated as much as possible. Flap monitoring is important as flaps can be salvaged by revision of the vascular anastomosis if thrombosis is detected early. Flaps are monitored by Dopplers placed by the nurses and physicians at 1-hour intervals for the first 2 days and 2-hour intervals for another 2 days. Specifically for hypopharyngeal flaps, implantable Dopplers placed directly on the vein can be very useful and give a continuous confirmation of vascular integrity. However, these also have their limitations, as they can become dislodged and fail to read, despite a healthy flap. If a skin island has been exteriorized, it is monitored for color, capillary refill, and bleeding after a needle prick or scratch. It must be kept in mind that the monitor island can be compromised due to issues with specific perforators, and the main flap may still be intact. In rare circumstances, direct laryngoscopy must be performed to assess the flap. More commonly, bedside ultrasound can be used if the Doppler studies are in doubt. Wounds are monitored for fistula development while in the hospital. If a patient develops signs of fluctuance and inflammation, drainage of an abscess early can prevent larger abscess formation and secondary tissue injury. Flap monitoring generally is reduced to twice daily after the 5th postoperative day, and patients can be ready for discharge by the 6th or 7th postoperative day.

It is important to ensure that patients and families are adequately instructed in care of the tracheostoma, and in some situations, placement in an extended care facility is necessary to ensure adequate care occurs. Failure to adequately care for the stoma can lead to airway obstruction and even death.

COMPLICATIONS

The majority of patients will develop at least a minor complication after hypopharyngeal reconstruction. The rate of pharyngocutaneous fistulization has been reported at approximately 31%. A pharyngocutaneous fistula can drain over major blood vessels and lead to vascular rupture, followed by flap necrosis, stroke, or death. Breakdown around the tracheostoma can also lead to vascular exposure, desiccation, and vascular rupture. Mortality after pharyngoesophageal repair has been reported as high as 10% but should be lower than this with proper patient selection, careful attention to detail, and the use of a cutaneous free flap rather than an enteric reconstruction.

Partial or complete necrosis of the flap can occur that will lead to massive pharyngocutaneous leakage if a secondary reconstruction is not rapidly performed. While rates of complete free flap failure are less than 5% in experienced hands, the group of patients undergoing hypopharyngeal reconstruction are typically compromised by malnutrition, prior radiation, poor peripheral circulation, and other issues, and the rate of vascular thrombosis may be higher in this group.

Other surgical risks include intraoperative injury of lower cranial nerves or carotid artery, chyle leak related to uncontrolled injury of the thoracic duct, stricture, dysphagia requiring a feeding tube, and intractable hypocalcemia. As in any major operation, general medical complications not directly connected to the surgical maneuvers can also occur, including deep venous thrombosis, pulmonary embolism, myocardial infarction, pneumonia, and renal failure.

RESULTS

Five-year survival for stage IV cancer of the hypopharynx treated with surgery followed by external beam radiation therapy has been reported to range between 30% and 50%. Palliation and local control are achieved in a larger percentage of patients. Functionally, patients are similar to other laryngectomies with regards to issues of speech rehabilitation, with the caveat that in some cases, pooled secretions in the reconstructed hypopharynx can make tracheoesophageal speech sound "wet" and difficult to understand. Many patients acquire quite good tracheoesophageal speech, and the "wet" voice is a greater problem after reconstruction with jejunum. Results with regard to deglutition are variable. Strictures can occur requiring dilation in up to 15% of patients. Furthermore, even if stricture is successfully avoided through superior surgical technique, lubrication and peristaltic function of the hypopharynx are lost after circumferential hypopharyngeal reconstruction with a forearm flap. Ingested nutrition moves through the repaired pharyngeal segment by gravity alone. Typically, patients wash meals down with fluids, using the tongue base to push food through the tubular reconstruction. While some patients can eat almost anything, some must restrict themselves to a full liquid or pureed diet.

PEARLS

- Unexplained continuous odynophagia, dysphagia, or otalgia for more than a month mandates direct laryngoscopy under general anesthesia.
- Initial endoscopy should focus on ruling out esophageal involvement beyond the esophageal inlet, fixation of cancer to the prevertebral fascia/muscle, and tracheal involvement, all of which could compromise subsequent resection and reconstruction.
- Careful informed consent should be obtained, and particularly in the less educated patient, repeated on multiple occasions, regarding the presence of a permanent tracheostoma, speech and swallowing difficulties after surgery, and the risk of healing problems, infection, vascular rupture, and tumor recurrence among other complications.
- During the scheduling period, attempts should be made to improve the patient's nutritional status, using liquid supplements and feeding tubes if indicated.

PITFALLS

- For emaciated, malnourished patients and those with significant comorbidities, the pectoralis major flap may be a preferred alternative, particularly if the subcutaneous tissue of the chest is thin and the patient is not extremely muscular.
- Patients who have failed their Allen test, who must have a different flap, are likely to prove to be vasculopathic in other parts of the body, and the surgeon should plan accordingly. Poor distal circulation can be anticipated in pedicled flaps, and atherosclerotic changes can be anticipated in donor vessels.
- If unexpected involvement of the prevertebral fascia is encountered, this fascia can be resected. While this portends a poor prognosis, an attempt can be made to strip the vertebral bodies, taking care to avoid the vertebral arteries inferiorly.
- Intraoperatively the surgeon should plan for a potential fistula and cover blood vessels with vascularized tissue whenever possible.
- Meticulous microvascular technique is necessary to achieve success.
- The surgeon should avoid prolonged use of vascular clamps. Precise suture placement under high magnification should be practiced, with careful observation to detect endothelial flaps, tears, and other subtle factors that could lead to thrombosis. Whenever possible, vessels should be cut back to areas away from atherosclerotic plaque or valves.
- If suturing through plaque, the surgeon should try to pass the needle from the lumen outward in order to avoid creating a separation of the endothelium that could subsequently lead to vascular dissection.
- The most important factor in flap success is vessel geometry.
- Meticulous pharyngeal closure is essential and should not be rushed.
- Exteriorized skin paddles should be separated from the internal flap by complete removal of dermis, as a dermal connection can facilitate fistulization.
- Careful postoperative monitoring for signs of local inflammation, and early drainage of abscess or fistula, reduce the risk of greater tissue injury or vascular thrombosis from fistula.
- Many local wound complications, including fistulas and breakdowns around the tracheal stoma, can be managed conservatively with local wound care. Heavily irradiated patients may benefit from hyperbaric oxygen therapy. The surgeon, however, must have a high index of suspicion regarding possible exposure of major blood vessels.

- If the trachea must be transected low in the mediastinum, significant attention should be paid to the protection of the carotid and innominate arteries and jugular and innominate veins. If necessary, additional flaps should be brought in.
- Issues with healing can occasionally occur late, even 4 to 6 weeks after surgery.

INSTRUMENTS TO HAVE AVAILABLE

- Head and neck surgical tray
- Sterile tourniquet
- Jeweler's forceps
- Micro needle holders
- 3 and 4 arterial and venous frame and single clamps
- Vascular bulldog clamps
- 9-0 nylon suture on V100-3 needle
- Synovis GEM microvascular anastomosis coupler

SUGGESTED READING

Varvares MA, Cheney ML, Gliklich RE, et al. Use of the radial forearm fasciocutaneous free flap and montgomery salivary bypass tube for pharyngoesophageal reconstruction. *Head Neck* 2000;22(5):463–468.

Marin VP, Yu P, Weber RS. Isolated cervical esophageal reconstruction for rare esophageal tumors. *Head Neck* 2006;28(9):856–860.

Andrades P, Pehler SF, Baranano CF, et al. Fistula analysis after radial forearm free flap reconstruction of hypopharyngeal defects. *Laryngoscope* 2008;118(7):1157–1163.

35 MANAGEMENT OF THE CHEEK DEFECT: CERVICOFACIAL ADVANCEMENT FLAP

Joseph A. Paydarfar

INTRODUCTION

Reconstructive options for defects of the cheek include healing by second intention, primary closure, skin grafting, advancement flaps, pedicled flaps, and free tissue transfer. The goals of reconstruction are to find the best skin color and texture match, maintain normal hair distribution, minimize noticeable incision lines, reconstruct within a facial subunit, and reduce the effects of scarring on adjacent structures such as the lower eyelid.

The cervicofacial advancement rotation flap is well suited for reconstructing a variety of postablative and traumatic defects of the cheek. The skin has excellent color, thickness and texture match, and when designed and implemented correctly, very acceptable scars are the result. There are a number of methods of elevating the cervicofacial flap depending on the size and location of the defect, patient factors, degree of laxity of surrounding skin, and the skill of the reconstructive surgeon. These approaches include using an anteriorly or posteriorly based flap, extending the elevation onto the chest (the so-called cervicothoracic or cervicopectoral flap), and elevating in a subcutaneous versus deep plane. For composite defects, this flap can also be used in combination with pedicled or free flaps.

HISTORY

A careful history is important in determining the optimal approach for reconstruction of the cheek defect. Specifically, a history of prior radiation and/or surgery to the face and neck, diabetes, malnutrition, autoimmune disease, and smoking should be obtained as these factors may impair healing and lead to flap necrosis. In addition, it is important to know if any other procedures are planned such as parotidectomy or neck dissection.

PHYSICAL EXAMINATION

A clear understanding of the anatomy of the flap is important to ensure that the vascular territory of the flap has not been compromised by prior therapy. The cervicofacial flap is vascularized by the facial artery, in particular the submental branch and the superficial temporal, as well as the transverse cervical, and suprascapular arteries. When elevation of the flap is carried onto the chest, additional arterial supply comes from perforators of the internal mammary artery. If a deep plane dissection is performed, the superficial musculoaponeurotic system (SMAS) layer as well as the platysma is included in the flap elevation. The SMAS lies deep to the subcutaneous adipose tissue superficial to the parotid fascia and is in continuity with the fascia investing the platysma muscle. The facial nerve, as it exits the stylomastoid foramen, travels through the parotid gland and is relatively safe as long as the gland is not entered. The nerve then emerges from the gland and travels deep to the muscles of facial expression. The frontal branch of the facial nerve runs just deep to the temporoparietal fascia about 3.5 cm from the external auditory canal as it traverses the zygoma. The marginal mandibular branch of the facial nerve runs deep to the platysma over the fascia that invests the submandibular gland. In the deep plane dissection, the retaining ligaments of the face, namely the zygomatic ligament that anchors the skin of the cheek to the inferior border of the zygoma and the mandibular ligament that anchors the skin overlying the mandible to the anterior aspect of the mandible will need to be divided in order to improve mobilization of the flap.

INDICATIONS

The cervicofacial flap is primarily used in the repair of posttraumatic or postablative cheek defects, although there are numerous other applications (Table 35.1). It is an ideal flap for skin resurfacing in the case of facial scarring secondary to trauma or burns, and likewise, it is well suited for repairing large defects created as a result of resection of cancer of the skin. Some of the original indications for this flap were for reconstruction of the orbit after exenteration as described by Beare in 1969 and repair of the lower lid as popularized by Mustarde. Conley described the use of the chest advancement flap based either laterally off of the thoracoacromial or lateral thoracic artery or medially off of the internal mammary perforators. Moore et al describe the use of this flap in conjunction with the pectoralis myofascial flap for coverage of defects of the neck as well as with the radial forearm flap for reconstruction of through-and-through buccal defects. If planned properly, harvest of the flap can be incorporated with the resection; for example, the incisions required for resection of a skin cancer extending into the parotid gland with neck dissection can be incorporated into the cervicofacial flap.

CONTRAINDICATIONS

There are no absolute contraindications to the use of this flap. The surgeon should be cautious in patients with a history of poor wound healing and smoking.

PREOPERATIVE PLANNING

A thorough medical history, in particular, a history of prior radiation to the face and neck, diabetes, malnutrition, autoimmune disease, and smoking should be obtained. Physical examination should make note of any facial nerve deficits, prior facial or neck incisions, cervical or parotid lymph adenopathy, extent of the tumor to be resected or defect to be reconstructed, and actinic changes of the skin. If the defect is being created for the treatment of malignancy, such as cancer of the skin, a delayed reconstruction may be of benefit so as to ensure that final tumor margins are negative. It is also important to know if other procedures such as parotidectomy or neck dissection will be required as this will also influence the timing of the reconstruction as well as the placement of incisions.

SURGICAL TECHNIQUE

The patient is placed in the supine position on the operating room table. Depending on the extent of resection and reconstruction as well as surgeon and patient preference, the procedure may be performed under general anesthesia or monitored anesthesia care.

A number of factors will determine the best reconstructive approach including the size, location and depth of the defect, the involved layers in the defect, the relationship between the defect and aesthetic units

TABLE 35.1 Defects Reconstructed with the Cervicofacial/Cervicothoracic Advancement–Rotation Flap
Cheek
Lower lip
Nasofacial groove
Nasolacrimal region
Oral commissure
Orbit
Preauricular region and postauricular region neck
Scalp
Temple

and subunits, as well as patient factors such as a history of smoking, autoimmune disease, or radiation therapy. The general principles of flap design and elevation are such that the flap to be inset should be under minimal tension and should require the least amount of resection of normal skin (i.e., for management of dog ears). The incisions should be made in a stepwise fashion, reassessing the extent of tissue rotation and suture line tension prior to each subsequent incision. Depending upon the size and location of the defect, an anteriorly based or posteriorly based flap may be elevated.

Anteriorly Based Flap

This flap is also referred to as the forward cervicofacial advancement flap or the inferiorly based cervicofacial advancement flap. A horizontal incision is made at the posterior–superior aspect of the defect along the inferior orbital rim, carried superiorly to the lateral canthus and then inferiorly into the preauricular crease. The incision is then carried inferiorly behind the earlobe and into the neck along the hairline. A back cutting incision may be required, and this may be placed in a crease in the neck. For larger defects, a cervicothoracic or cervicopectoral flap may be used. In this case, the incision along the hairline is carried inferiorly into the lower neck, staying 1 to 2 cm posterior to the anterior border of the trapezius, then creating a curvilinear incision that runs lateral to the acromioclavicular joint, stays along the lateral edge of the pectoralis muscle and then extends medially on the chest, parallel to the clavicle. The medial incision is usually placed at the level of the third intercostal space (or just above the areola in males) although it may be carried down to the costal margin if needed.

The flap is elevated superficial to the SMAS layer and parotideomasseteric fascia in the subcutaneous plane thereby avoiding the branches of the facial nerve. If the flap elevation is carried inferiorly, it can be elevated superficial or deep to the platysma. With elevation deep to the platysma, dissection should be kept in the subplatysmal plane to minimize the risk of injury to the marginal mandibular branch of the facial nerve. If dissection is carried onto the chest, elevation is in the plane deep to the deltoid and pectoralis fascia. Care should be taken to avoid injury to the internal mammary perforators, which arise about 2 cm lateral to the lateral border of the sternum.

As the flap is advanced into the defect in question, the edges are trimmed accordingly. A standing cone deformity will normally occur at the medial–inferior incision line usually in the melolabial groove; the greater the rotation of the flap, the larger the deformity. This can be addressed primarily once the flap is inset. Closure of the donor site is usually achieved primarily and occasionally by V-Y advancement or with skin grafting. Placement of a suction drain will minimize hematoma or seroma formation especially when more extensive dissection is carried out.

Posteriorly Based Flap

This flap is also referred to as the reverse cervicofacial advancement flap or laterally based cervicofacial advancement flap. This rotation advancement moves redundant skin from the jowl and neck superiorly into the cheek defect. The incision starts along the anterior–inferior aspect of the defect and is carried inferiorly either through or parallel to the nasolabial crease and then lateral to the oral commissure. The incision can then be carried inferiorly over the mandible into the neck. The incision may then be made in one of three ways: (1) An anteriorly directed back cutting incision may be made in a submental neck crease; (2) the incision may be carried inferiorly as a vertical midline incision and then posteriorly along a neck crease parallel to the mandible toward the sternocleidomastoid muscle and superiorly to the earlobe/mastoid; and (3) the vertical midline incision may be extended inferiorly on the chest and then extended laterally above the areola and into the axilla.

Elevation and inset of the posteriorly based flap is similar to the anteriorly based flap. When elevating posteriorly, it is critical to discontinue undermining when within 2 to 3 cm of the ear thereby avoiding possible injury to the superficial temporal artery. Closure of the donor site can be achieved primarily as with the anteriorly based flap, although occasionally a V-Y advancement or skin graft is necessary.

Deep Plane Elevation

The cervicofacial advancement-rotation flap as described above is a random pattern flap. As such, there is concern that necrosis of the edges may occur especially with larger flaps. The likelihood of necrosis of the flap is higher among smokers. A deep plane approach has been advocated by some authors in order to improve the vascularity of the flap. Born out of the deep plane rhytidectomy technique, this flap is elevated deep to the SMAS layer but superficial to the facial muscles. The preauricular/pretragal incision is elevated in the subcutaneous plane for about 2 cm and then into the plane deep to the SMAS layer. The dissection also includes the adipose tissue of the cheek. As the dissection is carried anterior to the parotid gland, the surgeon should be careful not to injure the branches of the facial nerve as they exit the parotid gland. Inferior elevation is carried out deep to the platysma muscle that is included with the flap. Staying just deep to the platysma will minimize the risk of injury to the marginal mandibular branch of the facial nerve. Injury to the frontal branch of the facial nerve in the temporal region can be avoided by carrying the dissection more superficially onto the temporoparietal fascia along the inferior border of the zygoma. Because the flap includes the SMAS layer, adipose tissue of the cheek, and platysma, it benefits from improved vascularity and greater ability to handle tension. Releasing the facial suspensory ligaments will improve mobility and transfer of the flap. Closure of the defect can be performed directly or with V-Y transfer.

Choice of Approach

When deciding on the anterior versus posterior approach, the size and location of the defect as well as the degree of rotation and resultant excision of the skin must be taken into account. As a rule of thumb, the anteriorly based flap is better suited for posterior and large anterior defects, while the posteriorly based approach is applied to small to moderately sized anterior defects. Boyette and Vural found that for defects medial to the lateral canthus, the ratio of height to width best determines the approach to minimize rotation and excision of normal skin. With this approach, defects with a larger horizontal dimension are managed with a posteriorly based flap, whereas for defects with a larger vertical component, the anteriorly based flap should be used.

The decision for using a subcutaneous or deep plane dissection will depend upon the size of the defect as well as the patients smoking history and other factors that may affect wound healing such as a history of radiation therapy, diabetes, or autoimmune disease. The subcutaneous flap is easier and quicker to elevate; the risk of injury to the facial nerve is minimal. However, there may be greater risk of necrosis of the edges, especially in larger flaps. The deep plane flap may be better suited for larger defects, especially in smokers; however, it is a more difficult dissection and introduces greater risk of injury to the facial nerve.

POSTOPERATIVE CARE

Routine incisional wound and drain care is appropriate. It is important that patients not be exposed to cigarette smoke as this may cause necrosis of a poorly perfused skin flap.

COMPLICATIONS

The most common complications associated with this flap are listed in Table 35.2. Distal necrosis of the flap edges is a concern, particularly with larger defects and in smokers and as such consideration should be given to the deep plane approach. However, with proper flap design and efforts to minimize tension, distal necrosis in smokers can still be avoided with subcutaneous elevation.

The other significant complication associated with the cervicofacial flap is ectropion. This occurs when the lower lid is displaced as a result of tension on the flap or gravitational pull. Older patients and those with resected or denervated orbicularis oculi muscle are at greater risk. To avoid this potential complication, when the flap is designed, the horizontal limb is curved superiorly above the level of the lateral canthus. When the flap is inset, it is imperative to secure the flap to the deeper tissues, if possible the periosteum of the lateral or inferior orbit, in order to direct suture line tension away from the lower eyelid and to the anchor point above the lateral canthus. Placement of sutures along the lower lid suture line last will also reduce the risk of ectropion. A canthopexy at the time of flap inset can also be performed.

Injury to the facial nerve is a greater risk with the deep plane dissection. During dissection over the parotid gland, the nerve is relatively safe as it travels through the gland; however, the nerve branches run in a superficial plane as they emerge from the gland anteriorly. Injury to the frontal branch of the facial nerve can be avoided by staying superficial to the temporoparietal fascia when the dissection reaches within 1 cm of the inferior border of the zygoma. By staying in a tight subplatysmal plane, injury to the marginal mandibular branch of the facial nerve can be avoided.

RESULTS

Results with this technique are often considered the best. I find that this technique provides reliable and reproducible results with excellent color and texture match to the adjacent native skin. Figure 35.1 demonstrates a

TABLE 35.2 Complications
Abnormal hair distribution
Facial nerve injury—hematoma
Lower lid edema
Residual standing cone deformity ("dog ear")
Skin edge necrosis—ectropion

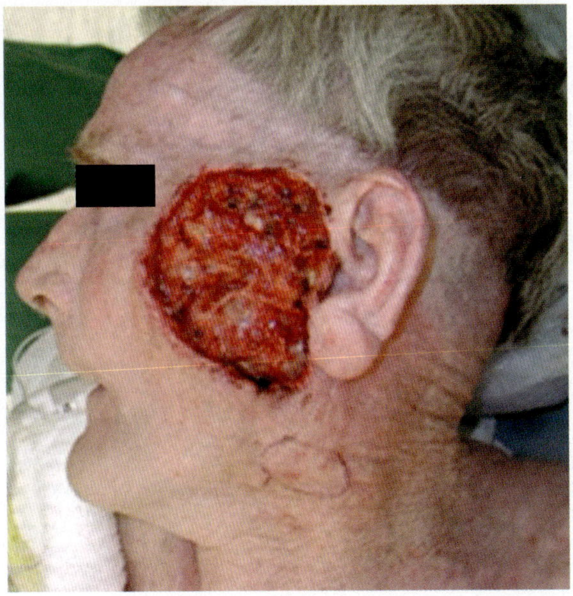

FIGURE 35.1
Cheek defect involving the full thickness of the skin.

defect that is amenable to this reconstructive approach. Figure 35.2 demonstrates the immediate postoperative results.

PEARLS

- Posterior defects should be reconstructed with an anteriorly based flap; small to medium anterior defects should be reconstructed with a posteriorly based flap.
- For large anterior defects, if the horizontal dimension is the larger dimension, an anteriorly based flap should be used; if the vertical dimension is the larger dimension, a posteriorly based flap should be used.
- Deep plane dissections may be advantageous for larger defects and in smokers or those with a history that predisposes to poor wound healing.
- Skin incisions made during flap elevation should be performed in a stepwise fashion, reassessing rotation and tension prior to each subsequent incision.
- Planning of the flap harvest incisions should take into account the extent of the resection portion of the operation.

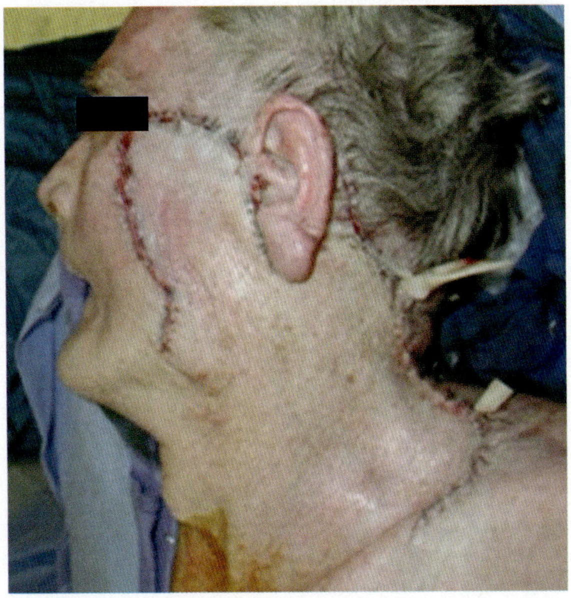

FIGURE 35.2
Anteriorly based cervicofacial rotation advancement flap used for reconstruction of large cheek defect following resection of an advanced cancer of the skin invading the parotid gland. Note how the incision follows the hairline inferiorly onto the clavicle.

PITFALLS

- Inset of the flap should be done to minimize tension along the lower eyelid. This can be partly achieved using deep anchoring sutures superior to the lateral canthus.
- Because the vascular supply to the flap can be compromised by vasoconstrictors, the patient should be restricted from tobacco use or contact with active smokers during the healing process to prevent necrosis.

INSTRUMENTS TO HAVE AVAILABLE

- Standard facial plastic surgical set

SUGGESTED READING

Juri J, Juri C. Advancement and rotation of a large cervicofacial flap for cheek repairs. *Plast Reconstr Surg* 1979;64(5):692–696.

Kroll SS, Reece GP, Robb G, et al. Deep-plane cervicofacial rotation-advancement flap for reconstruction of large cheek defects. *Plast Reconstr Surg* 1994;94(1):88–93.

Menick FJ. Reconstruction of the cheek. *Plast Reconstr Surg* 2001;108(2):496–505.

Moore BA, Wine T, Netterville JL. Cervicofacial and cervicothoracic rotation flaps in head and neck reconstruction. *Head Neck* 2005;27(12):1092–1101.

Austen WG, Parrett BM, Taghinia A, et al. The subcutaneous cervicofacial flap revisited. *Ann Plast Surg* 2009;62(2):149–153.

Boyette JR, Vural E. Cervicofacial advancement-rotation flap in midface reconstruction: forward or reverse? *Otolaryngol Head Neck Surg* 2011;144(2):196–200.

36 MANAGEMENT OF THE CHEEK DEFECT: FREE FLAP RECONSTRUCTION

Douglas B. Chepeha

INTRODUCTION

To prepare for free flap reconstruction of the cheek, a history that involves discussion of the patient's objectives will affect donor site choice. Depending on the patient's body habitus and skin color, different sites will affect the degree that the skin paddle of the transplant will blend with the recipient site. I use the subscapular/thoracodorsal system or the lateral arm as donor sites. Careful assessment of prior surgery, past or future radiation planning, orbital function, ocular function, position of the corner of the mouth, facial nerve function, and depth of the planned defect is important. The cheek consists of three lamellae that, in total, are quite thin; the skin/subcutaneous tissue, the superficial muscle aponeurotic system (SMAS), and the buccinator/buccal mucosa. It is important to address all three lamellae, be sure to maintain the suspension of the corner of the mouth, and support the lower eyelid (Figs. 36.1 and 36.2). For tumors that involve more than one layer and/or perineural invasion is a concern, MRI and CT are an important component of preoperative assessment and planning. When assessing the patient for cheek reconstruction, it is important to consider local tissue. A free tissue transfer should be used for patients who have inadequate local donor tissue, have involvement of at least two lamellae of the cheek, will develop ectropion, or will not be able to maintain the position of the corner of the mouth.

HISTORY

As with any history, the assessment has to take into account prior treatment, the extent of the defect, and the patient's goals relative to what the reconstructive intervention can accomplish. If the patient had a significant radiation or smoking history, the likelihood of a wound complication or late tissue atrophy increases. Therefore, a thicker, higher volume reconstruction may require customization of the flap or choice of an alternative donor site. Prior trauma or surgery to possible donor sites needs to be assessed. It is best to have a primary and secondary donor site discussed with the patient prior to the surgery. It is important to know about prior surgery or trauma to the site to understand the risk to the facial nerve, for example, prior local excision, parotid procedures, local flaps, facelift, facial trauma, or idiopathic facial nerve weakness. It is important to take a history about prior eye surgery or trauma, because this is an adjacent subunit and can be impacted by cheek reconstruction. It is important to support the lower eyelid with the reconstruction. If there is a preexisting ectropion, or the cheek defect extends to the eyelid subunit, an oculoplastics consultation should be considered.

PHYSICAL EXAMINATION

Assessment of the extent of the disease is essential for the surgeon to plan the defect, help prepare for tissue transplantation, and help to educate the patient. In the case of prior trauma, burns, or surgery, the degree of contracture of the involved subunits is important to assess to allow for compensation with skin paddle design.

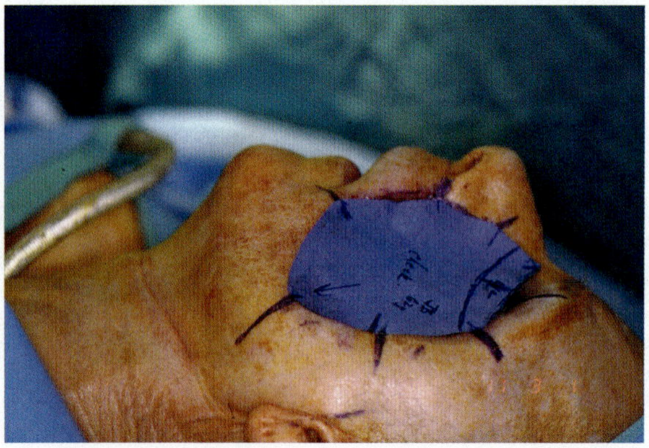

FIGURE 36.1 This is a 62-year-old woman who has undergone resection of a maxillary sinus squamous cell carcinoma (SCC) that involved the cheek subunit. This is an intraoperative view of the left lateral face. The *blue* paper template has been made for the external skin paddle. Eight marks have been placed on the template for transfer to the donor site to facilitate the inset. The defect includes all three lamellae of the cheek. The angle of the mouth requires suspension of the modiolus. The nerve to the upper lip orbicularis oris was stimulated and was felt not to require additional nerve grafting.

The goal of the assessment is to determine the extent and depth of the cheek subunit involvement. Specifically, assessment of the involvement of the adjacent eyelid and nasal subunits, the involvement of the deeper lamellae of the cheek that include the SMAS, the facial nerve, the buccinator muscle, the parotid duct, and the buccal mucosa. Bimanual palpation is helpful to assess the depth of tumor involvement. Intraoral examination of the buccal mucosa is good for assessing the extent of intraoral involvement. Palpation of the infraorbital rim is good for assessing lid mobility and deep extension. Observing the face in repose in addition to eye closure, angle of mouth elevation, and lip closure is useful to determine SMAS or facial nerve involvement. Testing of cheek sensation is useful for determining involvement of the infraorbital nerve.

INDICATIONS

Local flaps such as cervical facial rotation flaps are the reconstruction of first choice for cheek defects. Microsurgical reconstruction of cheek defects is for patients who have inadequate local donor tissue for a local rotational, advancement, or interpolation flaps. These situations arise when there has been extensive tissue loss such as in burns, trauma, or necrotizing fasciitis, in situations where the defect is deep and the essential elements of the SMAS, facial nerve, lower eyelid, and/or the buccal mucosa have been lost. The goals of cheek reconstruction are to prevent ectropion, maintain the position of the corner of the mouth, restore the soft tissue contour of the midface, prevent rotation and contracture of the nose into the reconstructed cheek, and maintain jaw opening by providing adequate intraoral lining.

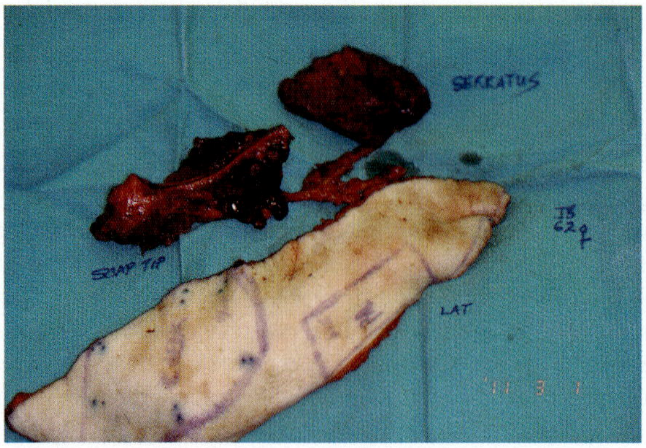

FIGURE 36.2 This is an elevated thoracodorsal artery scapular tip flap (TDAST). Three paddles have been elevated from the donor site. The cheek portion of the skin paddle is shown on the lower left of the image, and the serratus muscle is shown on the upper right of the image. The cheek skin template has been outlined, and the remainder of the skin paddle will be deepithelialized. The additional skin paddle will be used to restore volume and resurface the posterior palate. The bone will be used to restore the malar eminence and orbital rim. The markings on the skin paddle can be seen; these will aid the inset at the recipient site.

CONTRAINDICATIONS

It is important to assess the local tissue options and not immediately move to a microsurgical option. There are few contraindications because patients tolerate cheek reconstruction well. As with any major surgical procedure, patients need adequate preoperative clearance.

PREOPERATIVE PLANNING

Radiology

The need for radiology varies greatly depending on the etiology of the defect, depth of the defect, and prior treatment. For superficial lesions, the need for preoperative imaging is limited. Imaging is important for patients with neoplastic disease extending to the SMAS, who have facial nerve weakness, who have had prior treatment, or whose disease crosses outside the cheek anatomic subunit, to anticipate the extent of the defect. CT scan with contrast is useful for assessment of the fascial planes of the SMAS, buccinator, pterygomandibular raphe, nasal facial groove, and the orbital septum. If there are facial nerve findings that are more extensive than the primary lesion would suggest, then an MRI can be helpful to assess perineural invasion. This would help anticipate the extent of nerve grafting that would be necessary. As with any reconstructive microsurgery case, the recipient artery and vein have to be a part of the reconstructive plan. If the patient had prior neck exploration or dissection, consideration of a CT angiogram to aid in identification of recipient artery can be helpful so that a donor site with adequate pedicle length can be chosen.

For cheek reconstruction, color and contour match are important when choosing the donor site. A patient's body habitus and skin color will affect the choice of donor site. Also, when choosing the adipose tissue used for contouring, it should be from a site that will not become ptotic when inset into the recipient site. For many patients, the lateral arm and the parascapular/latissimus site provide the best color match, are good for contouring, have fewer problems with ptosis, and are my first choice sites. The lateral arm is also a good donor site for nerve grafts, particularly the posterior antebrachial cutaneous nerve (PACN) of the forearm. Despite these advantages, the lateral arm site has a very short, very small-caliber pedicle and will rarely reach past the facial or occipital artery recipient sites and, for this reason, is less commonly used. The parascapular/latissimus donor site has a longer, larger caliber pedicle, has well-compartmentalized adipose tissue, and good skin color match, but the harvest is from the lateral thorax, and this makes the elevation more difficult when the extirpation is being performed. To overcome this, I place the patient in a semidecubitus position for the extirpation and reconstruction.

The most commonly used donor site for cheek defect reconstruction is the anterolateral thigh (ALT) donor site because it has a long, large-caliber pedicle, is easy to harvest during the extirpation of the cheek, and is at least second best for many of the reconstructive challenges of cheek reconstruction. The color match of the ALT is not as good as that of the lateral arm or the parascapular site, but it offers a long pedicle that is particularly valuable for patients who have a "vessel poor" neck. If the ALT donor site is thin, volume issues are easily addressed by elevating a larger skin paddle that can be deepithelialized to obtain adequate volume. The vastus lateralis of the ALT donor site can be used to aid in the reconstruction of intraoral defects; otherwise this donor site is best elevated as a muscle sparing or perforator-based transplant so that the volume is not left distorted by muscle that will eventually atrophy. The rectus abdominis donor site is not commonly used because of poor color match and ptosis. The forearm is useful in thin defects or after tissue expansion prior to transfer. For defects that include the zygomaticus muscles and are extensive, the corner of the mouth needs to be suspended statically or dynamically. The latissimus dorsi muscle sparing flap with a slip of neuromyogenous serratus for suspension of the corner of the mouth is a useful intervention. Decision making with respect to facial reanimation is addressed in other chapters. For extensive cheek and intraoral defects, two skin paddles are required. In these cases, the thickness of the skin paddle has to be considered because the cheek is thin and care has to be taken to choose the donor sites to ensure that the two skin paddles together do not produce an excessively bulky reconstruction.

I perform nerve grafting if the facial nerve branches that supply the orbicularis oris or the zygomaticus muscles are sacrificed. In these cases, the posterior, lateral, or medial antebrachial cutaneous nerve (MACN) of the forearm is used as the donor site because the branching pattern allows for a single proximal anastomosis and multiple distal anastomoses. As mentioned previously, involve oculoplastics if there has been prior surgery on the eyelid or there is concern that the patient will have ectropion postoperatively.

SURGICAL TECHNIQUE

Prior to excision of the cheek defect, a template is fashioned that is the same size as the extirpated tissue. Approximately six to eight tacking sites are marked out around the circumference of the defect and are also transferred to the template for transfer to the donor site. This improves the accuracy and speed of the inset. If there is concern about ectropion, the template can be enlarged in the area of the lower eyelid to help prevent ectropion. The template is traced out on the donor site taking into consideration the axis of the pedicle. The template is helpful because it prevents distortion of the face after inset.

Pincushioning is a problem with cheek reconstructions. To help reduce this late complication, the deep portion of the transplant is pulled past the excision line. This maneuver is accomplished with five to six bolster sutures that are placed around the defect to stretch the deep tissue of the skin paddle into the defect. The 2-0 monofilament nonabsorbable suture is used in a half horizontal mattress technique. This suture is passed through the recipient site skin about 1.5 cm from the edge of the excision, then into the deep adipose tissue of the transplanted skin paddle, and then back out through the skin of the recipient site with about 7 mm of travel from where the suture was initially passed. The two ends of the suture are crossed inside a 10 French bolster, and the ends are tied over the bolster with minimal to moderate tension. This approach is thought to help the deep tissue of the transplant slide under the recipient tissue and minimize dead space in a manner that deep sutures are not entirely able to address. Deep 4-0 interrupted resorbable monofilament suture to the adipose tissue, a second interrupted layer to the subdermal tissue, and a third layer in a subcuticular running technique are also used.

To maintain the position of the mouth, it is important to address the SMAS layer. A determination needs to be made with respect to partial versus total resection of the components of the SMAS that support the angle of the mouth and contribute to oral competence. For the cases where the SMAS is partially resected and critical neuromuscular elements are intact, the cut edges of the muscle or the fascia should be tacked back together with a 4-0 monofilament resorbable suture on a small taper needle. Often, the partially resected SMAS cannot be fully reapproximated without producing facial distortion. In these cases, return the partially resected SMAS to its anatomic position and tack it to adjacent intact SMAS. If there is not adjacent SMAS and there is a gap, then use the suture to bridge the resected tissue without reapproximation. The scar from the underside of the skin paddle of the transplanted tissue will scar to the anatomically positioned SMAS and help maintain the remaining SMAS in anatomic position. If the zygomaticus support to the angle of the mouth is resected, the modiolus needs to be supported statically or dynamically. For patients undergoing autogenous transplantation, fascia can be harvested from an adjacent compartment at the donor site or a dynamic neuromuscular unit can be used to provide suspension, and these techniques are covered in another chapter (Fig. 36.3). When performing oral commissure suspension, the anchorage to the zygoma should be secure; plate and screws should be used if necessary. I suspend in the anatomic position of the zygomaticus and use some minor overcorrection.

Attention to the lower eyelid is important so that the patient does not develop ectropion as a late effect. The skin paddle should be designed with excess skin and subcutaneous tissue pushing the lid superiorly. The skin paddle should be securely tacked into the circumference of the cheek defect before closing the lid site. The first two sutures in the area of the lid should be toward the lateral then medial canthus. This should produce a soft tissue sling under the lower lid. Then the deep portion of the transplanted skin paddle should be tacked to the orbital rim starting centrally in the midpupillary line. To prevent contraction of the lower lid, temporary sutures can be placed in the lower lid and taped to the forehead.

Few patients need the facial nerve grafted because the facial nerve courses deep to the SMAS. As a result, the end organ (SMAS) is resected before the facial nerve is resected. There are exceptions, patients who require nerve resection for perineural invasion or patients who have an intact but denervated orbicularis oris. For these cases, nerve grafting can be of some benefit. My donor site of choice is the arm. The PACN, the

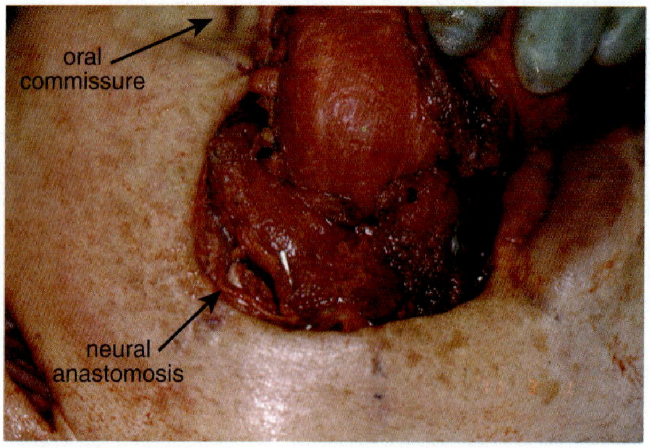

FIGURE 36.3 This is an image of the left lateral face. The right side of the image is cranial, and the left side of the image is caudal. The commissure can be seen at the top of the image. The serratus muscle is seen crossing the defect from the modiolus to the malar eminence to support the commissure, and the neural anastomosis can be seen in the inferior/posterior aspect of the defect. The skin paddle is reflected anteriorly, exposing the deep surface. The thin sheet of latissimus muscle can be seen on the deep surface from the muscle sparing elevation.

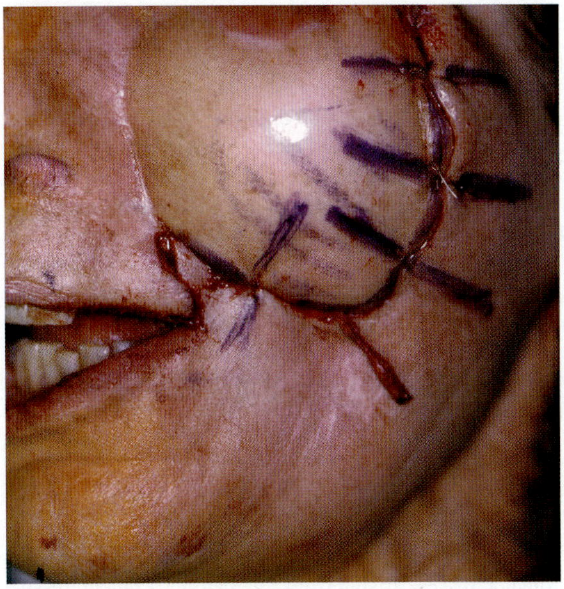

FIGURE 36.4
This image is of the left lateral face. The upper part of the image is cephalic and the lower part of the image is caudal. This is an image from revision surgery 10 months after chemoradiation. There has been atrophy and contracture of the orbicularis oris, and this has reduced lip height. In addition, the lip is longer on the operated side than on the unoperated side. The modiolus is adequately suspended. There is an incision on the lip, and an advancement flap from lateral to medial has been performed along the expected location of the nasolabial crease. The desired result of increasing lip height and decreasing lip length is achieved. In addition, the preauricular cheek skin has been advanced from lateral to medial to reduce the size of the transplanted skin paddle.

MACN, or the lateral antebrachial cutaneous nerves (LACNs) are used. The PACN is harvested when elevating a lateral arm skin paddle for transplant. The nerve fibers are located over the muscle belly of the digastric in Camper' fascia. If the arm is not being used as a free tissue donor site, then a curvilinear incision can be made between the brachioradialis and flexor carpi radialis from a side just distal to the antecubital fossa to approximately two-thirds down the forearm to harvest the MACN or LACN. The incision is made to the depth of Camper fascia, and the MACN nerve can be identified and selected for the appropriate branching pattern. A scalpel is used distally that incorporates the fascia so as not to cause wallerian degeneration in the smaller fibers. The LACN can be identified laterally, coursing with the cephalic vein in Camper fascia. This area can be accessed with a scissor spread toward the cephalic vein where the LACN will be colocated. The LACN tends to be larger and has fewer branches. The nerve anastomosis is performed with an operating microscope and 8-0 nonabsorbable monofilament suture. Three simple sutures are placed. If there is not a clear distal neurovascular bundle, then the nerve is drawn into, for example, the orbicularis oris muscle with a suture and left buried within the muscle belly.

The parotid duct may be excised with the cheek defect. For patients who do not have xerostomia and have a functioning parotid gland, there are two alternatives. The duct can be clipped, and the parotid will undergo involution. If the parotid is a functioning gland, I use a small vein graft to reconstruct the duct. An interrupted suture technique is used with an 8-0 nonabsorbable monofilament suture with the assistance of an operating microscope. If the ampulla was excised, the remaining terminus of the duct can be tacked to the margin of the buccal defect with 6-0 monofilament, nonabsorbable suture using a taper needle (Figs. 36.4 and 36.5).

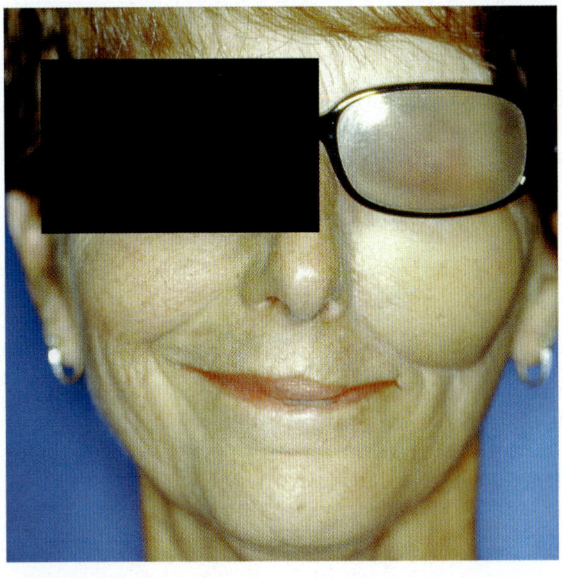

FIGURE 36.5
This is an 18-month posttreatment image. The modiolus is in an acceptable position. The cutaneous portion of the lower lateral cheek skin paddle still needs to be reduced and the skin paddle overall needs some debulking. The overall facial symmetry is good. The nose has not rotated into the defect although the patient will need a nasal spreader graft on the left. Because of concerns about long-term contracture, the nasal ala would not be repositioned for several more years.

POSTOPERATIVE MANAGEMENT

All patients have Silastic suction drains placed in the base of the defect. Drains are removed if drainage is less than 30 mL in a 24-hour period. If there is a buccal defect, a suction drain is placed in a dependent location adjacent to the buccal closure that runs parallel to the pedicle and nerve grafts but does not cross these structures. If the patient has undergone resection of the buccal mucosa with the cheek defect, the patient takes nothing by mouth for the first week if he or she has not undergone prior radiation treatment. For patients who have undergone prior chemoradiation, depending on postoperative healing, a period of 2 to 4 weeks should pass before resuming oral intake. During this time, the patient should undergo oral care that can include three times daily oral irrigation with half and half normal saline and 3% hydrogen peroxide. For compliant patients, brushing of the teeth is desirable to improve oral hygiene. The patient remains in hospital for approximately 6 to 8 days and is seen weekly with speech pathology and nursing during the early postoperative period. Should the free flap dehisce, the area is reapproximated with monofilament suture. Three postoperative doses of antibiotics and deep venous thrombosis (DVT) prophylaxis until the patient is ambulating are routinely administered.

COMPLICATIONS

The most common early complications are hematoma or abscess arising from a hematoma. I am aggressive about taking the patient back to the operating room, irrigating the wound, protecting the nerve grafts if present, and reclosing. To prevent hematoma, I place a face lift dressing or place transbuccal mattress sutures using a 2-0 nonabsorbable monofilament run through 10 French Silastic bolsters.

There are a number of late complications that relate to positioning of the adjacent anatomic subunits such as the lower eyelid, lip, oral commissure, and nasal ala. There can also be complications that relate to the bulk of the transplanted skin paddle or difficulties with color match or pincushioning. In my opinion, the best treatment of these complications is prevention. It is important to try to address the issues of the reconstruction with the initial inset, particularly if the patient has undergone or planned for adjuvant radiation since revision surgery can be difficult. The most important structures to deal with during the initial reconstruction are the lower eyelid, the suspension of the commissure, optimization of the remaining SMAS system, and facial nerve grafting. The late revisions that are easier to manage are reduction of transplanted skin paddle bulk, advancement of local cheek tissue to reduce the surface area of the transplanted skin paddle, and resection of the denervated lip to improve symmetry of the oral commissure.

RESULTS

The results with free flap reconstruction of the cheek are generally excellent. The limitations such as skin color, skin texture, and bulk represent the most significant challenges. Debulking and flap augmentation following the initial healing can result in an excellent functional and aesthetic outcome.

PEARLS

- Choose the donor site that has the best color match and the least chance for ptosis to improve blending of the reconstruction into the face.
- Match the size and shape of the skin paddle to the defect to reduce dysmorphism.
- Stretch the deeper adipose layer into the defect with bolsters to reduce pincushioning.
- Support the lower eyelid to prevent ectropion, to protect the cornea, and to have excess tissue available for any revision which may become necessary.
- Carefully reconstruct the remaining SMAS because very acceptable results can be obtained with careful reconstruction of the local muscle aponeurotic system.

PITFALLS

- Because the position of the corner of the mouth is the most important functional and esthetic consideration, failure to support the oral commissure can result in significant functional and cosmetic deformity.
- In spite of the finest reconstructive techniques, the failure to perform a nerve graft at the time of the initial reconstruction may hinder the achievement of an acceptable reconstructive result.

INSTRUMENTS TO HAVE AVAILABLE

- Major head and neck set
- Marking system for templating the defect
- Ruler to assist in positioning of the oral commissure
- Operating microscope for vessels, nerve, and duct

SUGGESTED READING

Jowett N, Mlynarek AM. Reconstruction of cheek defects: a review of current techniques. *Curr Opin Otolaryngol Head Neck Surg* 2010;18(4):244–254.

Menick FJ. Discussion: simplifying cheek reconstruction: a review of over 400 cases. *Plast Reconstr Surg* 2012;129(6):1300–1303.

Rapstine ED, Knaus WJ II, Thornton JF. Simplifying cheek reconstruction: a review of over 400 cases. *Plast Reconstr Surg* 2012;129(6):1291–1299.

37 RECONSTRUCTION OF THE SCALP: LOCAL FLAPS

Mark K. Wax

INTRODUCTION

There are many options available in the reconstruction of scalp defects, each with its own indications, advantages, and disadvantages. The scalp can be challenging to reconstruct due to the inelasticity and thickness of the tissues. In comparison to the soft tissues of the rest of the head and neck, aging seems to make the tissue of the scalp less elastic and mobile. The ability to primarily reconstruct or entrain tissue from adjacent areas may not be easy. The primary goals of reconstruction of the scalp are to cover exposed bone (preventing desiccation and osteomyelitis), limit distortion of surrounding landmarks (eyebrows, ears, hairline), and provide an acceptable aesthetic outcome. To achieve optimal cosmetic results, significant attention should be paid to preservation of the normal hairline, directionality of hair growth, and well-disguised scars. For all malignant lesions, confirmation of negative margins should be obtained prior to definitive reconstruction and ease of continued surveillance for recurrent tumor should be considered. Reconstruction of the scalp requires a clear understanding of the anatomy and characteristics of the tissue. This will allow for proper preoperative planning and reconstruction.

Layers of the SCALP

The scalp consists of five layers, represented by the SCALP mnemonic. S, skin; C, subcutaneous tissue; A, galea aponeurosis; L, loose connective tissue; and P, pericranium (Fig. 37.1). The scalp is the thickest skin of the body. The skin and connective tissue are firmly adherent to the galea aponeurosis, which makes the skin inelastic. The subcutaneous layer contains the vasculature, nerves, and hair follicles. The galea aponeurosis is the strength layer of the scalp and consists of a thick, inelastic, fibrous sheet spanning between the frontalis muscle anteriorly, the occipitalis muscle posteriorly, and the temporoparietal fascia laterally. The loose connective tissue layer deep to the galea aponeurosis is an avascular plane that allows for mobility of the scalp and is the ideal plane of dissection for elevating flaps. The pericranium is the periosteum of the skull and is tightly adherent to the bone. This layer serves as a well-vascularized bed for skin grafts and can form granulation tissue if allowed to heal by second intention.

Mobility of the SCALP

The scalp is much less mobile than the soft tissue of the face. This makes primary closure and reconstruction with local flaps more difficult in comparison. The tissue laxity differs depending on the location in the scalp. The vertex is the least mobile, while the parietal regions have the greatest mobility. This is important to factor into the reconstructive plan as defects in the parietal region may be amenable to primary closure or local flap reconstruction, while the vertex may require skin grafting, tissue expansion for larger flaps, or free tissue expansion.

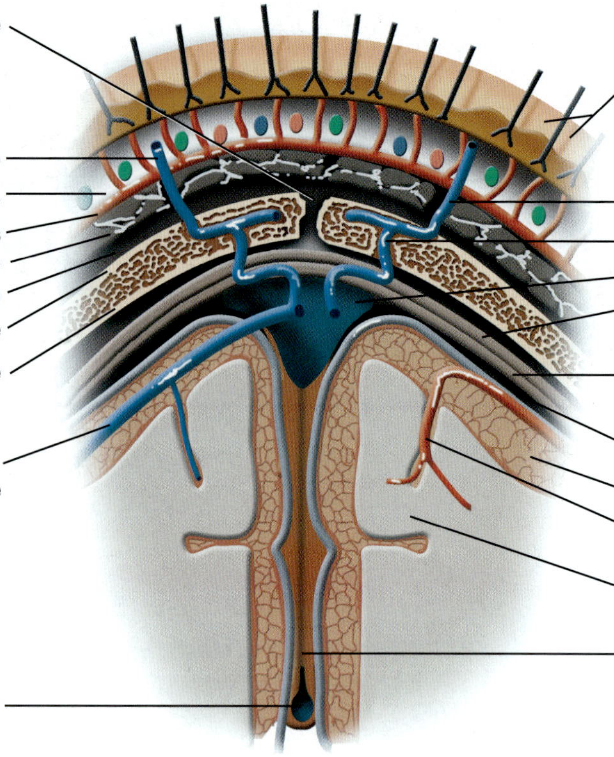

FIGURE 37.1 This schemata demonstrates the five layers of the scalp.

Vasculature of the SCALP

The vasculature of the scalp consists of five paired vessels from both the internal and external carotid arteries that form a rich anastomotic plexus centrally and are located in the deep subcutaneous layer just superficial to the galea aponeurosis. Anteriorly the scalp is perfused by paired supraorbital and supratrochlear arteries. These are the terminal branches of the internal carotid artery as it passes through the orbit. The supraorbital artery passes through the supraorbital notch, while the supratrochlear artery travels through the orbit and pierces the orbital septum in the same vertical plane as the medial edge of the eyebrow. The lateral scalp is perfused by two branches of the external carotid artery, the superficial temporal and postauricular arteries. The superficial temporal artery travels in a vertical direction within the temporoparietal fascia just anterior to the tragus and bifurcates into the frontal branch anteriorly and the parietal branch posteriorly. The posterior scalp is vascularized by paired occipital arteries. The occipital artery pierces the trapezius muscle just superior to the nuchal line and travels in the deep subcutaneous layer until it forms anastomoses with surrounding vessels. The venous drainage of the scalp corresponds to the named arterial vessels and subsequently drains into the common facial, external jugular and internal jugular veins. Understanding the location of these vessels is imperative when designing local and regional flaps as they should be pedicled off one or two vessels to ensure an adequate blood supply to perfuse the distal aspect of the flap.

Nerves of the SCALP

There are eight nerves that supply sensation to the scalp, four anterior to the auricle and four posterior. The nerves supplying sensation to the anterior scalp originate from the trigeminal nerve and include the supraorbital (V1) and supratrochlear nerves (V1) and zygomaticotemporal (V2) and auriculotemporal (V3) nerves. The supraorbital nerve travels with the supraorbital artery through the supraorbital foramen and divides into the superficial and deep branches. The supratrochlear nerve passes above the trochlea and exits the orbit medial to the supraorbital notch. The nerve then pierces the corrugator muscle and the frontalis muscle and travels to supply sensation to the central forehead and medial upper eyelid.

The zygomaticotemporal nerve exits the facial skeleton at the zygomaticotemporal foramen, travels through the temporalis muscle, and pierces the temporalis fascia above the zygomatic arch to innervate the skin of the temple. The auriculotemporal nerve travels through the parenchyma of the superficial parotid gland and exits posteriorly over the zygomatic arch. The nerve then travels superiorly in the temporoparietal fascia to innervate the tragus, anterior portion of the ear, and the posterior temple. The four nerves supplying sensation posterior to the auricle include branches of the cervical plexus, which includes the great auricular (C2 and C3), greater occipital (C2 and C3), lesser occipital (C2), and third occipital (C3). These nerves have been found to communicate freely with one another.

HISTORY

When determining the appropriate method of reconstruction, there are multiple questions that must be asked. A thorough history must be obtained to determine the patient's desires in regards to aesthetic outcomes. It is important to get a full past medical history with specific attention to comorbidities that may delay wound healing, such as diabetes mellitus, chronic immunosuppression, smoking, or the risk of postoperative bleeding from taking anticoagulants, aspirin, or herbal supplements.

An important factor to consider is whether there has been any previous surgery or radiation to the scalp. Many patients will have been previously treated. Either surgery or radiation will affect the ability to use local tissues in the reconstruction. If the defect is a result of the excision of a malignant lesion, the type of cancer, confirmation of negative margins, and risk for recurrence are important to determine prior to reconstruction.

PHYSICAL EXAMINATION

A thorough examination of the head and neck should be performed with a detailed evaluation of the primary defect and surrounding tissue. When evaluating the primary defect, it is necessary to note the characteristics of the defect itself as well as the surrounding tissues. Determining the size and location of the defect and the mobility of surrounding tissue will help to determine if the defect is amenable to primary closure or reconstruction with a local flap. The quality, thickness, presence of hair, and the location of nearby landmarks will dictate what local flap design options are available. The exposure of bone or dura is important to note, and these defects should be reconstructed appropriately to avoid desiccation and infection. A thorough assessment and documentation of facial nerve function is important to note as is sensation to the surrounding tissues. If the defect is secondary to malignancy, the scalp and face should be evaluated for other suspicious lesions, and the parotid glands and neck should be palpated to identify possible metastatic lymph nodes.

INDICATIONS

The indications for reconstruction of the scalp include any defect that cannot be closed primarily. An algorithm is detailed below.

CONTRAINDICATIONS

There are no absolute contraindications to reconstruction of a scalp defect, as all scalp defects should be repaired. An open conversation should be held with the patient and his or her family discussing the goals of the procedure, expected functional and aesthetic outcomes, and risks associated with the procedure.

PREOPERATIVE PLANNING

Methods of reconstruction include many options including healing by secondary intention, skin grafts, primary closure, local tissue flaps, regional tissue flaps, and free tissue transfer. There are limitations and advantages to each technique, and careful consideration is needed to determine the ideal method for reconstruction, based on the size and location of the defect and the patient's desires and ability to tolerate extensive surgery. In general, the simplest technique that gives the desired functional and cosmetic outcomes should be chosen.

SURGICAL TECHNIQUE

Second Intention

With this method, the wound is covered with a nonadherent dressing and allowed to slowly granulate. It is important to have vascularized tissue upon which granulation tissue will grow. Ideally, bone is covered with a minimum of pericranium. If bone is exposed and lacking pericranium coverage, then the outer cortex of the skull can be drilled down to the diploic space that will provide a vascular bed for granulation tissue to form. A second option is to cover the exposed bone with a pericranial or temporoparietal tissue flap, based on a vascular pedicle. The primary advantage of this technique is the quickness of the procedure. Disadvantages of secondary intention are the prolonged period of time while the wound is granulating. With large defects, it can take months of local wound care until the area is healed. Frequent use of ancillary personal is required to assist in the care of the wound. Alopecia of the healed wound and relative thin skin make the area susceptible to trauma. Frequent wound breakdown is common and bothersome to the patient. The area must be protected from any trauma.

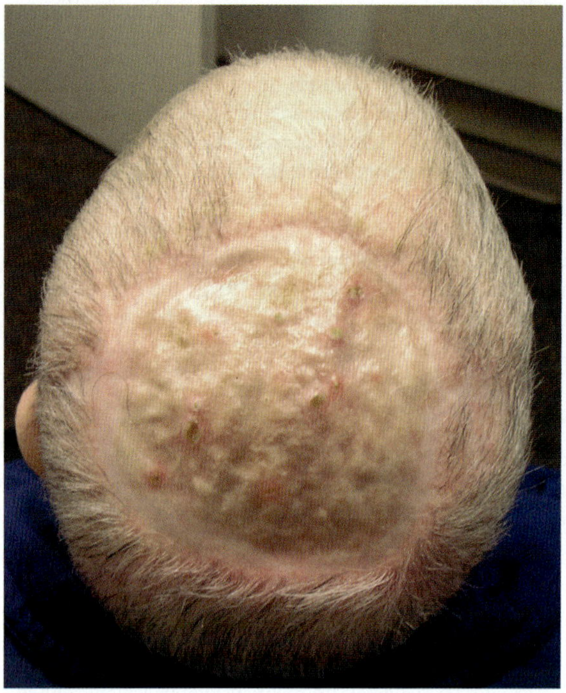

FIGURE 37.2
This patient had a large area of the scalp resected with reconstruction with a split-thickness skin graft. The graft has healed well and can be seen to be quite thin. The areas of redness are local areas that have broken down due to trauma. These will heal, but inevitably other areas will break down.

Split-/Full-Thickness Skin Grafts

Split-thickness and full-thickness skin grafts are options for closing a wide range of scalp defects. These grafts must be placed onto a bed of well-vascularized tissue, which includes periosteum, granulation tissue after delay in closure, mobilized pericranial or musculofascial flaps, or after drilling off the outer cortex of the skull. It is important to remember that this is not an acceptable reconstructive option if radiation therapy has been given or is planned postoperatively. The negative aspects of skin grafts include alopecia, insensate skin, risk for ulceration or breakdown with mild trauma, poor color match, and often a depressed and an undesirable aesthetic outcome (Fig. 37.2).

Primary Closure

These defects are typically transformed to an elliptical shape with the long axis perpendicular to the plane of maximum laxity, and wide undermining is required in the subgaleal plane. Typically, this option is used for defects less than 4 cm in diameter. If the defect is near the anterior hairline, an M-plasty may be performed to prevent exposed incisions into the non–hair-bearing areas. When possible, this method is simple and typically gives the best cosmetic outcome with similar tissue and proper directionality of hair follicles. This method should not be used if significant tension must be applied to close the wound.

Local Flaps

Local tissue transfer from surrounding skin is a major method of scalp reconstruction for small to medium-sized defects. This technique can offer both excellent function and aesthetic outcomes when primary closure is not possible. This follows the principle of "replace tissue with like tissue." Tissue flaps should be properly designed to minimize tension on the wound closure, maintain blood flow, and create ideal aesthetic outcomes. Local flaps can be used to reconstruct defects measuring up to approximately 50 cm^2. When local flaps are used together with split-thickness skin grafts, it has been reported that large defects up to 150 cm^2 can be reliably closed. The skin grafted defects are then reconstructed with secondary procedures after the wound has healed. When reconstructing larger defects, it is important to create a tissue flap with a wide base that is dependent on one or more major arteries. The handheld Doppler probe can help to identify the course of the vascular pedicles of these flaps.

Advancement Flaps

Advancement flaps are mobilized by sliding the elevated flap in one direction toward the primary defect. This is done best with areas of redundant skin or increased elasticity. The surrounding tissue is undermined in order to close the defect and decrease tension on the wound closure. The subgaleal loose connective tissue plane on the scalp allows for easy, avascular undermining. The site of greatest tension is the distal edge of the skin flap.

There are multiple types of advancement flaps: Unipedicle, bipedicle, V to Y, Y to V, and island. This method of closure is ideal for reconstruction of small scalp defects in patients with mobile scalp tissue. For large scalp defects, advancement flaps are suboptimal due to the lack of elasticity of the scalp.

Pivotal Flaps

Pivotal flaps are the most frequently used type of scalp reconstruction. These are moved toward the primary defect by pivoting around a fixed point at the base of the skin pedicle. There are multiple types of pivotal flaps for the scalp: Rotation, transposition, and interpolated flaps. It is better to close a moderately sized scalp defect with multiple rotation flaps (2 to 3) rather than just one. Multiple flaps decrease the size of each individual flap, as they will all share in providing tissue to cover the defect. Closure of the secondary defects may be easier as they will not be as large if multiple flaps are used. With all pivotal flaps, a standing cutaneous deformity will be present at the base of the skin pedicle after it is rotated into place. Caution should be used when deciding to excise the standing cutaneous deformities to keep from narrowing the base and compromising the blood supply. Often the standing cutaneous deformity can be left in place as it will flatten out with time and offer an acceptable cosmetic appearance without further excision (Fig. 37.3A–C). The flap is usually elevated in a subgaleal plane. Once enough scalp has been elevated to allow for closure, the wound is closed in two layers. I use a 3-0 suture that lasts 1 to 2 months for the deep layer and a fast-absorbing suture for the skin. Drains are not needed as the scalp lies on the bone of the skull and collections of fluid are rare.

Rotation Flaps

Rotation flaps have a curvilinear configuration and are designed so that the flap is placed immediately adjacent to the defect. Often the primary defect is modified to a triangular shape to aid with inset of the flap. The

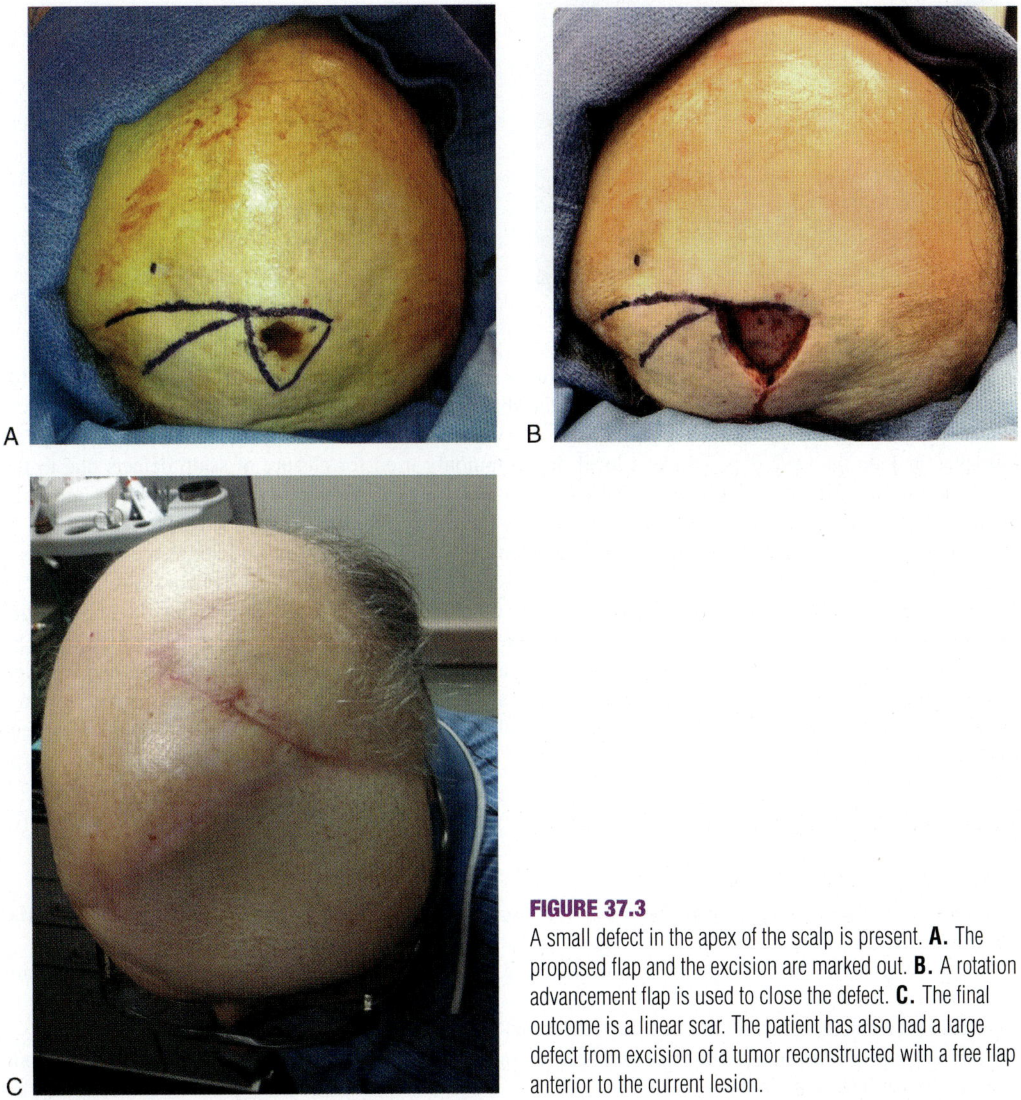

FIGURE 37.3
A small defect in the apex of the scalp is present. **A.** The proposed flap and the excision are marked out. **B.** A rotation advancement flap is used to close the defect. **C.** The final outcome is a linear scar. The patient has also had a large defect from excision of a tumor reconstructed with a free flap anterior to the current lesion.

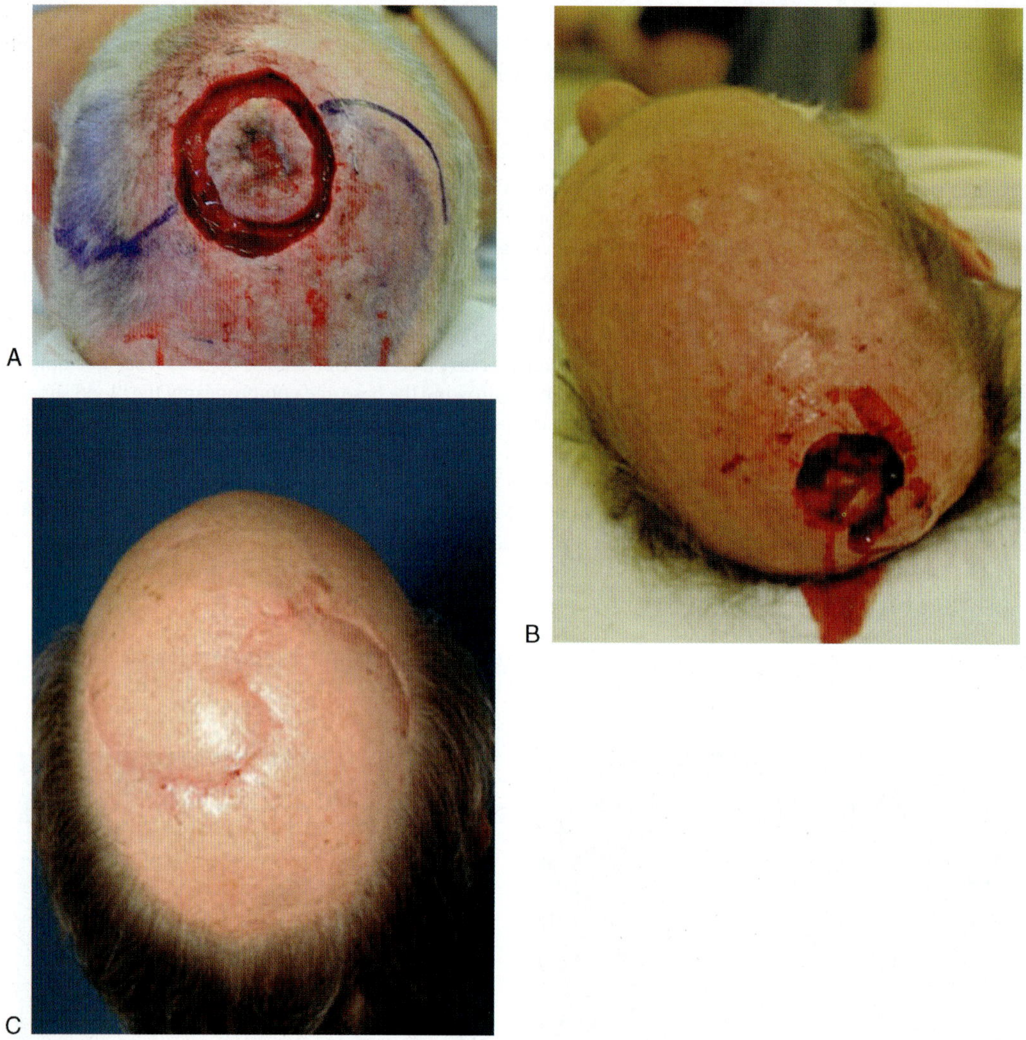

FIGURE 37.4
A. The defect here is circular and is to be closed with two curvilinear advancement/rotation flaps. **B.** The flaps have been elevated and rotated to meet in the middle of the defect. **C.** The end result is a curvilinear scar that is straight in the middle.

proposed length of the rotation flap should be four times the width of the primary defect (4:1). This is great for closure of scalp defects given the convex shape of the skull and the inelastic nature of the galea aponeurosis.

Examples include the O–T flap. This is a local flap commonly used for closure of scalp defects due to the simple design and reliability. This technique entails bilateral curvilinear rotation flaps rotated around individual pivot points. Using more than one rotational flap allows for a decrease in the length of the incision as tissue laxity is recruited from opposite sides of the defect. The primary defect is modified to a circular defect. In the **O–T** configuration, the flaps are rotated in opposite directions, and the final incisions resemble a "T" (Fig. 37.4A–C). The **O–Z** configuration is designed for rotation in the same direction so that the final closure resembles a "Z." This is also referred to a "yin yang" flap due to the appearance of the initial flap design. The flap is usually elevated in a subgaleal plane. The wound is closed in two layers in all of these flaps once enough scalp has been elevated to allow for closure. I use a 3-0 suture that lasts 1 to 2 months for the deep layer and a fast-absorbing suture for the skin. Drains are not needed as the scalp lies on the bone of the skull and collections of fluid are rare.

Algorithm for Surgical Management

Defects of the Anterior Scalp:

- Careful attention should be given to reconstruction of the anterior scalp to minimize distortion of the hairline.
- Defects involving both the scalp and forehead should be reconstructed as two separate defects to maintain the hairline.
- For bald patients, incisions should be oriented parallel to, and when possible, within existing rhytides.
- When designing rotational flaps, orient secondary dog-ears toward the parietal and occipital scalp regions where they will be less obvious.

Options for Managing Small Defects (<2 cm^2)

- Primary closure

Options for Managing Moderate-Sized Defects (2 to 25 cm^2)

- Local flaps
  - Along hairline: advancement flap or rotation flap
  - Hair-bearing scalp: O to Z flap

Options for Managing Large-Sized Defects (>25 cm^2)

- Temporoparietal occipital flap to recreate anterior hairline
- Non–hair-bearing scalp: large rotation advancement flap based on occipital artery ± skin grafting to close donor site.

Options for Managing Extreme-Sized Defects (>50 cm^2)

- Orticochea flap
- Free flap

Defects of the Parietal Scalp

Defects in this region are the easiest to close primarily due to the mobility of the scalp in this region.

Options for Managing Small-Sized Defects (<2 cm^2)

- Primary closure

Moderate-Sized Defects (2 to 25 cm^2)

- Local flaps
  - Rotation or advancement flaps (All dog-ears should be positioned posteriorly where they are less noticeable)

Options for Managing Large-Sized Defects (>25 cm^2)

- Orticochea flaps may be difficult to design in this region to allow adequate coverage. Consider skin grafts with secondary reconstruction and tissue expansion.

Options for Managing Extreme-Sized Defects (>50 cm^2)

- Free flap

Defects of the Occipital Scalp:

Defects in this region of the scalp are less noticeable and can be easily camouflaged with longer hair.

Options for Managing Small-Sized Defects (<2 cm^2)

- Primary closure

Options for Managing Moderate-Sized Defects (2 to 25 cm^2)

- Local flaps
  - Rotational flaps/advancement flaps
    - Dissection and undermining can be carried over the trapezius and splenius capitis muscles to allow for increased tissue mobility.

Options for Managing Large-Sized Defects (>25 cm^2)

- Orticochea flap
- Regional flaps: trapezius myocutaneous or pedicled latissimus dorsi myocutaneous flap

Options for Managing Extreme-Sized Defects (>50 cm^2)

- Orticochea flap
- Microvascular free flap

Defects of the Vertex:

There is limited mobility of the vertex of the scalp and primary closure may not be possible for even small defects. Wide undermining and galeatomies are often needed to recruit sufficient skin laxity from surrounding tissue.

Options for Managing Small-Sized Defects (<2 cm^2)

- Primary closure
- Pinwheel rotational flaps
  - This can recreate the natural spiral hair growth pattern that occurs at the vertex

Options for Managing Moderate-Sized Defects (2–25 cm^2)

- Local flaps
  - O to Z rotational flaps

Options for Managing Large-Sized Defects (>25 cm^2)

- Large rotation advancement flap based on occipital artery ± skin grafting to close donor site.

Options for Managing Extreme-Sized Defects (>50 cm^2)

- Free flap

POSTOPERATIVE MANAGEMENT

The primary goal of postoperative care is to promote proper healing and survival of the flap or skin graft. Common complications include hematoma, infection, wound dehiscence, loss of flap or graft, poor flap design, and unwanted scarring. Prevention of postoperative bleeding and hematoma begins in the operating room with adequate hemostasis. Hematomas are most common in the first 48 hours after surgery. In scalp reconstruction, these are very rare.

All skin grafts should have a secure pressure dressing to prevent shearing or hematoma formation under the graft, which will lead to necrosis. To prevent infection, adherence to sterile technique during the procedure is imperative.

Excess tension on skin incisions should be avoided to prevent wound dehiscence and excess scarring. Careful wound monitoring by the patient or family is important, and any change in appearance or delayed healing should be reported to the surgeon. The patient and family should be educated regarding the expected healing process, proper wound care, and potential complications.

COMPLICATIONS

Complications range from wound breakdown to flap tissue necrosis. Complications are generally rare and most can be managed with debridement and local wound care.

RESULTS

The results with each of the techniques reviewed herein are generally excellent. I find that each of the techniques requires a proficiency that is gained through experience, but the results in most patients are excellent.

PEARLS

- The reconstructive method should be tailored to the patient's needs.
- Adequate injection of local anesthesia with epinephrine should be used to help to provide hemostasis and may assist with hydrodissection.
- Dissection is to be performed in the subgaleal layer. Avoid trauma to hair follicles in the subcutaneous layer.
- Large flaps should be based on one to two arterial perforators to ensure adequate perfusion.
- Scalp incisions should be closed in two layers.

PITFALLS

- Alopecia and scarring may result from excess tension on the wound closure.
- Mechanical creep and galeatomies will help to decrease wound closure tension.
- Avoid excision of dog-ears until after scalp has healed. When possible, place dog-ears on the posterior aspect of the scalp where they are less noticeable

INSTRUMENTS TO HAVE AVAILABLE:

- Head and neck surgical tray
- Hemostatic scalp clips

SUGGESTED READING

Orticochea M. New three-flap reconstruction technique. *Br J Plast Surg* 1971;24(2):184–188.

Vecchione TR, Griffith L. Closure of scalp defects by using multiple flaps in a pinwheel design. *Plast Reconstr Surg* 1978;62(1):74–77.

Frodel JL Jr, Ahlstrom K. Reconstruction of complex scalp defects: the "Banana Peel" revisited. *Arch Facial Plast Surg* 2004;6(1):54–60.

Kruse-Lösler B, Presser D, Meyer U, et al. Reconstruction of large defects on the scalp and forehead as an interdisciplinary challenge: experience in the management of 39 cases. *Eur J Surg Oncol* 2006;32(9):1006–1014.

Mehrara BJ, Disa JJ, Pusic A. Scalp reconstruction. *J Surg Oncol* 2006;94(6):504–508.

38 RECONSTRUCTION OF SCALP DEFECT: LATISSIMUS DORSI FREE FLAP

Keith E. Blackwell

INTRODUCTION

Multiple factors need to be considered when selecting a technique for reconstruction of defects of the scalp. As it is a hair-bearing region, aesthetic considerations favor reconstruction using local hair-bearing tissues whenever possible. The frontal, parietal, and occipital scalp offer considerable soft tissue laxity that facilitates repair by means of primary closure and local flaps when compared to defects arising at the vertex of the scalp, where there is less soft tissue laxity. At the vertex, wide subgaleal undermining, galeal relaxing incisions, and tissue creep allow for primary closure of defects as wide as 5 cm. Local rotation, advancement, and transposition flaps are useful for reconstruction of larger defects. Defects of up to 50 cm^2 at the vertex of the scalp can be reconstructed using bilateral laterally based advancement flaps combined with a posteriorly based rotational flap.

If a scalp defect has intact periosteum, the wound can be left open to heal by secondary intention or a skin graft can be used on the periosteum, and the rigid nature of the underlying calvarium helps to prevent distortion of the wound by scar contraction. Biologic dressings such as Integra and wound vacuums can be applied in cases in which the periosteum is absent to promote formation of granulation tissue and thereby facilitate healing by second intention or skin grafting. These methods, however, will result in compromised aesthetic results due to alopecia, cavity of the wound, and unpredictable pigmentation of the healed wound.

Wound repair by primary closure and local flaps may be impossible or ill-advised in cases when prior therapies using surgery and radiation therapy make local tissues unreliable for reconstruction of defects that otherwise might be repaired using local tissues. Unfortunately, this is a common situation, with one prior large series of scalp reconstructions reporting that 65% of patients had undergone prior scalp surgery and 44% of patients had undergone prior radiation therapy. Among patients undergoing microvascular flap reconstruction of the scalp, Van Driel et al. reported prior scalp reconstructive surgery in 80% of patients and prior scalp radiation in 50% of patients.

Associated defects of the calvarium and dura need to be carefully considered when thinking through options for reconstruction of scalp defects. Attempting to repair a wound under tension using local tissues over an alloplastic cranioplasty or in a patient with a dural repair carries a high risk of wound dehiscence that can result in cranioplasty extrusion and/or cerebrospinal fluid leak. In cases where local tissues cannot reliably be used for reconstruction of defects of the temporal and occipital scalp, the inferior island trapezius flap has proven to be a reliable method of reconstruction. However, when the defect involves the parietal or frontal scalp, free tissue transfer is often needed when local tissues prove to be inadequate, as the arc of rotation provided by regional flaps is insufficient to reach defects that extend to the vertex of the scalp or to the forehead.

While radial forearm flaps, rectus abdominis flaps, anterolateral thigh flaps, and omental flaps are also useful for scalp reconstruction, many series have reported that latissimus dorsi flaps are the most commonly used free flaps for reconstruction of scalp defects (Table 38.1). The latissimus dorsi free flap offers many desirable attributes for scalp reconstruction, including a large volume of soft tissue that can be combined with other subscapular system flap components for reconstruction of very large or complex defects, a long vascular pedicle that usually can reach recipient vessels without using vein grafts, and limited long-term flap donor site morbidity.

TABLE 38.1 Use of Latissimus Dorsi Flaps and Incidence of Complete Free Flap Necrosis in Series of Scalp Reconstructions that Relied Predominantly on Latissimus Dorsi Free Flaps

Series	O'Connell et al. 2011	Oh et al. 2011	Tseng et al. 2009	Van Driel et al. 2010	Ioannides et al. 1999	McCombe et al. 2002	Wang et al. 2007
Number of free flaps	68	18	71	84	31	32	24
Number (%)	46	11	45	38	25	13	9
Total flap necrosis	0%	0%	1.5%	6.0%	3.2%	6.3%	0%

General Concepts

The latissimus dorsi flap can be used as a myofascial flap or as a myocutaneous flap for reconstruction of scalp defects (Fig. 38.1). It is critically important to consider the nature of the scalp defect when planning the design of a latissimus dorsi flap for scalp reconstruction, as the nature of the defects of the scalp skin, calvarium, and dura all have a significant impact on flap design. For soft tissue defects of the scalp where there is not a full-thickness defect of the calvarium, a myofascial flap combined with a skin graft often results in the best possible aesthetic reconstruction (Fig. 38.2). As they are harvested from a sun-protected donor site, myocutaneous latissimus dorsi flap often are pale in color, so they result in a poor color match for native scalp skin, especially when used in the common situation of patients with scalp skin cancers, who invariably have significant chronic actinic damage to their scalp skin. In addition, the flank skin is very thick, and the skin paddle of a latissimus dorsi myocutaneous flap is often too bulky to restore an appropriate scalp contour. This often results in a pin-cushioned appearing scalp reconstruction (Fig. 38.3). As a broad, thin muscle that will undergo postoperative denervation atrophy when inset over the rigid infrastructure of an intact calvarium, latissimus dorsi myofascial flaps often produce superior aesthetic results with regard to the thickness and contour of the resulting scalp reconstruction, and the color match of a skin-grafted myofascial flap is often superior to that achieved using a latissimus dorsi myocutaneous flap.

In situations where there is a scalp skin defect occurring in conjunction with a full-thickness defect of the calvarium, a latissimus dorsi myocutaneous flap may be the best option. In this situation, the increased thickness of the flap helps to camouflage contour defects of the skull in patients who have small calvarial defects. Many patients with larger defects of the calvarium will undergo cranioplasty reconstruction using nonvascularized bone grafts or alloplastic materials. In this situation, scalp reconstruction using a myofascial flap is ill-advised, as there will be a risk of cranioplasty extrusion after a myofascial flap becomes very thin due to postoperative denervation atrophy. The risk of cranioplasty extrusion may be reduced in patients with thick myocutaneous flap reconstructions, although the aesthetics of the resulting reconstruction are usually compromised.

Myocutaneous flaps may be preferred for reconstruction of scalp defects that occur in conjunction with defects of the dura. This is the case because it is difficult to achieve a watertight closure of the scalp skin defect when using a myofascial latissimus dorsi flap that is resurfaced with a skin graft, thereby increasing the risk of a postoperative cerebrospinal fluid leak that can lead to meningitis. In this situation, the use of a myocutaneous latissimus dorsi flap may lessen the risk of cerebrospinal fluid leak by allowing for a watertight scalp wound closure, thereby increasing the safety of the reconstruction at the expense of the aesthetic results.

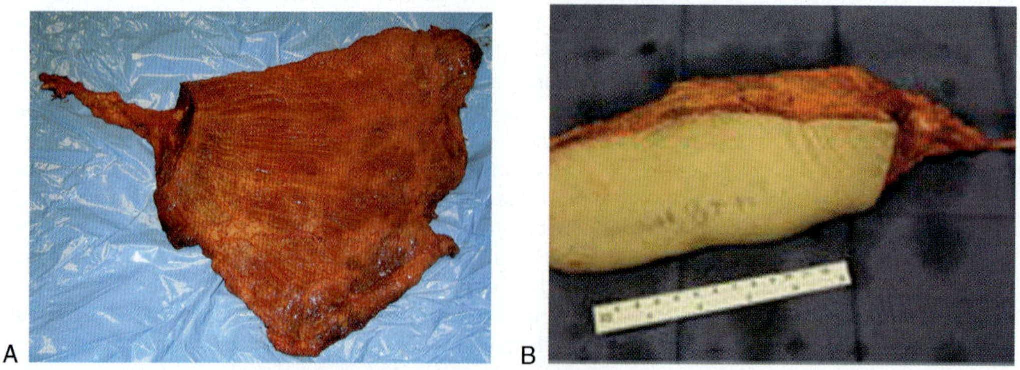

FIGURE 38.1
A. Latissimus dorsi myofascial flap. **B.** Latissimus dorsi myocutaneous flap.

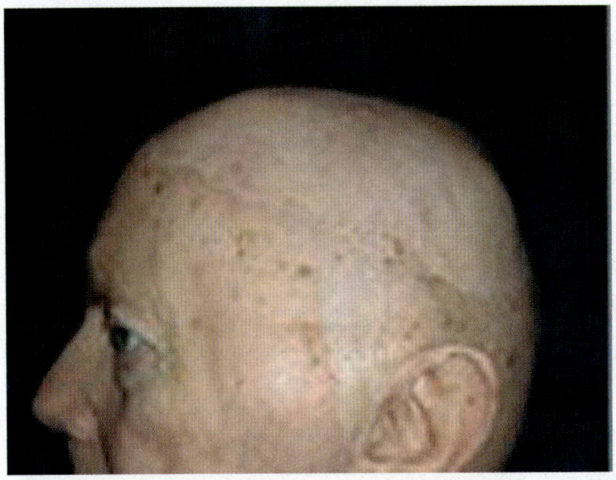

FIGURE 38.2
Two-year postoperative appearance of scalp reconstruction using latissimus dorsi myofascial flap with meshed split-thickness skin graft.

Multiple other flap components that are perfused by the subscapular vascular pedicle are available for transfer with the latissimus dorsi muscle in patients with large or complex defects of the scalp. When the soft tissue defect of the scalp is larger than what can reliably be resurfaced using a latissimus dorsi flap, additional soft tissue components can be incorporated, including the serratus anterior muscle that is perfused by the serratus anterior branch of the thoracodorsal artery, and the parascapular and scapular fasciocutaneous flaps that are perfused by the circumflex scapular artery. Using these additional soft tissue components, even near-total defects of the scalp can be reconstructed using a single subscapular system "megaflap" (Fig. 38.4). Osseous reconstruction of the calvarium can be accomplished using vascularized ribs, which are perfused either by the serratus anterior branch of the thoracodorsal artery or by the perforating branches from the intercostal blood vessels. In addition, a vascularized graft of the lateral border of the scapula and scapular tip can be transferred based upon the circumflex scapular vessels or the angular branch of the thoracodorsal vessels. Vascularized thoracolumbar or serratus anterior fascia can be used for reconstruction of associated defects of the dura.

Identification of the borders of the latissimus dorsi muscle is usually a straightforward endeavor using visible and palpable landmarks. The latissimus dorsi muscle is a broad thin muscle that covers most of the lower back from the inferior tip of the scapula to the iliac crest (Fig. 38.5). The anterior border of the latissimus dorsi muscle is an important landmark that is usually identified early during the flap harvest procedure and is a key landmark with regard to identifying the flap's vascular pedicle. The anterior border of the latissimus dorsi muscle can be palpated in thin patients by asking patients to press their hands against their hips. The location of the anterior border of the latissimus dorsi muscle can also be estimated drawing a line from the humerus in an inferior direction toward the ipsilateral iliac crest at approximately the midaxillary line.

HISTORY

With regard to the patient's history, because free tissue transfer provides the advantage of transferring well-vascularized tissue to a recipient site, the condition of the recipient site is important. Any history of prior radiation may impede healing. This should be elicited in the history to prepare the patient for the potential for wound healing problems. A history of prior surgery or trauma to the donor site(s) may eliminate the use of this flap.

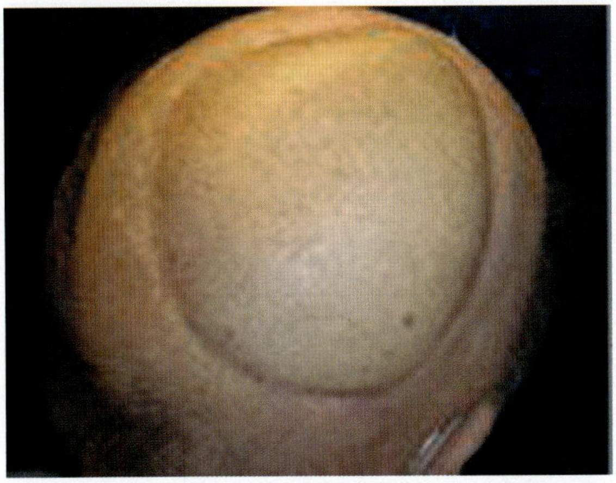

FIGURE 38.3
Five-year postoperative appearance of scalp reconstruction using latissimus dorsi myocutaneous flap with duraplasty and titanium mesh cranioplasty.

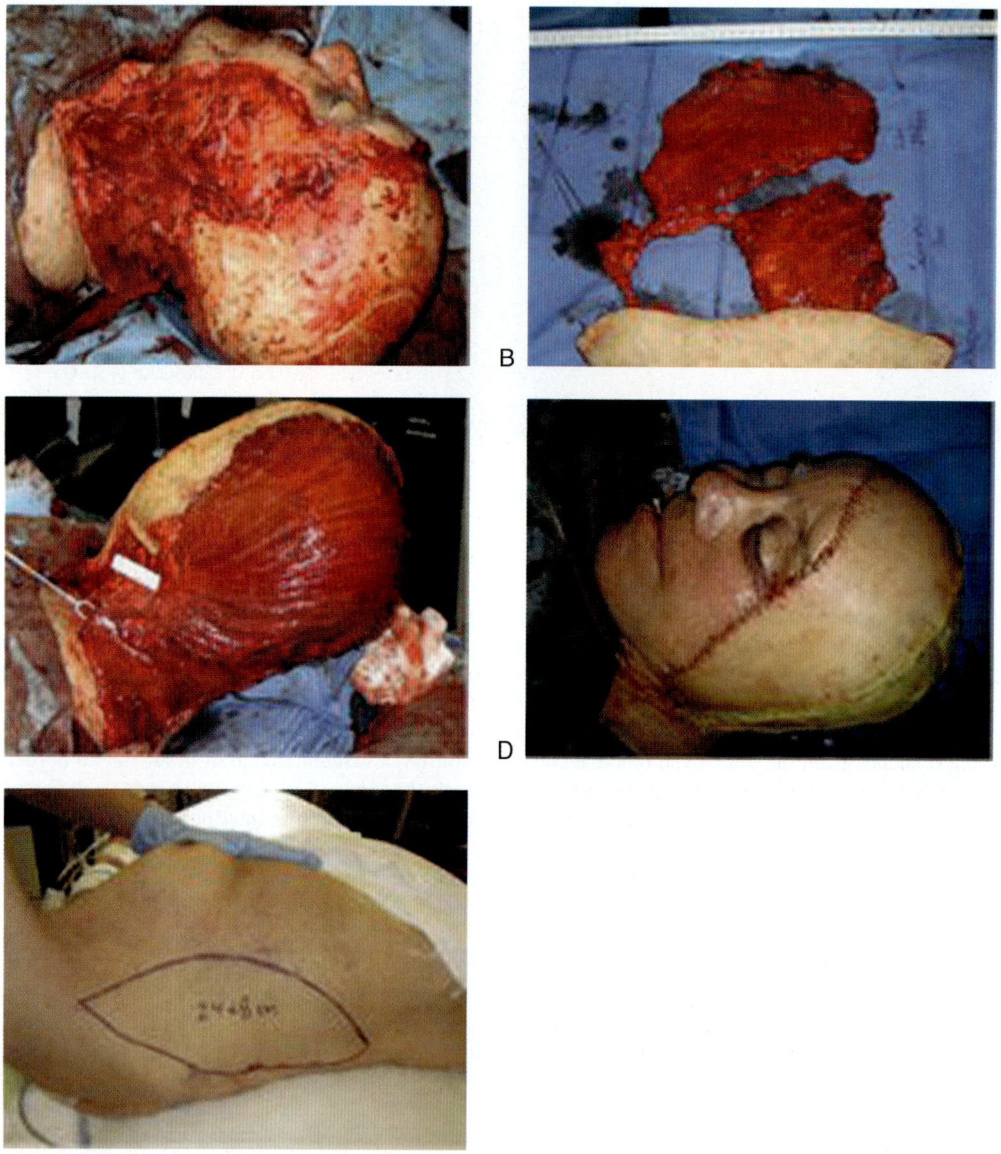

A B C D E

FIGURE 38.4 **A.** Defect of the left cheek, forehead, and subtotal resection of scalp sparing only the right temporal scalp after excision of angiosarcoma. **B.** A latissimus dorsi myofascial—serratus anterior myofascial—parascapular fasciocutaneous flap allows for single-flap reconstruction of this large defect. **C.** The latissimus dorsi myofascial—serratus anterior myofascial flap components are used to resurface temporal, parietal, and occipital calvarium. **D.** The parascapular fasciocutaneous flap component is used to resurface the cheek and forehead defect. **E.** The myofascial flaps have been covered with a meshed split-thickness skin graft.

PHYSICAL EXAMINATION

The physical examination should include an examination of the recipient site and the donor site. In many cases, the patient will have sustained the scalp defect as a result of excision of skin cancer. It is important to assess both sites for skin cancers that may have been missed or incompletely excised. The condition of the recipient site should also be evaluated to anticipate the potential for wound healing complications. The donor site must be examined to rule out previous trauma or surgery in this tissue.

INDICATIONS

Latissimus dorsi free flaps are indicated for reconstruction of scalp defects that cannot reliably be reconstructed using local tissues, skin grafts, or regional flaps. As previously discussed, this indication varies according to the size of the defect in different regions of the scalp as determined by laxity of the scalp tissue, the location of the defect with regard to the utility of regional flaps as determined by their arc of rotation,

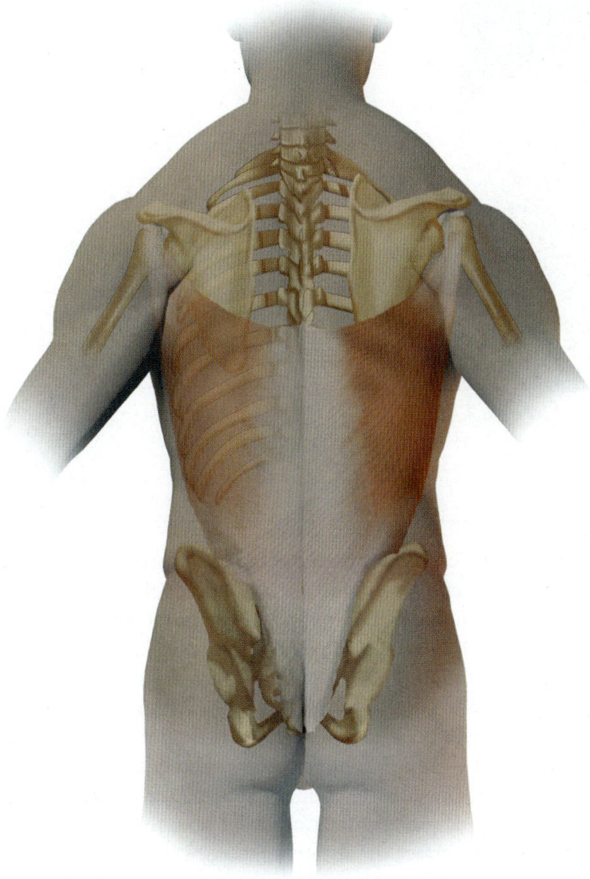

FIGURE 38.5
The latissimus dorsi muscle. The latissimus dorsi muscle is a broad thin muscle that covers most of the lower back from the inferior tip of the scapula to the iliac crest.

prior therapies that affect the reliability of local and regional flaps, and the nature of associated defects of the calvarium and dura.

CONTRAINDICATIONS

Prior surgeries that might have adversely affected the integrity of the thoracodorsal vascular pedicle need to be recognized. In this regard, the most common prior surgeries to consider include prior axillary lymph node dissection and prior thoracotomy. In these patients, preoperative flap angiography or an alternative flap donor site should be considered. In addition, use of a large skin paddle can produce a restrictive pulmonary defect caused by tight primary closure of the flank skin after latissimus dorsi flap harvest, so large myocutaneous flaps should be used with caution in patients with limited pulmonary reserve. In this situation, the flap donor site can be repaired with a skin graft, but skin graft healing is notoriously slow due to a shearing effect on the skin graft caused by respiratory motion of the flap donor site.

PREOPERATIVE PLANNING

The magnitude of the defect and nature of associated defects of the calvarium and dura need to be considered in planning to use a myofascial or myocutaneous latissimus dorsi flap and when considering the need to incorporate other osseous and soft tissue components that are perfused by branches of the subscapular blood vessels.

Patient positioning should be planned to allow for simultaneous two-team surgery at the flap donor site and in the head and neck whenever possible. Subscapular system flaps that incorporate the latissimus dorsi muscle and overlying flank skin, the serratus anterior muscle, the parascapular fasciocutaneous flap, and vascularized ribs can be harvested with the patient in a supine position, with slight elevation of the ipsilateral shoulder, or with the patient in a full decubitus position, thereby allowing simultaneous two-team surgery in all cases that require scalp reconstruction (Fig. 38.6). Flaps that include the lateral border of the scapula bone or the scapular fasciocutaneous skin paddle usually require intraoperative positioning in a full lateral decubitus position, with the patient's position supported by a beanbag. This patient positioning may still allow simultaneous two-team surgery in patients with pathologies of the posterior or lateral scalp.

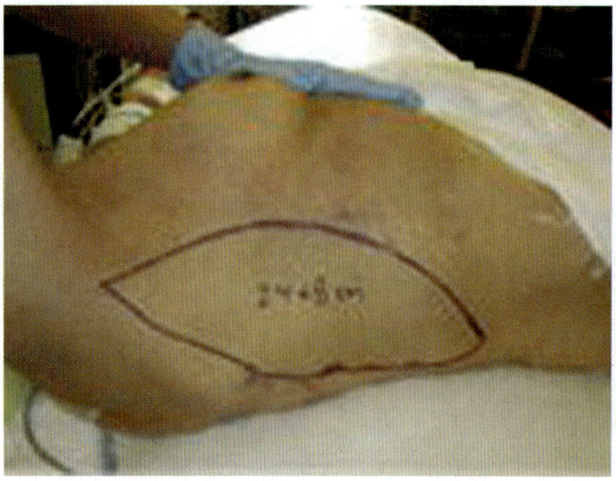

FIGURE 38.6
It is a common misconception that lateral decubitus positioning is necessary to harvest free flaps based upon the subscapular vascular pedicle. Flaps that are perfused by the thoracodorsal vessels including the latissimus dorsi and serratus anterior muscles are easily harvested with patients positioned in a supine position.

SURGICAL TECHNIQUE

Instruct the anesthesiologist and nurses not to place arterial or intravenous lines in the upper extremity on the side of the flap donor site, as this upper extremity will be prepped and draped into the field so that the arm position can be adjusted during flap harvest. Place a beanbag on the operating room table even if it is anticipated that flap harvest will be done in the supine position. This will allow for lateral decubitus repositioning if necessary. If flap harvest is done in the supine position, place an armrest on the operating room table on the side of the flap donor site. This supports the arm and shoulder position to prevent a traction injury to the brachial plexus.

While endoscopic flap harvest has been described, myofascial latissimus dorsi flaps are more often harvested using an open technique. A longitudinal incision that is placed along the anterior border of the latissimus dorsi muscle is made, and the anterior border of the latissimus dorsi muscle is exposed. The anterior border of the latissimus dorsi muscle is elevated off the underlying serratus anterior muscle and rolled posteriorly. The thoracodorsal vascular pedicle is identified on the deep surface of the latissimus dorsi muscle, about 4 cm posterior to the anterior border of the latissimus dorsi muscle. The vascular pedicle enters into the hilum of the latissimus dorsi muscle at a distance of about 12 cm inferior to the insertion of the latissimus dorsi muscle into the humerus. The vascular pedicle is then traced superiorly through the axilla up to the takeoff of the subscapular vessels from the axillary vessels. During this dissection, branches of the vascular pedicle including the serratus anterior branch, the angular branch, branches to teres major muscle, and the circumflex scapular vessels are encountered. These side branches of the vascular pedicle are ligated unless they are supplying additional osseous or soft tissue flap components that are to be incorporated into the flap for reconstruction of large or complex defects. Flap harvest is then completed by elevating the superficial surface of the latissimus dorsi muscle from the overlying flank skin and then detaching the insertions of the latissimus dorsi muscle from the ilium inferiorly, from the vertebrae posteriorly, and from the humerus superiorly.

When a myocutaneous flap is needed, an oval flap skin paddle is often designed overlying the anterior border of the latissimus dorsi muscle. The width of the flap skin paddle is determined by the width of the scalp skin defect and also by pinching the flank skin to determine how much flank skin can be removed while allowing for primary closure of the flank donor site wound. The amount of flank skin that can be removed while allowing for primary closure of the resulting flank skin defect usually varies from 8 to 10 cm in width. In cases where a myocutaneous flap is needed but the width of scalp defect exceeds 8 to 10 cm, a wider flap skin paddle can be harvested, but skin graft reconstruction of the flank donor site with possible delayed healing for the flap donor site should be anticipated. The length of the flap skin paddle is determined by the length of the scalp skin defect and the distance of the scalp defect from the recipient vessels that will perfuse the free flap. Skin paddles that are centered only over the middle and inferior thirds of the latissimus dorsi muscle are prone to experience distal marginal skin paddle necrosis, so in all cases, the skin paddle should be designed to incorporate skin that is overlying the superior third of the latissimus dorsi muscle, where cutaneous perforators to the skin paddle are plentiful. In cases where the defect cross the vertex of the scalp and the flap recipient vessels are located in the neck, the most proximal portion of the flap skin paddle is either deepithelialized or incorporated into a preauricular or postauricular incision to enhance perfusion to the most distal aspect of the skin paddle.

The scalp defect should be widely undermined in a subgaleal plane before latissimus dorsi flap insetting, and the peripheral edges of the latissimus dorsi muscle should be tacked to the galea or pericranium at least a few centimeters away from the skin edges of the scalp defect. A second layer of flap insetting is then done from the edges of the scalp skin defect to the superficial myofascial component or to the skin paddle of the flap so that the scalp skin overlaps the myofascial component that has been inset to the periosteum or galea (Fig. 38.7). This two-layer overlapping flap insetting reduces the risk of a wound dehiscence that might result in calvarial or cranioplasty exposure, and the risk of cerebrospinal fluid leak is reduced in cases where there is an associated defect of the dura.

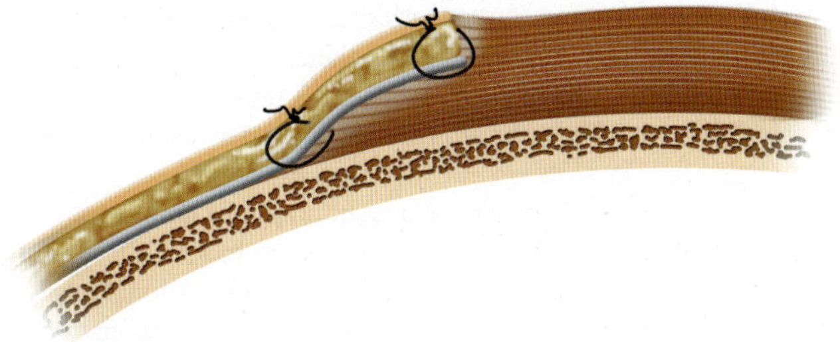

FIGURE 38.7
A two-layer, overlapping "vest-over-pants" flap insetting reduces the risk of scalp wound dehiscence that can lead to exposed cranium, exposed cranioplasty, or cerebrospinal fluid leak.

Superficial temporal blood vessels can be used to perfuse the flap if they are of suitable caliber to match the vascular pedicle of the flap. In many patients, the superficial temporal artery at the level of the root of the zygomatic arch is of suitable caliber to match the caliber of the subscapular or thoracodorsal artery, but the caliber and quality of the superficial temporal vein is more variable and will usually determine whether the superficial temporal vessels can be used as recipient vessels. When the superficial temporal vessels prove to be unsuitable, then recipient vessels in the upper neck are used to perfuse the flap, and the flap's vascular pedicle is passed through a preauricular or postauricular subcutaneous tunnel, or the vascular pedicle can be brought through the cheek wound if a parotidectomy has been done in conjunction with removal of regional lymph nodes. In most cases, the vascular pedicle of the flap is long enough to reach recipient blood vessels in the upper neck without the need to extend the length of the vascular pedicle using vein grafts.

POSTOPERATIVE MANAGEMENT

Flaps should be monitored for postoperative vascular compromise. My preference is to monitor flaps using transcutaneous Doppler stethoscope assessment of the flap's arterial inflow, with the Doppler checks being done by the nursing staff on an hourly basis that is equal to the postoperative day number. In addition, myocutaneous flaps are monitored by observation of the color and turgor of the flap's skin paddle. I have observed an incidence of free flap failure of less than 1% with this postoperative flap monitoring protocol.

Skin-grafted myofascial flaps are covered with a Xeroform dressing that is stapled to the wound edges at the conclusion of surgery. This dressing is moisturized with Bacitracin ointment on a twice a day basis to prevent it from drying. The Xeroform dressing that is placed at the time of surgery is removed 5 to 7 days after surgery, and daily Xeroform dressing changes are then instituted until the skin-grafted muscle as fully epithelialized. A regimen of daily scalp wound care for 4 to 8 weeks after surgery is often needed in patients who have myofascial flaps resurfaced with split-thickness skin grafts (Fig. 38.8).

In cases where there is no defect of the dura, the scalp wound is drained with a subgaleal 10-mm flat Jackson-Pratt drain that is positioned so that it does not compress the flap's vascular pedicle. When a dural defect is present, the scalp wound is not drained in order to lessen the risk of cerebrospinal fluid leak.

Prolonged high-output drainage from the flank donor site is common, and indwelling flank closed suction drains are sometimes needed for a long as 3 weeks after surgery to prevent seroma formation at the flank donor site. As length of hospitalization in patients who have uncomplicated recoveries after surgery is frequently 5 to 7 days, hospital discharge with an indwelling flank drain is necessary in some patients. Lipa and Butler proposed application of an aerosolized fibrin sealant to the flap donor site to reduce the risk of prolong flank wound drainage.

Myocutaneous latissimus dorsi free flaps often result in a bulky-appearing reconstruction that may benefit from a revision procedure to improve the contour of the flap. However, care must be taken to try to preserve

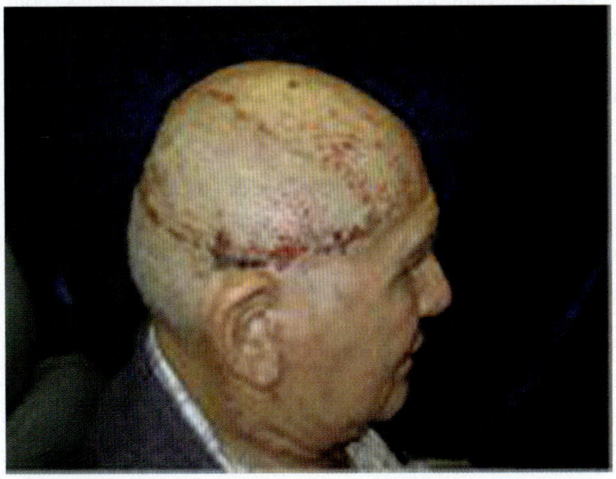

FIGURE 38.8
Two-week postoperative appearance of a scalp reconstruction using a latissimus dorsi myofascial flap with a meshed split-thickness skin graft. Full epithelialization of the meshed skin graft frequently takes 4 to 8 weeks.

the integrity of the flap's vascular pedicle during secondary revision surgeries, as neovascularization of the flap may be very slow and incomplete with large volume flaps, especially when there is a history of radiation therapy. I have treated a patient who suffered near-total necrosis of a latissimus dorsi myocutaneous flap that was used for scalp reconstruction when flap debulking done 9 months after free flap transfer resulted in injury to the flap's vascular pedicle.

Reconstructed hair-bearing regions of the scalp will suffer from alopecia after latissimus dorsi flap reconstruction. Small to moderate areas of alopecia in patients who have not had radiation can be successfully managed by tissue expansion of adjacent hair-bearing scalp or by follicular unit hair transplantation. However, many patients who undergo resection of advanced skin cancers of the scalp that require free flap reconstruction also undergo wide-field scalp radiation therapy, which makes them poor candidates to undergo tissue expansion, and there is frequently little hair-bearing scalp tissue left to serve as a follicular unit transplant donor site after the completion of surgery and radiation therapy. In these patients, camouflaging the defect with a wig or hat is often the best option for management of the resulting alopecia.

COMPLICATIONS

Free Flap Failure

Like any microvascular free tissue transfer, complete free flap necrosis can occur, usually during the early postoperative period and usually secondary to thrombosis of the flap's vascular pedicle.

Scalp Wound Dehiscence

Scalp wound dehiscence is a serious complication that can result in exposure of the calvarium, cranioplasty exposure, and/or cerebrospinal fluid leak. Small dehiscences can often be managed using local wound care, but large or complicated dehiscences may need more complex revision surgery, including a second free flap in some cases.

Flap Donor Site Morbidity

The shoulder and upper extremity position needs to be supported during latissimus dorsi flap harvest in order to avoid a traction injury to the brachial plexus. The long-term donor site morbidity after harvest of a latissimus dorsi flap is often quite acceptable. Litung and Peck reported that shoulder disability after latissimus dorsi flap harvest diminishes with time, and most patients regain a normal shoulder range of motion and report no occupational limitations or interference with sporting activities. However, Russell et al. reported frequent change in occupation, household activities, and sporting activities after latissimus dorsi flap harvest.

RESULTS

The risk of complete flap necrosis in series of microvascular flap reconstruction of the scalp that relied predominantly on latissimus dorsi flaps ranges from 0% to 6% (Table 38.1). Recipient blood vessel selection reported in some of these series is summarized in Table 38.2. The incidence of vein grafts that were needed to lengthen the vascular pedicle varied from 3% to 7%. Van Driel et al. reported a significantly increased incidence of scalp wound healing complications including partial and total flap necrosis in patients who needed vein grafts.

O'Connell reported five cases of scalp wound dehiscence among 68 free flap scalp reconstructions. Four healed by secondary intention, but one patient with a major dehiscence required a second free flap. Afifi et al. reported scalp wound dehiscence in 5 of 13 cases of microvascular flap reconstruction of the scalp in patients who underwent free flap reconstruction of the scalp in conjunction with cranioplasty. Those authors concluded

TABLE 38.2 Recipient Vessels Used to Perfuse Free Flaps in Series of Scalp Reconstructions that Relied Predominantly on Latissimus Dorsi Free Flaps

Series	O'Connell et al. 2011	Tseng et al. 2009	Van Driel et al. 2010
Superficial temporal recipient vessels	0%	18%	60%
Cervical recipient vessels	100%	72%	40%

that primary cranioplasty using acrylic implants should be avoided in patients who have contaminated surgical wounds. Lipa and Butler advocated a two-layer overlapping "vest-over-pants" flap insetting to reduce the risk of scalp wound dehiscence.

O'Connell reported that myofascial latissimus dorsi flaps used in conjunction with skin grafts were the most useful method for free flap reconstruction of scalp defects, being used in 86% of cases. Oh et al. reported increased patient satisfaction with regard to durability and well-fitting wigs in patients who underwent scalp reconstruction with skin-grafted myofascial latissimus dorsi free flaps. Van Driel reported improved color match, contour, overall aesthetic result in patients with skin-grafted muscle flaps versus fasciocutaneous flaps, although this difference in outcome did not reach statistical significance.

PEARLS

- Latissimus dorsi flaps are the most common type of free flap used for microvascular flap reconstruction of scalp defects.
- Myofascial latissimus dorsi flaps that are resurfaced with a skin graft provide the optimal aesthetic result of reconstruction.
- Myocutaneous latissimus dorsi flaps may be indicated in cases of alloplastic cranioplasty reconstruction to reduce the risk of cranioplasty extrusion.
- Myocutaneous latissimus dorsi flaps may be indicated in cases where there is a defect of the dura to lessen the risk of cerebrospinal fluid leak.
- Latissimus dorsi flaps can be combined with other soft tissue and osseous flaps that are also perfused by the subscapular vascular pedicle to allow for single-flap reconstruction of very large or complex defects of the scalp.
- The long thoracodorsal vascular pedicle usually reaches superficial temporal or cervical recipient blood vessels without the need to perform a vein graft.
- Latissimus dorsi flaps are very reliable for reconstruction of scalp wounds, and long-term donor site morbidity is frequently acceptable.
- When harvesting a large volume latissimus dorsi flap, leave the humeral insertion of the latissimus dorsi muscle attached to the humerus until the flap is ready to be moved up to the scalp defect.
- In patients in whom a skin graft is needed in conjunction with a myofascial flap, it is my preference to design a myocutaneous flap with an elliptical skin paddle that has a width of approximately 7 cm overlying the anterior border of the latissimus dorsi muscle. A dermatome is used to harvest a split-thickness skin graft from the flap skin paddle at the beginning of the flap harvest, and the resulting deepithelialized flap skin paddle is subsequently excised and discarded. The resulting 7-cm-wide flank donor site wound is closed primarily in a tension-free closure, and skin graft donor site morbidity is thereby avoided since the skin graft donor site is excised and discarded. Skin grafts are expanded using a 3:1 skin graft mesher to cover large scalp skin defects. Nonmeshed skin grafts are often used for reconstruction of smaller defects to avoid a fish net stocking appearance of the healed skin graft, and additional split-thickness skin grafts are harvested from the thigh as needed (Fig. 38.9).
- At the beginning of the flap insetting, the latissimus dorsi muscle tendon that was detached from the humerus should be tacked down to deep fascia in the cheek or upper neck in a position where the geometry of the flap's vascular pedicle relative to the recipient vessels is suitable for microvascular anastomosis. This will prevent the vascular pedicle from retracting superiorly and becoming too short for anastomosis during flap insetting.

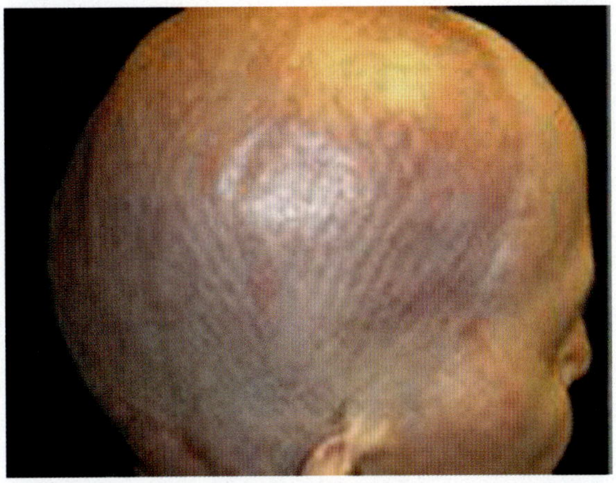

FIGURE 38.9
Nine-month postoperative appearance of a scalp reconstruction using a latissimus dorsi myofascial flap combined with a meshed split-thickness skin graft. The meshed split-thickness skin graft has a fish net stocking appearance, so nonmeshed skin grafts should be used in patients who do not plan on wearing a wig or a hat.

PITFALLS

- Large-volume latissimus dorsi flaps that are commonly used to reconstruct large scalp defects are very heavy. The weight of the flap can cause a traction or avulsion injury to the flap's vascular pedicle after the flap harvest dissection is completed but before the flap is transferred to the scalp defect.
- Myofascial latissimus dorsi flap often require large skin grafts for restoration of an epithelial surface. This can create additional donor site morbidity at the skin graft harvest site.
- During flap insetting into the scalp wound, there is a tendency for the latissimus dorsi muscle to contract and become foreshortened, which pulls the flap's vascular pedicle superiorly and can adversely affect vessel geometry for microvascular anastomosis.

INSTRUMENTS TO HAVE AVAILABLE

- Standard head and neck surgical set
- A rib tray including Doyen periosteal dissectors
- Reciprocating and oscillating saws
- Monopolar and bipolar electrocauteries
- Hemoclips
- Dermatome
- Utrasonic shears (Harmonic Focus, Ethicon Endo-Surgery, Cincinnati, OH)

SUGGESTED READING

Cho BC, Lee JH, Ramasastry SS, et al. Free latissimus dorsi muscle transfer using an endoscopic technique. *Ann Plast Surg* 1997;38:586–593.

Frodel JL Jr, Ahlstrom K. Reconstruction of complex scalp defects: the "Banana Peel" revisited. *Arch Facial Plast Surg* 2004;6:54–60.

Hierner R, Van Loon J, Goffin J. Free latissimus dorsi flap transfer for subtotal scalp and cranium defect reconstruction: report of 7 cases. *Microsurgery* 2007;27:425–428.

Blackwell KE, Rawnsley JR. Aesthetic considerations in scalp reconstruction. *Facial Plast Surg* 2008;24:11–21.

Afifi A, Djohan RS, Hammert W, et al. Lessons learned reconstructing complex scalp defects using free flaps and a cranioplasty in one stage. *J Craniofac Surg* 2010;21(4):1205–1209.

39 RECONSTRUCTION OF THE LATERAL SKIN DEFECT

Frederic W.-B. Deleyiannis

INTRODUCTION

Defects of the skin involving the lateral neck and/or scalp present a challenge to the reconstructive surgeon that begins with addressing the question of whether the expected defect can be treated in a staged, reconstructive approach or whether an immediate, single-stage reconstruction is the primary priority. Staged reconstruction often provides the optimal method of reconstruction since tissue expansion can be used to expand regional flaps/tissue to replace the missing skin or scalp with similar, regional tissue. When acute coverage is needed, skin grafts and regional flaps are available depending on the site of the defect, the available blood supply, and the underlying structures that are exposed after the resection such as exposed bone, periosteum, and the great vessels. Free flaps, in particular the anterolateral thigh free flap, are often the first choice for large defects of the lateral neck (Fig. 39.1). This chapter focuses on the selection of regional flaps, particularly combined with tissue expansion, for the reconstruction of lateral neck and scalp defects. The morbidity of regional flaps is also considered, especially in regard to the creation of donor site scars (i.e., alopecia) and donor defects. The potential complications associated with tissue expansion are also discussed.

HISTORY

The majority of defects involving loss of the skin of the neck or scalp are usually the result of the resection of cancers of the skin, trauma, or burns. For cancer of the skin, reconstruction is initiated once surgical margins are clear. This often can be accomplished in a delayed manner, such as within a few days after Mohs surgery, or more immediately in the operating room after frozen sections are negative. Traumatic loss of the scalp, unless the underlying dura is exposed, should be reconstructed with the goals of minimizing the number of scalp incisions, creating a stable wound that will allow eventual expansion of the scalp tissue, and placing any incisions necessary for acute coverage so that they do not interfere with the blood supply of regional flaps (Fig. 39.2) or the secondary placement of tissue expanders. Prior radiation therapy to the surgical field can negatively affect local wound healing. Thus, in addition to understanding the TNM stage of the cancer, the surgeon should obtain the history of any previous treatment with radiation therapy and anticipate the possible need for postoperative radiation therapy.

PHYSICAL EXAMINATION

The physical examination should focus on defining the extent of the defect. The following questions should be addressed:

- What are the expected dimensions (i.e., surface area and volume) of the defect?
- What critical underlying structure will be exposed (i.e., bone, periosteum, vessels, facial nerve)?

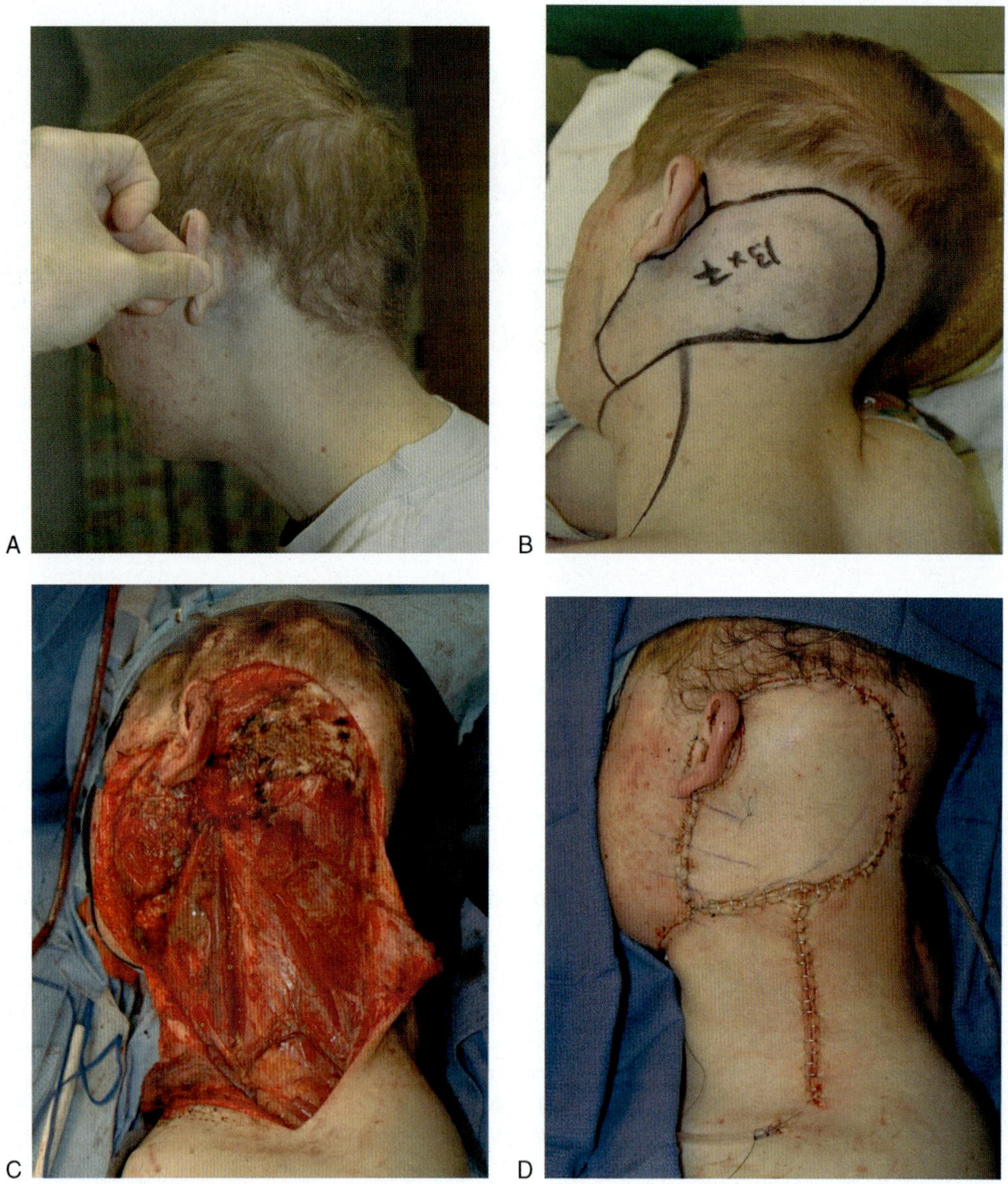

FIGURE 39.1 Lateral neck reconstruction with an anterolateral thigh free flap. **A.** A 17-year-old male with melanoma. **B.** Planned skin resection. **C.** Resection. **D.** Reconstruction with anterolateral free flap.

- What regional blood supply will remain after the resection (i.e., what identifiable arteries will be resected, such as the superficial temporal, supraorbital, facial artery) that would support regional flaps?
- Will a neck dissection be needed, and if so, where will the incisions for the neck dissection be placed so that they do not interfere with flap design?

INDICATIONS

The indications for reconstruction of the lateral neck defect are any defect that cannot be closed primarily or where the risk of skin breakdown and great vessel exposure is significant.

CONTRAINDICATIONS

Free tissue transfer is often a better choice for reconstruction if the surgical site has received prior radiation. Comorbidities, such as severe cardiovascular or peripheral vascular disease, may guide one to choose a regional flap instead of a microvascular flap. Transposing or rotating regional flaps that have been previously in an irradiated field likely place the reconstruction at risk for wound dehiscence. In a similar manner, if a surgical extirpative site is expected to receive postoperative radiation therapy, regional flaps or free flaps

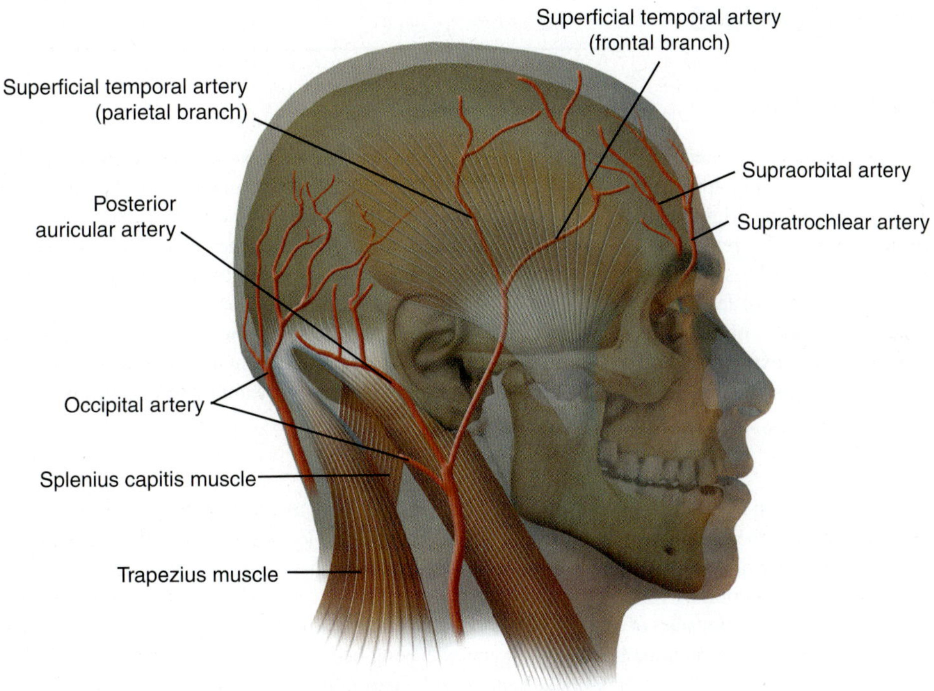

FIGURE 39.2 Regional blood supply for scalp reconstruction. Scalp flaps should be designed to capture regional axial blood supply in their base. Optimal, secondary reconstruction usually requires tissue expansion.

(vs. the use of skin graft) likely reduce the risk of osteoradionecrosis since the bone is being covered with well-vascularized tissue.

PREOPERATIVE PLANNING

Once the extent of the expected defect has been anticipated and defined, preoperative planning now involves determining the various ways to reconstruct the defect with an understanding of the respective requirements, advantages, and disadvantages of each method (Table 39.1). Whether the defect is caused by a malignant lesion (i.e., cancer of the skin), a benign lesion (i.e., nevus), or a traumatic injury will also affect the choice of reconstruction. Methods of reconstruction will include staged excisions, adjacent tissue transfer (i.e., rotation–advancement flaps with a random blood supply), regional flaps, regional flaps combined with tissue expansion, and free flaps. To ensure the greatest vascularity, one should design the chosen regional flap so that its base contains a regional artery. This can be confirmed with a Doppler examination if there is any doubt about the regional blood supply.

TABLE 39.1 Methods of Reconstruction

Reconstruction	Requirements	Advantages	Disadvantages
• Staged excision	Benign lesion	All incisions (i.e., scars) within area of lesion	Multiple surgeries
• Split-thickness skin graft	Vascularized bed	Simplicity, large supply of skin	Poor regional color and texture match, contracture
• Regional flaps	Flap based on named regional artery	Similar tissue replacing missing tissue	Possible donor defect, possible limited ability to rotate into defect
• Tissue expansion	Staged surgery	Expansion of regional tissue to allow the design of larger regional flaps	Two additional operations (one for TE replacement and one for removal and flap advancement)
• Free flaps	Microvascular expertise	Multiple flap options to reconstruct most defects	Technically demanding, lengthy operations

SURGICAL TECHNIQUE

Staged Excisions

Staged excisions are most suited for large benign lesions, usually congenital nevi, of the neck or scalp. The first surgery involves removing approximately 60% to 80% of the original lesion and placing the entire excision within the borders of the original lesion. For lesions of the neck, one should try to place the final orientation of the scar in a natural skin crease (Fig. 39.3). After the first surgery, some spreading of the scar can be expected.

The advantages of a staged excision should be compared to the possibility of doing tissue expansion. Many staged excisions of lesions of the scalp will be associated with some scar alopecia at the closure site. Thus, tissue expansion is often offered as an additional way to remove the lesion with the possibility of less scar spreading. However, expansion requires approximately 2 to 3 months between surgeries while the expander is being inflated, and some patients either do not want or cannot make weekly appointments for expansions.

Skin Grafts

Skin graft reconstruction of the neck or lateral scalp is usually done only as a temporizing measure. Skin grafts are placed acutely with the goal of creating a healed wound but with the long-term expectation that they will be removed and replaced with local tissue (Fig. 39.4). Grafts are usually harvested as split-thickness grafts with an approximate thickness of 0.014 inch in adults. In children, grafts are thinner with thicknesses that ranging from 0.008 to 0.014 inch. Because of the similar color match, the scalp is an excellent source of skin grafts for the face or neck. Skin grafts must be placed on an underlying bed of well-vascularized tissue. Periosteum will support a split-thickness skin graft. Cranial bone must be partially decorticated to allow granulation prior

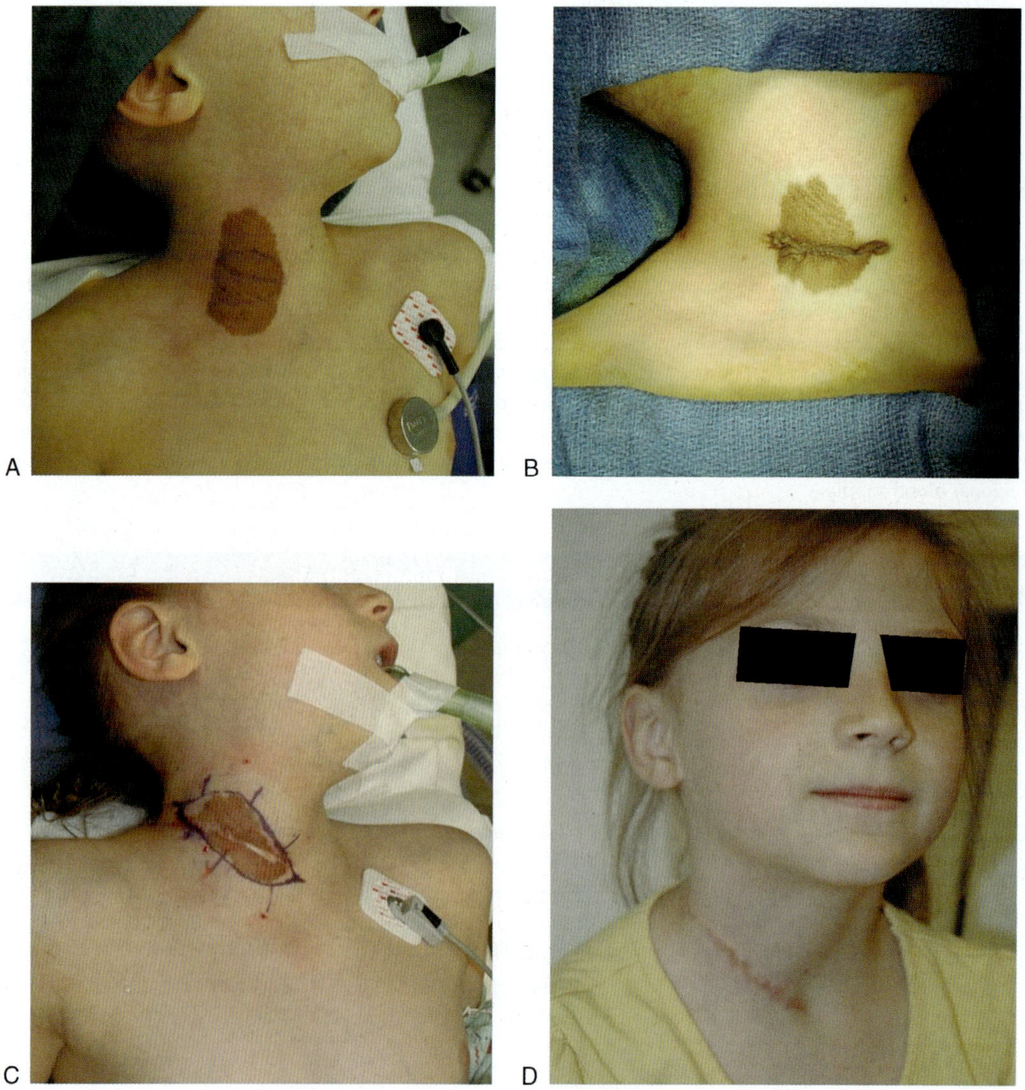

A B C D

FIGURE 39.3
Staged neck excision. **A.** Vertically oriented nevus to be excised in stages. The goal is to place the final closure in a natural skin crease. **B.** First stage. **C.** Six months after first stage. **D.** One month after second stage.

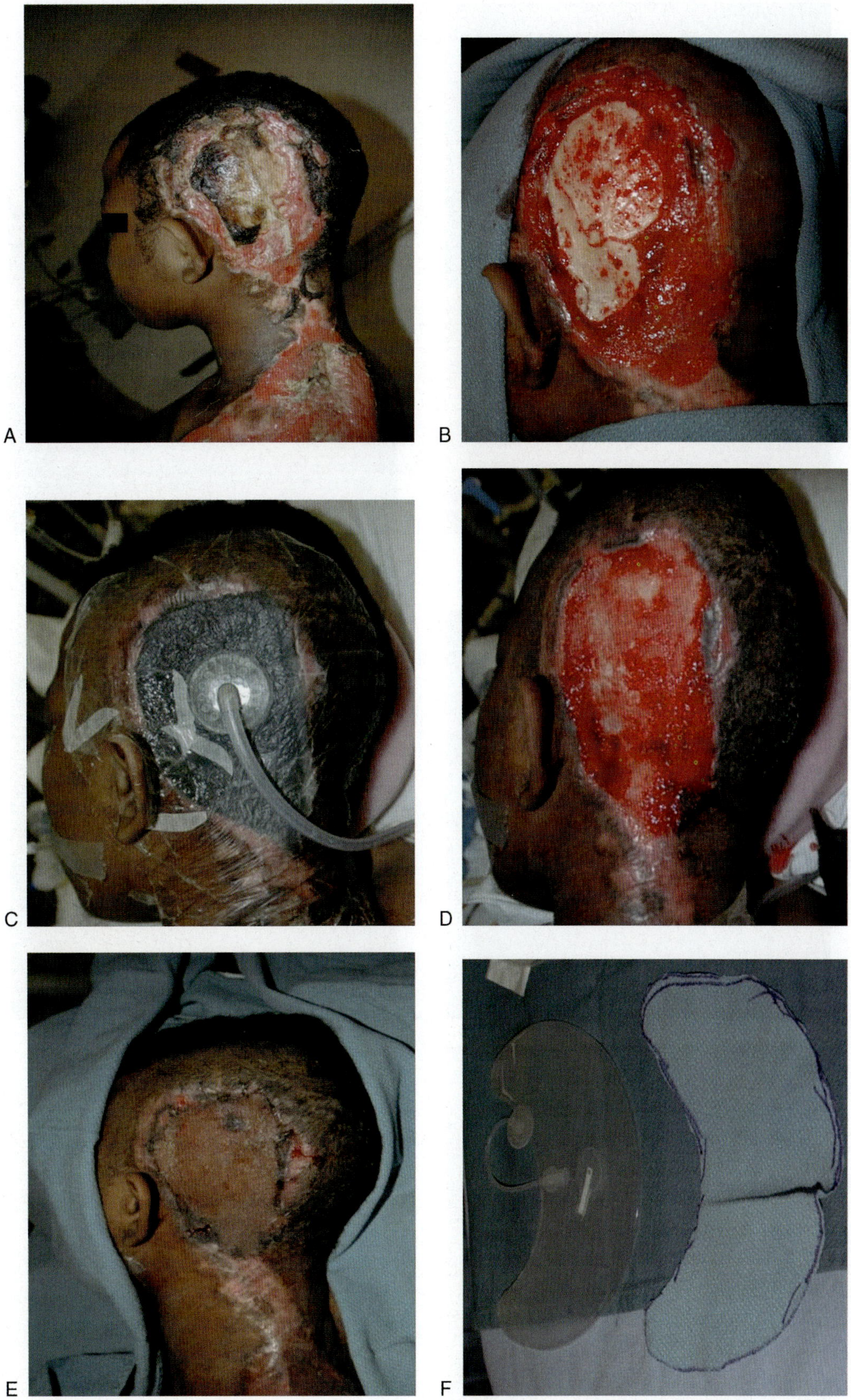

FIGURE 39.4 Multistage scalp reconstruction with skin grafts, VAC, and expanded scalp flaps. **A.** Full-thickness burn of lateral scalp to bone. **B.** Outer table drilled to allow cortical bleeding. **C.** VAC in place. **D.** Three weeks of VAC therapy. **E.** One week after split thickness skin graft. **F.** Tissue expander to be placed with template.

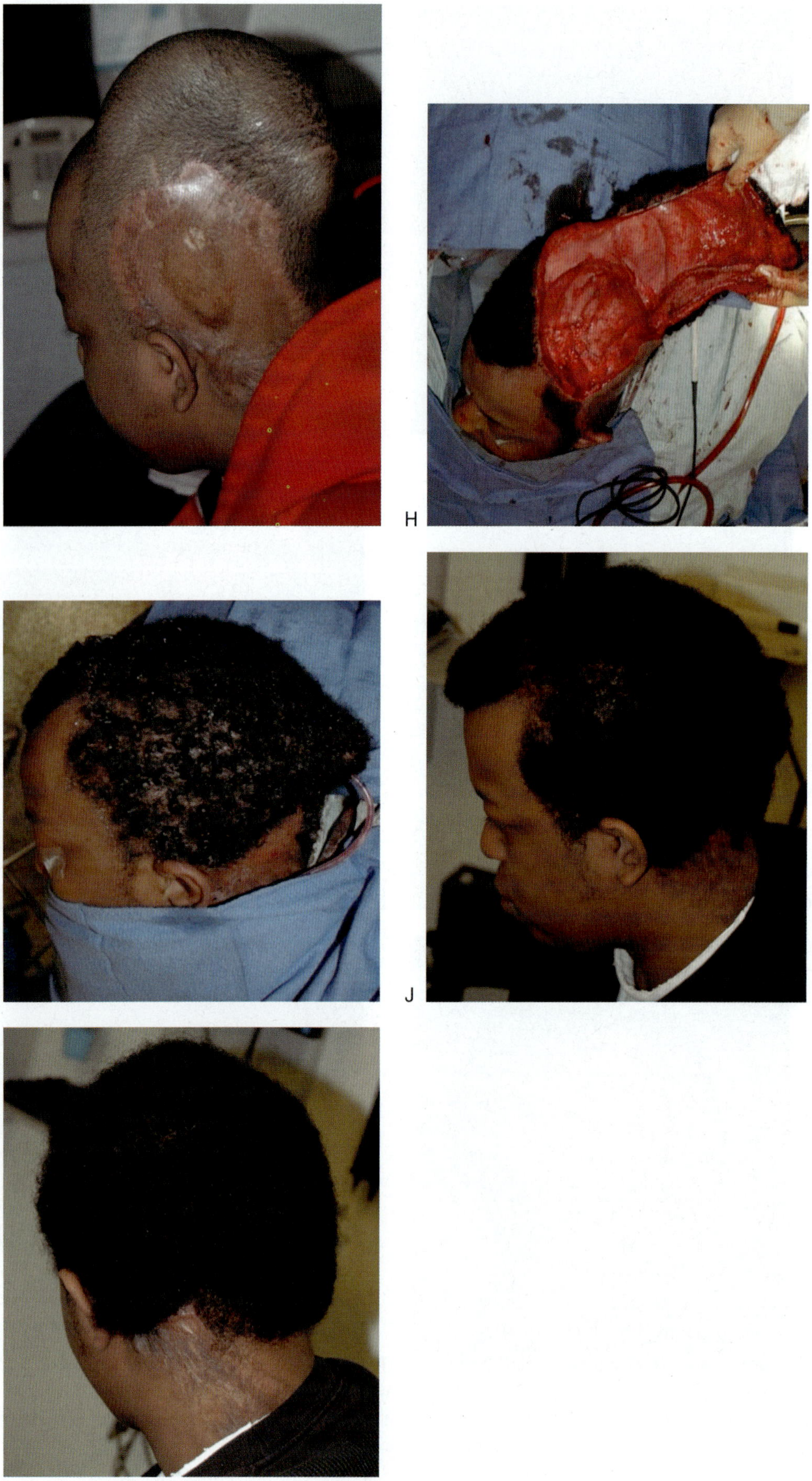

FIGURE 39.4
(*Continued*) **G.** After 2 months of expansion. **H.** Tissue expander removed with scalp flap raised. **I.** Scalp flap rotated to replace excised skin graft. **J.** Lateral view, 3 years postinjury. **K.** Posterior view, 3 years postinjury.

to placing a skin graft. A vacuum-assisted closure (VAC) can be used to promote granulation tissue prior to placing a skin graft (Fig. 39.4). For scalp defects once the skin graft has healed and there is no longer an open wound, tissue expanders are placed with the goal of replacing the skin grafts with the surrounding scalp once it has been expanded.

Regional Flaps

Regional flaps of the lateral skull are designed on the regional blood supply, in particular the supraorbital, superficial temporal, and/or postauricular artery (Fig. 39.2). These are rotation–advancement or transposition flaps that are designed to cover the defect. At the same time, their movement often leaves a donor defect that needs skin grafting (Fig. 39.5). Large, overlapping scalp flaps, such as "pinwheel" or "banana peel" (Orticochea flaps), require undermining most of the scalp and incising large areas of scalp. Defects can be closed with these flaps, but large areas of scar alopecia may also be a long-term outcome (Fig. 39.6). Figures 39.5 and 39.6 demonstrate two patients immediately closed with scalp flaps. In each case, the scalp wound was acutely closed, but these cases also demonstrate the potential morbidity of the donor defect created by the transposition or rotation of scalp flaps.

Other pedicled flaps, such as the lower trapezius island musculocutaneous flap, can reach posterior and lateral scalp defects. The flap may be mobilized by pedicling it solely on the transverse cervical artery and vein. The arc of rotation may be increased by placing the skin paddle more caudal. If the skin paddle of the flap is placed over the lower portion of the trapezius and within the territory of the latissimus, then the dorsal scapular artery and vein should be preserved. The dorsal scapula artery and vein pass between the rhomboid minor and major to supply the caudal portion of the trapezius muscle. Trapezius flaps have a number of relative disadvantages. These include potential loss of the spinal accessory nerve, inability to use these flaps if the transverse cervical artery has been sacrificed in a neck dissection, the occasional need to skin graft the donor

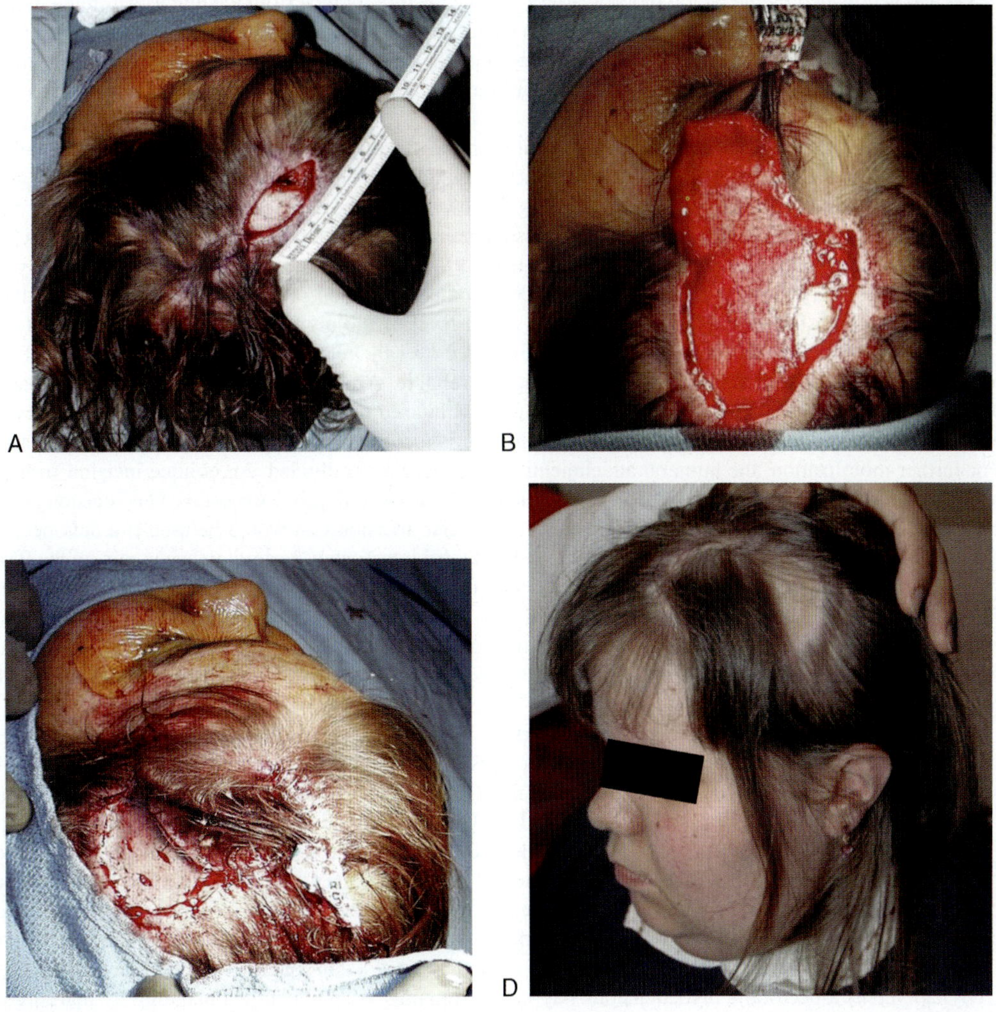

FIGURE 39.5 Anterior scalp with donor site. **A.** Exposed craniotomy burr hole after resection of a squamous cell carcinoma. **B.** Anteriorly based scalp flap raised to cover defect/burr hole. **C.** Donor site closed with skin graft. **D.** One year after reconstruction with skin graft.

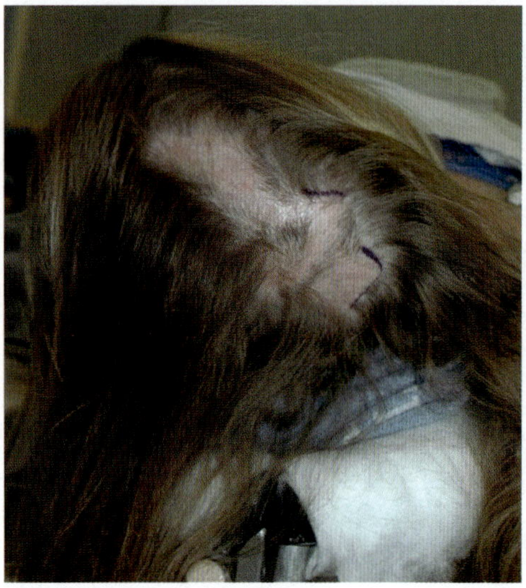

FIGURE 39.6
Alopecia after scalp rotation flaps. Vertex and parietal scar alopecia after raising two large (pinwheel) scalp flaps to close an area of excised cutis aplasia.

site, and special positioning to harvest the flap. The use of trapezius flaps has almost been completely replaced by fasciocutaneous free flaps, in particular the anterolateral thigh free flap (Fig. 39.1).

Regional flaps for lateral and posterior–lateral neck reconstruction primarily consist of pectoralis, cervicodeltopectoral (CDP), deltopectoral, and pedicled scapular flaps. The pectoralis major myocutaneous (PMM) flap is the most frequently used myocutaneous flap in head and neck reconstruction. The blood supply of the PMM flap is provided by the lateral thoracic artery and the pectoral branch from the thoracoacromial artery, a branch of the subclavian artery. The pectoral branch passes deep to the clavicle through the clavipectoral fascia at approximately the junction of the medial two-thirds with the lateral one-third. It then takes an oblique course deep to the pectoralis muscle and gives off muscular branches that supply the muscle and pierce the muscle to supply the overlying skin.

The PMM flap should be designed on the anterior chest wall to conform to the size and shape of the defect. To ensure that the length of the musculovascular bundle will be adequate to reach into the oral cavity, one should fabricate a template of the flap with surgical towel cut to the anticipated size and length. The point of rotation of the flap can be designed as superior as the point of exit under the inferior edge of the clavicle of the pectoral branch of the thoracoacromial artery. If the PMM flap is to be mobilized this far superiorly, the lateral thoracic artery must be divided. This may compromise the blood supply of the flap in some patients. Under most circumstances, the PMM flap begins at the level of the nipple and is carried inferiorly to the lower borders of the rib. The skin paddle may be extended over the rectus sheath, but these portions of skin are supplied by a random vascular pattern and are less reliable. After the incisions around the skin paddle are carried through the subcutaneous tissue, the muscle is incised medially from its sternal attachments and elevated off of the chest wall. The neurovascular bundle is identified by direct visualization and palpation. For further mobilization, the humeral attachments of the muscle are divided. An oblique incision from the superior, lateral edge of the skin paddle to the axillae can be used to improve exposure. This incision should be located approximately at the site of an inferior transverse incision that would be used if a deltopectoral flap was being designed. By not dividing the second and third intercostals perforators when raising the PMM flaps and by not incising the skin supplied by the second and third intercostals perforators, one still has the future option of using an ipsilateral deltopectoral flap. The donor area from the PMM flap can be closed primarily, leaving little chest deformity. The pectoralis muscle can be employed without the cutaneous portion of the paddle. In this way, the flap is far less bulky. A split-thickness skin graft can be applied directly to the muscle.

My approach for a CDP flap begins with marking the skin resection for tumor removal in conjunction with the neck incision used for the anticipated neck dissection so that the neck incisions used by the ablative surgeon will not disrupt the design of a CDP flap (Fig. 39.7). A standard transverse neck incision may prevent incorporation of the cervical component of the CDP flap. In the neck, the incisions for the CDP flap typically follow the anterior border of the trapezius muscle and proceed laterally to medially on the chest below the third intercostal perforator from the internal maxillary artery (the traditional site of the inferior chest wall incision of the deltopectoral flap). The entire skin island between the inferior aspect of the defect and the chest wall incision is transferred in continuity. The use of CDP flap for lower face or neck reconstruction provides for a better skin quality match compared to a distant or free flap. My decision to use a CDP flap versus a pectoralis myocutaneous flap is based mainly on preoperative planning by marking the anticipated skin defect and determining with a surgical towel cut into a template of the CDP flap whether the flap will rotate sufficiently to close the defect. By placing the skin island of a pectoralis flap inferior to or

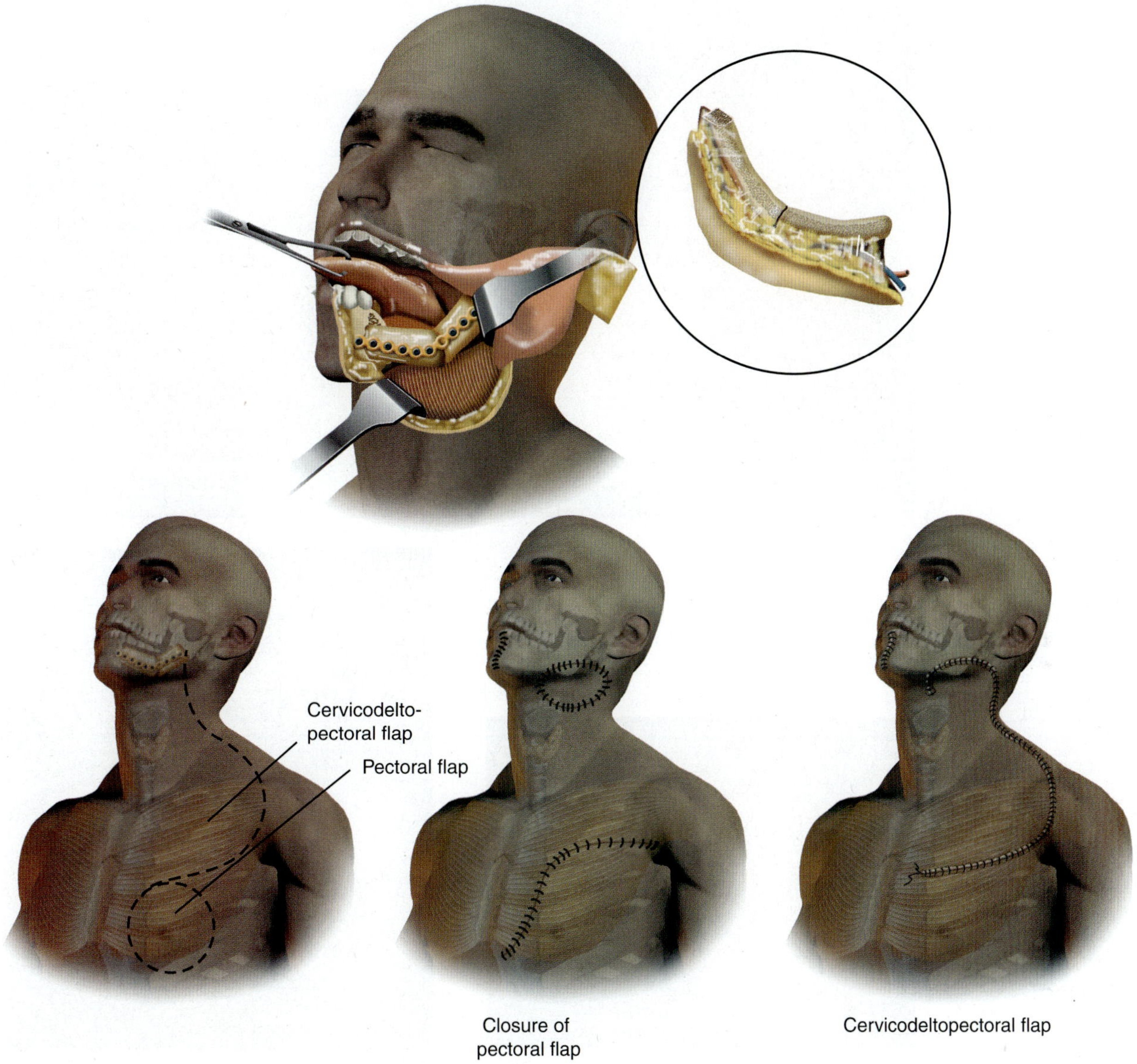

FIGURE 39.7 Design of CDP and pectoralis flaps. Skin incisions for CDP and pectoralis major flaps. The defect includes a cutaneous, cervical resection. Lower left: closure with a PMM flap; Lower right: closure with CDP flap.

in continuity with the chest wall incision of the CDP flap and by preserving the second and third intercostal perforators during the pectoralis flap harvest, one can safely raise both a CDP and pectoralis flap (Figs. 39.7 and 39.8).

The branching pattern of the circumflex scapular artery and vein permits the harvest of a number of fasciocutaneous flaps. The scapular flap is based on the horizontal cutaneous branch of the circumflex scapular artery. The parascapular flap is based on the descending cutaneous branch of the circumflex scapular artery. These flaps are routinely harvested as free flaps, but they can also be used as pedicled flaps for posterior–lateral neck defects, especially if they are tissue expanded prior to their transposition. Figure 39.9 demonstrates one such case where a preexpanded scapular flap was combined with a preexpanded deltopectoral flap for a large posterior–lateral neck defect. First, a deltopectoral flap was designed on the right chest; Doppler ultrasound was used to identify the internal mammary perforators between the second and third intercostal spaces. Back cuts were then made along the deltopectoral groove and along the anterior aspect to where the expander capsule was located. This allowed the flap to rotate 90 degrees and to close the neck defect anteriorly and laterally to the level of the trapezius muscle. The patient was then placed in the left lateral decubitus position, and the scapular flap was designed. Doppler ultrasound was used to identify the circumflex scapular artery in the triangular fossa. A large pedicled, scapular fasciocutaneous flap was then raised. A back cut along the rim of the capsule of the expander extending to the posterior axillary line allowed the flap to rotate 90 degrees to close the remaining defect. All donor sites were then closed primarily.

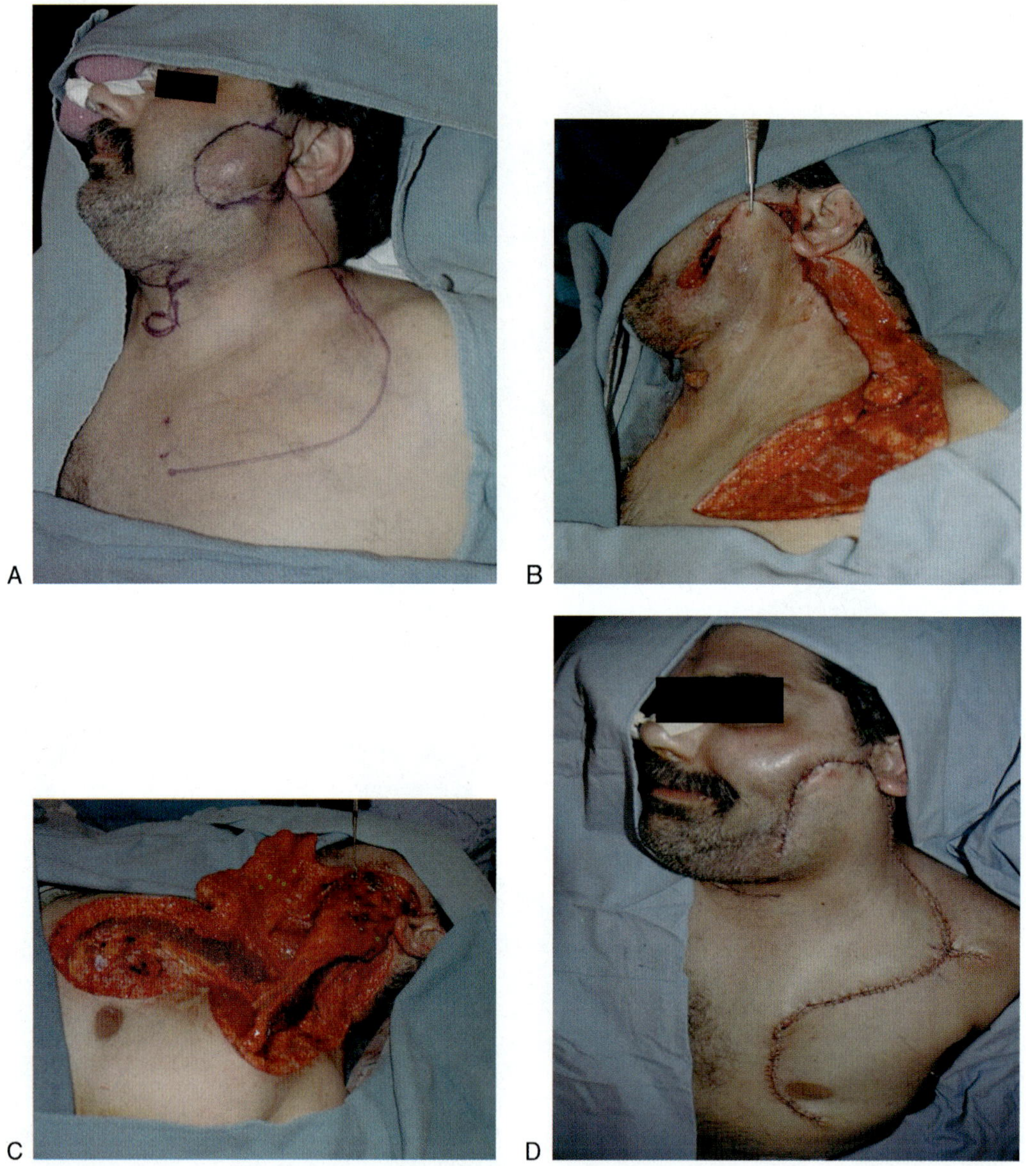

FIGURE 39.8 Cheek and lateral neck reconstruction with a CDP and pectoralis flap. **A.** Resection of skin, parotid, and lateral mandible for cancer of the parotid gland. **B.** CDP flap raised; blood supply from internal mammary artery perforators. **C.** Inset of pectoralis muscle flap; skin paddle removed; adipose tissue and muscle of flap provide bulk restoration for the cheek. **D.** Closure with rotation of the CDP over the pectoralis flap.

Tissue Expansion

Tissue expansion allows for adjacent transfer of sensate tissue to repair defects while maintaining skin color and texture. In 2004, Hurvitz et al. reviewed pediatric cervicofacial tissue expansion and showed an overall complication rate of 30.8% with the highest complication rate affecting the neck area. Previous studies have shown similar results and have postulated that the neck region carries a higher complication rate secondary to shearing forces from the wide range of motion of the neck along with the thin tissue envelope in the skin of the neck. The most common complication is exposure followed by infection. Tissue expansion requires careful surgical planning, often multiple visits for serial expansion, and meticulous care of the site of expansion. Therefore, it is important that the family is well advised and is able to be compliant with the postimplantation care.

Tissue expansion is traditionally advocated for use with advancement flaps; however, in more difficult and larger areas of reconstruction, the use of an expanded transposition flap (Fig. 39.9) plays a powerful role in improving final contour, decreasing risk of anatomic distortion, improving scar position, and lowering the risk of contracture.

POSTOPERATIVE MANAGEMENT

Drains are typically left in place until their output is less than 30 mL over 24 hours per drain. If skin grafts have been placed over periosteum or on cortical bone that has granulated, a bolster (or VAC sponge used as a bolster) is sewn in place for 5 to 7 days. Skin grafts that have been placed on muscle flaps are covered only with Adaptic and antibiotic cream. Bolsters are not used because of the possibility of compressing the circulation of the underlying flap.

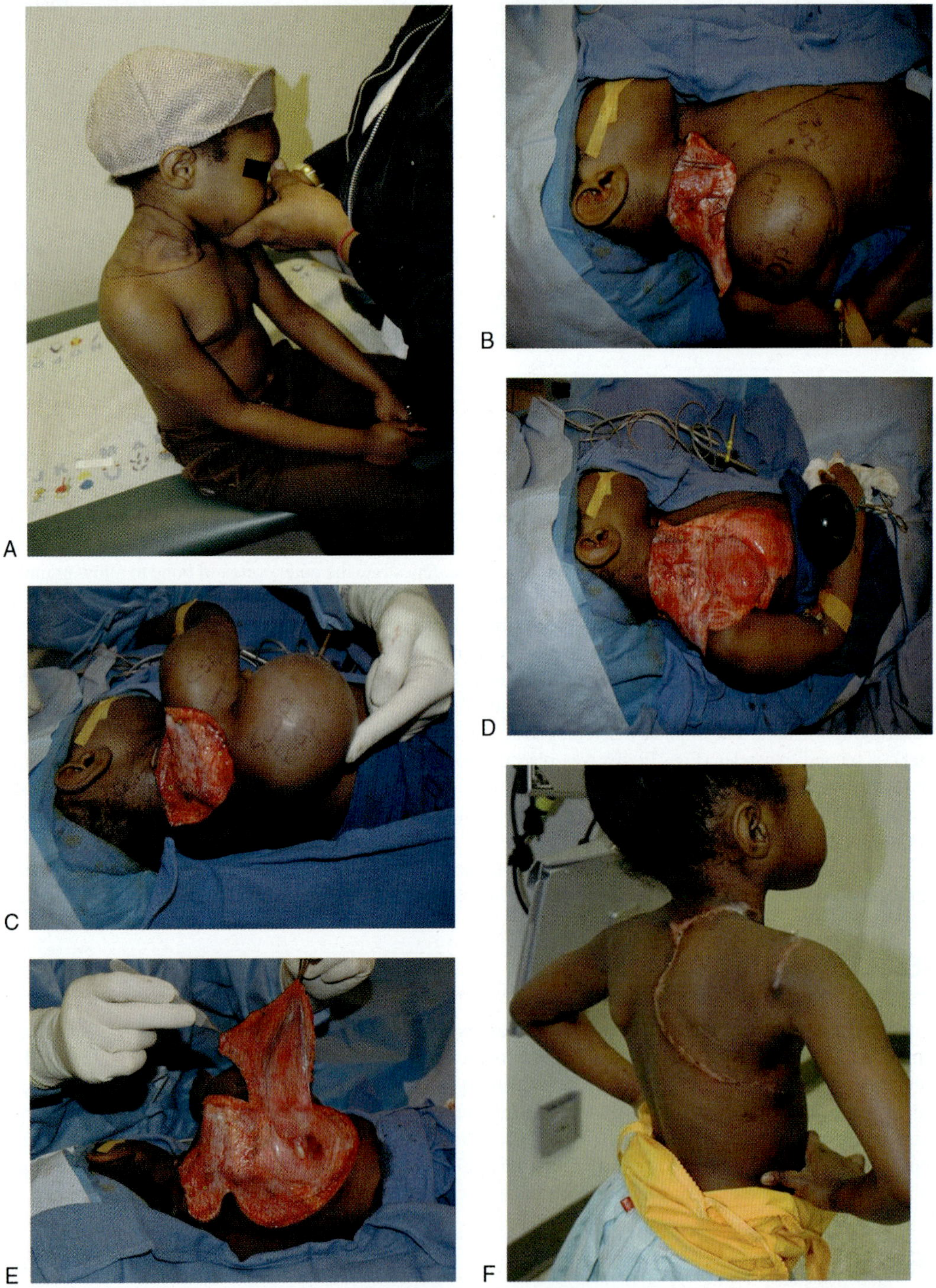

FIGURE 39.9 Tissue expansion of deltopectoral and scapular flaps. **A.** Five-year-old with massive dermatofibrosarcoma. The expected resection of neck skin, platysma, and trapezius fascia is outlined. **B.** Expanded deltopectoral flap. **C.** Expanded, pedicled scapular flap. **D.** Tissue expander removed deltopectoral flap being rotated. **E.** Scapular flap being rotated. **F.** Six weeks post-op: posterior view.

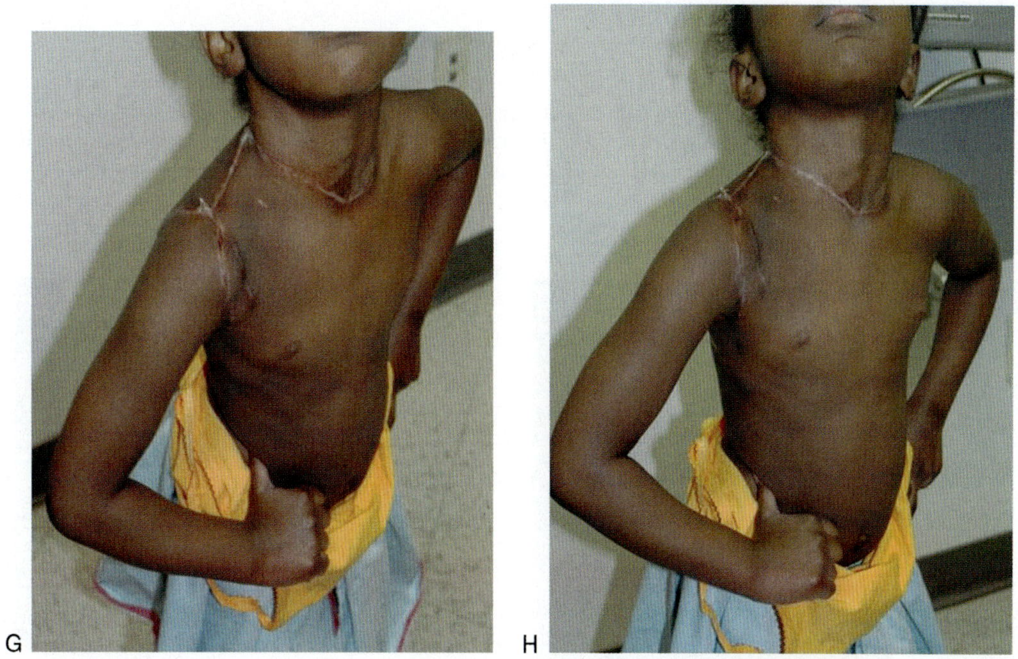

FIGURE 39.9 (*Continued*) **G.** Six weeks post-op: lateral view. **H.** Six weeks post-op: anterior view.

COMPLICATIONS

The most common complication of the transposition of any regional flap will be loss of the distal tissue of the flap due to inadequate perfusion or venous congestion. To decrease this complication, regional flaps should be designed to incorporate at least one named artery in the base of the flap. A skin graft will not take if the recipient bed is not well vascularized. For exposed bone, if possible, fenestrate the outer cortex of bone to allow granulation tissue to cover the entire wound bed before applying a skin graft.

As a tissue expander progressively expands, the risk of extrusion is highest at the site used for implantation. Therefore, avoid placing incisions used for implant placement directly within atrophic scars or within skin graft sites. As an example, the patient in Figure 39.4 suffered one complication of implant extrusion when the incision for expander placement was placed just a few millimeters medial to the skin graft site in the left temporal area. The implant was removed after it became exposed. At a subsequent operation (1 month later), a second expander (Fig. 39.4F) was placed through an incision on the contralateral scalp. The site for this incision was chosen at the site where the back cut for flap transposition was anticipated. The scalp immediately adjacent to the skin graft was also not undermined so that the expander would not put pressure on this site as it expanded.

Scalp flaps can be associated with scar alopecia. The use of tissue expansion prior to the excision of lesion can reduce the risk of alopecia because the wound can be closed with less tension.

RESULTS

Defects of the lateral scalp and/or neck have a variety of etiologies. Whether the etiology is a malignant tumor, benign tumor, or trauma, the goals of reconstruction are to create an aesthetically acceptable, healed wound and to introduce the least amount of morbidity with the reconstruction. Skin graft reconstruction, regional flaps that may be tissue expanded, and free flaps are all methods of reconstruction with which the surgeon must be comfortable and have experience. Discussing the advantages and disadvantages of these approaches with the patient prior to extirpation is important so that the final reconstructive result is acceptable to the patient and that the patient's postoperative expectations match the reconstructive outcomes.

PEARLS

- Anticipate the extent of the defect prior to tumor extirpation. If scalp or large areas of cervical skin are to be excised, question whether tissue expansion could serve a role in the reconstruction.
- If a CDP flap is to be used for reconstruction, any neck incision used for a neck dissection should be incorporated into the design of the flap.

- If a split-thickness skin graft is to be used, consider harvesting a skin graft from the scalp due to the better color match and the minimal morbidity. The donor site is first infiltrated with a tumescent solution (i.e., saline with 1:500,000 epinephrine). Scalp skin graft can be harvested with a thickness as thin as 0.005 to 0.007 inch.
- Regional scalp flaps should be designed to capture a named artery in the base of the flap.
- A tissue expanded flap can often provide greater versatility for reconstruction (i.e., greater movement) if harvested as a transposition flap (i.e., with back cuts along the expander capsule), instead of as an advancement flap.
- Pedicled flaps, in particular the scapular flap, can be converted to a free flap if the pedicle of the flap prevents adequate movement of the flap for reconstruction.
- A bulky musculocutaneous flap can be debulked by not including the overlying skin paddle and subcutaneous tissue. The pedicled muscle is then skin grafted.

PITFALLS

- Skin grafts placed on cortical bone will not survive. This can be avoided by removing the outer layer of the cortical bone and allowing the area to granulate prior to placement of the skin graft.
- Expanders placed next to skin grafts are at risk for extrusion. Decrease the risk of this complication by choosing an incision for expander placement away from the skin graft site.
- Scalp flaps that are transposed into defects will leave a donor defect. Anticipate how the donor defect will be reconstructed (i.e., skin graft), and question whether the scalp flap can be designed so its transposition allows the donor defect to be placed in a less visible location on the scalp.

INSTRUMENTS TO HAVE AVAILABLE

- Standard head and neck surgical set
- Dermatome
- Tissue expander equipment

SUGGESTED READING

Orticochea M. New three-flap scalp reconstruction technique. *Br J Plast Surg* 1971:24:184.

Lynch JR, Hansen JE, Chaffoo R, et al. The lower trapezius musculocutaneous flap revisited: versatile coverage for complicated wounds to the posterior cervical and occipital regions based on the deep branch of the transverse cervical artery. *Plast Reconstr Surg* 2002;109(2):444–450.

Deleyiannis FWB, Carolyn C, Lee E, et al. Reconstruction of the lateral mandibulectomy defect: management based on prognosis and the location and volume of the soft tissue resection. *Laryngoscope* 2006;116(11):2071–2080.

Deleyiannis FWB, Dunklebarger J, Russavage J, et al. Reconstruction of the marginal mandibulectomy defect: an update. *Am J Otolaryngol* 2007;28(6):363–366.

Rebelo M, Ferreira A, Barbosa R, et al. Deltopectoral flap: an old but contemporaneous solution for neck reconstruction. *J Plast Reconstr Aesthet Surg* 2009;62(1):137–138.

40 THE ANTERIOR SKULL BASE DEFECT

Paul Donald

INTRODUCTION

The harvesting and placement of the pericranial flap has become the keystone technique in the reconstruction of the anterior skull base following resections of intracranial/extracranial tumors. During the coronal incision of the scalp for the anterior craniotomy, the pericranium is carefully preserved.

Usually, the floor of the anterior cranial fossa and often the cribriform plate, as well as adjacent dura, have been removed as part of the exenteration procedure (Fig. 40.1). The reconstruction dictates that the dura is closed, establishing a watertight seal, and that some form of lining of the subcranial exenteration cavity is placed. The interposition of some type of firm, resilient vascularized tissue is required to reinforce the dural repair as well as to serve as a nutrient bed for a split-thickness skin graft or free flap. The pericranial flap best serves these needs.

HISTORY

In the taking of the history, it is important to note whether the patient has had prior craniotomy and if he or she has been treated with radiation in the past to the anterior cranial fossa. This is not an uncommon experience in patients with recurrent meningioma or a patient with a prior history of surgery and radiation for cancer of the ethmoid or maxillary sinus with intracranial penetration. The past history of a frontal craniotomy makes the harvest of a pericranial flap at this site extremely difficult and sometimes impossible.

A history of prior irradiation will jeopardize not only the survival of the flap but also the viability of the underlying cranial bone. The use of some form of free vascularized tissue to line the subcranial cavity is often mandated in these cases to establish a good blood supply to these compromised tissues.

PHYSICAL EXAMINATION

Examination of the defect will determine if the pericranial flap is the appropriate donor site. The blood supply to the flap should be evaluated to assure that it is intact and that the flap is well vascularized. There should be no evidence of prior surgery, trauma, or radiation to the donor site. The width of the flap should be wider than the expected cranial floor defect. Finally, before beginning the flap reconstruction, the dural reconstruction should be examined to assure that it is watertight to decrease the potential for CSF leakage.

INDICATIONS

The pericranial flap is indicated for central defects of the skull base.

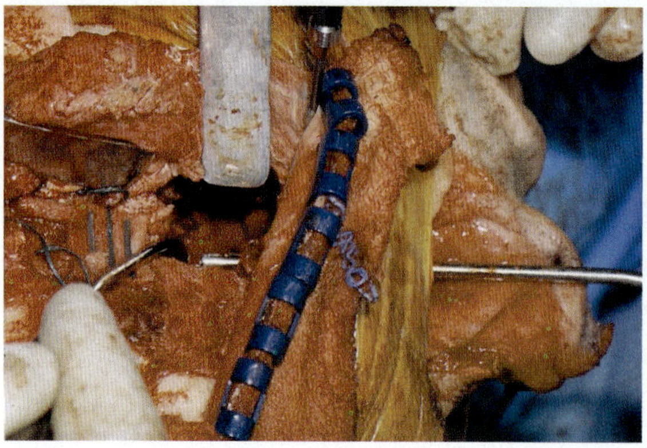

FIGURE 40.1
Exenteration defect following anterior skull base resection requiring a three-layer reconstruction.

CONTRAINDICATIONS

Contraindications to the pericranial flap include when the flap vascularity has been compromised by injury to the blood supply or in some previously radiated patients, the flap may not be hearty.

PREOPERATIVE PLANNING

Unless a prior craniotomy has been performed, there is little preoperative planning. If a prior craniotomy has been performed and the pericranial flap has been previously used for a reconstruction of the central skull base, I prepare for the possibility of a free flap for reconstruction. A free flap reconstruction is the only alternative because a temporalis flap will not reach the midline.

SURGICAL TECHNIQUE

Under general anesthesia, the patient usually has a tracheostomy done, to prevent postoperative tension pneumocephalus, and the head is place in a padded Mayfield headrest. The anterior aspect of the hair is usually shaved in order to prevent hairs from prolapsing into the wound at the time of closure at the end of the procedure. The scalp incision is outlined in methylene blue in a curvilinear fashion from the anterior–superior aspect of the auricle over the vertex of the skull running about 2 cm behind the hairline to the opposite side (Fig. 40.2). Injection of the scalp along the incision line is then done with a solution of ½% Xylocaine with 1 in 20,000 epinephrine.

The coronal scalp incision is then made with a scalpel usually one side at a time, taking great care to avoid incising the pericranium. Periodic gentle blunt elevation in the depths of the incision with the back of the scalpel handle will allow easy identification of the area of the pericranium. Hemostasis is secured along the edges of the scalp incision by the placement of Raney clips and the use of the bipolar cautery. The elevation of the scalp flap proceeds toward the brows taking care not to make holes in the underlying pericranium. As the more posterior elevation of the flap proceeds over the temporalis muscle, care is taken to incise a semilunar portion

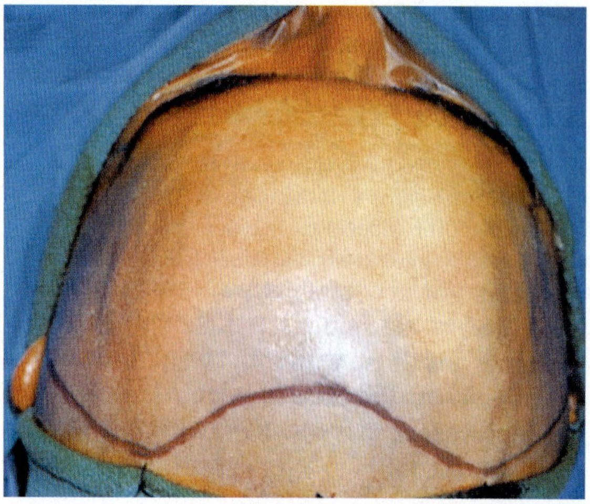

FIGURE 40.2
Scalp incision outlined.

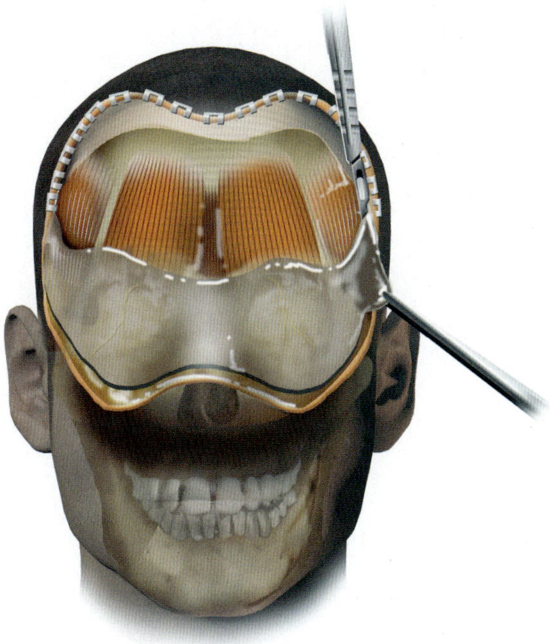

FIGURE 40.3
Semilunar flap of superficial and deep temporalis fascia kept adherent to the skin to protect the frontal branch of the facial nerve.

of superficial temporal fascia keeping it attached to the scalp (Fig. 40.3). This will protect the temporal branch of the facial nerve as the flap elevation proceeds anteroinferiorly.

The flap elevation stops at the brows. Care is taken not to injure either the supraorbital or supratrochlear vessels as they emerge from their respective foramina in the region of the brows as they provide the vascular pedicle for the pericranial flap. Dissection is directed superiorly where a retrograde elevation under the scalp posterior to the coronal incision will provide additional length to the pericranial flap. Paired vertical incisions are made in the pericranium each at the lateral extremities of the flap and carried under the retrograde part of the elevated scalp. They are then connected over the vertex. The width of the flap will be predicated on the anticipated width of the defect. The pericranial incisions are carried down to the lateral brows. The pericranium is then carefully separated with a Langenbeck dissector from the underlying calvarium from under the superior extension of the scalp flap down to the brows (Fig. 40.4). A four-by-four gauze sponge soaked periodically in saline is placed over the pericranial flap as it lies against the raw undersurface of the coronal scalp flap while the resection part of the procedure is carried out.

An alternative to constructing the pericranial flap in this fashion, especially when the width of the defect in the cranial floor is hard to predict, is to keep the pericranium attached to the scalp flap to be separated from its undersurface at a width necessary to cover the defect after the resection; this is done by elevating the retrograde part of the pericranial flap first, and then, once the site of the scalp incision is reached, the vertical incisions in the pericranium are made on the calvarium as the elevation of the scalp flap proceeds inferiorly. The pericranium is elevated from the underlying skull over the width of this flap, and the more lateral elevation is between the galea and the pericranium.

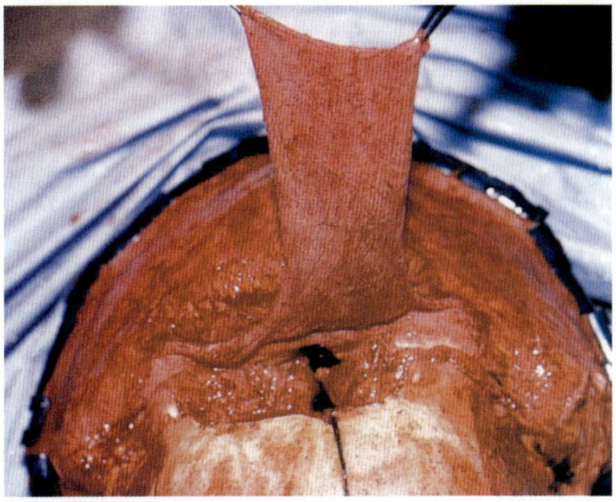

FIGURE 40.4
Pericranial flap elevated.

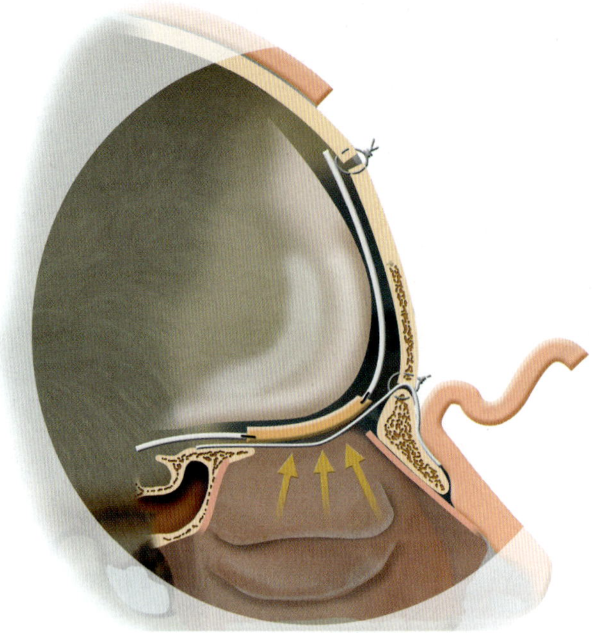

FIGURE 40.5
Pericranial flap tucked into position.

POSTOPERATIVE MANAGEMENT

At the completion of the resection, there is an eventration in the anterior fossa floor. Bleeding is stopped from any brain tissue and dural resection is repaired usually with temporalis fascia or fascia lata. The pericranial flap is now turned 90 degrees on its vascular pedicle and placed over the defect in the cranial floor (Fig. 40.5). It is important to bridge the entire bony gap with tissue left over to tuck between the bone of the planum sphenoidale and the dura. It is important to extend the flap beyond the area of the repaired dural defect. Thus, the flap goes from its pedicle on the brow, over the inferior aspect of the craniotomy cut, across the intact portion of the anterior floor at the anterior limit of the resection, across the open resection site over the dural graft to finally be tucked between the bone remaining at the posterior limit of the dissection and the dura.

One of the biggest problems in the placement of the flap is to fix it to the posterior aspect of the anterior fossa floor in the area of the sphenoid sinus. The surest way is to place several drill holes in the bone and then parachute in the end of the flap. This is augmented by the use of tissue glue.

Nasal packing is placed for 5 days, and the patient is monitored for CSF leak. Antibiotics are administered while the nasal packing is in place.

COMPLICATIONS

Complications include CSF leak, meningitis, and pneumocephalus. I take care to make sure that positive pressure nasal ventilation is avoided at all cost to prevent pneumocephalus.

RESULTS

The results with this form of reconstruction are generally excellent. The flap and technique are reliable and reproducible.

There are some advocates of the pericranial flap that state that including the galea is essential to preserve a healthy blood supply. The problem with this technique is that the blood supply to the forehead skin may be compromised especially in someone who has had prior radiation. In using the pericranial flap without including the galea in well over 150 patients, I have had only one flap slough. This was in a man who insisted on smoking during the immediate postoperative period. First, the skin graft sloughed and then the pericranial flap died. This produced a brain fungus of the frontal lobe that required resection and the placement of a radial forearm free flap over the defect.

PEARLS

- To avoid the potential for compromise of the flap's blood supply, a strip of bone at the inferior aspect of the craniotomy flap is removed (Fig. 40.6).

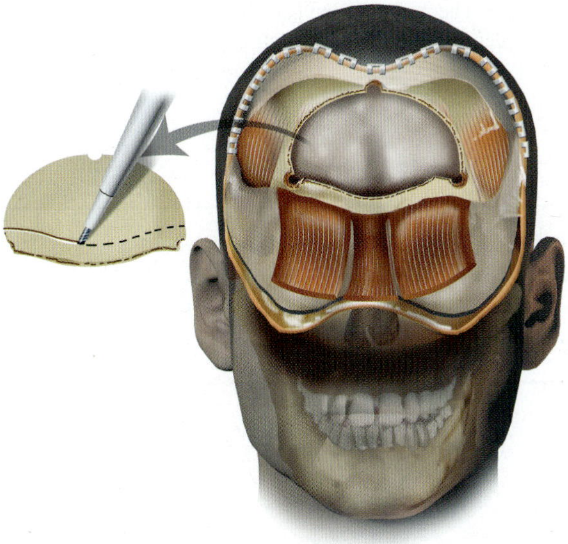

FIGURE 40.6
Bar of bone is cut from the inferior aspect of the cranial bone flap to relieve any compression on the pedicle of the pericranial flap.

- On some occasions, the frontal bone is involved with tumor as is the orbit requiring orbital exenteration and resection of a portion of the frontal calvarium including the vascular supply on one side to the projected pericranial flap. Even a wide flap will survive on a single pedicle, from the opposing side as demonstrated in Figure 40.7. This patient had a large portion of frontal lobe dura removed as well as the frontal bone on the left side that included both the supraorbital and supratrochlear arteries as part of a craniofacial resection for a squamous cell carcinoma of the frontal and ethmoidal sinuses. The flap survived on a single contralateral vascular pedicle and the patient is alive and free of cancer 14 years postoperatively.
- If a prior craniotomy has been done and the pericranium is of poor quality, the donor site can be constructed from a temporalis fascial flap pedicled on the superficial temporal artery whose pericranial extension goes across the vertex posterior to the prior craniotomy.
- My preference for reconstruction of anterior skull base resections is dural grafting, pericranial flap, and a split-thickness skin graft to line the cavity. The rationale for this is that the bulk of the free flap, especially if an anterolateral thigh flap or latissimus dorsi flap is used, will obscure the appearance of a local recurrence. Neither MRI nor CAT scanning will reveal an early recurrence. Unfortunately, even PET scans are

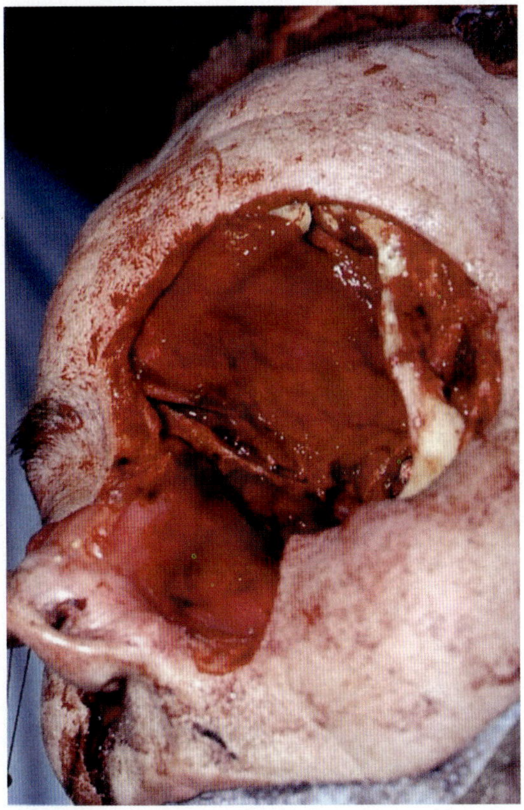

FIGURE 40.7
Large pericranial flap pedicled on only one supraorbital and supratrochlear artery from the side opposite the defect.

not entirely reliable in detecting early recurrent disease. The notion of the patient having had the "ultimate operation" and that any further intervention for early recurrence is hopeless is clearly nonsense. Early detection is the key to successful salvage.

PITFALLS

- The pedicle of the flap may be pinched when the craniotomy bone flap is returned to its position and fixed in place if a small cutting tool such as the Midas Rex drill is used to do the craniotomy.

INSTRUMENTS TO HAVE AVAILABLE

- Standard head and neck surgical set
- Osteotome
- Periosteal Freer

SUGGESTED READING

Zanation AM, Snyderman CH, Carrau RL, et al. Minimally invasive endoscopic pericranial flap: a new method for endonasal skull base reconstruction. *Laryngoscope* 2009;119(1):13–18.

Patel MR, Shah RN, Snyderman CH, et al. Pericranial flap for endoscopic anterior skull-base reconstruction: clinical outcomes and radioanatomic analysis of preoperative planning. Neurosurgery 2010;66(3):506–512; discussion 512.

Zhang FG, Tang XF, Hua CG, et al. Anterior skull base reconstruction with galeal-frontalis-pericranial flap based on temporalis myofascial flap. *J Craniofac Surg* 2010;21(4):1247–1249.

41 TEMPORALIS MUSCLE FLAP AND TEMPOROPARIETAL FASCIA FLAP

Eric M. Genden

INTRODUCTION

Prior to the introduction of free tissue transfer, local and regional flaps represented the primary source of tissue for reconstruction of the lateral skull base. While free tissue transfer has supplanted many of the unreliable local flaps, the temporalis muscle flap (TMF) and temporoparietal fascia flap (TPFF) remain popular donor sites for reconstruction of the skull base. These donor sites provide a reliable source of well-vascularized tissue that can be used to reconstitute dural defects, fill soft tissue defects, or support the brain in the case of a cranial defect.

The TPFF was initially described more than a century ago. It is a thin, highly vascular layer of connective tissue immediately deep to the subdermal fibroadipose tissue of the scalp. The TPFF is continuous with the occipitofrontalis and galea superiorly, and below the zygomatic arch, it extends into the superficial musculo-aponeurotic system (Fig. 41.1). Deep to the TPFF is a loose areolar layer that separates the TPFF from the deep temporal fascia. The blood supply to the TPFF is the superficial temporal artery. The vascular pedicle provides a rich vascular network to the flap but also limits the arch of rotation. Although the flap can be rotated to cover the lateral aspect of the skull base, it will not reach the central skull base.

Like the TPFF, the TMF is a reliable, myofascial flap that was also described more than a century ago. The vascular supply is the deep temporal artery, which originates from the internal maxillary artery (Fig. 41.2). The temporalis muscle lies deep to the temporoparietal fascia. It is a broad, radiating muscle that arises from the temporal fossa and from the deep surface of the temporal fascia. Its fibers converge inferiorly to form the tendon, which passes deep to the zygomatic arch and inserts into the medial surface of the coronoid process. The flap can be raised up and pedicled only on the coronoid process. This improves the arc of rotation to reach the paramedian aspect of the skull base.

I find that these flaps provide an excellent source of well-vascularized tissue that can be used for skull base reconstruction. They are reliable, and the donor site is well tolerated.

HISTORY

There are several important issues that must be considered when taking a history. The first relates to prior surgery. The advantage of the TPFF and the TMF is that they are often preserved in spite of prior surgery. As part of the history, it is important to determine if the patient has had prior cranial base surgery that may have compromised the pericranial flap. In such a case, the TPFF or TMF may be used for reconstruction of the lateral skull base. A careful history will often determine if the pericranial flap has been previously used for reconstruction. A second aspect of the history relates to the blood supply of these two flaps. The TPFF receives its blood supply from the superficial temporal artery and vein. In contrast, the TMF receives its blood supply from the deep temporal artery and vein. In the former case, if the external carotid artery has previously been ligated, the TPFF will not be viable. In the latter case, if the internal maxillary artery has been previously sacrificed, then the blood supply to the TMF will be compromised. A history of previous trauma to the donor site should be sought.

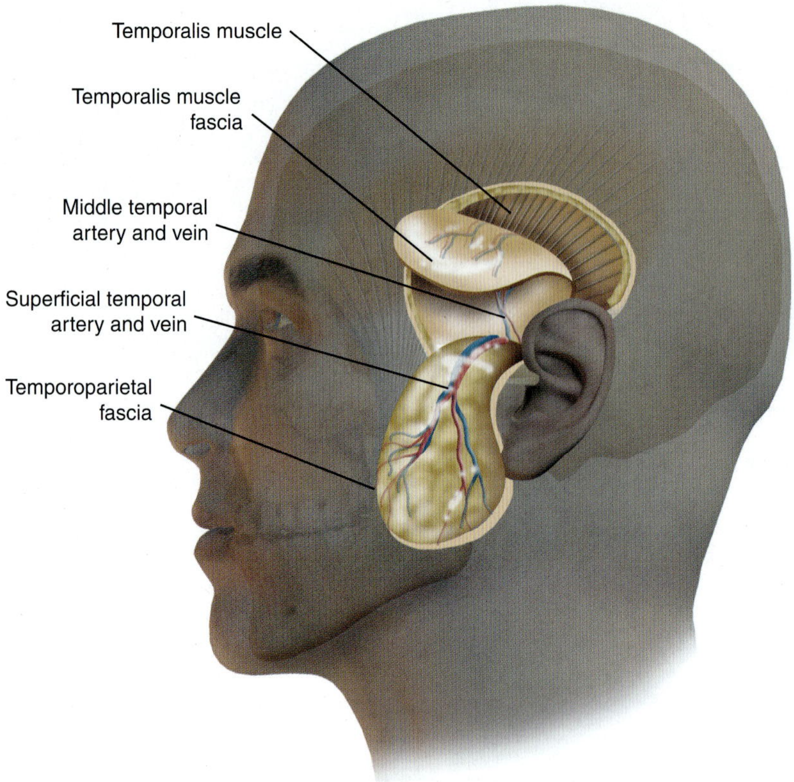

FIGURE 41.1
The temporoparietal fascia is a superficial vascularized tissue flap that is located immediately deep to the subcutaneous tissue of the scalp. The temporalis muscle is found deep to the temporalis muscle fascia.

PHYSICAL EXAMINATION

The physical examination should be directed toward an evaluation of the external carotid artery and the lateral skull base region. Evidence of scarring or prior surgery should be carefully noted to determine if there has been a compromise in the blood supply to the temporalis muscle or temporal parietal fascia. Physical examination should also include a careful evaluation of the defect. While both the temporal parietal and the temporalis flaps are well vascularized, the arc of rotation and reach to the midline is limited. Both flaps are ideal for lateral temporal bone and lateral cranial base defects; however, they are not well suited for medial defects of the cranial base.

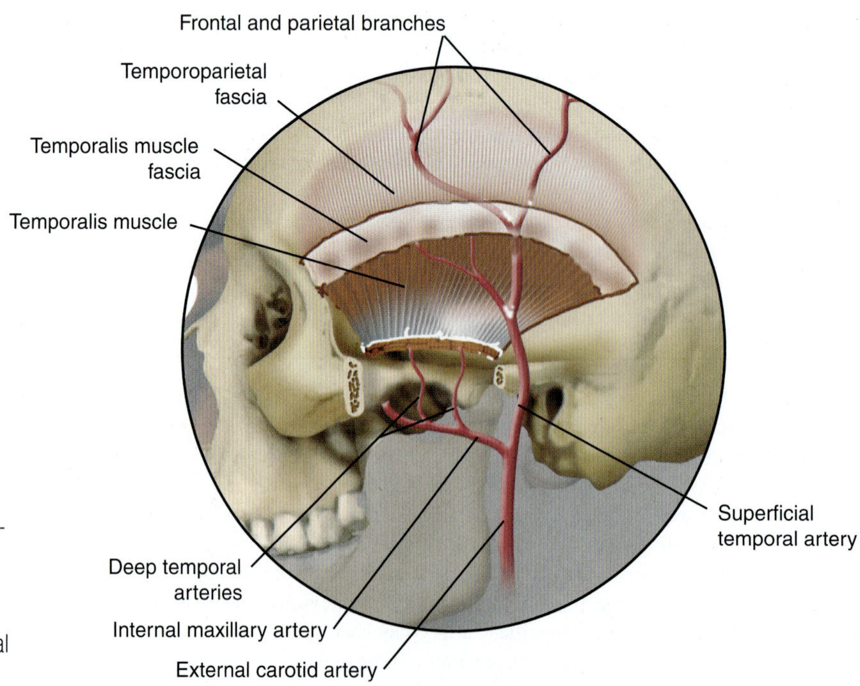

FIGURE 41.2
The vascular supply to the TPFF is the superficial temporal artery and vein; however, the vascular supply to the TMF is the deep temporal artery derived from the internal maxillary system.

INDICATIONS

The indications for the TPFF and TMF are for defects of the lateral skull base. The TPFF is a well-vascularized flap that is ideal for reconstitution of defects of the dura. In contrast, the TMF is bulky but well vascularized. I tend to use the TPFF in cases where dural reconstruction is required. I reserve the TMF for defects that require restoration of bulk.

CONTRAINDICATIONS

The contraindications to the use of these flaps relates to the blood supply. In cases where the internal maxillary artery or external carotid artery had been sacrificed, the use of the temporalis and TPFFs is contraindicated.

PREOPERATIVE PLANNING

The preoperative planning begins by understanding the size, location, and the characteristics of the defect. Because of the limited arc of rotation and reach, defects of the lateral temporal bone, mastoid, orbitocranial segment, and the orbit are best suited for these flaps. I often Doppler the superficial temporal vascular system at some point preoperatively because there is a small proportion of patients who will have a vascular anomaly wherein the superficial temporal vein is not well developed. Although this vascular anomaly is rare, I like to know this before embarking on the harvest. Additionally, Doppler examination also assures me that the vascular system has not been compromised during prior surgery.

SURGICAL TECHNIQUE

The Temporoparietal Fascia Flap

This flap is harvested through a vertical incision with distal "Y" incision to provide optimal access to the underlying fascia, vascularized pericranial bone graft, and, if necessary, a vascularized skin paddle (Fig. 41.3). The fascia of the flap lies immediately deep to the subcutaneous tissue of the scalp. As a result, careful dissection is required to separate the subcutaneous skin of the scalp from the underlying fascia (Fig. 41.4). Careful attention to the superficial temporal artery and vein are necessary to prevent injury to the vascular

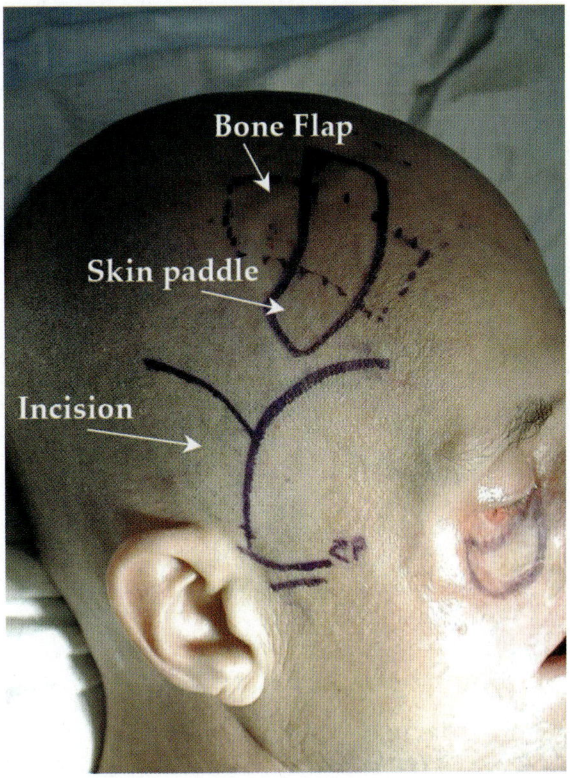

FIGURE 41.3
The flaps are accessed via a "Y" incision made on the lateral aspect of the parietal scalp. This provides access to the TPFF, TMF, and, if required, a vascularized skin flap and/or a vascularized pericranial bone graft.

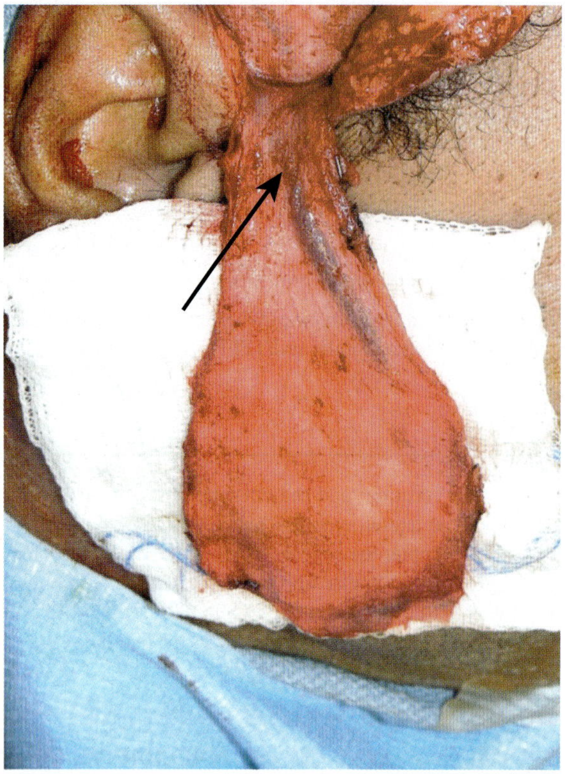

FIGURE 41.4
The temporoparietal fascia is a superficial vascularized tissue flap that is located immediately deep to the subcutaneous tissue of the scalp. In this photo, the TPFF and the vascular supply are seen through the incision.

supply of the flap. The flap can be raised as far as necessary to obtain a flap that is an appropriate size. Once the temporal parietal fascia is exposed (Fig. 41.5), the peripheral incision is made and dissection between the underlying fascia and the deep temporalis fascia is developed.

The TPFF/TMF system is versatile and provides the opportunity to harvest a composite graft composed of a vascularized skin paddle with or without a vascularized cranial bone graft (Fig. 41.6). Composite grafts are useful for orbital reconstruction when a bone graft is indicated to support the orbit and skin is required to address a contracture ectropion (Fig. 41.7). Alternatively, the TPFF can be used as a sling to support the orbit (Fig. 41.8).

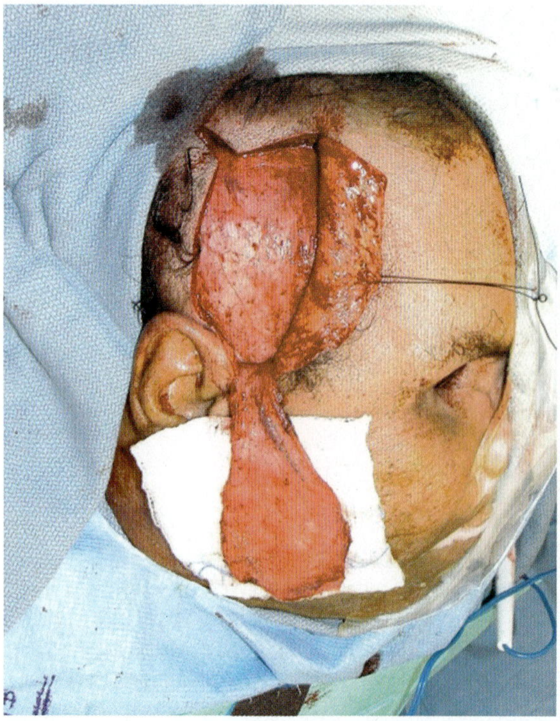

FIGURE 41.5
The TPFF is rotated inferiorly, and the temporalis muscle fascia is exposed.

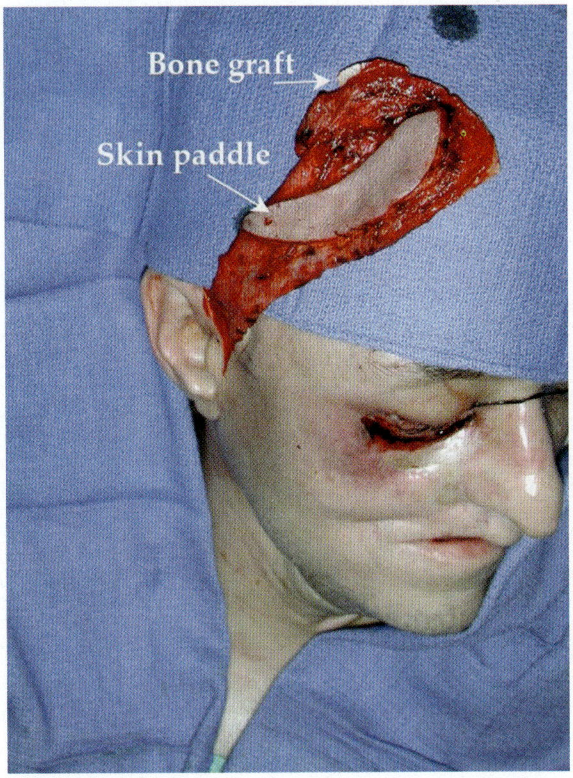

FIGURE 41.6
The photo demonstrates a TPFF–bone–skin composite graft to be used for orbital reconstruction.

POSTOPERATIVE MANAGEMENT

Postoperatively, I place a suction drain and leave that in place for 1 to 2 days. I close the wound with staples because sutures are often difficult to remove in the hair-bearing areas of the scalp.

COMPLICATIONS

Complications are rare; however, when harvesting the TPFF, if you elect to use cautery, alopecia may result from damage to the hair follicles. Cautery can be used, but I would recommend a low setting. If the scalp flaps are too thin, another complication is necrosis of the distal skin edges. For this reason, I use the "Y" design incisions to prevent wound necrosis as a result of compromised blood supply. Finally, when harvesting the

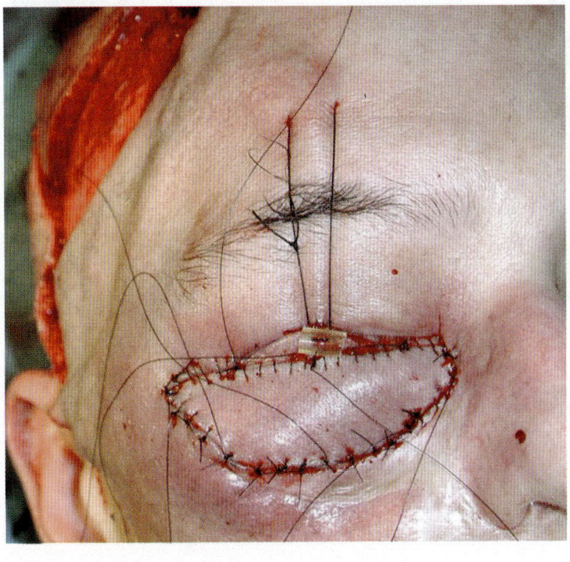

FIGURE 41.7
The composite flap can be positioned such that the skin augments the infraorbital deficiency while the vascularized bone graft is used to support the orbit. This technique is particularly useful in the radiated tissue bed.

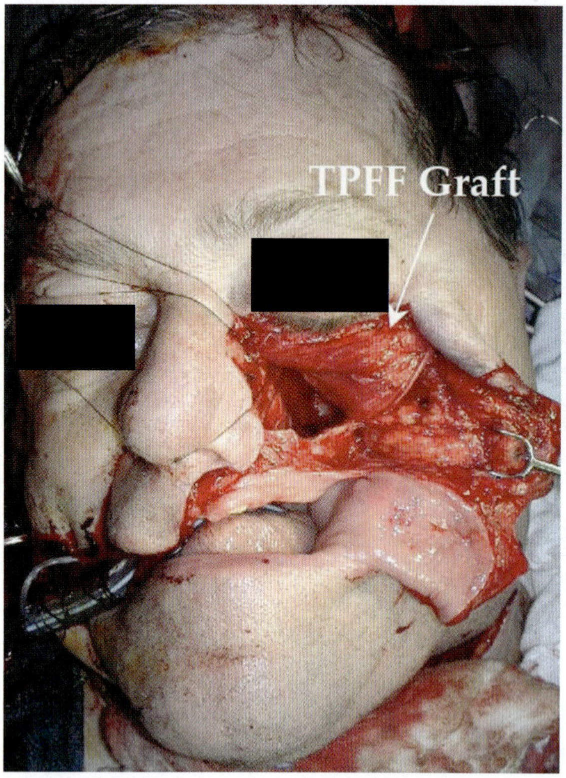

FIGURE 41.8
The TPFF can also be used as a sling to support the orbit.

temporalis muscle, the loss of muscle volume can result in a hollowing defect of the parietal scalp. I typically raise the TPFF as a separate flap when I plan to use the TMF so that I can use the TPFF to fill the muscle donor defect.

RESULTS

The results using this flap have been excellent. Both flaps are reliable because of the axial pattern blood supply. They provide an excellent bed for skin grafting and coverage of a radiated defect (Fig. 41.9A–D).

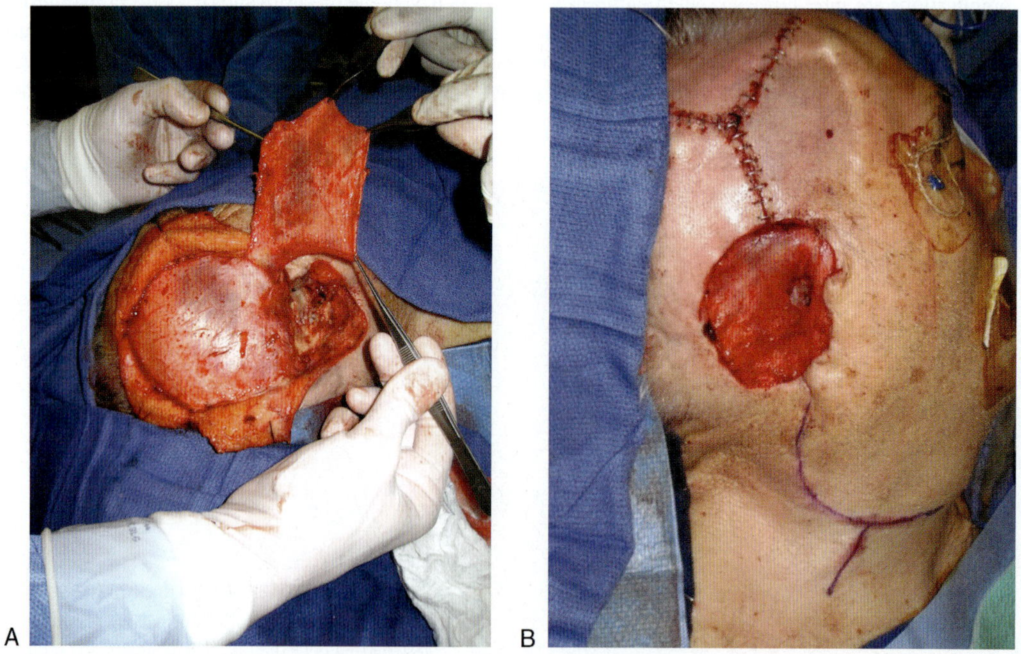

FIGURE 41.9
A. This photo demonstrates the TPFF being raised for coverage of a radiated auriculectomy and mastoid defect. **B.** The graft can be used to cover the defect, and a preformation can be made to preserve an external canal.

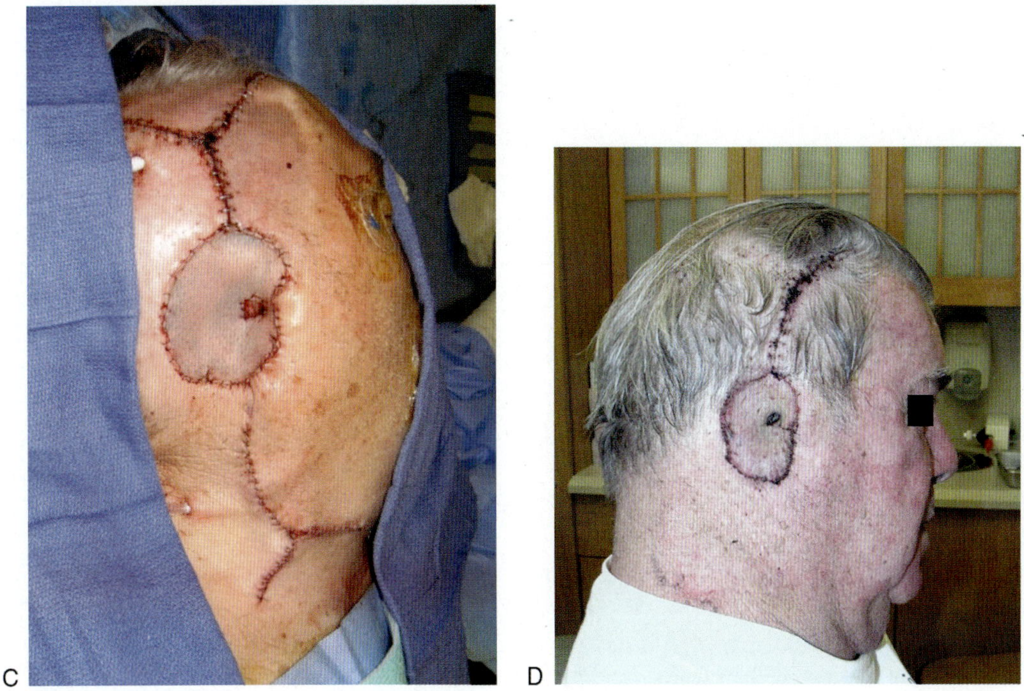

FIGURE 41.9 (*Continued*) **C.** A skin graft is placed over the TPFF. **D.** One-week postoperative evaluation demonstrates the healing graft. This bed will be prepared for osseointegrated implants and an auricular prosthesis.

PEARLS

- The TPFF has a distinct reach limited by the arc of rotation; however, the TMF arc of rotation can be increased by removing a segment of the zygoma or by transecting the coronoid attachments.
- The TPFF is ideal for soft tissue coverage of a nonhealing mastoid cavity.
- The TPFF can be used to fill in the donor defect left following harvest of the TMF.
- The TMF is ideal for reconstructing orbital defects following orbital exenteration.

PITFALLS

- The TPFF is thin and richly vascular. The initial incision through the scalp should be performed with care so as not to injure the nourishing vessels.
- Raising the TPFF with a cautery may result in alopecia.
- If you are planning to transect the coronoid process to increase the TMF arc of rotation, be careful not to injure the vascular pedicle that lies deep to the muscle.

INSTRUMENTS TO HAVE AVAILABLE

- Standard head and neck surgical tray
- Reciprocating saw if a coronoid release is planned.

SUGGESTED READING

Marzo SJ, Leonetti JP, Petruzzelli GJ, et al. Closure of complex lateral skull base defects. *Otol Neurotol* 2005;26(3):522–524.

Smith JE, Ducic Y, Adelson RT. Temporalis muscle flap for reconstruction of skull base defects. *Head Neck* 2010;32(2): 199–203.

Collar RM, Zopf D, Brown D, et al. The versatility of the temporoparietal fascia flap in head and neck reconstruction. *J Plast Reconstr Aesthet Surg* 2012;65(2):141–148.

42 THE RECTUS ABDOMINUS FREE FLAP AND ITS VARIATIONS

Terry A. Day

INTRODUCTION

Major resections involving the lateral skull base present a complex challenge to the reconstructive surgeon. Over the past 30 years, advances in free tissue transfer techniques have improved both the safety of resection of the skull base and the quality of functional and cosmetic outcomes. Moreover, improvements in reconstructive methods have allowed for more comprehensive oncologic resection of advanced tumors of the skull base. Extensive resections involving the lateral skull base entail an array of reconstructive requirements, including the establishment of physiologic and structural separation between the neurocranium, the splanchnocranium, and the aerodigestive compartments; tissue volume replacement and contouring; and functional rehabilitation. Free tissue transfer of the abdominal musculature and its associated fasciocutaneous tissue are key techniques in reconstruction of the lateral skull base. This chapter presents an overview of the development and technical aspects of reconstruction of the lateral skull base using muscular, fascial, and cutaneous elements of the abdominal wall.

Characterization of Lateral Skull Base Defects

Defects of the base of the skull may be classified based on a system proposed by Irish and colleagues, which divides the base of the skull into three regions for the purpose of categorizing reconstructive requirements. Tumors arising in Region II tend to be centered on the infratemporal and pterygopalatine fossae and commonly feature extension through skull base foramina into the middle cranial fossa transversing the pterygoid muscular plane. Region III tumors most commonly originate from the temporal bone with extension into the middle or posterior cranial fossae. Broadly categorized, resection of the lateral base of the skull can encompass ablation of an array of anatomic features, including the lateral temporal bone, the infratemporal fossa, auricle, external auditory canal, masticatory musculature, and cranial nerves. Resulting defects therefore may entail multiple deficits, including insufficient dural coverage, exposure of the internal carotid artery, cavernous sinus or sigmoid sinus, cranial nerves with associated functional deficiencies, and loss of afferent sensory inputs. The most common etiologies for large defects of the base of the skull include extensive cutaneous malignancies, often involving the auricle or external auditory canal; neoplasms of the temporal bone; malignancies of the parotid with deep extension; tumors of the maxillary sinuses with invasion of the pterygopalatine or infratemporal fossae; carcinoma of the nasopharynx; and soft tissue sarcomas arising from the masticatory musculature. Tumor ablation involving the lateral base of the skull may entail extensive resections involving adjacent structures, such as orbital exenteration, auriculectomy, maxillectomy, palatectomy, or mandibulectomy, further complicating the reconstructive endeavor (Fig. 42.1).

In the 1960s, the development of local reconstructive flap techniques marked the opening of the modern era of skull base surgery. During the next two decades, innovations in regional flap techniques facilitated the adoption of more comprehensive resections of the skull base, but surgical complications remained prevalent. Since the 1980s, technical advancements in microsurgical techniques have facilitated broad adoption of free

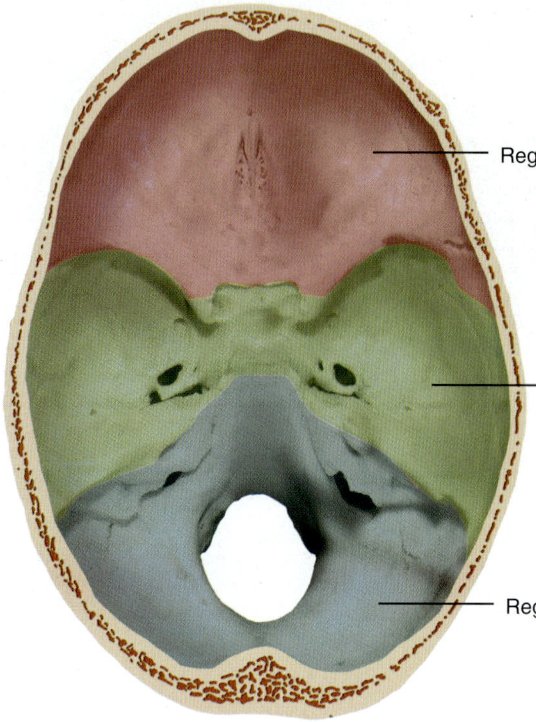

FIGURE 42.1
Skull base defects by region.

tissue transfer as the favored approach to reconstruction of the large defects of the base of the skull. Advantages to free tissue transfer approaches to reconstruction of the lateral base of the skull include the large volumes of tissue available for restoration of contour and obliteration of dead space, the location of donor sites outside irradiated fields, and the presence of well-vascularized tissue that is robust enough to withstand adjunctive radiotherapy and is well suited to the maintenance of effective separation between intra- and extracranial compartments. The development of free flap techniques for reconstruction of the base of the skull has allowed for the performance of increasingly extensive and complex resections. In many cases, functional and aesthetic outcomes in the reconstruction of major defects of the base of the skull may be achieved by combining both locoregional and free flaps in the design of tailored reconstructions.

Free tissue transfer techniques have emerged as the approach of choice for repair of defects of the lateral base of the skull given that effective reconstruction typically requires transfer of large volumes of tissue with aggressive contouring. The distal aspects of local and pedicled flaps, which are most susceptible to failure, are most frequently used in achieving coverage of critical defects. Given the dire consequences of flap loss in this region, the need for reliable coverage of the base of the skull has favored the increasing adoption of free transfer techniques over local or pedicled alternatives. Pedicled flaps, in general, are unlikely to provide adequate coverage for defects of the lateral temporal bone extending above the level of the external auditory canal or infraorbital rim. Whereas pedicled or local flap repairs required multilayer closure with fascial or pericranial grafts for dural repair and pedicled muscle flaps employed for bulk, a rectus abdominis myocutaneous free flap can provide both significant tissue bulk and vascularized lining for dural repair or reinforcement. The interposition of a vascularized layer of tissue yields a more robust partition that resists spread of infection, heals more effectively in a radiated bed, and better withstands adjunctive radiotherapy. A combined rectus muscle and fascial flap allow for one-stage repair of these defects even in patients with gross infection or osteomyelitis. Maintenance of intact vascularization in free tissue obliteration of defects of the skull base also facilitates enhanced delivery of antibiotics or chemotherapeutic agents to the wound site.

HISTORY

In evaluating patients under consideration for rectus flap harvest, it is critical to obtain a complete surgical history with particular attention to any previous abdominal procedures. Caution should be employed with regard to patients who have undergone prior abdominal surgery, particularly inguinal hernia repair. The patient's performance status should be noted, and the overall suitability of the patient for performance of free tissue transfer should be assessed. Key considerations include factors that could adversely impact microvascular tissue transfer, such as coagulation disorders, severe vascular disease, and autoimmune disease. Moreover, adverse influences on wound healing such as smoking and poorly controlled diabetes should be identified. The patient's nutritional status should be assessed and appropriate management of perioperative nutrition undertaken.

PHYSICAL EXAMINATION

Preoperatively, the patient should be examined for abdominal scars. Prior abdominal incisions can compromise the abdominal flaps due to disruption of native vasculature. Moreover, violation of the rectus sheath during prior intra-abdominal surgery or elevation of an abdominal skin flap in the performance of abdominoplasty may increase the risk of formation of a postoperative abdominal hernia. Evidence of a previous Kocher incision is particularly concerning, as the entire thickness of the rectus abdominis has likely been divided. Preoperative arteriography may be employed to ensure vascular sufficiency of potential donor vessels. Body habitus is also a critical factor in selecting appropriate candidates for use of the rectus flap in lateral skull base reconstruction. Obese patients may not be suitable because of excessive tissue bulk, inadequate blood supply, or lipodystrophy. The risk of necrosis of adipose tissue is higher in obese patients when superiorly based flaps are used; thus, inferiorly based pedicles may be preferable in such patients. Performance of the “pinch test” yields a rough estimate of the extent of abdominal tissue that can be excised without undue tension on the abdominal closure.

INDICATIONS

Initially used exclusively as a pedicled rotational flap, the rectus abdominis was first employed as a free tissue transfer for breast reconstruction in the 1970s. Subsequent evolution of the technique entailed the development of muscle-sparing and perforator-based approaches. Advantages of the rectus flap in amelioration of defects of the lateral base of the skull include the following: Lengthy vascular pedicle; soft tissue bulk for effacement of cranial contour defects; anatomically distant from ablative site; little donor site morbidity in appropriately selected patients; potential for use of multiple skin islands; relative ease of harvest and reliable vasculature (Table 42.1). Harvest of the abdominal flaps may be performed concurrently with head and neck ablation. The incisions for these flaps tend to heal favorably and may be well camouflaged within the waistline. Remaining abdominal musculature is generally sufficient in maintaining capacity for abdominal flexion.

Weber, Kim, and Wax have proposed an algorithm for selecting donor sites for reconstruction of the base of the skull by the size of the defect and its location. They consider rectus abdominis flaps to be most suitable for reconstruction of large defects of the lateral base of the skull or maxillectomy defects, with the anterolateral thigh flap as an alternative for smaller lateral defects requiring less bulk. Rosenthal and colleagues described a classification system for describing defects of the lateral temporal bone and base of the skull. Under this system, Class I defects are limited in scope, encompassing mostly preauricular skin, partial auriculectomy, and parotidectomy defects. Class II defects involve significant resection of the lateral temporal bone with middle ear obliteration. Class III defects also include total auriculectomy with or without resection of the parotid gland. Among these categories, the authors characterized Class III defects as being most suitable for reconstruction with a rectus flap.

Defects of the lateral base of the skull present an array of reconstructive imperatives. Reconstructive objectives may be broadly categorized as physiologic/structural, functional, and cosmetic. Table 42.2 delineates the specific imperatives to be considered in lateral skull base reconstruction. Among these diverse reconstructive goals, the establishment of an effective partition between the neural compartments and the aerodigestive tract is an overriding priority. Separation of these compartments is even more critical when large dural defects are involved or when healing is likely to be compromised by infection or irradiation.

Small to moderate defects of the lateral base of the skull may be suitable for reconstruction using locoregional or pedicled flaps such as temporoparietal fascia or pericranial flaps with or without calvarial bone grafts. However, local flaps have insufficient pedicle length and soft tissue bulk for the reconstruction of large defects. Moreover, the tissues most suitable for local flap reconstruction of defects of the lateral base of the skull, including galea, pericranium, temporoparietal fascia, and temporalis musculature, are often compromised during the ablative procedure.

TABLE 42.1 Advantageous Features of Rectus Flaps for Reconstruction of Lateral Skull Base Defects
Lengthy vascular pedicle
Location remote from resection site
Minor donor site morbidity
Potential for multiple skin paddles
Relative ease of harvest
Reliable vascular pedicle
Soft tissue bulk for reconstruction of contour defects

TABLE 42.2 Reconstructive Goals in Addressing Lateral Skull Base Defects

Amelioration of dead space
Coverage and protection of the central nervous system (CNS)
Coverage of major cervical and cranial vasculature
Establishment of a vascularized partition between aerodigestive and CNS compartments
Functional rehabilitation
Maintenance of a barrier to ascending infections
Prevention of CSF leakage
Prevention of pneumocephalus
Relining of mucosal surfaces
Restoration of tissue volume and contour
Support of dural and orbital structures

In most cases of resection of the lateral base of the skull, placement of an adequate volume of soft tissue with comprehensive dural coverage obviates the need for reconstruction of osseous defects. However, specific circumstances may require reconstruction with osseous flaps, bone grafts, or alloplastic implants. Such measures are more likely to be required in extended resections involving the orbitomaxillary structures or mandible. Indications for repair of osseous defects include the following: (1) Very large defects predisposing to gross cerebral herniation; (2) extensive defects of the roof of the orbit risking development of pulsatile enophthalmos; (3) large defects of the orbital or nasal wall; (4) large contour defects not amenable to repair with soft tissue alone; and (5) defects involving the maxilla, mandible, or glenoid fossa likely to interfere with occlusion or mastication.

CONTRAINDICATIONS

With the exception of abdominal scarring that precludes harvest of the rectus abdominis flap, there are no strict contraindications to this option for reconstruction. It is reliable for most defects of the lateral base of the skull.

POSTOPERATIVE PLANNING

In designing a rectus flap, important surface landmarks include the umbilicus, the anterior iliac spine, the symphysis pubis, the linea alba, and the caudal margins of the fifth, sixth, and seventh costal cartilages. The presence of significant diastasis rectus, most common in multiparous females, should be noted. In addition to increasing the risk of abdominal wall herniation, diastasis recti may also necessitate modification of flap design. Multiple flap designs can be employed based on specific reconstructive needs, although consideration should be given to incorporating as much of the periumbilical perforator distribution and subdermal plexus vasculature as possible given particular design constraints. Major perforators should be demarcated preoperatively. This can generally be performed using a handheld Doppler at the time of surgery. However, preoperative imaging using either color flow Doppler or multiphase abdominal CT imaging may also be helpful; obtaining these studies preoperatively is particularly useful if a perforator-based rather than a myocutaneous flap is planned.

SURGICAL TECHNIQUE

Anatomical Considerations

The rectus abdominis originates from the symphysis pubis and pubic crest and inserts on the fifth, sixth, and seventh costal cartilages. The arcuate line traverses the rectus abdominis at the midpoint between the umbilicus and symphysis—approximately 4 to 6 cm superior to the pubis. The extent of the rectus abdominis lying cephalad to the arcuate line is completely ensheathed in thick rectus fascia formed by the division of the internal oblique aponeurosis into anterior and posterior leaflets. Caudal to the arcuate line, the fascia of the internal oblique arises superficially to form the deep layer of the anterior rectus sheath, and the posterior rectus muscle is covered by transversalis fascia only. Longitudinally, the rectus abdominis is transected in the midline by the linea alba. Transversely, it has three tendinous inscriptions that are contiguous with the anterior rectus sheath, and it is thus separated into six muscular compartments. The entire length of the rectus abdominis musculature from xiphoid to pubis is potentially available for harvest and free transfer as a myocutaneous flap.

The rectus abdominis muscle features two dominant vascular pedicles, the deep inferior and superior epigastric arteries, along with an extensive arcade of perforators. The deep inferior epigastric artery (DIEA) originates from the external iliac artery approximately 1 cm cephalad to the inguinal ligament with an orientation toward the wall of the lateral rectus. As it ascends within a plane between the transversalis fascia and conjoint tendon superficially and the peritoneal fascia, the DIEA gently curves in a medial direction. It passes superficially to the arcuate line and then deep to the rectus abdominis within the posterior rectus sheath. It typically divides into lateral and medial branches. The lateral branch tends to be larger and often features anastomotic continuity with the deep superior epigastric artery (DSEA). The average caliber of the DIEA is 2.7 mm at its origin and 2.0 mm at the point where it penetrates the rectus sheath in its posterolateral aspect; typical pedicle length is 7 cm.

The DSEA is derived from the internal mammary artery at roughly the level of the sixth intercostal space. It descends superficial to the plane of the transverse thoracic muscle, running between its origins on the costal margin and xiphoid. It subsequently pierces the fascial envelope of the rectus and then arborizes within an intramuscular plane superficial to the posterior rectus sheath. The DSEA features an average caliber of 2.1 mm at its point of origin where it separates from the musculophrenic artery and 1.9 mm where it enters the deep surface of the rectus sheath. The DIEA is the largest artery of the abdominal wall, with a caliber (2.5 to 3.8 mm) that is generally twice that of the DSEA, and it is the preferred vessel for standard free transfer of a rectus myocutaneous flap. Both the DSEA and the DIEA are accompanied by consistent venae comitantes. Although venous drainage into the venae comitantes typically crosses the midline, the venae comitantes alone may be insufficient to prevent vascular congestion if the flap features significant contralateral extension. In these circumstances, harvest and incorporation of the superficial inferior epigastric vein (SIEV) decrease the risk of venous congestion and partial loss of the flap (Fig. 42.2).

The DIEA and the DSEA both contribute to a rich anastomotic network within the intramuscular plane and give off multiple perforators that travel though the rectus musculature toward the abdominal surface. As they emerge from the anterior rectus sheath, these perforators communicate with the subdermal plexus. An extensive watershed area exists between the DSEA and DIEA arcades above the level of the umbilicus. It is this watershed distribution, along with the shared territory of the subdermal plexus, that allows for versatility in using either DSEA or DIEA vessels as flap pedicles. Circumferentially, the subdermal plexus overlying the rectus musculature communicates via a system of choke vessels with multiple other regions of subdermal perfusion, including those distributions arising from the superficial superior and inferior epigastric arteries, the superficial circumflex arteries, and the intercostal vasculature. This extensive network of subdermal plexus vasculature allows for great variability for cutaneous flap design, with the potential for incorporation of adjacent angiosomes beyond those directly nourished by harvested perforators. Reliability of adjacent angiosome utilization can be increased by delayed flap elevation, which promotes dilation of the choke vessels prior to flap harvest.

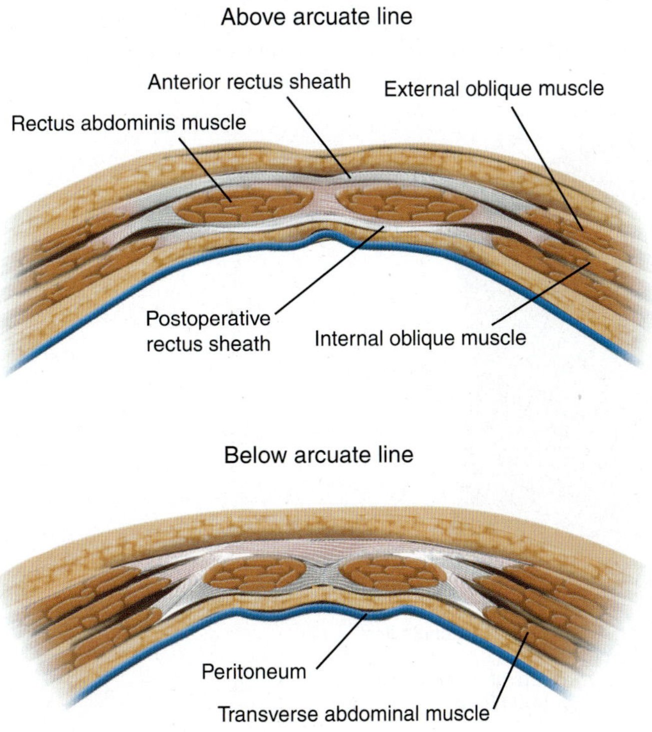

FIGURE 42.2
Cross-sectional view of the vascular and muscular anatomy of the abdomen above and below the arcuate line.

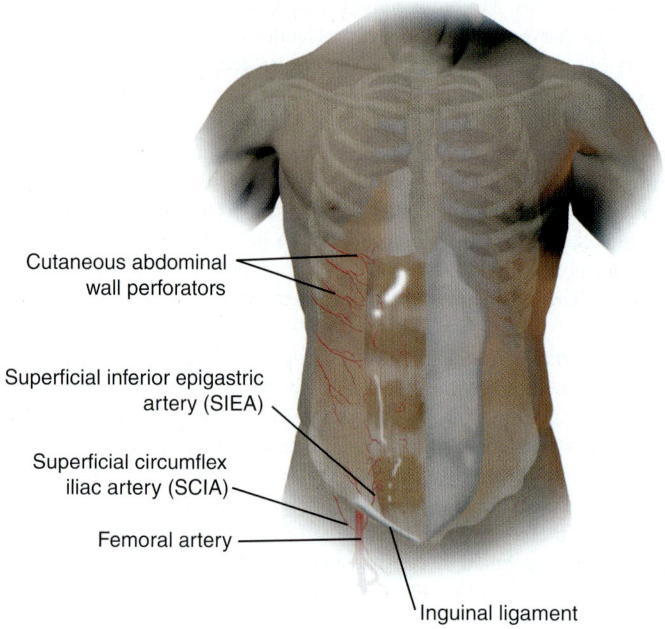

FIGURE 42.3
Cutaneous perforators of the abdominal wall.

The deep inferior epigastric perforator (DIEP) flap is based upon a constellation of periumbilical perforators emerging from the DIEA. There are typically five or six such large-caliber vessels (>0.5 cm in diameter). The largest periumbilical perforator is typically encountered lateral to or just caudal to the level of the umbilicus. While the course and orientation of these periumbilical perforators is highly variable, most emerge within 10 cm of the umbilicus and can be easily localized preoperatively with a handheld Doppler. If a territory is mapped in a half-circle shape extending out laterally and inferiorly around the umbilicus with a 6-cm radius, the major periumbilical perforators will be encompassed within this area in 90% of cases. Although DSEA-based flaps may be designed that incorporate the periumbilical perforators, they are generally less favored due to the fact that the perforators derive directly from the DIEA or its branches while their connection to the DSEA vascular arcades are attenuated by the periumbilical watershed anastomoses (Figs. 42.3 and 42.4).

Additional blood supply to the lower area of the abdominal wall is derived from the superficial inferior epigastric artery (SIEA). The SIEA diverges from the common femoral artery, typically at a point 2 to 3 cm caudal to the inguinal ligament. However, the arterial course of the SIEA varies widely, and the SIEA is minor or absent in roughly one-third of patients. The SIEA traverses the femoral triangle, crossing the inguinal ligament roughly at its midpoint, and then ascends the abdominal wall within the subcutaneous layer, with its course becoming more superficial as it approaches the periumbilical area. Branches of the SIEA anastomose widely with both the main periumbilical perforators and the arterial network of the subdermal plexus. The average diameter and length of SIEA are 1.6 mm and 5 cm, respectively.

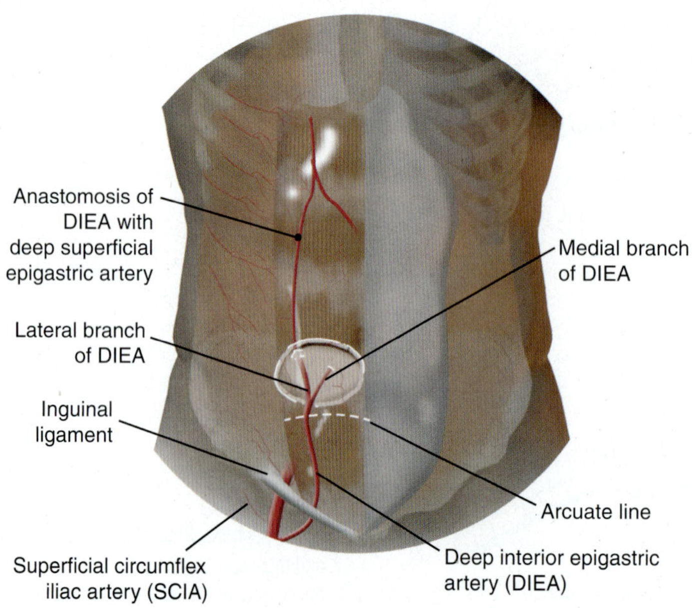

FIGURE 42.4
Distribution and localization of periumbilical perforators.

The superficial circumflex iliac artery (SCIA) is also derived from the femoral artery. Sharing of a common trunk by the SIEA and SCIA is a frequent anatomic variation. Most commonly, the SCIA diverges from the superficial femoral artery at a point approximately 3 cm caudal to the inguinal ligament and ascends in a trajectory roughly parallel to the inferior border of the inguinal ligament toward the anterior superior iliac spine (ASIS). Upon reaching the level where it traverses the sartorius, the SCIA tends to split into superficial and deep branches. The relative sizes of the superficial and deep SCIAs are highly variable. A series of perforators are emitted by both the superficial and deep systems. The SCIA is typically accompanied by paired venae comitantes.

The Rectus Abdominis Myocutaneous Flap

Multiple flap designs may be employed in the harvest of a myocutaneous rectus abdominis free flap, including the vertical rectus abdominis myocutaneous flap (VRAM), the transverse rectus abdominis muscle flap, and thoracoumbilical variations. Each of these flap designs uses the DIEA pedicle and should be fashioned such that the base is centered upon the rich perforator arcade of the periumbilicus. The standard VRAM flap is begun with a longitudinal incision extending from the level of the superior tendinous insertion superiorly to the inguinal ligament inferiorly. The upper portion is straight and centered over the midpoint of the ipsilateral rectus musculature in a transverse dimension. Below the level of the anterior–superior iliac spine, the incision is gently flared out laterally over the inguinal region so as to remain centered over the DIEA pedicle. Electrocautery is then used to deepen the incision through the subcutaneous plane and the anterior rectus sheath. Excision of rectus sheath below the arcuate line should be avoided, as leaving rectus sheath intact below this level decreases the risk of the subsequent development of a ventral hernia.

The two edges of the split anterior rectus sheath are then retracted laterally to allow for exposure of the bulk of the ipsilateral rectus musculature. Dissection is carried inferiorly until exposure of the rectus abdominis origin at the pubis is achieved. The attachment of the muscle is carefully divided and the caudal end of the muscle retracted superiorly, revealing the underlying DIEA pedicle. The pedicle is dissected caudally and may be followed until its divergence from the external iliac artery. Division of the DIEA at this level provides an average of 10 cm of pedicle length. Once the pedicle is divided and protected, harvest of the muscle is performed in accordance with flap design, with the muscle preferentially divided along its fascial borders or tendinous inscriptions (Table 42.3; Fig. 42.5).

Muscle-Sparing Variations

The era of reconstruction using muscle-sparing abdominal flaps began in 1989 with Koshima and Soeda's description of the DIEP flap. The primary advantage of the DIEP over traditional rectus flaps was that by sparing the bulk of the rectus musculature, the risk of postoperative abdominal wall weakness and herniation was reduced. Although the DIEP flap entails only skin and subcutaneous tissue, harvest still requires incision of the anterior rectus sheath and dissection through the abdominal wall musculature. With the advent of the superior–inferior epigastric artery flap, complete sparing of the abdominal musculature was achieved. A more recently described abdominal free flap, the SCIA flap, also spares dissection of both the rectus musculature and its fascial sheath. Woodworth and colleagues presented a series of head and neck reconstructions performed using muscle-sparing variations on DIEP, SIEA, and SCIA flaps. Advantages of these flaps included reduced morbidity of the donor site, a predictable volume of tissue transfer, and the favorable cosmetic result of a low-set transverse abdominal scar. The average size of the head and neck defect repaired was 74.5 cm^2. There were no postoperative abdominal hernias (Fig. 42.6).

TABLE 42.3 Characteristics of DIEA-based Rectus Abdominis Myocutaneous Free Flaps
DIEA diameter = 3.5 mm (3–5 mm)
DIEA length = 7 cm (6–8 cm)
DIEV diameter = 4 mm (2–5 mm)
DIEV length = 6 cm (4–8 cm)
Skin island length = 13 cm (10–20 cm)
Skin island width = 25 cm (20–40 cm)
Skin island thickness = 2.5 cm (1–6 cm)
Muscle thickness = 1.5 cm (0.7–2 cm)

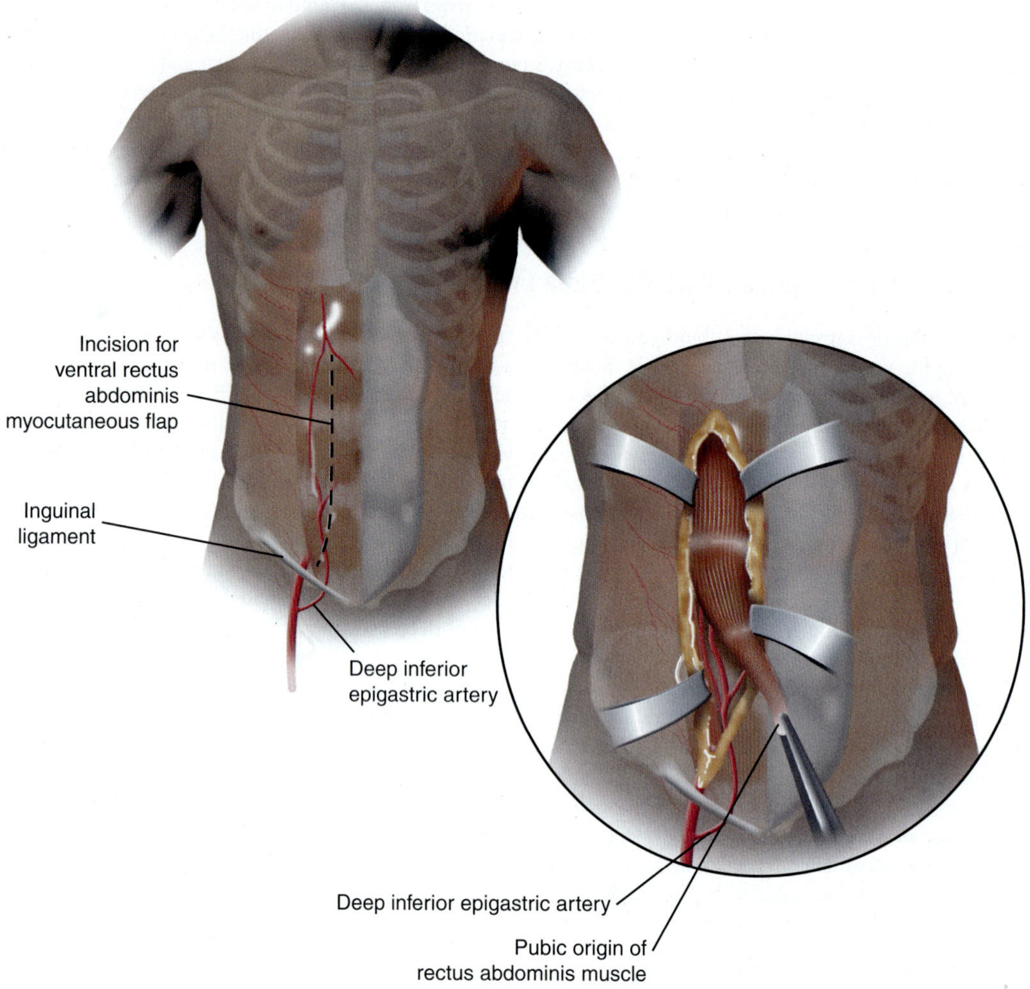

FIGURE 42.5 Dissection of the pubic origin of the rectus muscle and identification of the DIEA pedicle.

Deep Inferior Epigastric Perforator Flap

Preoperatively, the locations of the primary umbilical perforators and the course of the SIEA and SIEV are confirmed with handheld Doppler and marked. As with the rectus myocutaneous free flap, differing size and orientations of the skin paddle may be employed depending on defect-specific reconstructive requirements, but the design must incorporate a portion of the periumbilical perforator region of the abdominal wall. DIEP flaps utilized for head and neck reconstruction are typically based on 1 to 3 perforators, with an average of 1.5 perforators employed. The skin incision is performed circumferentially. Dissection is then carried down to the deep fascial layer. Generally, flap elevation begins at the most lateral or inferior aspects of the flap depending on the orientation of the skin paddle. As elevation progresses toward the periumbilicus, care is taken to identify and preserve the major perforators as they exit the anterior rectus sheath. The SIEV, which typically courses in a paramedian orientation approximately 4 to 5 cm lateral to the linea alba, should also be identified and preserved, as it may be useful in maintaining adequate venous drainage of large flaps. Up to three large-caliber perforators are then selected for preservation. Small, longitudinally oriented openings in the anterior rectus sheath allow for egress of the large perforators. The desired perforators are freed from the anterior rectus fascia with releasing incisions of the rectus sheath and then progressively followed through the rectus muscle using intramuscular dissection. In most cases, perforators can be freed by simply enlarging the natural disruptions in the fascial wall, which surround the perforators by inserting one blade of a small scissors and then splitting the fascia above and below to create a 2- to 3-cm longitudinally oriented fascial opening. A small cuff of rectus tissue is preserved around each perforator. Other perforators are then ligated, and the flap is progressively released from the anterior abdominal wall until it is tethered only by the preserved perforators. Separation of muscle fibers in their longitudinal plane allows for dissection of the perforators with only minimal damage to the surrounding rectus musculature. Segmental innervation of the rectus abdominis should be preserved when possible.

Perforators are followed down toward their origin from the DIEP vessels with ligation of small muscular branches. As dissection of the pedicle progresses, adjacent perforators may join into common vessels. Dissection is continued until appropriate pedicle and caliber length are obtained in accordance with the

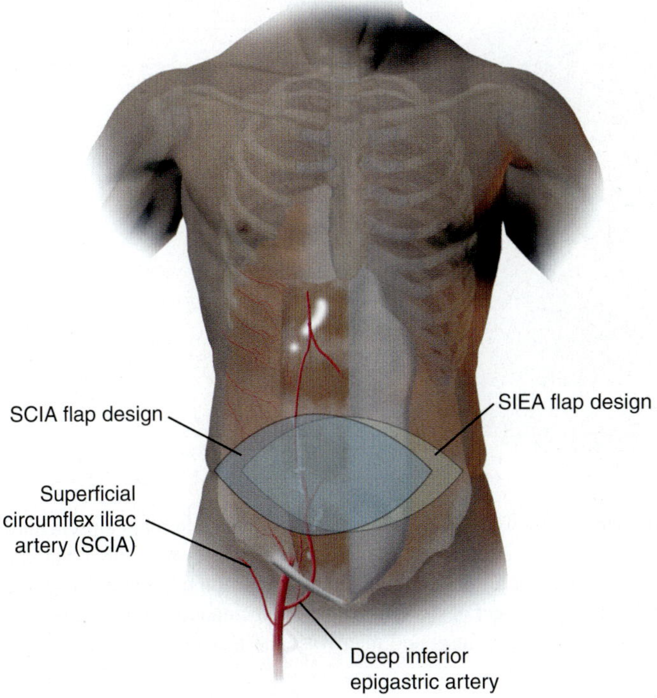

FIGURE 42.6
SCIA, SIEA, and DIEA designs.

reconstructive requirements. Typical pedicle length is greater than 10 cm. If further pedicle length is required, incision of the inferior rectus sheath can facilitate tracing of the pedicle all the way back to the origin of the DIEA vessels. The perforators selected for the pedicle are then ligated and separated from surrounding DIEP vasculature with division of any anastomotic connections to the superior epigastric arcade. The perforator-based pedicle is then delivered through the previously fashioned apertures in the overlying rectus musculature and the anterior fascia (Figs. 42.7 and 42.8).

Superior–Inferior Epigastric Artery Flap

Preoperatively, the position of the SIEA, the SIEV, and the periumbilical perforators should be delineated with a Doppler. Initial elevation of the flap proceeds in a suprafascial plane, with early identification of the SIEA at the midpoint of the inguinal ligament. The caliber of the vessel should be assessed; if the SIEA is absent or features a diameter less than 1 mm, consideration should be given to conversion to conversion to a DIEP flap. Among patients in whom the SIEA is small or absent, the periumbilical perforators tend to be larger—making use of the DIEP flap more advantageous in such settings. If the SIEA is judged to be adequate, it can be carefully dissected to its takeoff from the femoral artery as needed, with division of the pedicle at a point where adequate caliber of the vessel and pedicle length have been achieved. Average SIEA pedicle length is 4 cm. The

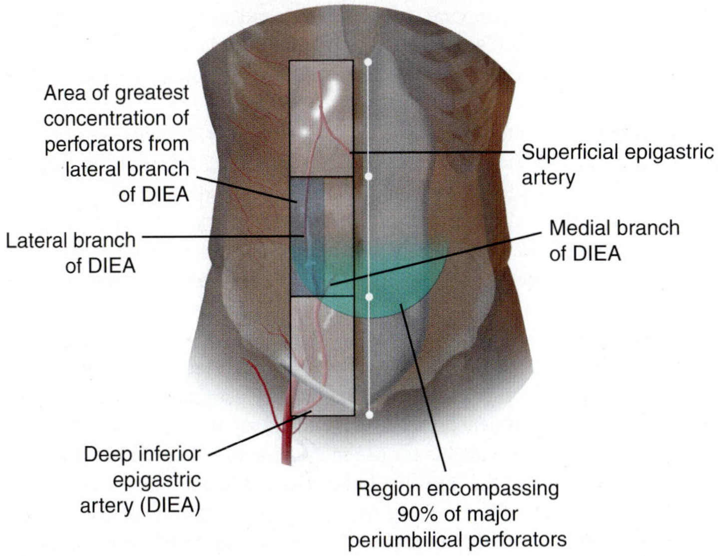

FIGURE 42.7
Preoperative marking of expected distribution of periumbilical perforators.

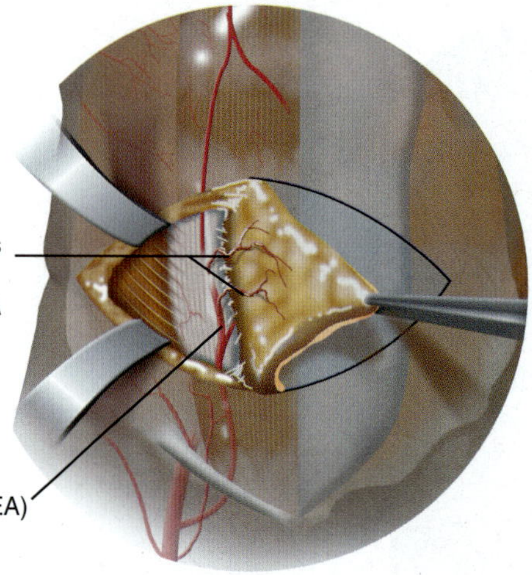

FIGURE 42.8 Elevation of flap with preservation and intramuscular dissection of perforators.

primary advantage of the SIEA flap as compared to the DIEP is the fact that the rectus abdominis musculature and the anterior rectus sheath are both left undisturbed. Disadvantages include a relatively small tissue volume and short pedicle length. Moreover, the SIEA is small or absent in a significant proportion of patients. Also, the fact that the SIEA pedicle emerges from the inferior aspect of the flap within a subcutaneous plane rather the deep surface of the flap can make orientation of the flap at inset and microvascular anastomosis more technically challenging, irrespective of relative pedicle caliber.

Superficial Circumflex Iliac Artery Flap

Preoperatively, the course of the SCIA inferior and parallel to the inguinal ligament from the femoral artery toward the ASIS and its major perforators are delineated and marked. The ASIS, inguinal ligament, and femoral artery are key anatomic landmarks. Flap design should encompass major SCIA perforators and the skin overlying the ASIS. Elevation of the flap is achieved in a suprafascial plane with careful preservation of major perforators. A dominant perforator is selected and traced back to the SCIA. Ideally, the superficial circumflex iliac vein (SCIV) should be dissected along with the venae comitantes, as the venae comitantes may be inadequate to provide sufficient drainage to avoid venous engorgement. Circumferential flap elevation is completed after the course of the selected SCIA perforator has been traced out. Dissection of the pedicle can be carried back to its takeoff from the femoral artery. Pedicle ligation and transfer should include the proximal SCIA and its venae comitantes along with a corresponding segment of the SCIV. Advantages of the SCIA flap include its thin profile, flexibility for folding and contouring, and the potential for rapid harvest. The major drawback to the flap is the small diameter of the SCIA, which may be 1 mm or less. In obese patients, the SCIA may be preferable to the DIEP and SIEA due to its less bulky relative volume and decreased risk of necrosis of adipose tissue.

Flap Inset

Options for arterial recipient vessels include superficial temporal, facial, lingual, and superior thyroid arteries. Priority may be given to preferential use of more cephalic vessels so as to preserve caudal options for possible future reconstructions. The superficial temporal vessels are a useful option based on their superior position and appropriate caliber.

The approach to dural repair varies depending on the size of the defect. If possible, primary dural repair yielding a watertight closure is optimal in protecting the dural contents from ascending infection. In the setting of large dural defects, grafts can be used, with preference given for autogenous grafts such as fascia lata or temporalis fascia. Alternatively, the fascial surface of the reconstructive free flaps may be used in patching dural deficiencies if defect and pedicle geometry allows. Free adipose tissue grafts harvested from the abdomen may be used to reinforce dural coverage in areas where defect dimensions make achievement of a tight dural seal difficult.

Following flap positioning to obliterate the defect, microvascular anastomosis is performed using standard techniques. Depending on the design of the flap and the characteristics of the defect, skin islands may be preserved as needed for cutaneous reconstruction. Other portions of the flap are deepithelialized. Any flap surfaces used in reconstruction of aerodigestive compartments should be meticulously deepithelialized to promote mucosal ingrowth. The fascial portion of the flap is suitable for use in creation of a watertight dural seal. If dura has been closed primarily, the fascial surface of the flap should be overlaid to reinforce a watertight repair. Alternatively, the fascial surface may be sutured directly to the free edges of the dura so as to obliterate directly the dural defect. The maintenance of an intact blood supply to the fascia is preferable to the use of a free rectus sheath fascial graft. If the complex dimensions of the defect require, the fascial portion of the flap may be pedicled on a sole perforator. The subcutaneous portion of the flap can also be positioned as a "cork" overlying the dural repair.

During inset, the flap should be carefully secured to the surrounding tissues to prevent the graft from falling away and compromising coverage of the base of the skull. The flap may be directly sutured to the adjoining temporalis musculature. Burr holes may be established in the bony cranial perimeter of the defect through which anchoring sutures may be placed to suspend and secure the flap. Suspension of the flap via drill holes placed around the craniectomy defect can facilitate secure placement of the free tissue transfer over the dura. If necessary, a channel may be drilled in the cranial wall to allow the vascular pedicle to drape away from the anastomotic site without undue kinking, torsion, or tension. When recipient vessels within the neck are used, the pedicle should be threaded into the neck through a tunnel between the angle of the mandible and the oral mucosa.

If the defect of the base of the skull extends to involve the orbit, the rectus myocutaneous flap may be employed in primary reconstruction of the orbit. If facial nerve resection is required for tumor extirpation, reanimation measures including the placement of gold or platinum weights in the upper lid, lid-tightening procedures such as wedge resection or canthoplasty, and static sling procedures may be performed in a single stage along with rectus flap reconstruction.

Primary closure of the donor site is preferred and is feasible in nearly all cases. If the rectus sheath was incised during flap harvest, it must be securely reapproximated. If significant rectus musculature is harvested or there is a sizable defect in the anterior rectus sheath, placement of a synthetic mesh as part of the donor site closure decreases the risk of postoperative hernia. Consideration should be given to placement of a lumbar drain and application of compressive dressing in circumstances where a reliable watertight dural seal has been impossible to establish. This measure counters the force of normal CSF pulsations, which will tend to promote dissection between tissue closure planes with a resulting increased risk of CSF leakage and susceptibility to ascending infection (Fig. 42.9).

Technical Innovations and Variations

Fasciocutaneous and perforator-based variations upon the rectus flap afford greater flexibility in reconstructive design, particularly in circumstances where less bulk is required. One key distinction between myocutaneous and perforator-based variations is that the perforator flaps allow for precise establishment of cranial and facial contours at the time of initial reconstruction without the expectation of significant atrophy as would occur with a myocutaneous flap. The degree of denervation atrophy likely to occur over time with the myocutaneous rectus flap is unpredictable, thus complicating decisions regarding the amount of bulk appropriate for initial reconstruction. Moreover, the absence of muscle bulk allows for more complex folding for three-dimensional reconstruction and increased independent mobility if multiple skin paddles are employed. Although muscle-sparing variations of the rectus flap have been widely adopted in the performance of breast reconstruction, their use in the reconstruction of head and neck defects is relatively new. DIEP and SIEA flaps have been shown to yield reduced morbidity at the donor site, length of stay, and hospital costs as compared to traditional myocutaneous rectus flaps in breast reconstruction. Recent published series of cases have also demonstrated the safety and effectiveness of muscle-sparing variants in head and neck reconstruction.

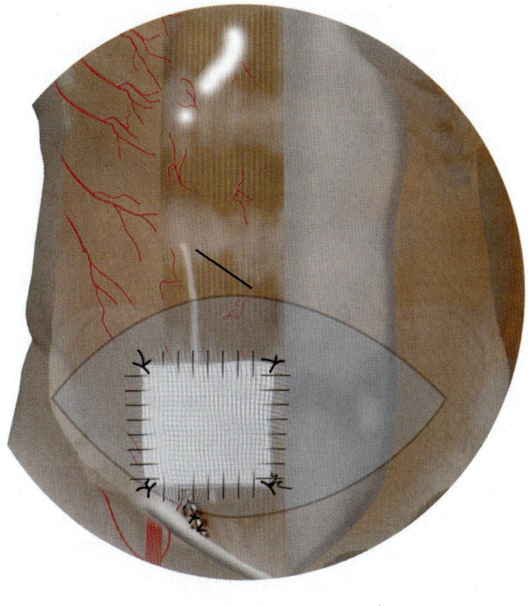

FIGURE 42.9
Closure of donor site with alloplastic mesh.

Although reconstruction of bony elements is not often required for reconstruction of defects of the lateral base of the skull, bony support may be desirable if defects extend to involve orbitomaxillary structures. In such cases, bone grafts from other sites such as the iliac crest may be incorporated into myocutaneous rectus free flaps prior to inset. Malar reconstruction may also be achieved using osteomyocutaneous composite free rectus flaps including a costochondral component. If bony elements are required for reconstruction, portions of the 7th, 8th, 9th, and 10th ribs, which derive their blood supply from their corresponding intracostal vessels, may be harvested in conjunction with abdominal flaps. These vessels are nourished primarily by the costomarginal artery, which features anastomotic connections with DSEA on the deep surface, allowing for incorporation of rib elements into the rectus flap. Free rectus flaps incorporating 7th to 10th rib elements have been successfully used in craniofacial reconstruction. Alternatively, vascularized bone can be incorporated into the DIEP flap with harvest of a portion of the superior pubic ramus, which receives arterial supply from the DIEP vessels. Use of the rectus abdominis as a free flap with efferent neural innervation as a one-stage procedure for reconstruction of facial defects with reanimation has been described, and the division of the rectus abdominis by tendinous inscription into multiple functional segments with separate neural fascicles holds the potential for complex facial reanimation.

POSTOPERATIVE MANAGEMENT

Postoperatively, patients should be admitted to an intensive care unit to monitor both the flap and the neurologic status. If the dural envelope was violated, a postoperative CT is indicated to evaluate for pneumocephalus. CSF leaks are an uncommon complication and generally resolve with lumbar drain decompression when they do develop. Neurosurgical consultation is necessary if a lumbar drain has been placed. Standard techniques for monitoring of free flaps should be employed with frequent flap checks in the immediate postoperative period. The neurologic status of the patient should be closely monitored for evidence of meningitis or other cerebral complications. Nutritional status should be optimized in the perioperative period to maximize healing. Manipulation of intraperitoneal contents during flap elevation may cause postoperative ileus, in which case enteral feeding must be temporarily suspended. Donor site care requirements are minimal, although strenuous activity should be limited until incision sites are well healed. Abdominal exercises should be deferred for several weeks.

COMPLICATIONS

Generally, I have found that complications are rare and typically are restricted to abdominal hernia. The closure of the donor site must be achieved with meticulous attention to the fascial closure, or the risk of hernia is high.

RESULTS

The results with the technique have been outstanding. In over 100 cases, I have has had excellent results. The anatomy and reliability are excellent. Free tissue reconstructions using the rectus abdominis myocutaneous free flap or its muscle-sparing variants are reliable techniques for ameliorating large defects involving the lateral base of the skull. The musculature of the abdominal wall and associated fasciocutaneous tissues can yield a large volume of highly vascularized tissue that can effectively protect neural elements of the base of the skull while also addressing complex associated functional and aesthetic deficits. Innovative techniques for the harvest and inset of abdominal flaps have been established that provide the reconstructive surgeon with tremendous flexibility in designing reconstructive procedures tailored to the specific needs of patients with defects of the lateral base of the skull.

PEARLS

- Achievement of a watertight dural seal and establishment of a physiologic barrier protecting the dural compartment is a critical factor in reconstruction of defects of the lateral base of the skull.
- In most cases, osseous elements are not required in reconstruction of the lateral base of the skull, and transfer of an adequate volume of vascularized soft tissue is sufficient.
- Muscle-sparing abdominal flaps such as the DIEP, SIEA, and SICA flaps provide greater flexibility for reconstruction of complex three-dimensional defects of the lateral base of the skull and minimize the risk of postoperative donor site complications.
- The rate of abdominal hernia following performance of a rectus myocutaneous free tissue transfer is low. However, placement of an alloplastic mesh during donor site closure should be considered in high-risk patients.

- Preoperative imaging with either color flow Doppler or CT may be helpful in ensuring adequate vascularity for free transfer of abdominal tissue and in identifying the locations and course of key perforator vessels.
- The major periumbilical perforators can generally be identified within a 6-cm radius of the umbilicus.
- Perforator-based abdominal flaps for reconstruction of the lateral base of the skull most commonly incorporate one to three periumbilical perforators. The largest perforator is typically located just lateral to the umbilicus, either directly on or slightly caudal to the transumbilical plane.
- Postoperative CSF leaks following free tissue reconstruction of lateral skull base defects are rare, and when they occur, they generally resolve rapidly with lumbar drain decompression.

PITFALLS

- Previous abdominal surgery is a relative contraindication to the use of the rectus abdominis flap or its variants in free tissue transfer.
- Perforator-based abdominal flaps may lack adequate bulk for amelioration of large defects of the lateral base of the skull.
- Significant volume loss will occur with transfer of a free rectus abdominis myocutaneous flap due to denervation atrophy, although the degree of loss is variable and difficult to anticipate.
- Ascending infection may lead to meningitis or other cerebral complications if sufficient insulation and partition of the neural compartment is not established.
- Abdominal flaps employed in reconstruction may be weighty, and secure attachment to the skull base may be challenging to achieve.
- Placement of a lumbar drain and application of compressive dressings should be considered if the dural seal is of questionable integrity.

INSTRUMENTS TO HAVE AVAILABLE

- Standard head and neck surgical set

ACKNOWLEDGMENT

I gratefully acknowledge the contributions of Barry T. Malin, MD MPP.

SUGGESTED READING

Gal T, Kerschner J, Futran D, et al. Reconstruction after temporal bone resection. *Laryngoscope* 1998;108(4 pt1):476–481.

Day T, Davis B. Skull base reconstruction and rehabilitation. *Otolaryngol Clin North Am* 2001;34(6):1241–1257.

Marchetti C, Gessaroli M, Cipriani R, et al. Use of perforator flaps in skull base reconstruction after tumor resection. *Plast Reconstr Surg* 2002;110(5):1303–1309.

Leonhardt H, Mai R, Pradel W, et al. Free DIEP-flap reconstruction of tumor related defects in head and neck. *J Physiol Pharmacol* 2008;59:59–67.

Rosenthal E, King T, McGrew B, et al. Evolution of a paradigm for free tissue transfer reconstruction of lateral temporal bone defects. *Head Neck* 2008;30(5):589–594.

43 FACIAL PARALYSIS

Elliott H. Rose

INTRODUCTION

Clinical characteristics of the totally or partially paralyzed face can be directly attributed to absence or weakness of the mimetic muscles of facial expression. The arborizing cranial nerve VII acts as the "electrical wiring" of the face (Fig. 43.1). Injury to the facial nerve, whether infectious, developmental, traumatic, or of tumor origin impacts the "targeted" facial muscles (Fig. 43.2) and creates very predictable functional and structural deficits based on specific innervation of the VII nerve branches as follows:

1. *Generalized facial laxity* related to atonicity of the deep foundation of the face (mimetic muscles and superficial aponeurotic system)—*VII nerve trunk*
2. *Upper lip immobility* (asymmetric smile with "shadowing" of the upper teeth) related to weakness of the lip elevators and zygomaticus major and minor muscles—*buccal* branch of the facial nerve
3. *Inadequate smile "spread"* (asymmetric smile) related to weakness of the risorius muscle—*buccal* branch of facial nerve
4. *Oral incompetence* (pursing, blowing, whistling, intraoral seal) related to weakness of the orbicularis oris sphincter—buccal branch of facial nerve
5. *Lower lip flaccidity* (drooling, speech impairment, chewing) related to paralysis of the depressor labii muscle—*marginal mandibular* branch of facial nerve
6. *Inspiratory collapse of nasal vestibule* (decreased nasal air flow, congestion) related to weakness of the levator labii superioris alaeque nasi muscle—*buccal* branch of the facial nerve
7. *Paralytic ectropion of the eyelids* (tearing, corneal exposure, lagophthalmos) related to weakness of orbicularis oculi muscle—*zygomatic* (*orbital*) branch of facial nerve
8. *Ptosis of the brow* (impaired upward gaze) related to paralysis of the frontalis muscle—*frontalis* branch of facial nerve

In view of the myriad of functional and structural deficits, successful reanimation of the paralyzed face is a lofty challenge to the reconstructive facial surgeon. The two defining objectives of any successful reanimation surgery are to achieve (1) static facial balance at rest and (2) symmetric, dynamic movement (preferably voluntary and spontaneous) by supplementation or substitution of the paralyzed muscles.

I have delineated methods of static rebalancing in my description of multiple applications of autogenous fascia lata slings in providing deep structural support of the facial foundation and correction of droopiness of the lips, eyelids, and nostrils.

Given the "symphony of motion" of the multiple mimetic muscles of facial expression, no single procedure can supplant the intricacies of motion/vectors needed for "natural" facial movement. The ideal situation, of course, is direct and/or interpositional nerve grafting of a recent facial nerve injury. Frequently, however, those repairs are neither feasible nor temporally suitable, and secondary reconstructive options need to be considered. In cases of partial paralysis or in older adults, regional muscle transfers (temporalis, masseter,

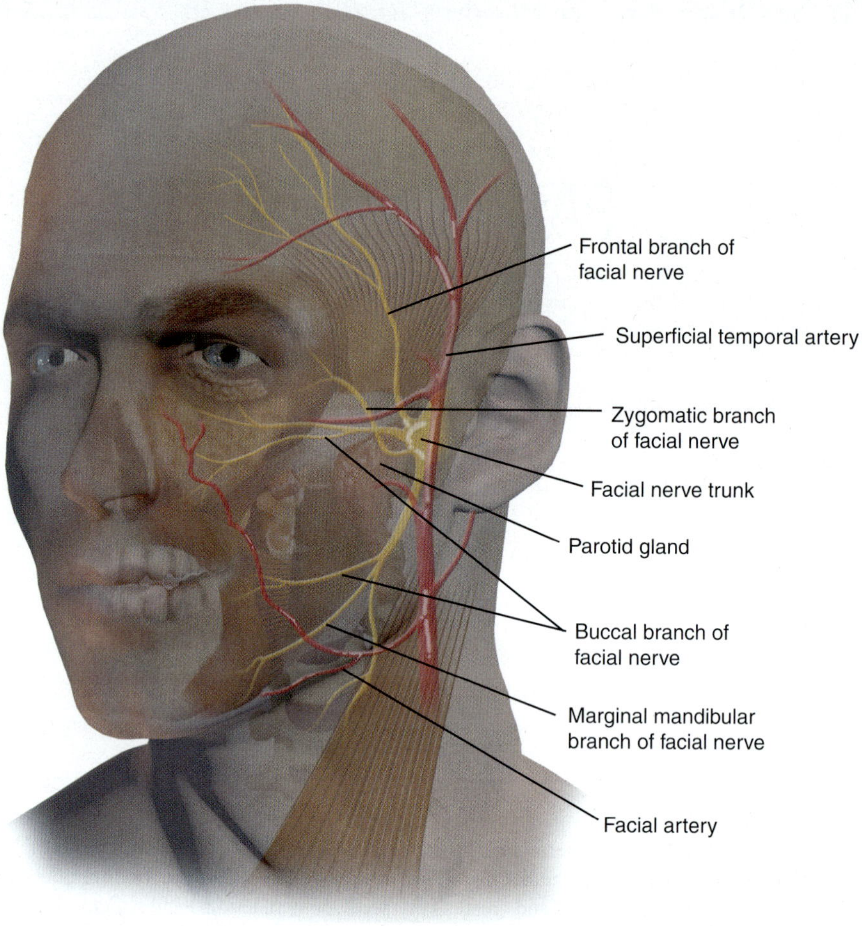

FIGURE 43.1
The arborizing VII cranial nerve acts as the "electrical wiring" of the face.

platysma, frontalis) are the procedures of choice. These procedures, although very effective, require lengthy neuromuscular retraining and may lack involuntary spontaneity. In younger patients, however, the preference is for facial nerve "specificity" by reinnervation from the contralateral facial nerve (via cross-facial nerve graft) into the distal branches of the injured facial nerve. Or, in long-standing facial paralyses where the target muscles have undergone "denervation atrophy," a substitute muscle is necessary to reanimate the paralyzed face (free gracilis muscle transfer). The focus of this chapter is on the use of cross-facial nerve grafts and microvascular free gracilis muscle flaps in achieving such dynamic motion.

The contemporary era of dynamic correction of facial palsy emerged with the introduction of the microvascular free transfer of the gracilis muscle by Harii in 1976 based on Tamai's earlier experimental (1970) and clinical work in the transfer of muscle as a vascularized unit. The initial gracilis transfer was neurotized by the ipsilateral V cranial nerve but, of course, required "triggering" by smiling or clenching the teeth (that concept is now being "recycled" by Manktelow and Klebuc's work using the branch to the masseter as the motor nerve). Usage of the contralateral normal facial nerve as a source of innervation was conceived by Scaramella (1970) and further refined by Smith and Anderl (1979). Gordon and Buncke showed in rhesus monkeys that heterotopic muscles could function adequately when motored by long interpositional nerve grafts. O'Brien in 1980 synthesized these concepts into an algorithm defining the clinical indications for cross-facial nerve grafting and free microvascular gracilis muscle transfers in long-standing facial paralysis. Other muscles, such as pectoralis minor, serratus anterior, extensor brevis, latissimus dorsi, and palmaris longus, have also been used as recipient muscles in facial reanimation. The gracilis muscle, however, is the most commonly used and, in my opinion, the easiest to work with and most predictable in outcome. The advantage of this approach is the ability to obtain synchronous and spontaneous bilateral facial expression and a more "natural" smile.

HISTORY

A careful history is elicited from the patient (or parents) confirming mode of onset, duration, and improvement (if any) since onset. In infants or toddlers with congenital facial paralysis, parents are questioned regarding problems during the pregnancy (infection, drug exposure, smoking, and eclampsia), positioning of the fetus, family history, and birth trauma (forceps delivery, small pelvic canal). If a hereditary etiology (i.e., CHARGE syndrome)

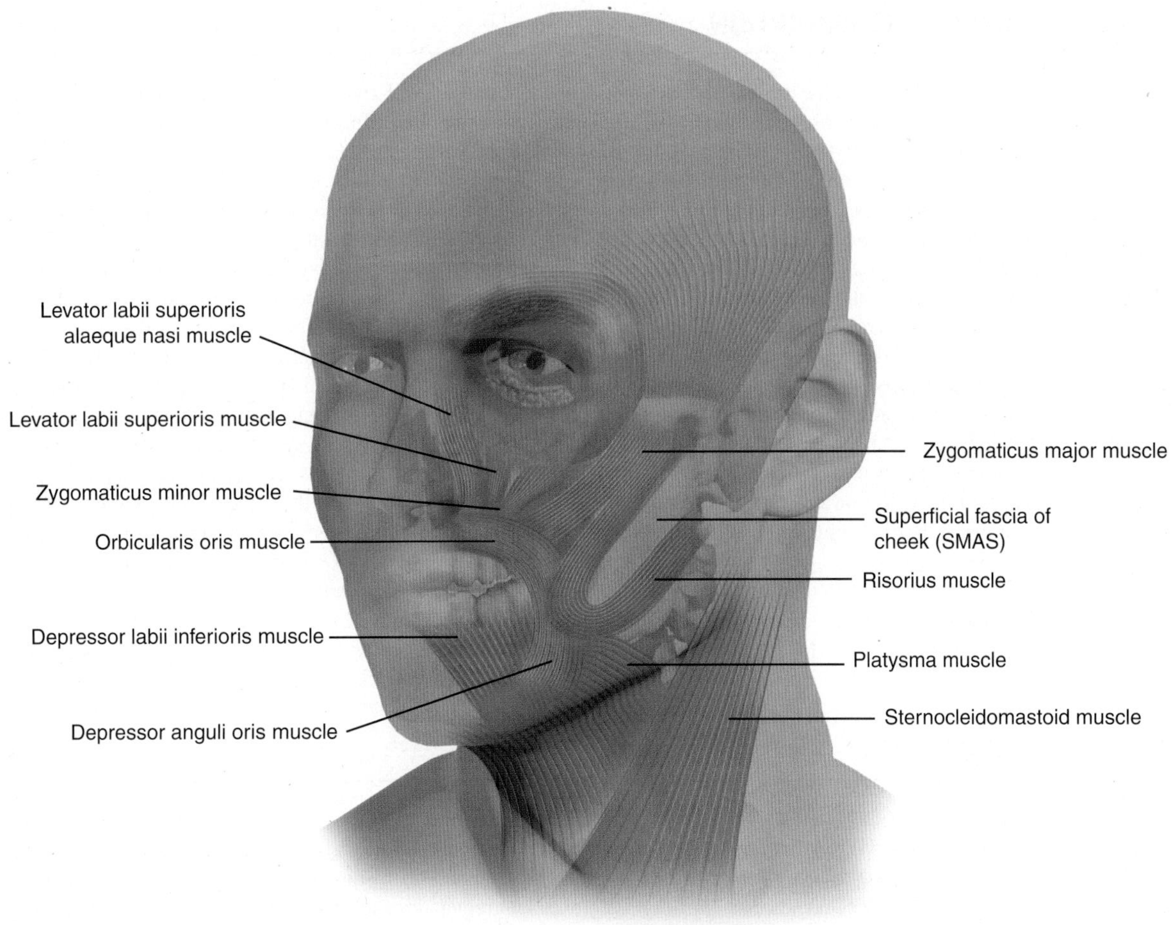

FIGURE 43.2 A facial nerve deficit creates generalized facial laxity related to atonicity of the deep foundation of the face, upper lip immobility, related to weakness of the lip elevators, zygomaticus major and minor muscles, and an inadequate smile "spread" related to weakness of the risorius muscle. Additionally, oral incompetence (pursing, blowing, whistling, intraoral seal) related to weakness of the orbicularis oris sphincter, lower lip flaccidity related to paralysis of the depressor labii muscle, and inspiratory collapse of nasal vestibule related to weakness of the levator labii superioris alaeque nasi muscle can occur. The upper face suffers from paralytic ectropion of the eyelids related to weakness of orbicularis oculi muscle and ptosis of the brow related to paralysis of the frontalis muscle.

is suspected, a geneticist should evaluate the family or siblings. A description of the timing of the onset (immediate or delayed), early treatment, and neurophysiologic testing should be obtained from the family.

In teens or adult patients, the etiology is usually more clear (intracranial or facial nerve trauma, developmental, acoustic neuroma, brain stem tumor, parotid tumor, Bell palsy, lymphangioma or hemangioma, or iatrogenic). Timing of the onset, early treatment, response to physical therapy or acupuncture, staging of return of facial function (timing of initiation of return and "plateau" of facial movement), prior testing (EMG/NCS or CAT scan), and neurologic, ophthalmologic, and speech evaluations should be elicited from the patient. Prior photos from family events are very helpful in assessing smile and facial expression. Work history and impact on social and professional interactions are helpful in understanding self-esteem issues and coping skills related to the functional disabilities. The final question in the assessment should be "Are you motivated to have your facial paralysis corrected?"

Functional problems associated with an established facial paralysis are fairly predictable (see clinical characteristics above). History related to periocular problems should include queries regarding visual impairment, corneal exposure, immobile brow, excessive tearing, impaired upward gaze, incomplete eye closure, and blepharospasm (synkinesis). Does the patient require taping, eye drops, or night time lubrication? Midface subjective findings include facial atonicity and flaccidity (while puffing cheeks); biting of the inside of the mouth, tongue, and lips; droopiness of the nostrils, cheek, and corner of the lip; difficulty with bolus management (oftentimes needing tongue to sweep food to healthy side); impaired chewing; inadequate oral seal while whistling, blowing, or sucking; and dribbling from the corner of the mouth while cup feeding or drinking through straw. Speech patterns affected are primarily the bilabial sounds—plosives (p's and b's) and phonemes (f's, w's, v's, and m's). Patients may complain of late-day lack of articulation, lower volume, or speech fatigability.

PHYSICAL EXAMINATION

Specific findings on physical examination are dependent on the level and extent of the lesion. In total or near total paralyses, the perioral, midface, and periocular regions are most affected. In milder cases, the patient may appear normal at rest; in more severe cases, droopiness and loss of muscle tone may be apparent (flatness of the nasolabial fold, loss of the nasolabial crease, elongation of the upper lip, sagging of the brow and corner of the eye, "open" eye). With animation, however, the discrepancies are much more visible. While smiling, there is asymmetry between the void and active side with an overpull by the healthy muscles. "Shadowing" of the upper teeth is noted (tooth exposure on the palsied vs. the healthy side is an easy measure of upper lip mobility). "Smile spread" is diminished on the affected side (measured by the distance between the midline tubercle and lateral commissure). The paralyzed lower lip is invaginated/inverted causing "shadowing" of the lower teeth. On inspiration, there is downward displacement of the affected nostril with snarling causing obstruction of the vestibular airway. Puckering and pursing of the lips are impaired, compromising the ability to create an intra-oral seal. With attempted lip approximation or puckering, there is usually a gap between the upper and lower lip allowing escape of air or fluids.

In the periocular region, the affected eyebrow is "flattened" having lost is arch and paralleling the supra-orbital rim. With upward gaze, there is a 1.0 to 1.5 cm discrepancy between the affected and healthy side. In residual Bell palsy or neuropraxic injuries within the intratemporal canal, intensive blepharospasm (synkinesis) may be "triggered" by the yawning, chewing, or clenching teeth. Extensive tearing (epiphora) may be noted in the affected "tear trough" (particularly when tilting the head) due to inadequate seal of the lower lid to the eyeball. In severe cases, lagophthalmos (gap) is noted between upper and lower lip with voluntary closure. The cornea is usually protected by automatic upward deviation of the globe with incomplete closure (Bell phenomenon). The blink reflex is often absent in lesions at the brain stem level.

INDICATIONS

Facial reanimation by cross-facial nerve grafting and gracilis muscle transfer is primarily an operation for *younger* patients. Axonal regeneration across an interpositional nerve graft tends to diminish with age and may be inadequate to neurotize the transferred muscle from a distant source. In my opinion, age 35 to 40 is the "cutoff" for cross-facial nerve grafting. Very excellent regional muscle transfers (temporalis and platysma) offer a "one-stage" facial reanimation with evidence of facial movement at 4 to 6 weeks postoperatively (albeit extensive neuromuscular retraining is necessary to "trigger" the transferred muscle). Most adults are not willing to wait the 1½ to 2 years necessary to experience spontaneous facial movement after microsurgical reconstruction utilizing the two-stage procedure. Regional muscle transfers (temporalis and platysma) are also the procedures of choice in the *partial* paralyses following Bell palsy, acoustic neuroma resection and trauma. In these patients, the risk of jeopardizing existing motion by splicing into intact facial nerve branches on the palsied side does not justify the more extensive microsurgical reconstruction.

CONTRAINDICATIONS

Elderly patients, particularly those with medical comorbidities, may not tolerate the lengthy operative times of the respective two stages and should be considered as candidates for static and/or regional muscle transfers.

PREOPERATIVE PLANNING

Initial evaluation should include CT imaging to rule out an intracranial lesion (acoustic neuroma, tumor, or vascular abnormality), skull fracture, or stenosis of the facial canal within the petrous portion of the temporal bone (in developmental facial paralysis). EMG/NCS studies determine the degree or localization of facial nerve neuropathy as well as strength of muscle motor action potentials. In longer-standing facial paralyses, the presence of fibrillations indicates potential viability of mimetic muscle (after neurotization) whereas "flat line" indicates denervation atrophy of the target muscles has occurred (not amenable to reinnervation). Photographs and videotapes in repose and while emoting (smiling, speaking, smirking, snarling, grimacing, puckering, sucking, blowing, closing eyes, looking upward) document facial asymmetry and aberrant speech patterns. Evaluation by a speech pathologist using the Frenchay Dysarthria Assessment delineates functional impairment of activities of daily living (chewing, swallowing, fluid management, lip seal, and bolus management) and critically analyzes alterations in speech articulation and clarity. Examination by a board-certified ophthalmologist inspects for conditions of paralytic ectropion, epiphora, brow ptosis, lagophthalmos, blepharospasm (synkinesis), and contralateral hyperactive frontalis, associated with facial palsy. All muscle activities are recorded on a 0–5 scale based on the Sunnybrook Facial Grading Scale. Asymmetric smile patterns are digitized and analyzed by facial recognition software comparing movement of fixed perioral landmarks on the palsied versus the healthy side.

SURGICAL TECHNIQUE

Two-stage cross-facial nerve grafting (with or without free gracilis transfer) is generally indicated in younger patients with complete palsy of the entire side of the face or an isolated sector of the face (i.e., perioral, periocular, midface, lower face, etc.). If the duration of the injury to the facial nerve is less than 2 years, the "target muscles" are still receptive to reinnervation (should be confirmed by EMG/NCS). That "window" may be extended to 2½ years in infants or children before denervation atrophy becomes permanent. Additional time can also be obtained by DC stimulation of the denervated muscles during the reconstructive period or incorporation of a "baby sitter" partial hypoglossal transfer as an interim step (Terzis). Time for axonal regeneration across the face (generally, 1 inch per month) must be accounted for in assessing total "denervation time." Multiple cross-facial nerve grafts may be employed to restore eye closure, midface movement, oral competence, and smile symmetry. In my experience, fine mimetic muscle movement (eye closure, nostril elevation, and lower lip eversion) can be achieved with direct cross-facial nerve grafting. Upper lip elevation (for creation of smile symmetry) usually requires the addition of a *mini-gracilis muscle* transfer to overcome the effects of gravity. In those cases, two buccal cross-facial nerve grafts are used—one for distal neurorrhaphy to the buccal branch on the injured side and the other to motor the gracilis transfer (Fig. 43.3). In long-standing facial paralyses, a single cross-facial nerve graft from the buccal branch is used to motor the gracilis transfer.

Cross-Facial Nerve Graft (Figs. 43.3 and 43.4)

A nasotracheal tube is passed through the nostril on the nonaffected side and anchored with a silk horizontal mattress suture to the nasal septum (Fig. 43.4A). Covering with a sterile drape allows the tube to be manipulated out of the way during the operative procedure. Short-acting paralyzing agents are used for induction. The anesthesiologist should check for muscle contractibility before mapping of the facial nerve. The surgical approach is through a face-lift incision on the *healthy* side with horizontal extension beneath the angle of the

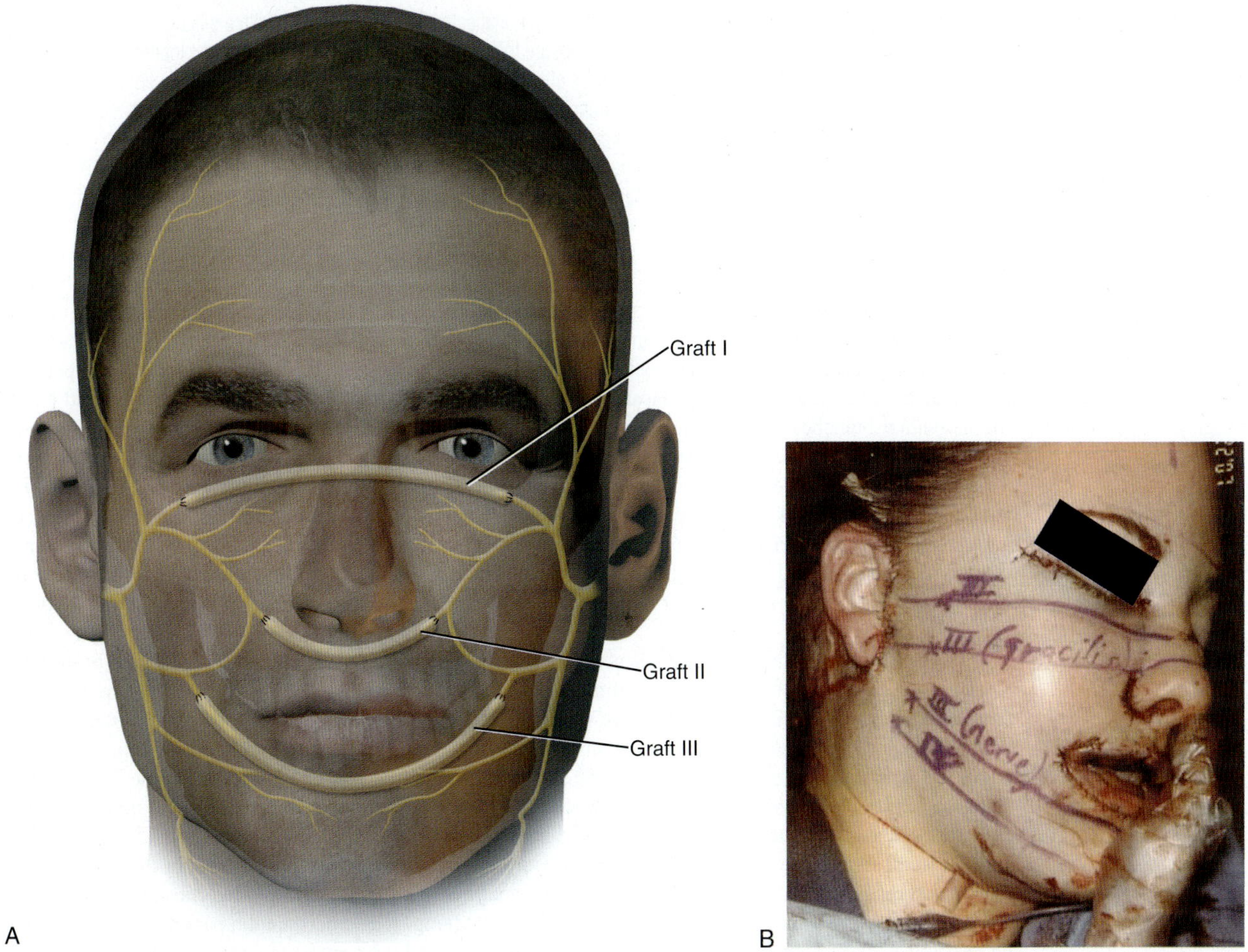

FIGURE 43.3 A. In select cases, one to four buccal cross-facial nerve grafts are utilized. **B.** Clinical photo outlining the gracilis position and the cross-facial nerve graft orientation.

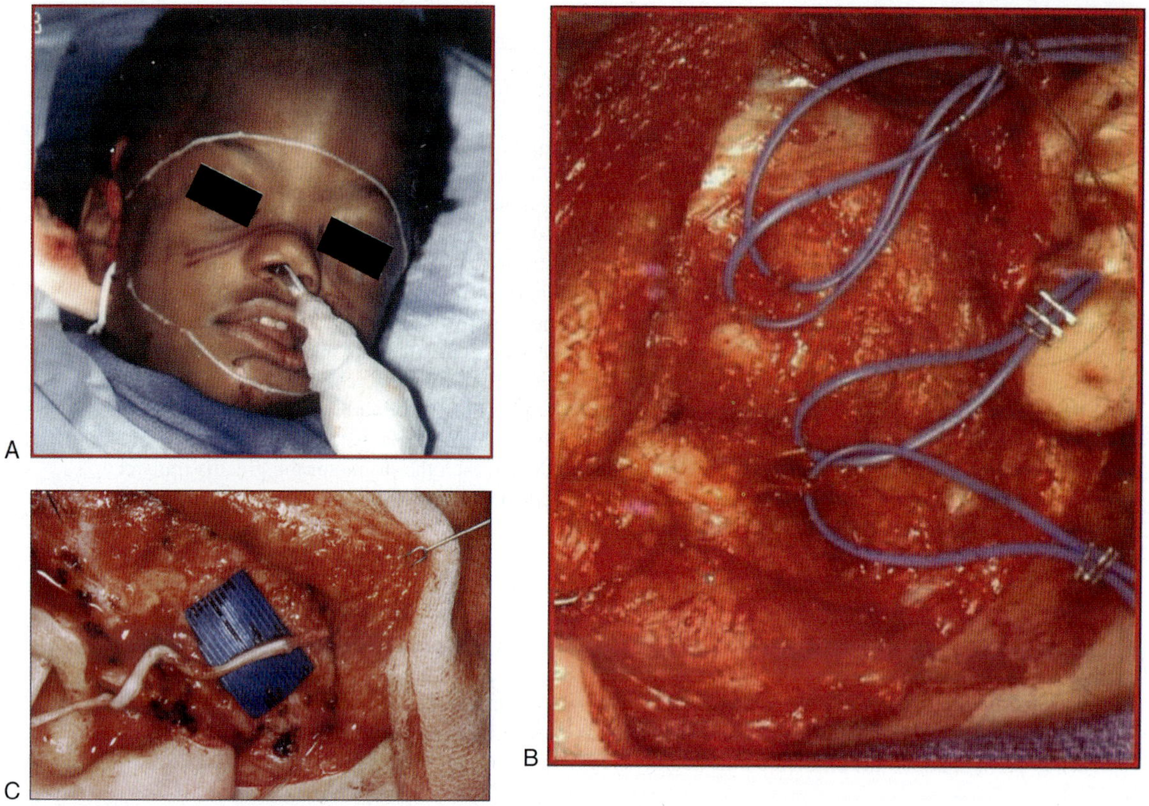

FIGURE 43.4 **A.** A nasotracheal tube is passed through the nostril on the nonaffected side and anchored with a silk horizontal mattress suture to the nasal septum. The grafts are oriented to ensure the appropriate length. **B.** Rubber vessel loupes are passed around the individually identified nerve branches. For ease of mapping identification, microhemoclips are placed on the vessel loupes to correspond with the specific facial nerve branch—1 for frontal, 2 for zygomatic (orbital), 3 for buccal, and 4 for marginal mandibular. **C.** The proximal neurorrhaphy is carried out under 40 to 50× magnification with 10-0 nylon on a 100-μm needle. Fascicles from the fresh end of the identified duplicate facial nerve branch are aligned with the proximal cut end of the sural nerve graft. Repair is by perineural placement of the sutures in a "watertight" closure around the nerve to preclude protruding of fascicles at the repair site.

mandible (Ridson type neck extension) to gain greater exposure. Soft tissue should be injected with a fresh epinephrine mixture of 1:100,000 concentration prior to dissection (Xylocaine or Marcaine should be avoided during mapping). The buccal flap is retracted and hemostasis obtained with the bipolar cautery. The superficial musculoaponeurotic system (SMAS) fascia is gently teased apart at the anterior margin of the parotid gland. The individual branches of the facial nerve are identified by microdissection in the periparotid region and stimulated with the handheld nerve stimulator (2 mV). Observation is made by the assistant for brow elevation, eye twitching, upper lip/nostril movement, and lower lip eversion. Rubber vessel loupes are passed around the individually identified nerve branches (Fig. 43.4B). For ease of mapping identification, microhemoclips are placed on the vessel loupes to correspond with the specific facial nerve branch—1 for frontal, 2 for zygomatic (orbital), 3 for buccal, and 4 for marginal mandibular. The largest branches are the ones selected as recipients for the sural nerve grafts. *Duplicates* of the individual nerve branches are confirmed prior to proximal nerve repair.

Harvesting of the sural nerve grafts is accomplished by a second team of surgeons. The length of the graft is determined by the number of cross-facial nerves needed (15 to 18 cm per graft). Generally, two grafts can be obtained per calf (maximum length 30 to 35 cm). A hockey-shaped incision is made 1 cm posterior to the lateral malleolus of the ankle. The retinaculum is released, and the sural nerve is dissected within the groove. Additional length can be obtained by extending the incision over the lateral foot to dissect the lateral dorsal cutaneous nerve. The nerve is traced proximally beneath the investing fascia of the calf. Serial transverse incisions are made on the posterior calf, and the nerve is delivered beneath the subcutaneous tunnel.

The sural nerves are "reversed," transposed to the recipient site, and "preset" within the face prior to microneural repair. A periauricular face lift incision is made on the palsied side and the cheek flap retracted to allow for placement of the fascia lata sling and SMAS tightening. A Kleinert tendon passer is used to deliver the respective nerves across the face (supraorbital, transnasal, and submental) from the healthy to the palsied side. Stab incisions are made in the frown lines, midline nose, and chin cleft and submentally to assist in passage of the nerve grafts. The distal end of each cross-facial nerve graft is delivered to the palsied side and attached to the deep SMAS with microclips, the number corresponding with the mapping of the nerve—1 for frontal, 2 for zygomatic (orbital), 3 for buccal, and 4 for marginal mandibular. A blue Prolene suture is used as a "tracer" interconnecting the fresh end of the distal nerve to an appropriate site on the cauda helix, tragus, or lobe of the ear.

One (buccal) to four cross-facial nerve (orbital, buccal × 2, marginal mandibular) grafts are inset and tagged. The operating microscope is brought into the field. Proximal neurorrhaphy is carried out under 40 to 50× magnification with 10-0 nylon on a 100-μm needle (Fig. 43.4C). Fascicles from the fresh end of the identified duplicate facial nerve branch are aligned with the proximal cut end of the sural nerve graft. Repair is by perineural placement of the sutures in a "watertight" closure around the nerve to preclude protruding of fascicles at the repair site. Felt-tip external skin markings are made of the position of the individual grafts on the face and documented photographically and numerically.

Axonal regeneration is monitored by advancing Tinel sign at monthly intervals postoperatively. The course of the nerve is tapped with fingertip or eraser tip to elicit a "shock." Distances of advancing Tinel are documented and dated on facial drawings contained within the chart. Regeneration across the face usually takes 6 to 9 months (1 inch per month). In toddlers in whom Tinel monitoring is not feasible, 6 to 7 months is the arbitrary time for secondary exploration. External DC stimulation may be used to stimulate the denervated facial muscles in the interval between the first and second stages.

At the second stage, the periauricular face lift incision on the palsied side is reopened and extended horizontally beneath the angle of the mandible (Ridson type neck extension). The blue "tracer" sutures are followed to the distal end of the cross-facial nerve. Corroboration of the specific nerve branch is confirmed by counting the microclips at the distal end of each nerve graft. The neuromata are resected, and frozen section biopsies are sent from the distal cut end of each graft to confirm axonal regeneration. Microdissection of the facial nerve branches on the palsied side is comparable to the opposite side by gently teasing away the SMAS fascia at the anterior parotid border. Distal neurorrhaphy is similar to the contralateral side as the distal end of the cross-facial nerve graft is microneurally repaired to the cut end of the distal branch of the facial nerve (or obturator nerve of the free gracilis transfer).

Moderately compressive dressings are applied circumferentially around the face. Patients are generally kept in the hospital 2 to 3 days after each stage. Diet is advanced from liquid to soft, and excessive facial expression is avoided for 10 to 14 days.

Free Gracilis Muscle Transfer (Figs. 43.5 and 43.6)

In long-standing paralyses where facial muscles have undergone permanent denervation atrophy, reinnervation by direct neurotization is not a viable option. In those cases, replacement of the target muscle is mandatory. A variety of options have been described by various authors—gracilis, pectoralis minor, latissimus dorsi, extensor digitorum brevis, serratus anterior, and palmaris longus. In my hands, the gracilis has proven to be the most reliable and predictable and has an excursion similar to the zygomaticus muscles to be replaced. Motor input is via the buccal cross-facial nerve graft from the contralateral side passed submentally or by an ipsilateral branch of the trigeminal nerve to the masseter (I prefer the former because of the specificity of motor nerve input and preclusion of neuromuscular retraining postsurgically; the latter is indicated in bilateral Mobius cases).

Anesthesia is once again delivered through a nasotracheal tube on the nonaffected side. The access to the cheek is via a face lift incision with Ridson neck extension on the palsied side. A large cheek flap is elevated at the level of the SMAS over the buccal cheek and premaxillary area. A counter incision is made just beneath the mucocutaneous border of the lateral third of the upper lip and slightly around the lateral commissure. The upper lip skin is teased away from the orbicularis oris with fine tenotomy scissors and undermined to the nasolabial crease. A tunnel is created interconnecting the lip and cheek flaps (through which the gracilis muscle will pass). The course of the facial artery and vein (or external jugular vein) is auscultated by a Doppler probe at the inferior border of the body of the mandible (junction of middle and posterior thirds). An incision is made transversely through the platysma muscle. The artery and vein are isolated and tagged with colored vessel loupes.

A separate surgical team harvests the gracilis muscle (usually on the contralateral side) through a vertical incision in the upper one-third of the inner thigh along the course of a line interconnecting the pubic tubercle to the medial malleolus of the knee. The investing fascia is split and the gracilis muscle dissected. The obturator nerve is dissected proximally for 7 to 8 cm. The arterial and venous leashes are traced laterally in the deep thigh to their origin from the profundus femoris vessels. The gracilis is debulked longitudinally in situ following stimulation of the fascicles of the obturator nerve to identify maximum locus of contraction (usually the lateral two-thirds). The resting length of the muscle is marked by placement of silk sutures at 5-cm intervals on the surface of the muscle prior to detachment. Perfusion of the muscle is verified and the muscle is stimulated again in situ to assure contractility.

The muscle is transposed to the recipient cheek and anchored proximally to the lateral zygomatic arch and deep temporal fascia with heavy Prolene suture. Orientation of the muscle is predetermined by the anatomy of the smile on the contralateral healthy side. The resting length of the muscle is preserved at the inset. Distal neurorrhaphy between the buccal cross-facial nerve graft and obturator nerve usually lies deep to the muscle and is performed prior to the final inset. The distal end of the muscle is brought through the lip incision and tapered

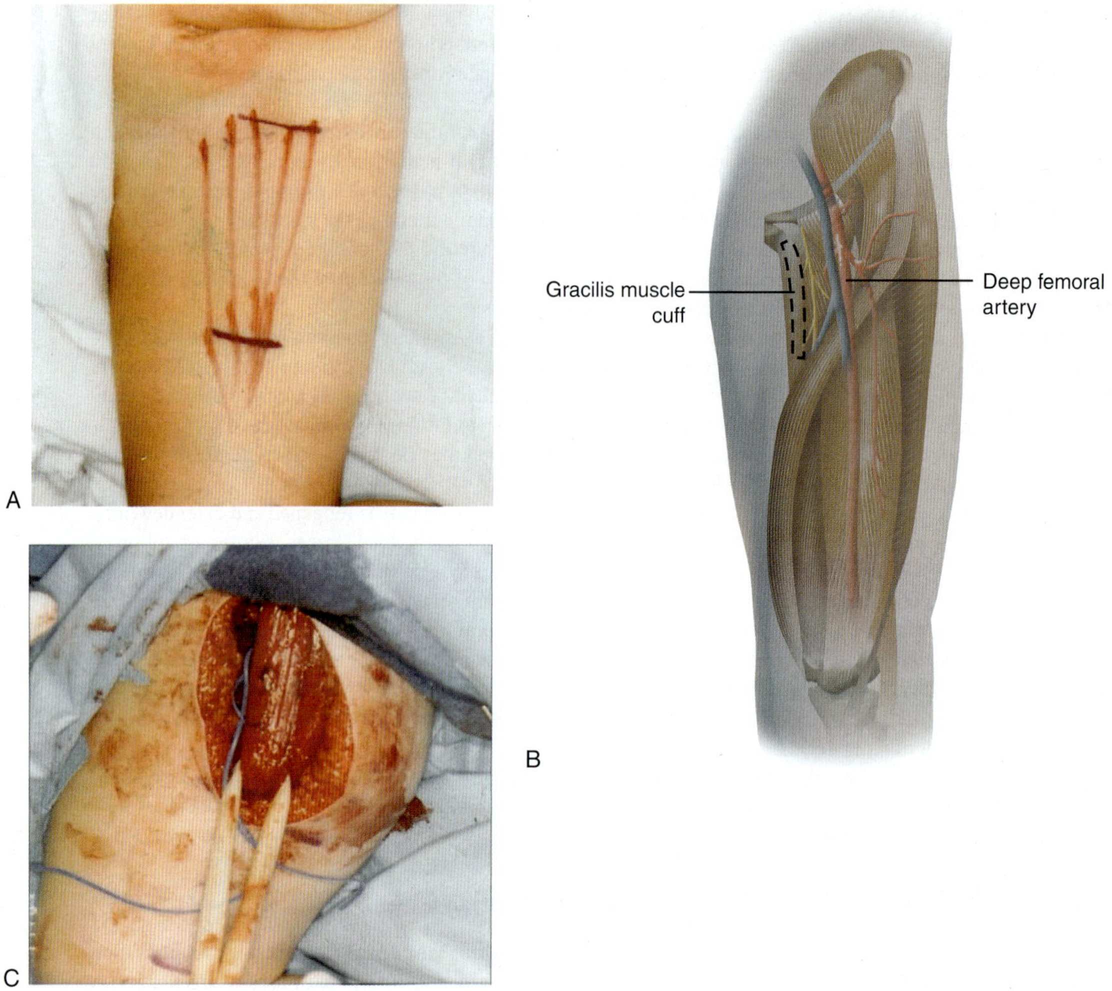

FIGURE 43.5 A. Harvest of the gracilis muscle (usually on the contralateral side) is performed through a vertical incision in the upper one-third of the inner thigh along the course of a line interconnecting the pubic tubercle to the medial malleolus of the knee. **B.** The arterial and venous leashes are traced laterally in the deep thigh to their origin from the profundus femoris vessels. **C.** The resting length of the muscle is marked by placement of silk sutures at 5-cm intervals on the surface of the muscle prior to detachment.

with the electrocautery. Muscle fibers are imbricated with vertical mattress Prolene sutures to the orbicularis oris muscle of the lateral third of the lip. Fibers of the lateral edge of the gracilis are sewn to the insertion of the fascia lata sling at the modiolus. If shortening of the upper lip element is necessary, it is trimmed on its inferior margin before closure of the incision at the mucocutaneous border. The nasolabial crease is recreated by placement of dermal sutures on the undersurface of the premarked crease and attached to the deep muscle. Standard vascular repairs are completed under the microscope prior to releasing the clamps. Anoxia time from muscle detachment to revascularization should be limited to less than 2 hours. Hemostasis is achieved and the cheek flap redraped and inset on the hemiface. A Jackson-Pratt drain parallels the muscle mass, and a small Penrose drain is placed along the inferior gutter. The nasotracheal tube is left overnight, and the patient is deeply sedated to prevent violent head motions during the first 24 hours postoperatively. Patency of the anastomoses is confirmed by hourly Doppler checks for the first 72 hours. Liquid diet is progressed to a soft diet by the 3rd or 4th day. Jaw activity and facial expressions are discouraged during the first couple of weeks.

POSTOPERATIVE MANAGEMENT

Rehabilitation is critical to the successful outcome of patients who have undergone facial reanimation. Toward that end, a comprehensive physical therapy protocol has been designed by the author and a PhD physical rehabilitation specialist. In the early stages post–muscle transfer (at 4 to 6 weeks), low-dose continuous phase E-stim is initiated to increase circulation and introduce E-stim to the patient. Electrodes are placed at the nasolabial fold and temporomandibular joint. Involuntary quivering (fasciculations) are usually observed at 2 to

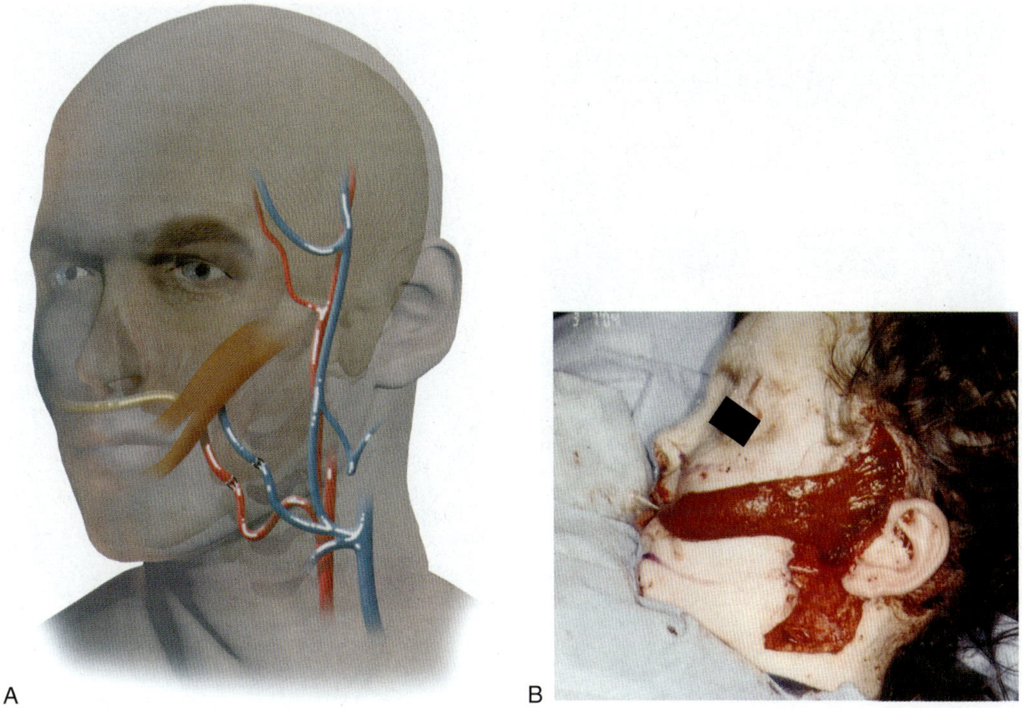

FIGURE 43.6 A. The muscle is transposed to the recipient cheek and anchored proximally to the lateral zygomatic arch and deep temporal fascia with heavy Prolene suture. Orientation of the muscle is predetermined by the anatomy of the smile on the contralateral healthy side. **B.** This photo demonstrates the orientation of the muscle. The attachments from the zygoma to the modiolus of the orbicularis.

3 months progressing to voluntary movements over the next 6 to 12 weeks. Increased interrupted pulse surface E-stim at increasing amplitudes is used during the active phase of muscle activity to boost strength of contraction. E-stim is supplemented by a home exercise program. As voluntary muscle activity reaches a plateau, E-stim should be tapered to prevent hypercontractibility. Patients are actively engaged in Biofeedback exercises in front of the mirror to "train" a symmetrical smile. The maximum spontaneous smile is usually achieved by 9 to 12 months. Most patients are able to achieve unilateral "specificity" over time. Frequent correspondence between the physical therapist and the surgeon is essential to monitor progress and adjust treatment modalities accordingly.

COMPLICATIONS

Patients are generally young and healthy and tolerate well the extensive anesthesia times (often 8 to 10 hours) of each operation. Postsurgical hematomas or take-backs for reexploration of thrombotic anastomoses are relatively rare (3% to 5%). Asymmetry due to excessive muscle fullness can be addressed by debulking of the gracilis by reelevating the skin flap of the cheek and recontouring the muscle mass (that is less of a problem now that the gracilis muscle is more aggressively debulked in situ prior to transfer). Corrections of overpull or underpull should be deferred for at least a year postsurgically until final muscle activity is determined. *Underpull* can be corrected by distal plication of the muscle or shortening of the fascia lata sling. In a few instances, a mini-temporalis turnover flap (regional muscle transfer) has been used to supplement the elevation of the upper lip. *Overpull* creates a more difficult challenge, particularly in children during rapid growth phases of the head/face. If release of the fascia lata sling at the modiolus fails to ameliorate the problem, reexploration and "slide" of the proximal gracilis muscle attachment may reduce tension and produce a more symmetric smile. Botox chemodenervation of the gracilis or contralateral lip depressor can effectively assuage minor imbalances. Secondary "refinements" are often necessary to address cosmetic concerns such as increased fleshiness of the lips, sharpness of the corner of the mouth, hypertrophic postsurgical scars, poor definition of the nasolabial crease, or droopiness of the corner of the mouth.

An area of approximately 5 to 6 cm of sensory loss on the lateral foot is to be expected in the donor site. This diminishes with time as the neurotization occurs from adjacent areas. Twenty-five percent to thirty percent of the patients report cold intolerance, scar tenderness, and minimal levels of discomfort, most of which resolves after a year. Minimal morbidity is experienced in the donor thigh.

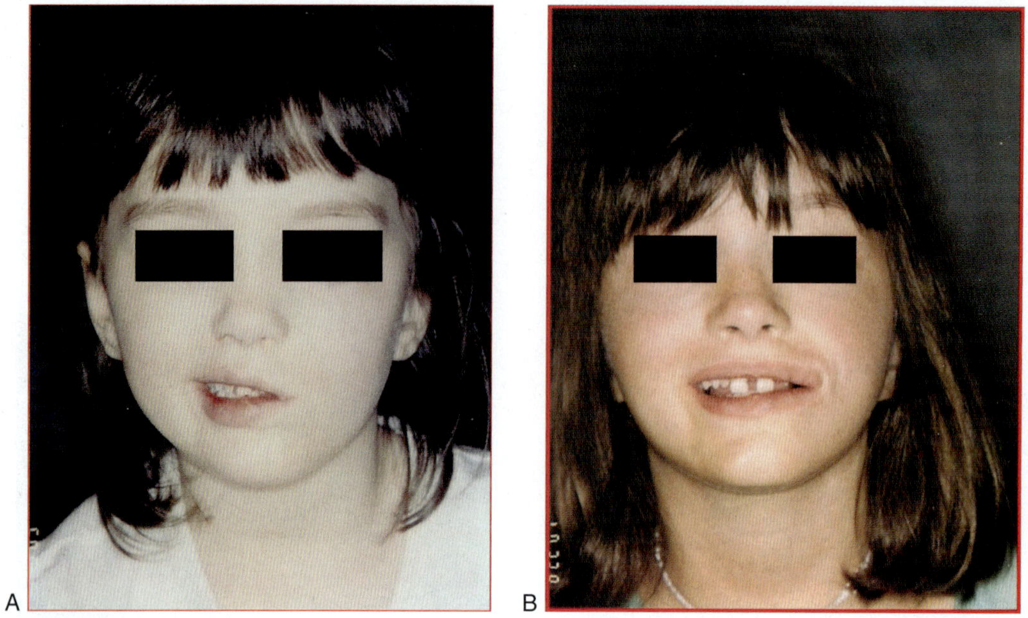

FIGURE 43.7 A. Six-year-old postresection of medulloblastoma of the posterior fossa. **B.** One year following cross facial nerve graft/gracilis transfer.

RESULTS

I have performed 46 cross-facial nerve grafts and 25 free gracilis transfers over the last 12 years. Case examples are shown in Figures 43.7, 43.8, and 43.9. Age range is from 18 months to 35 years old. Most common etiologies are congenital (developmental or birth trauma) or following tumor ablation (acoustic neuroma or brain stem). Most patients achieved nearly full symmetry in repose and 75% to 100% of dynamic smile restoration (documented by postoperative photos, videos, and smile recognition software). Development of physiologic activities of daily living (cup feeding, drinking through a straw, chewing, fluid retention) have been restored postsurgically. In toddlers (<4-year-old), feedback from the speech therapists and parents has confirmed that speech patterns have developed at normal landmarks and have not required specialized retraining as

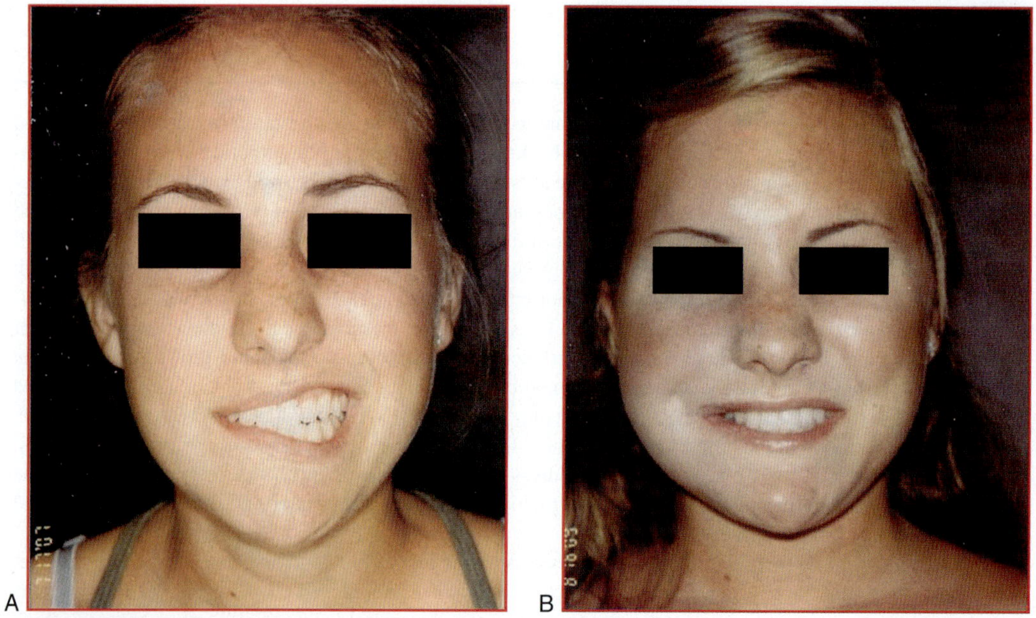

FIGURE 43.8 A. Sixteen-year-old postresection of golf ball size acoustic neuroma. **B.** Post-op after cross facial nerve grafts × 4 and free gracilis transfer.

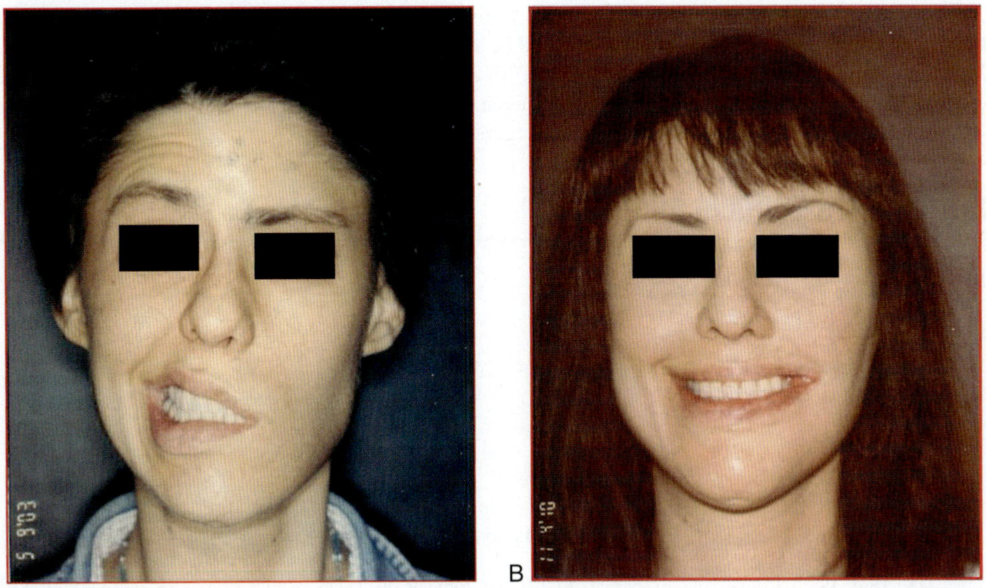

A B

FIGURE 43.9 **A.** Twenty-eight-year-old post resection of a medulloblastoma. **B.** Postoperative smiling after cross facial nerve grafts × 4 and free gracilis transfer.

is so characteristic of children operated at older ages after poor speech patterns and altered facial expressions have developed.

PEARLS

- Careful preoperative evaluation is critical in designing the most appropriate approach for facial reanimation.
- Patients should be advised preoperatively of the lengthy rehabilitation and the "time frame" (at least 18 to 24 months) before voluntary muscle activity is observed.
- Patients (or parents) must be "active participants" in the rehabilitation process.
- Nasotracheal intubation places the tube away from the operative site.
- Inset of a *primary* fascia lata sling at the first stage of reconstruction allows for immediate restoration of facial balance in repose and counteract the "overpull" of the contralateral healthy muscles.
- Fine mimetic muscle movement (eye closure, nostril elevation, lower lip eversion, etc.) can be achieved with direct cross-facial nerve grafting.
- Cross-facial nerve grafts should be "preset" within the face prior to microneural repair. This avoids disruption of the microneural repair during manipulation of the nerve.
- Cross-facial zygomatic (orbital) grafts are passed supraorbitally. Cross-facial buccal (for fine mimetic muscles) grafts are passed transnasally. Cross-facial margin mandibular (for lower lip paralysis) is passed submentally.
- Cross-facial buccal (for motor of gracilis) is passed across the chin.
- Microhemoclips at distal end of nerve grafts and blue "tracer" sutures are critical in identification at the second-stage procedure when scarring has encompassed the nerve graft.
- Biopsy of the fresh end of the distal nerve graft at the second stage confirms axonal regeneration.
- Orientation of the gracilis muscle is best achieved by harvesting from the *contralateral* side.
- Free gracilis muscle should be placed at normal length at inset (confirmed by sutures at 5-cm intervals on surface).

PITFALLS

- Cross-facial nerve grafting should be avoided in "older" patients since axonal regeneration falls off precipitously by the fourth or fifth decade.
- Cross-facial nerve grafting should be avoided in adult patients with partial paralysis since "splicing" end to end into intact functioning facial nerve on the palsied side may jeopardize existing muscle motion.
- Do not "sell" the more complex microsurgical procedures (cross-facial nerve grafting and free gracilis transfer) to adult patients, since generally, they do not have the tolerance for two major reconstructive procedures and the extensive time (2 years) before facial motion is visualized.

- Always prepare patients of the need for additional "refinement" surgery. Do not fall into the trap of "you told me it would only take two procedures and I would be smiling."
- Make sure patients have "reasonable expectations" of aesthetic and functional outcome. Avoid young, "narcissistic" patients who expect "perfection." If necessary, have prospective patients speak with other patients who have undergone similar facial reanimation surgeries.

INSTRUMENTS TO HAVE AVAILABLE

- Facial plastics surgical tray
- Tendon stripper
- Microscope
- Microsurgical instruments
- Kleinert tendon passer

SUGGESTED READING

Chun JK. Facial reanimation and smile reconstruction. In: Rose EH, ed. *Aesthetic facial restoration*. Philadelphia, PA: Lippincott-Raven, 1998:251–262.

Griebie MS, Huff JS. Selective role of partial XI-VII anastomosis in facial reanimation. *Laryngoscope* 1998;108 (11 Pt 1):1664–1668.

Takushima A, Harii K, Asato H, et al. Neurovascular free-muscle transfer for the treatment of established facial paralysis following ablative surgery in the parotid region. *Plast Reconstr Surg* 2004;113(6):1563–1572.

Rose EH. Autogenous fascia lata grafts: clinical applications in reanimation of the totally or partially paralyzed face. *Plast Reconstr Surg* 2005;116(1):20–32

Terzis JK, Konofaos P. Nerve transfers in facial palsy. *Facial Plast Surg* 2008;24(2):177–193.

Gousheh J, Arasteh E. Treatment of facial paralysis: dynamic reanimation of spontaneous facial expression-apropos of 655 patients. *Plast Reconstr Surg* 2011;128(6):693e–703e.

Note: Page numbers in *italics* denote figures; those followed by 't' denote table.